ESSENTIALS OF GROSS ANATOMY

Berhanu Kindu

ALLIED
HEALTH
PRESS

Essentials of Gross Anatomy

Author: **Berhanu Kindu**

Allied Health Press
4164 Lakeshore Road
Burlington ON L7L 1A4
Canada
www.alliedhealthpress.com
Email: orders@arclereducation.com

ISBN: 978-1-77956-774-1

Allied Health Press publishes wide variety of books and eBooks. For more information about Allied Health Press and its products, visit our website at www.alliedhealthpress.com

ABOUT THE AUTHOR

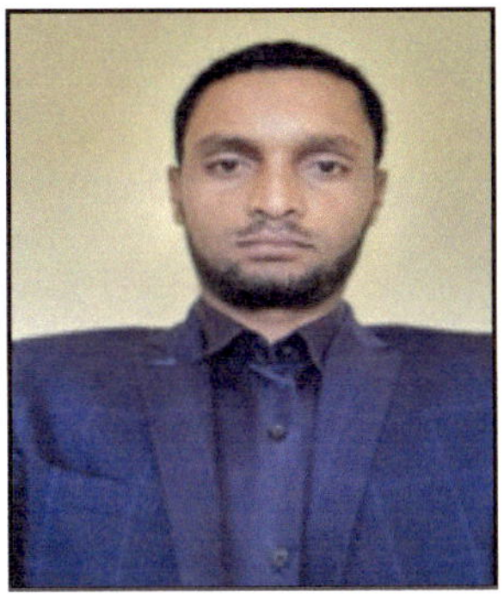

Berhanu Kindu Ashagrie, lecturer and researcher of Human Anatomy at Debre Tabor University, Ethiopia. He has been working in Debre Tabor University since 22 September, 2018 as a lecturer and researcher of Human Anatomy, Histology, Embryology and other related fields of science. Since then, he has been publishing research articles, review manuscripts, and teaching materials in health science and related fields of science.

He graduated with Bachelor's degree from Debre Markos University in Public Health (BSc) and Master's degree from University of Gondar (one of the top legendary universities in Ethiopia) in Human Anatomy (MSc).

Brief Table of Contents

Getting Started with This Book

Chapter Openers

A list of Chapter Outline is presented providing a brief Introduction to what will be covered in the chapter.

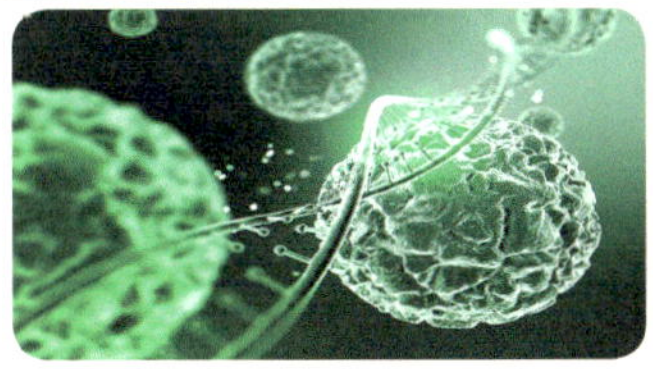

Introduction

Often referred to as the science of life, biology is a broad field of study aimed at comprehending the several kinds of life on Earth, from tiny creatures to sophisticated multicellular entities. Comprising several subfields, including molecular biology, ecology, and evolutionary biology, each of which advances our knowledge of living systems, this field clarifies the mechanisms controlling life events, including development, reproduction, and interaction with the surroundings, which is the central goal of biology. Moreover, biology fills in the void between the natural sciences and medicine by offering a necessary understanding of health, illness, and the interactions between organisms and their environments. Dealing with urgent global issues such as climate change, biodiversity loss, and new diseases depends on an awareness of these complex biological interactions, therefore highlighting the critical part biology plays in modern civilization. Fundamentally, biology explores and tests ideas about the living world using the scientific method. Through methodical observation and experimentation,

LEARNING OBJECTIVES

After studying this chapter, you will be able to:

1. Discuss the scientific method in biology;
2. Explain the cell theory;
3. Discuss the genetics and heredity;
4. Evolution and natural selection;
5. Focus on ecology and ecosystems;
6. Learn about human biology;
7. Evaluate the plant biology;
8. Explain the microbiology;
9. Focus on current trends in biology.

1.1. The Scientific Method in Biology

Learning Outcome

1. Describe the steps of the scientific method;
2. Focus on hypothesis formation;
3. Learn about experimental design.

Learning Outcomes

The beginning of each section of every chapter contains a set of Learning Outcomes that inform students of concepts they should understand. These outcomes help students understand what they should be able to do if they have mastered the material in that section.

Test Your Knowledge

Throughout each chapter, Test Your Knowledge cues you to note which topics have been covered and to self-test your understanding of the material presented.

Test Your Knowledge

1. Explain why correlation does not imply causation in scientific experiments.
2. How does the scientific method help reduce the influence of personal opinions in research?

Chapter Summary

The Summary Section appear at the end of each chapter and summarize main concepts covered throughout the chapter. These points provide key concepts in an engaging and meaningful way.

Summary

The investigation of biological principles highlights the importance of a comprehensive view of life by reflecting the intricate interactions that occur within living systems. The complexity of biology goes beyond individual species or systems, as this essay highlights; it also includes the interactions that mold ecosystems and affect biodiversity. Researchers can conduct in-depth analyses of metabolomic data using sophisticated technologies like MetaboAnalyst, which offer insights into the molecular mechanisms underlying these interactions. As demonstrated by the developments in MetaboAnalyst, for example, the integration of diverse omics data promotes a thorough understanding of metabolic pathways and helps identify important biological markers necessary for research on development and disease (Chong et al., 2018). Additionally, the phenomenon of ecological invasions is a key component of biological research and a vital field of study. The introduction of non-native species into unfamiliar habitats has significant ramifications and calls for multidisciplinary management strategies. Examining the origins and effects of these biological incursions, invasion science has become a crucial field that highlights the need to comprehend ecological dynamics and community interactions. As interest in biological invasions increases, new findings are emerging that put conventional ecological theories and practices to the test. The importance of incorporating various scientific viewpoints is shown by this developing discipline, which also highlights how invasive species shape ecosystems and advances our knowledge of ecological resilience (David et al., 2013). When taken as a whole, these discoveries from invasion science and metabolomics highlight the value of multidisciplinary biology research. Fostering cross-disciplinary collaboration and utilizing technological breakthroughs to improve our comprehension of intricate biological interactions are crucial as we look to the future of biological research. In addition to deepening our understanding of the complexities of life, this method lays the groundwork for tackling urgent environmental issues. Future studies can ensure the continued relevance of biology in a world that is constantly changing by acknowledging the interconnection of biological systems and opening the door to creative solutions that support sustainability and biodiversity conservation. We might imagine a thorough comprehension of life that serves both academia and society at large through ongoing investigation and integration of scientific knowledge.

Knowledge Assessment

The chapter includes material designed to review and reinforce each content. It includes Critical Thinking Questions to help test of your understanding of information presented in the chapter and Short answer Questions to review your understanding of the key concepts presented in the chapter.

Critical Thinking Questions

1. **Who is known as the "Father of Modern Biology"?**
   a. Aristotle
   b. Charles Darwin
   c. Gregor Mendel
   d. Louis Pasteur
2. **What is the basic unit of life?**
   a. Atom
   b. Molecule
   c. Cell
   d. Organism
3. **Which branch of biology studies the interaction of organisms with their environment?**
   a. Genetics
   b. Ecology
   c. Physiology
   d. Botany
4. **Which macromolecule is the main source of energy for living organisms?**
   a. Proteins
   b. Lipids
   c. Carbohydrates
   d. Nucleic acids
5. **DNA is primarily responsible for which function in living organisms?**
   a. Energy production
   b. Protein synthesis
   c. Storing genetic information
   d. Regulating body temperature

Short Answer Questions

1. What is biology, and why is it important to study biology?
2. What are the three main domains of life, and how are they different from one another?
3. Define homeostasis and give an example of how it works in living organisms.
4. What is the cell theory, and why is it fundamental to biology?
5. How do autotrophs and heterotrophs differ in the way they obtain energy?
6. What is the scientific method, and how is it applied in biological research?
7. Discuss how biology helps address global challenges such as climate change, disease, and food security.
8. Explain the levels of biological organization from the smallest unit to the largest. Provide examples at each level.
9. Describe the relationship between structure and function in biology, giving specific examples from cells or organs.
10. How has the discovery of genetics shaped our understanding of inheritance and variation among organisms?

Supplementary Materials

Key Terms: A list of key terms is given for quick reference

KEY TERMS FROM THIS CHAPTER

Annotation enrichment analysis	Biological structure	Cell
Cell theory	Cellular structure	Ecology
Ecosystems	Genetics	Human biology
Microbiology	Natural selection	Organism
Plant biology		

Further Resources: Recommendations for additional readings, websites, and multimedia resources.

References

1. Argelaguet, R., Velten, B., Arnol, D., Dietrich, S., Zenz, T., Marioni, J. C., Buettner, F., et al. (2018). Multi-omics factor analysis—A framework for unsupervised integration of multi-omics data sets. *Molecular Systems Biology, 14*. https://doi.org/10.15252/msb.20178124.
2. Bacher, S., Blackburn, T. M., Essl, F., & Genovesi, P. (2017). *Socio-Economic Impact Classification of Alien Taxa (SEICAT)*. https://core.ac.uk/download/286567949.pdf (accessed on 8th March 2025).
3. Barnett, R., Brace, S., Cucchi, T., & Dobney, K. (2013). *Divergent Evolutionary Processes Associated with Colonization of Offshore Islands*. https://core.ac.uk/download/20664364.pdf (accessed on 8th March 2025).

Detailed Table of Contents

CHAPTER 2

Upper Limb 31

CHAPTER 3

Lower Limb 65

CHAPTER 4

CHAPTER 5

Thoracic Wall and Breast 125

CHAPTER 6

Lungs and Pleura 159

CHAPTER 12

CHAPTER 13

CHAPTER 14

CHAPTER 15

LIST OF FIGURES

LIST OF ABBREVIATIONS

AC	Abdominal Cocoon
ACDF	Anterior Cervical Decompression and Fusion
ACE	Angiotensin-Converting Enzyme
ACL	Anterior Cruciate Ligament
ADL	Activities of Daily Living
AI	Artificial Intelligence
AR	Augmented Reality
ARDS	Acute Respiratory Distress Syndrome
AS	Ankylosing Spondylitis
ASIA	American Spinal Injury Association
AV	Atrioventricular
AWS	Abdominal Wall Service
CAD	Coronary Artery Disease
CAP	Community-Acquired Pneumonia
CBL	Case-Based Learning
CBME	Competency-Based Medical Education
CE CT	Contrast-Enhanced Computed Tomography
CHF	Congestive Heart Failure
CIPN	Chemotherapy-Induced Peripheral Neuropathy
CMF	Craniomaxillofacial
CMR	Cardiovascular Magnetic Resonance
CNS	Central Nervous System
CO_2	Carbon Dioxide
COPD	Chronic Obstructive Pulmonary Disease
CPP	Chronic Pelvic Pain
CPT	Continuous Performance Test
CRT	Cardiac Resynchronization Therapy

CSF	Cerebrospinal Fluid
CT	Computed Tomography
DIEA	Deep Inferior Epigastric Artery
DTI	Diffusion Tensor Imaging
DVF	Digital Video Fluoroscopy
EAT	Eating as Treatment
EBUS	Endobronchial Ultrasound
EBV	Epstein-Barr Virus
ECG	Electrocardiogram
EEG	Electroencephalography
EIH	Exercise-Induced Hypoalgesia
EIT	Electrical Impedance Tomography
ELR	Elastin-Like Recombinamer
EMG	Electromyography
ENT	Ear-Nose-Throat
ESLP	Ex Situ Lung Perfusion
ESP	Erector Spinae Plane
FMA	Foundational Model of Anatomy
FNAC	Fine Needle Aspiration Cytology
FRP	Flexion-Relaxation Phenomenon
GERD	Gastroesophageal Reflux Disease
GIUS	Gastrointestinal Ultrasound
GM-CSF	Granulocyte/Macrophage Colony-Stimulating Factor
GSV	Great Saphenous Vein
HDV	Hepatitis Delta Virus
hFABP1	Human Liver Fatty Acid Binding Protein
HNC	Head and Neck Cancer
HPB	Hepato-Pancreatic-Biliary
HPV	Human Papillomavirus
HRQOL	Health-Related Quality of Life
IBS	Irritable Bowel Syndrome
ICS	International Continence Society
IH	Incisional Hernias
ILD	Interstitial Lung Disease
IMA	Inferior Mesenteric Artery
IMH	Intramuscular Hemangioma

IONM	Intraoperative Neurophysiological Monitoring
IPA	Internal Pudendal Artery
IRA	Innate Response Activator
IUGA	International Urogynecological Association
IVD	Intervertebral Disc
iVR	Immersive Virtual Reality
LAM	Levator Ani Muscle
LBP	Low Back Pain
LDH	Lumbar Disc Herniation
LEC	Lifting Energy Consumption
LI	Lifting Index
LIHR	Laparoscopic Inguinal Hernia Repair
LPP	Lumbo Pelvic Pain
LVAD	Left Ventricular Assist Device
MEG	Magnetoencephalography
MFPP	Myofascial Pelvic Pain
M-GAN	Multi-Channel Generative Adversarial Network
MR-DTI	Magnetic Resonance Diffusion Tensor Imaging
MRI	Magnetic Resonance Imaging
MSK	Musculoskeletal
NAC	Nipple-Areola Complex
NET	Neuroendocrine Tumor
NOTES	Natural Orifice Transluminal Endoscopic Surgery
NPV	Negative Pressure Ventilation
NSAID	Non-Steroidal Anti-Inflammatory Drug
NTE	Neural Tissue Engineering
OASIS	Obstetric Anal Sphincter Injuries
OH	Orthostatic Hypotension
OPCAB	Off-Pump Coronary Artery Bypass
OPSCC	Oropharyngeal Squamous Cell Carcinoma
OSAS	Obstructive Sleep Apnea Syndrome
OSCC	Oral Squamous Cell Carcinoma
PAD	Peripheral Artery Disease
PCFP	Pericruciate Fat Pad
PCL	Posterior Cruciate Ligament
PCOS	Polycystic Ovary Syndrome

PET	Positron Emission Tomography
PFD	Pelvic Floor Disorder
PFM	Pelvic Floor Muscle
PMPS	Post-Mastectomy Pain Syndrome
PNS	Peripheral Nervous System
POP	Pelvic Organ Prolapse
PPV	Positive Pressure Ventilation
PSSE	Physiotherapeutic Scoliosis-Specific Exercises
PTA	Peritonsillar Abscess
PTH	Parathyroid Hormone
PV	Perforator Vessels
QoL	Quality of Life
RRN	Relational Reasoning Network
RSA	Reverse Shoulder Arthroplasty
SA	Sinoatrial
SAMP8	Senescence-Accelerated Mouse-Prone 8
SBO	Small Bowel Obstruction
sEV	Small Extracellular Vesicle
SMA	Spinal Muscular Atrophy
SMA	Superior Mesenteric Artery
SO_2	Sulfur Dioxide
SPL	Sternopericardial Ligament
SRS	Stereotactic Radiosurgery
SSEH	Spontaneous Spinal Epidural Hematoma
SSI	Surgical Site Infection
SUI	Stress Urinary Incontinence
TBNA	Transbronchial Needle Aspiration
TEP	Totally Extraperitoneal Herniorrhaphy
TEVAR	Thoracic Endovascular Aortic Replacement
TFL	Tensor Fascia Lata
TJM	Thrust Joint Manipulation
TMJ	Temporomandibular Joint
TNBC	Triple-negative breast cancer
TNFα	Tumor Necrosis Factor Alpha
TSA	Total Shoulder Arthroplasty

UTI	Urinary Tract Infection
VALI	Ventilation-Associated Lung Injury
VATS	Video-Assisted Thoracoscopic Surgery
VLNT	Vascularized Lymph Node Transfer
VNS	Vagus Nerve Stimulation
VR	Virtual Reality
WCST	Wisconsin Card Sorting Test

PREFACE

Anatomy is the foundation of all medical and health professions. Gross anatomy deals with the structure and organization of body structures apparent to the naked eye and is the basic information required for understanding function, appreciating normal variation, and detecting pathological change. Through the examination of organs, muscles, bones, and vessels in cadaveric dissection, prosected specimens, imaging studies, and three-dimensional models, students acquire a spatial awareness that underlies clinical decision-making. Starting from basic landmarks and moving towards complicated regional organization, gross anatomy covers the gap between theoretical knowledge and clinical practice. This approach provides students with observation skills and descriptive terms to enable them to provide correct descriptions regarding body structures within a classroom, lab room, or practice environment. Highlighting the interdependence of tissues and organs, this course positions students to confidently interpret diagnostic images, conduct physical examinations, and conduct surgery.

Essentials of Gross Anatomy offers a detailed yet concise introduction to human anatomy, aiming at both novice learners and those requiring a quick overview. The academic textbook masterfully combines simple language with elaborate illustrations, providing a uniform treatise that correlates anatomical facts with their clinical relevance. Anatomical terminology is put into perspective in the book, enhancing memorization through careful repetition and visual reinforcement. There are brief captions for each illustration that point out important points, and clinical correlations that show their applicability to patient care.

The structure of *Essentials of Gross Anatomy* puts complicated information at your fingertips. The textbook is organized into 15 chapters and each chapter addresses a particular anatomical region or topic. Chapter 1 presents the background by defining anatomical terminology, describing body planes and movements, and outlining imaging modalities. Chapters 2 and 3 cover the upper and lower limbs, respectively, and include osteology, musculature, neurovascular supply, and common anatomical variations that affect function. Chapters 4 through 8 address the thoracic cavity and contents: Chapter 4 gives the boundaries of the thorax and the organization of bones, muscles, and joints; Chapter 5 is on the thoracic wall and breast, emphasizing surface anatomy and lymphatic drainage; Chapter 6 addresses lungs and pleura, including the bronchial tree and pleural reflections; Chapter 7 is on the heart and pericardium, with chambers, valves, and coronary circulation; Chapter 8 is on the mediastinum, describing compartments and the passage of major structures such as the esophagus, trachea, and great vessels. Chapters 9 and 10 shift to the abdominal region: Chapter 9 discusses the anterior abdominal wall and inguinal region, highlighting fascial layers, neurovascular pathways, and locations of hernias; Chapter 10 takes a trip through the peritoneal cavity and abdominal viscera, detailing the digestive organs, their vascular supply, and clinical points such as referred pain. Chapter 11 turns to the pelvis and perineum, describing the pelvic floor muscles (PFMs), reproductive organs, and the neurovascular components necessary for an understanding of childbirth and the maintenance of urinary continence. Chapter 12 moves to the head and skull, providing a comprehensive description of the cranial bones, sutures, and foramina through which vessels and nerves pass. Chapter 13 continues with the brain and cranial nerves, detailing the cerebral hemispheres, brainstem, and twelve pairs of nerves facilitating sensory and motor activities. Chapter 14 presents a review of the neck and cervical viscera with particular attention to the hyoid apparatus, thyroid gland, pharynx, larynx, and vasculature enveloped by the carotid sheath. Chapter 15 then proceeds with the back and vertebral column, explaining vertebral anatomy, posture-maintaining muscles, and the spinal cord with meningeal coverings. Key clinical points in these chapters highlight the need for accurate anatomical knowledge in diagnosis, surgical procedures, and emergency medical interventions.

This book is primarily aimed at students of medicine, dentistry, nursing, and the allied health professions of physical therapy, occupational therapy, and radiologic technology. It aims to be an undergraduate anatomy study guide for your anatomy classes, dissection laboratory work, and licensure examination review. Instructors can find it appropriate for core text or supplementary use, thanks to its logically organized design and pedagogic figures that enhance both lecture presentations and independent study assignments. Beyond its value to students and instructors, *Essentials of Gross Anatomy* is also a useful reference for residents, clinicians, and other professionals who need a quick review of regional anatomical principles. This book is intended to strengthen core knowledge and continuing professional development by emphasizing the most important structures and clinical correlation, thereby guiding readers to precise comprehension of anatomical relationships and confident application in patient care.

INTRODUCTION TO GROSS ANATOMY

1

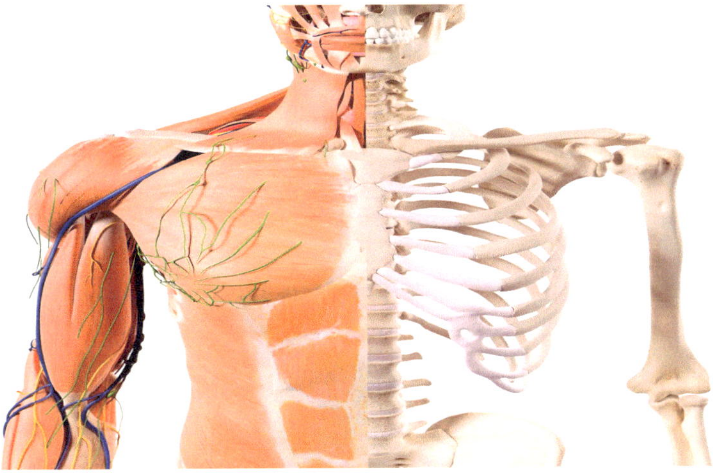

LEARNING OBJECTIVES

After studying this chapter, you will be able to:

1. Discuss the anatomical terminology
2. Focus on major organ systems
3. Explain the techniques in gross anatomy
4. Learn about the clinical relevance of gross anatomy

Introduction

Understanding the complex makeup of the human body lies at the core of many scientific and medical disciplines, requiring a firm foundation in gross anatomy. This branch of anatomy is concerned with the examination of body structures visible to the naked eye, bridging the gap between microscopic cellular studies and whole-body functional analysis. The study guides practitioners to determine the organization and interrelationship of organs, tissues, and systems required for clinical application and research. In biomechanics, for example, knowledge of gross anatomical structures is the foundation of modeling processes that mimic human movement and predict physical response to applied forces (Ronald, 2013). Gross anatomy's basic concepts also underpin disciplines that involve careful examination of tissues and organ systems to assess physiological or pathological status (Bolon, 2023). Establishing these basic anatomical tenets allows learners and practitioners to construct a comprehensive image of body structure and function that is essential for health sciences advancement.

Definition of Gross Anatomy

Understanding the structural organization of the human body lies at the heart of numerous medical and scientific specialties, particularly those involved with surgical and diagnostic procedures.

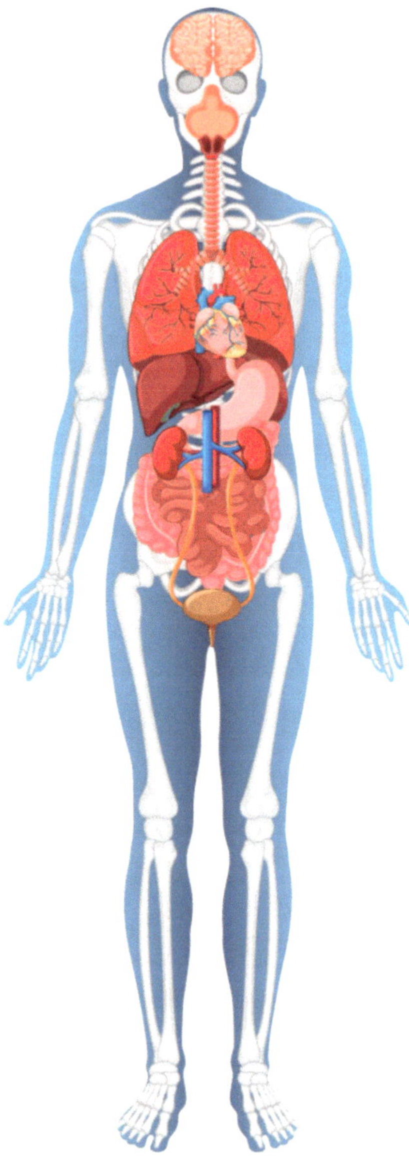

Figure 1.1. Definition of gross anatomy.

Source: Freepik. (n.d.). *Anatomical Structure of Human Body*.

Gross anatomy, in this context, can be described as the examination of anatomical structures that can be identified only with the naked eye, as contrasted with microscopic anatomy, which requires magnification to visualize. This anatomical discipline is the basis for understanding the spatial relationships and function of tissues and organs that are essential for effective treatment interventions such as surgical resection or image-guided intervention. For example, precise knowledge of gross anatomical landmarks is crucial in interventions such as tumor ablation, where accurate localization enhances treatment effects and minimizes complications (Ahmed et al., 2014). Similarly, in the treatment of complex diseases such as osteosarcoma, gross anatomical knowledge facilitates successful removal and recognition of gross disease and guides adjunctive therapies (Douglas et al., 2017). Gross anatomy, hence, provides an essential basis for clinical practice and research aimed at improving patient care and therapeutic outcomes (Figure 1.1).

Importance of Gross Anatomy in Medicine

Understanding the structural plan of the human body remains essential to effective medical practice, as it is the foundation upon which diagnostics, surgery, and therapeutic interventions are based. Herophilus and Vesalius, visionaries of the past, established the paradigm for the central role of dissection in unraveling the complexities of human anatomy that have continued to influence contemporary medical education and practice (In-Kim et al., 2024). This general knowledge enables clinicians to interpret complex imaging modalities and perform invasive procedures safely. Moreover, the recent advances in prenatal diagnostics, such as targeted fetal neurosonography, point to the importance of extensive knowledge of anatomy in order to diagnose and treat central nervous system (CNS) malformations early in gestation, thereby improving patient outcomes (Paladini et al., 2021). With advances in technology, medicine keeps expanding, yet gross anatomy remains a core discipline that bridges the gap between basic science and the clinical setting with an emphasis on obtaining adequately qualified educators and resources to ensure quality anatomical education (In-Kim et al., 2024).

Historical Background of Gross Anatomy

The history of gross anatomy has been pivotal to medical science development, changing over centuries from rough observation to scientific investigation. Early underpinnings were laid down by the ancient Egyptians and Greeks, both through experiential practice and philosophical reflection of the human form. During the Renaissance, pioneers like Andreas Vesalius transformed anatomical knowledge by giving preference to firsthand dissection and observation, sweeping away long-standing misconceptions inherited from antiquity. This shift was a move towards evidence-based research, highlighting the importance of real-world experience in understanding physical structures.

The evolution of anatomical studies has been enhanced even more by integrating modern technologies and methodologies, which makes it simpler to perform more complex analyses of biological systems. While contemporary research relies increasingly on computerized resources and bibliometric data analysis to map scientific advancement correctly, these advances are built on the previous groundwork laid by gross anatomy as a discipline that is dedicated to the study of the human body at depth (Husaeni et al., 2021). That history leads us to infer the ongoing applicability of gross anatomy both in education and clinical practice (Faruqi et al., 2017).

Differences between Gross and Microscopic Anatomy

The comprehension of human anatomy entails the recognition of various levels of structural organization, each providing new information regarding the body's complexity.

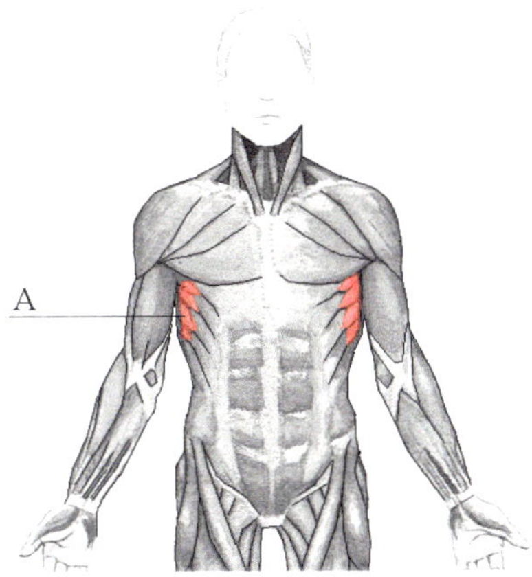

Figure 1.2. Differences between gross and microscopic anatomy.

Source: By Padawane - de commons, CC BY-SA 3.0, https://commons.wikimedia.org/w/index.php?curid=2472746

Gross anatomy, which deals with structures visible to the naked eye such as organs and organ systems, is exposed by microscopic anatomy, revealing cellular and tissue-level organization that provides the basis for these macroscopic structures. Gross anatomy is performed by direct observation and incision into the body, permitting a clearer appreciation of spatial relationships of structures, essential for clinical practice and surgery. Microscopic anatomy employs techniques like histology to examine cells and tissues, yielding valuable information on function and pathology not obtainable by gross examination. This disparity is a reflection of the complementary nature of the two disciplines; gross anatomy provides the gross context within which microscopic information becomes pertinent, casting further light on physiological function and disease pathology. Although not anatomy-specific, fields of research such as investigations into marine mammal physiology or gut microbiome demonstrate the relevance of microscopic observations to describe sub-surface-induced biological responses within complex organisms (Nguyen et al., 2015; Tara et al., 2023) (Figure 1.2).

Overview of Anatomical Terminology

It is critical to learn gross anatomy's basic vocabulary to accurately describe the structures of the human body and their approximate locations. Anatomical terminology provides for standardized language, free from ambiguity, to be used in communication among students and healthcare providers. These include directional terms such as anterior and posterior, planes of section such as transverse and sagittal, and relative position terms that are extremely crucial in the positioning of structures in living and dissected bodies. Knowing these terms heightens awareness throughout imaging technique interpretation, which has become increasingly integrated into anatomy learning with the aid of tools like augmented reality (AR) and virtual dissection websites that integrate radiology and gross anatomy education (Bork et al., 2019). Moreover, the appreciation of the historical evolution of anatomical descriptions emphasizes the importance of precise terminology, given how early medical discoveries, like those for oral cancer, depended significantly on proper anatomical references to identify pathological changes (Inchingolo et al., 2020). Thus, anatomical terminology is the linguistic foundation for effective anatomical learning and clinical practice.

Methods of Studying Gross Anatomy

Advances in technology and pedagogical paradigms have made a profound influence on learning gross anatomy. Traditionally grounded in cadaveric dissection, which provides invaluable three-dimensional access to human anatomy, anatomical education today includes multimedia material and virtual reality to enhance the learning experience. The emergency shift to remote learning during the COVID-19 pandemic further raised the call for innovative online resources, and institutions responded with virtual dissection videos, review slides, and other online resources to supplement the limited availability of physical specimens (Georga et al., 2020). These resources address multiple learning styles and promote self-directed learning, necessary in contemporary curricula that prioritize flexibility and productivity. For instance, multimedia learning modules that include video dissections of the brain narrated by experts with quiz-like review materials have been found to achieve high student satisfaction and better knowledge of neuroanatomy (Matthew et al., 2020). Such hybrid models where experiential learning is combined with digital learning give comprehensive approaches that not only preserve essential anatomical knowledge but also supplement evolving pedagogic needs (Figure 1.3).

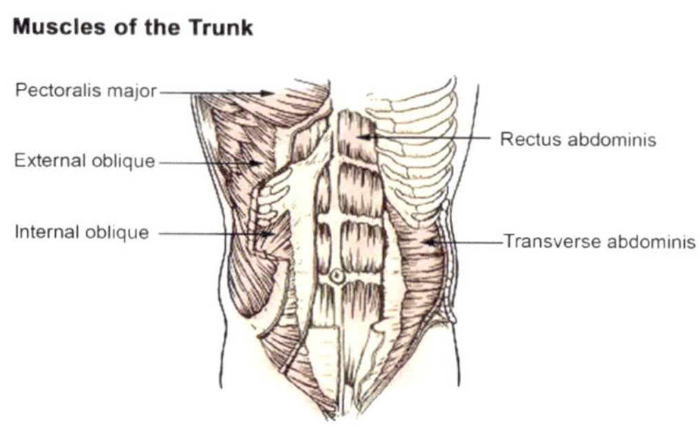

Figure 1.3. Methods of studying gross anatomy.

Source: Public Domain, https://commons.wikimedia.org/w/index.php?curid=789657

Role of Dissection in Learning Gross Anatomy

The mastery of the body's complex spatial relationships and intricate structures is essential to medical students, and this level of comprehension is best realized through the direct experience of dissection. Working with cadaveric material exposes learners to the three-dimensional arrangement of tissues and organs in a fashion that cannot be fully replicated by two-dimensional pictures or computer models. Dissection not only produces anatomical knowledge but also sharpens the required skills such as close observation, hand dexterity, and judgment which are a must in professional practice. Technology-based substitutes have gained popularity, yet dissection has remained an anatomy learning cornerstone because of its non-replicable experiential value and imparting professional working attitudes toward handling patients and the human body. However, recent global developments have challenged access to cadaver dissection, validating its worth as well as the need for supplementary resources in anatomy education (Franchi, 2020; Pushpa et al., 2023).

Ethical Considerations in Anatomical Studies

Throughout history, anatomical practice has been intricately associated with evolving ethical concerns that reflect the values of the time. Early anatomical dissections depended predominantly on the bodies of executed convicted criminals or unclaimed corpses, often without consent or consideration for human dignity, and this led to controversies and even secret practices such as grave robbing (Bhattacharjee & Ghosh, 2023). This dense history raises the need for modern anatomy to embrace humanistic values deferential to donor agency and ethical acquisition. Such present advances as 3D print models offer potential substitutes for cadaver use that overcome ethical and access difficulties (Sami et al., 2024). By including the use of cutting-edge technology and a commitment to ethical standards, education in gross anatomy can honor previous teachings and promote respect for human life, safeguarding the pursuit of knowledge from diminishing moral responsibility. The balance is essential to the building of responsible, caring medical professionals tomorrow.

Applications of Gross Anatomy in Clinical Practice

Gross anatomy mastery is crucial for effective clinical practice, particularly in surgical disciplines where precise knowledge of body structure may greatly influence patient outcomes. Such a history as that of developing surgical approaches, e.g., the refinement of radical hysterectomy, demonstrates how integrating precise anatomical knowledge and surgical technique can reduce such complications as hemorrhage and nerve damage to enhance recovery and patients' quality of life (QoL) (Yabuki, 2020).

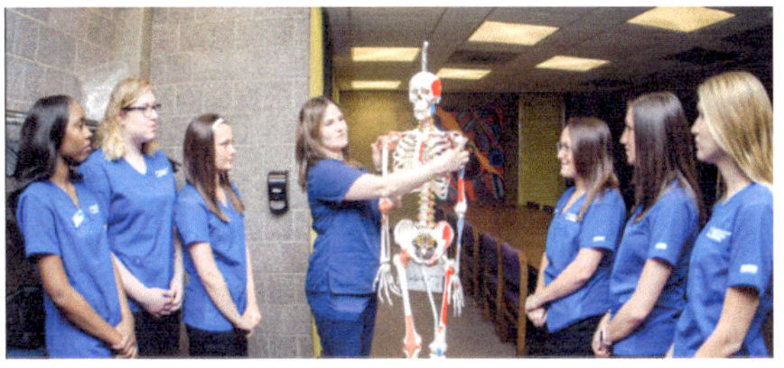

Figure 1.4. Applications of gross anatomy in clinical practice.

Source: Verve College. (2019). *How Studying Anatomy and Physiology Offers a Rewarding Career*.

Moreover, gross anatomy provides the foundation for medical professionals to interpret images, perform physical examinations, and perform interventions with confidence. It is not merely applicable to surgery but also to diagnostics and emergency medicine, where immediate recognition of anatomical landmarks can be life-saving. The recent challenges posed by inadequate hands-on anatomical training due to global health crises highlight the imperative for ongoing strong anatomical education to effectively prepare future clinicians such that they can apply anatomical principles practically and ethically in the management of patients (Franchi, 2020) (Figure 1.4).

1.1. Anatomical Terminology

Learning Outcome

1. Discuss the Anatomical position and directional terms
2. Explain the Planes of the body: sagittal, coronal, and transverse
3. Focus the Body cavities: dorsal and ventral
4. Learn about Regions of the body: quadrants and regions
5. Describe the Terminology for movements: flexion, extension, etc.
6. Explain the Anatomical landmarks and their significance
7. Focus on Common abbreviations in anatomy
8. Identify Importance of standardized terminology in communication
9. Know Challenges in learning anatomical terminology

Acquiring the vocabulary of any scientific discipline is important for effective communication, particularly in medicine, where precision is imperative. Terms related to anatomy provide the foundation upon which the structures of the human body are described in gross anatomy and are assigned official names that minimize confusion among healthcare providers. The Terminologia Anatomica, which was accepted as the official nomenclature in 1998, made international consent and accuracy in terms of anatomy possible and has been indispensable in classroom and clinical settings. Although its longtime supremacy has prevailed, new advances in the medical sciences and technology reveal niches that call for periodic revision and expansion of this nomenclature with more specific definitions, especially for clinically significant structures. Efforts to update Terminologia Anatomica address the dynamic nature of anatomical nomenclature and the need to keep abreast of evolving educational demands and simplification of complexity to new students. Such initiatives aim to enhance comprehension and reduce errors, advancing better interdisciplinary collaboration (Kachlík et al., 2020; Pawe et al., 2023).

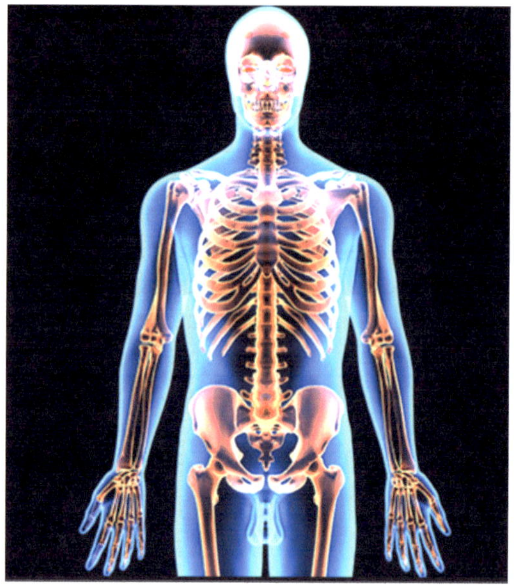

Source: Ideal Spine. (2019). *Anatomical Illustration of the Human Skeletal System with Glowing Overlay*.

1.1.1. Anatomical Position and Directional Terms

It is essential to understand the spatial position of the human body in gross anatomy because it creates precise communication among medical professionals. The communication is founded on the anatomical position, a standard reference posture in which the body is upright and oriented forward with the arms at the sides and palms facing outward, feet parallel and flat on the floor, and head and eyes directed straight ahead. This is the reference point from which directional descriptions are defined. Terms such as superior and inferior describe locations above or below a reference point, while anterior and posterior describe the front and back of the body, respectively. Medial and lateral describe closeness to the midline, as in inner relative to the outer position, which is fundamental in organ position and location of injury description. Proximal and distal terms similarly describe the relative distance from the trunk along an arm. Understanding these concepts makes it possible to accurately describe thermal applications in medical treatments, such as localized hyperthermia for oncological treatment, which depend on accurate anatomical localization to function effectively (Kok et al., 2020). Second, familiarity with direction terms also increases awareness of neurological tracts, such as those in complex basal ganglia circuits (Milardi et al., 2019) (Figure 1.5).

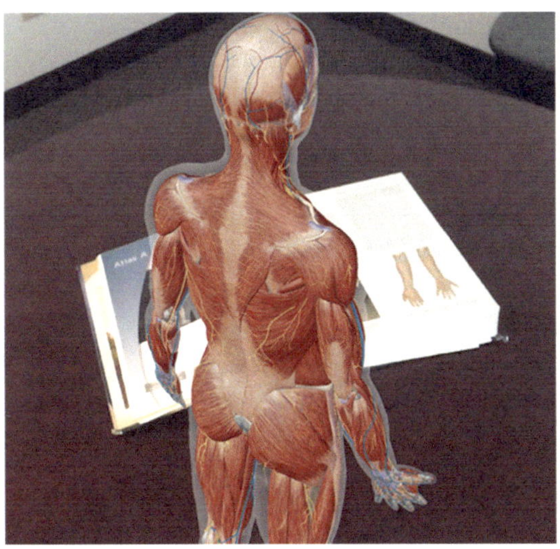

Figure 1.5. Anatomical position and directional terms.

Source: Visible Body. (n.d.). *Augmented Reality Anatomy Model Over Textbook*.

1.1.2. Planes of the Body: Sagittal, Coronal, and Transverse

The anatomy of humans requires a precise system for describing the locations and orientations of body structures. These systems are supplied by the body's three principal planes: sagittal, coronal, and transverse. The sagittal plane divides the body into left and right portions, facilitating detailed examination of bilateral symmetry and medial-lateral relationships. The coronal plane separates the body into anterior and posterior sections, facilitating the study of front and back anatomical structures. Lastly, the transverse plane separates the body into superior and inferior sections, which is convenient for cross-sectional study and imaging modalities. Competency in these planes is also essential for accurate diagnostic imaging and surgical planning, as in fetal neurosonography where the use of multiple planes ensures a detailed assessment of the central nervous system (CNS) (Paladini et al., 2021). Similarly, standardized use of the planes plays a significant role in the grading of spinal pathologies to maintain consistency in clinical reporting and research (David et al., 2014).

1.1.3. Body Cavities: Dorsal and Ventral

A knowledge of the organizational structure of the body is central to learning its complex anatomy and physiology. One of the distinguishing features is the division of the body cavities, which offer protection and housing for vital organs. The dorsal cavity, located along the posterior midline of the body, comprises the cranial cavity housing the brain and the vertebral cavity with the spinal cord. In contrast, the ventral cavity, being anterior, is separated into the thoracic and abdominopelvic cavities that are utilized to accommodate organs such as the heart, lungs, digestive organs, and reproductive organs. These provide spaces for separation and protection of organs while enabling their specialized functions to take place in restricted environments. Advanced imaging technologies like iodine contrast-enhanced computed tomography (CE CT) have allowed improved visualization of such cavities, demonstrating exquisite soft-tissue detail necessary for anatomical research and medical diagnosis (Paul et al., 2016). Research in model organisms like Drosophila illuminates organogenesis and cavity function, revealing evidence of evolutionary conservation between species (Berrak et al., 2016) (Figure 1.6).

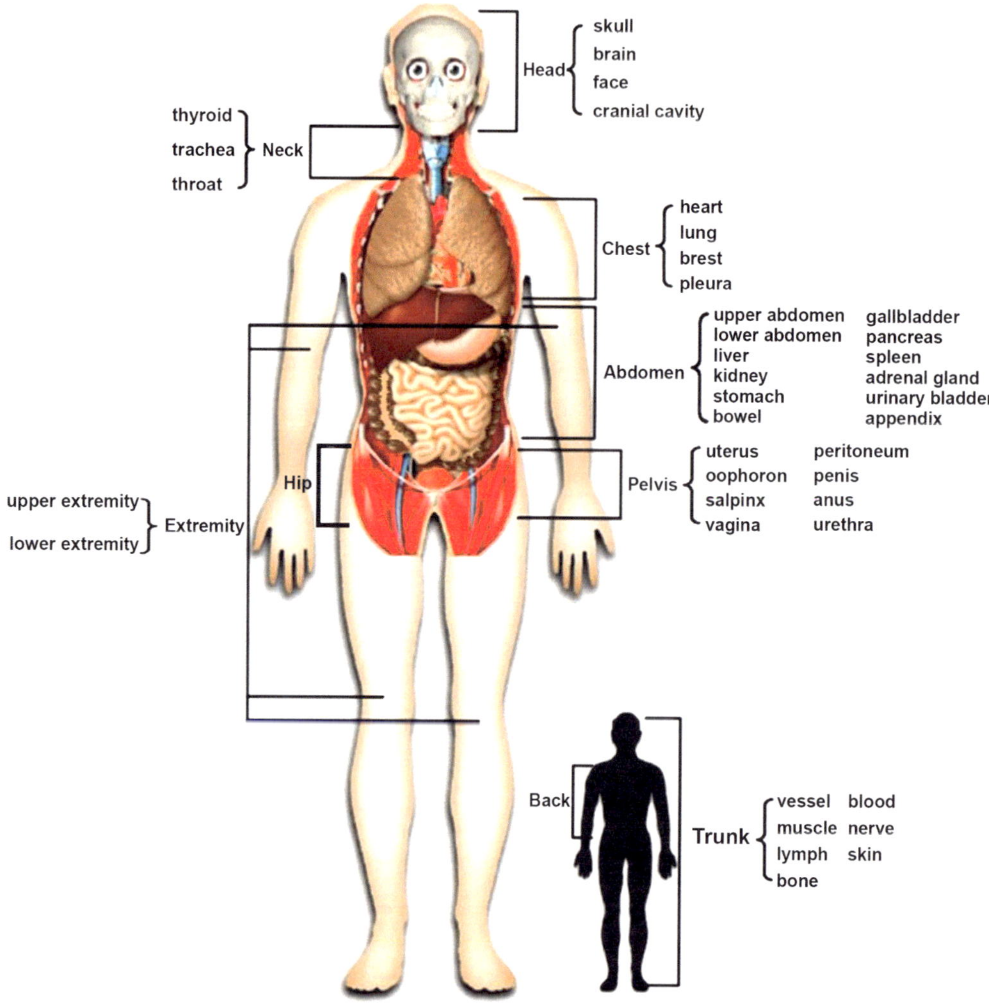

Figure 1.6. The organizational framework of the human body.

Source: Wang, Y., Fan, X., Chen, L. *et al.* Mapping anatomical related entities to human body parts based on wikipedia in discharge summaries. *BMC Bioinformatics* **20**, 430 (2019). https://doi.org/10.1186/s12859-019-3005-0

1.1.4. Regions of the Body: Quadrants and Regions

It is important to know the human body's organization so that anatomical locations can be properly identified and a common terminology employed by health practitioners. One such fundamental aspect in the organization of the body is the separation of the body into quadrants and regions, which form a reference point for clinical assessment and communication. The abdominopelvic cavity is typically divided into four quadrants—right upper, left upper, right lower, and left lower—allowing the identification of signs or abnormalities related to specific organs of those areas. More precise is the division into nine regions, like the epigastric, umbilical, and hypogastric regions, etc., that allow precision in the diagnosis and localization of structures within. Such regional divisions correspond very closely to underlying anatomy and physiology, enhancing both educational understanding and clinical skills. Advances in imaging and endoscopic procedures validate the importance of a thorough knowledge of body regions to be able to travel through intricately branching anatomical corridors successfully (Richard et al., 2021; Vural et al., 2021).

1.1.5. Terminology for Movements: Flexion, Extension, Etc.

Understanding the language of describing the body movements is crucial in gross anatomy, presenting a precise framework for communication throughout the profession. Flexion and extension are simple but fundamental movements whereby flexion refers to the bending of a joint that decreases the angle between two body parts and extension refers to straightening or opening out of that angle. These terms are all contained within one group that includes abduction, adduction, rotation, and circumduction, all labels for different directions and planes of motion essential to both clinical and educational settings. The accuracy that such nomenclature provides makes it possible to describe and analyze human movement accurately, with significant implications in medical education, rehabilitation, and emerging technologies like wearable robotic suits that aim to improve motor function (Xiloyannis et al., 2021). Moreover, systematic anatomical syllabi reinforce learning of these terms by dental and medical students so that they can have a comprehensive understanding required for patient care (Matthan et al., 2020) (Figure 1.7).

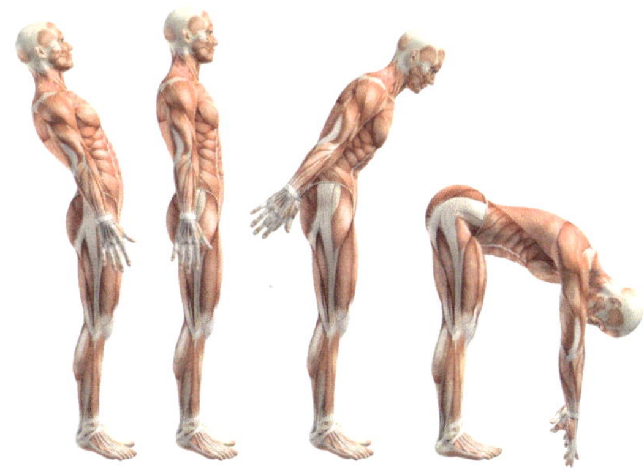

Figure 1.7. Terminology for movements.

Source: Yoga Teacher Central. (2017). *Illustration of Muscular Anatomy During Forward Bending Movement.*

1.1.6. Anatomical Landmarks and their Significance

Identification of the precise location and relationship of anatomical landmarks is crucial in clinical practice and medical education, for such references guide surgical interventions and add diagnostic precision. For example, the complex organization of the circumferential fascia of the rectum, including Denonvilliers' fascia and the rectosacral fascia, provides vital landmarks that allow surgeons to avoid injury to important neurovascular bundles during the process of rectal surgery, as exemplified by the signification of dissection 1 cm above the reflection of the peritoneum to protect surrounding tissues (Wang et al., 2024). The functional and symbolic attributes of anatomical landmarks extend their structural roles. In learning settings, the incorporation of digital storytelling about hand anatomy allows students to personally connect with anatomical features, which supplements their learning of anatomy and its relationship with daily life and therapy (Nation et al., 2025). Anatomical landmarks are thus critical pointers that not only facilitate precise medical procedures but also supplement the general comprehension of human anatomy.

1.1.7. Common Abbreviations in Anatomy

In gross anatomy, most abbreviations are necessary for effective and clear communication between students and healthcare professionals. Such abbreviations, e.g., "R" for right, "L" for left, "ant" for anterior, and "post" for posterior, allow for the avoidance of redundancy and the minimization of description of anatomical structures and their positions.

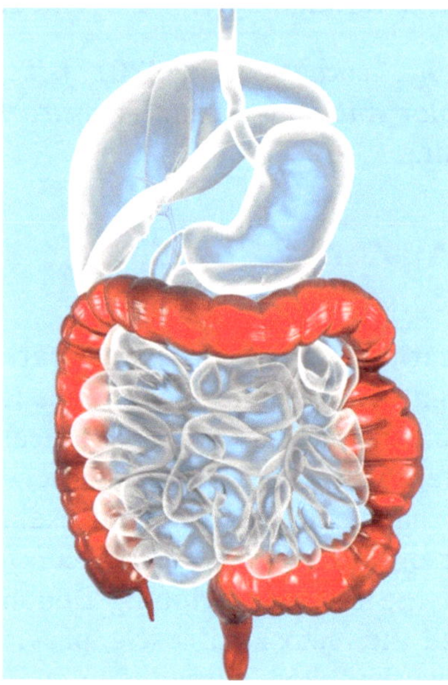

Source: AAPC. (n.d.). *Illustration of the Human Digestive Tract Highlighting the Large Intestine.*

Standard abbreviations also facilitate the reading of anatomical drawings, medical reports, and academic work so that uniformity can be established across situations. Knowledge of these abbreviations also allows speedy comprehension without compromising accuracy, which is critical in clinical procedures where speed and accuracy must be ensured. Despite their utility, abuse can lead to confusion and emphasizes the need for rigorous training and standard guidelines for anatomical terminology. This reflects broader activity in the medical sciences to codify and share things, such as the development of guidelines and protocols for greater clarity and fewer errors (Paul et al., 2017; Erd Fő et al., 2018).

1.1.8. Importance of Standardized Terminology in Communication

Effective communication in gross anatomy is in great measure based on the use of standardized terminology for precision and simplicity. Anatomically diverse structures, and between species variability necessitate an overlapping term to ensure uniformity to combat ambiguity as well as enhance cross-disciplinary collaboration. As an example, Uberon, a cross-species ontology, offers a rigorously structured framework that unites over 6,500 anatomical classes of species-independently, supporting effortless comparison and data integration between human and model organisms, which is critical for translational research and education (Mungall et al., 2012). Similarly, in clinical contexts, such as image-guided tumor ablation, the consistency in terminology and reporting criteria is the most important aspect of delineating procedures, imaging findings, and treatment outcomes correctly so that accuracy in communication between physicians and researchers is maximized (Ahmed et al., 2014). It not only improves mutual understanding but also accuracy in diagnostic and therapeutic procedures, finally leading to better patient care and advancing anatomical knowledge.

1.1.9. Challenges in Learning Anatomical Terminology

The subtle terminology of anatomy presents profound challenges to students entering the field of gross anatomy. The extensive list of technical terms, many of which come from Latin and Greek, can be intimidating to students and inhibit learning. This degree of linguistic sophistication is compounded by the fact that not only must terms be memorized, but also grasped must be the spatial and functional relationships that they represent. Moreover, sporadic exposure and limited practical application hinder retention, thus students find it difficult to integrate terminology into clinical reasoning effectively. Innovative pedagogies that foster engagement and active learning, such as interactive presentations and innovative pedagogies, have been promising in surmounting these issues by fostering more understanding and recall (Singh et al., 2019). However, beyond pedagogical approaches, structural obstacles such as an absence of diagnostic facilities in some regions limit students from visualizing and contextualizing anatomical terms to the highest degree (Fleming et al., 2021). These connected issues must be addressed to establish proficiency in anatomical terminology, which forms the foundation of effective communication in clinical practice (Figure 1.8).

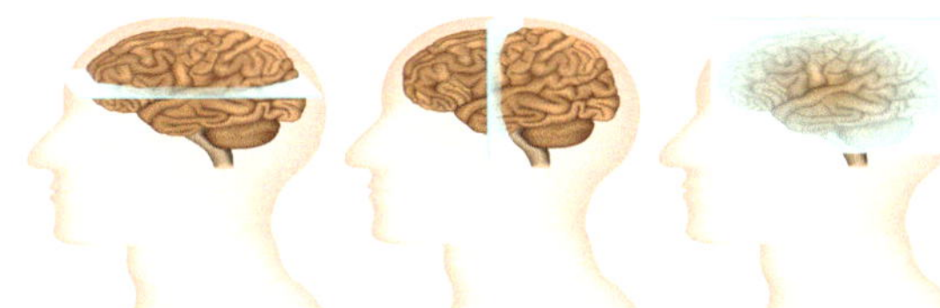

Figure 1.8. The complex language of anatomy presents significant obstacles for students entering the field of gross anatomy.

Source: ProProfs. (n.d.). *Anatomical Terminology Showing Different Brain Section Planes.*

Test Your Knowledge

1. Differentiate between the dorsal and ventral body cavities in terms of location and the major organs they contain.
2. Define flexion and give an example of a joint where it occurs.
3. What is the opposite of flexion? Describe it with an example.

1.2. Major Organ Systems

Learning Outcome

1. Give an overview of the human body's organ systems
2. Discuss the skeletal system: structure and function
3. Explain the muscular system: types of muscles
4. Know the circulatory system: heart and blood vessels
5. Focus on the respiratory system: anatomy of breathing
6. Discuss the digestive system: organs and their functions
7. Understand the nervous system: central and peripheral components
8. The endocrine system: hormonal regulation
9. The urinary system: kidney and excretory functions

Knowledge of the human body requires a close examination of its major organ systems, which perform critical functions to sustain life. The systems, including the cardiovascular, respiratory, nervous, musculoskeletal (MSK), and digestive systems, among others, operate in a complex interdependence that supports homeostasis and overall health. The cardiovascular system, for example, delivers blood to provide oxygen and nutrients and to remove waste products, whereas the nervous system coordinates body responses and sensory data. Gross anatomy provides descriptive information on such systems by examining their structure and spatial relations in the body. In addition, the overlap between visual and pragmatic learning methods such as interactive workshop sessions and the dissection of cadavers enables more knowledge of the organization and operation of such systems through a kinesthetic learning experience of reaffirmation of theoretic facts (Barbie, 2018). Precise recording of organ systems augmented by expert pathological studies further sharpens our knowledge of their disease and health (Bolon, 2023).

1.2.1. Overview of the Human Body's Organ Systems

A comprehensive understanding of the intricacy of the human body is not whole without studying the interconnected organ systems that sustain life. These systems, including the circulatory, respiratory, digestive, nervous, and MSK systems, collaborate to maintain homeostasis, facilitate movement, and allow for cognitive processes. For example, the circulatory system supplies essential nutrients and oxygen to tissues, while the respiratory system manages the gas exchange required for cellular respiration. The nervous system regulates body functions through electrical impulses, showing the integration necessary for responsiveness and survival. Covering these systems in gross anatomy gives the macroscopic view necessary for medical and biological sciences. Emerging knowledge of specialized anatomical barriers, such as the blood-brain barrier, indicates the complexity of organ systems and protection, influencing pharmacological strategies and treatment regimens (Erd Fő et al., 2018). Such a systems approach is not just required for the understanding of normal function but also for pathological conditions encountered in the clinical setting (Tara et al., 2023).

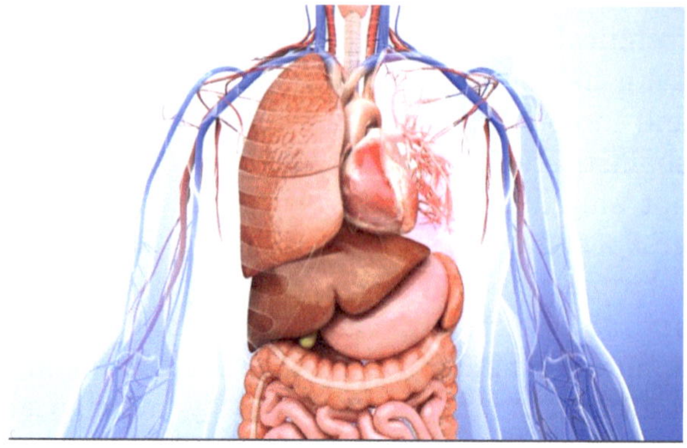

Source: ACC Trust. (2023). *Illustration of Human Internal Organ Systems Including Cardiovascular, Digestive, and Respiratory Systems.*

1.2.2. The Skeletal System: Structure and Function

The structure of the human body heavily relies on the interaction among multiple structural systems, of which the skeletal system ranks the highest. This structure not only provides mechanical support and protection for organs but also facilitates movement through its articulation with the muscles. Composed primarily of bone tissue, cartilage, ligaments, and joints, the skeletal system is extremely complicated in both its macroscopic and microscopic structure. Bone tissue is dynamic, constantly remodeling to meet physiological demands and providing space for bone marrow in which hematopoiesis occurs. The sheer cellular nature of the skeleton reflects general cellular organization within the human body and suggests the importance of quantitative and qualitative cellular research to account for tissue function (Bianconi et al., 2013). Moreover, cadaveric dissection remains a crucial pedagogical tool in the teaching of gross anatomy, with an unmatchable understanding of skeletal morphology and clinical relevance that cannot be fully imitated through the use of digital or alternative learning materials (Ghosh, 2016). Such a dual focus on function and structure underpins the skeletal system's central role in human anatomy.

1.2.3. The Muscular System: Types of Muscles

It is essential to know the fundamental distinctions between muscle types to comprehend the function of the muscular system within gross anatomy. The human body possesses three primary types of muscles: skeletal, cardiac, and smooth muscle. Voluntarily controlled and attached to bones, skeletal muscles facilitate movement and posture. Cardiac muscle, only found in the heart, contracts involuntarily through rhythmic contractions that are critical for blood circulation. Smooth muscle, found in the walls of internal organs and blood vessels, is likewise involuntary, regulating such movements as digestion and blood flow. Both muscles have unique structural and functional characteristics, respectively, to match the respective functions, reflective of the complexity of body systems. Advances in medical imaging and non-invasive technologies have improved visualization and understanding of muscle function and dysfunction at multiple levels (Rossini et al., 2015; Levi et al., 2019). The data are priceless for anatomical education and clinical practice and underscore the integral role of muscular system in human physiology.

1.2.4. The Circulatory System: Heart and Blood Vessels

The complex interaction of heart action and vascular dynamics serves to underscore the circulatory system's central position in gross anatomy. The heart is an energetic pump that displaces oxygen-rich blood through an enormous network of arteries, veins, and capillaries, bringing the necessary exchange of vital nutrients and gases to the rest of the body. Knowledge of this system in detail demonstrates how disruptions such as fulminant myocarditis can severely jeopardize cardiac output and cause multi-organ failure, which supports the need for early intervention and advanced care in late-stage heart failure treatments (Robb et al., 2020). Moreover, blood vessel growth and upkeep via angiogenesis remains the basis of physiological development and disease conditions and is regulated by numerous biochemical and mechanical parameters that can be analyzed using numerous bioassays (Nowak et al., 2018). Thus, research on the heart and blood vessels provides essential information regarding both their structural properties and their kinetic functions in sustaining life (Figure 1.9).

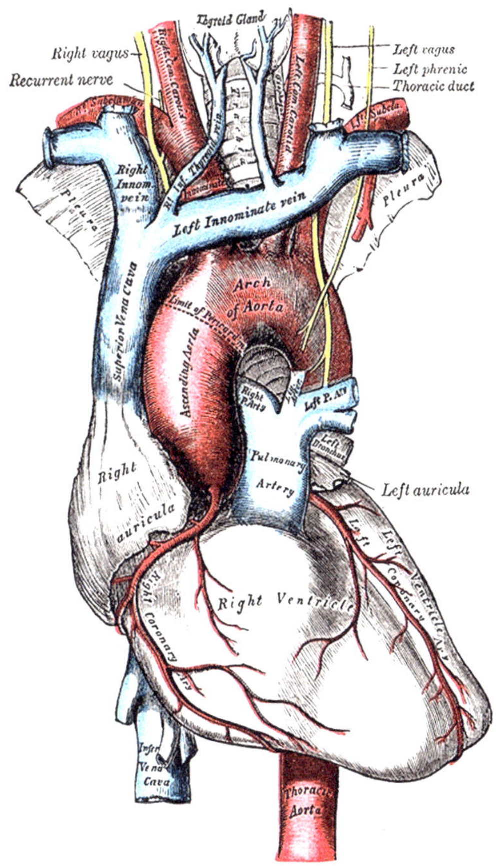

Figure 1.9. The circulatory system: heart and blood vessels.

Source: By Henry Vandyke Carter - Henry Gray (1918) Anatomy of the Human Body (See "Book" section below)Bartleby.com: Gray's Anatomy, Plate 505, Public Domain, https://commons.wikimedia.org/w/index.php?curid=425709

1.2.5. The Respiratory System: Anatomy of Breathing

Comprehension of the body's structural intricacy involves a thorough analysis of the systems that perform life-sustaining functions, especially those that allow for respiration. The respiratory system includes the nasal cavity, pharynx, larynx, trachea, bronchi, and lungs, all of which participate in the mechanism of breathing through the provision of airflow and exchange of gases. Mechanics of breathing entail the coordinated motion of the diaphragm and intercostal muscles to create pressure gradients for air entering and leaving. Gross anatomy focuses on integrating components, demonstrating how structural characteristics allow for functional effectiveness, such as branching bronchioles for maximum surface area for oxygen uptake. While imaging modalities like cardiovascular magnetic resonance (CMR) primarily help in cardiovascular evaluation, the same techniques are important to respiratory anatomy visualization for clinical and instructional purposes (Fratz et al., 2013). Technological advancement in imaging helps in further improvement in the comprehension and management of respiratory and associated thoracic structures, which testifies to the importance of anatomy in medical treatment (Laura et al., 2007).

1.2.6. The Digestive System: Organs and their Functions

The complexity of the human body is shown in the highly organized framework of its organ systems, each with significant roles in sustaining life. The digestive system is one of these systems and is designed to transform food consumed into vital nutrients and energy cells require. This device is made up of a sequence of specialized organs, including the mouth, esophagus, stomach, small and large intestines, liver, pancreas, and gallbladder, each having distinct but complementary functions. The stomach initiates protein digestion through enzymic activity and continuous acidity, followed by the small intestine, which continues nutrient absorption with the help of enzymes from the pancreas and bile from the liver. The large intestine is concerned with water absorption and the formation of feces to be eliminated. Understanding these organs' anatomical contacts and physiological activity not only throws light on human health but also allows for comparative perspectives from model systems, including the fruit fly, Drosophila melanogaster, whereby shared organ functionality emphasizes conserved molecular processes across morphological differences (Berrak et al., 2016). Understanding in this context highlights the value of anatomical and functional awareness within broader biomedical contexts (Lebow & Chen, 2016).

1.2.7. The Nervous System: Central and Peripheral Components

An understanding of the complex coordination of body functions necessitates a close examination of the central and peripheral nervous systems. These two co-operate to modulate the sensory input to the body and the motor output. The CNS, i.e., the brain and the spinal cord is the common center where the information is processed and the response decided. On the contrary, PNS comprises nerves running outside the CNS. These allow the body to communicate with the brain. In spite of the progress in neuroscience, peripheral nerve regeneration is still a major clinical problem, with recovery from injury usually being slow and incomplete, and fewer than half of the patients having satisfactory motor or sensory return. This deficiency is a reflection of a gap between the theoretical understanding of nerve physiology and the present surgical ability in the repair of nerves (Grinsell & Keating, 2014). Meanwhile, developments in non-invasive brain stimulation have widened the study and therapeutic instruments used, opening up neural pathways and treatments for neurological disorders (Rossini et al., 2015). All these aspects bring out the complexity of nervous system structure and function within gross anatomy (Figure 1.10).

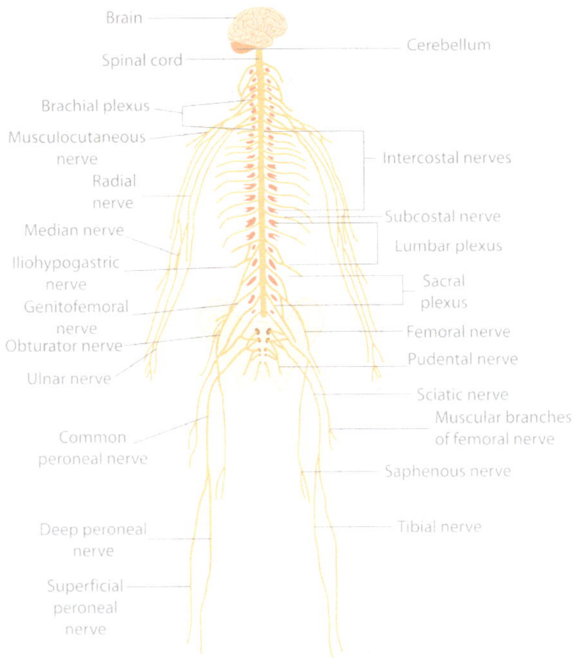

Figure 1.10. The nervous system.

Source: By Own work, CC BY 3.0, https://commons.wikimedia.org/w/index.php?curid=10187018

1.2.8. The Endocrine System: Hormonal Regulation

The subtle interaction of body functions in human anatomy largely relies on a rich tapestry of chemical signaling pathways. Of these, the endocrine system is the vital part of homeostasis by the provision of hormones into the bloodstream directly. Hormone regulation governs all from metabolism and growth to stress response and reproduction, a testament to its central position in gross anatomy study. This body's endocrine glands, such as the thyroid, adrenal, and pituitary, respond to feedback mechanisms that precisely fine-tune hormone levels to meet the needs of the body. Changes in hormone balance have been associated with a variety of diseases, including metabolic disorders related to circadian disturbance, as seen among shift workers, pointing to the dynamic interaction between environment and endocrine function (Luciana et al., 2010). Further, novel evidence is uncovering that endocrine-disrupting chemicals may have some effect on neurodevelopmental disease, implying the extensive reach of hormonal regulation over traditional physiological boundaries (Lyall et al., 2017).

1.2.9. The Urinary System: Kidney and Excretory Functions

The kidneys' complicated function extends beyond mere waste removal, playing a major role in systemic homeostasis and metabolic equilibrium. Within the urinary system, the kidneys are extremely sophisticated excretory organs that filter blood selectively to remove waste products and excess substances while retaining essential nutrients and electrolytes. This dynamic regulatory process not only assists in urine production but also influences blood pressure, acid-base balance, and red blood cell production. New imaging technologies, such as dual energy computed tomography (CT), have enhanced the diagnosis of renal calculi, a common urinary tract pathology, by identifying stone composition and assisting in correct clinical interventions (Montatore et al., 2023). Moreover, kidneys indirectly facilitate general physiological functions, like fertility, by managing micronutrient balance, like selenium, and this emphasizes their systemic relevance (Mojadadi et al., 2021). Renal structure and excretory mechanisms are thus fundamental to gross anatomy, with a focus on the multi-functionality of the kidney in human physiology.

Test Your Knowledge

1. What are the two components of the peripheral nervous system (PNS)?
2. How does the somatic nervous system differ from the autonomic nervous system?

1.3. Techniques in Gross Anatomy

Learning Outcome

1. Discuss the Dissection Techniques and Best Practices
2. Focus on Imaging Techniques: X-Rays, CT, and MRI
3. Describe the 3D Modeling and Virtual Anatomy
4. Know Cadaveric Studies and their Educational Value
5. Understand Comparative Anatomy: Learning From Other Species
6. Discuss the Anatomical Atlases and Resources
7. Explain the Role of Technology in Modern Anatomy Education
8. Identify Challenges in Teaching Gross Anatomy
9. Learn about Future Trends in Gross Anatomy Research

Advances in anatomical research methodology have significantly enhanced the precision and level of information in gross anatomy. Dissection remains a fundamental technique, providing direct visualization and haptic appreciation of the complexity of body structure. Supplementing traditional dissection, imaging technologies such as magnetic resonance imaging (MRI) and CT offer non-surgical means to investigate anatomical relationships *in vivo* and hence bridge the gap between surface anatomy and internal tissue. Further, computational approaches inherent in digital equipment geared for the analysis of neural signals, even as they find mainstream application within neurophysiology, show embedding of computational methods into anatomical investigations, further marking the inter-disciplinary facet of anatomy studies nowadays (Gramfort et al., 2013). Also, knowing dynamic change in temporal correlations in neural networks via advanced imaging dictates functional correlations in anatomy, promoting dynamic information over static snapshots (Elena et al., 2012). All these techniques are used to provide comprehensive knowledge of gross anatomy, and both educational work and clinical practice in the field are advantaged by them (Figure 1.11).

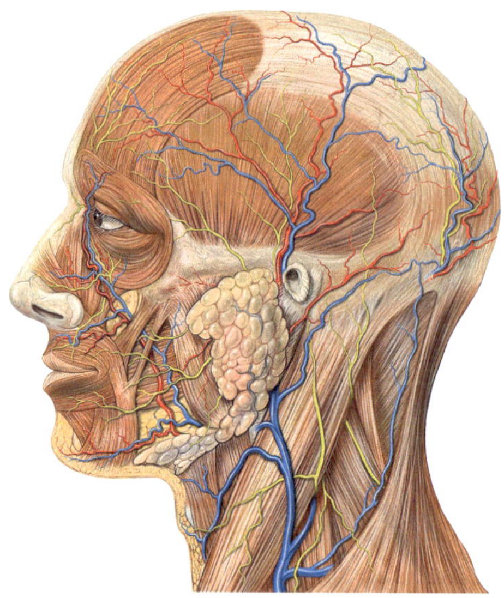

Figure 1.11. Techniques in gross anatomy.

Source: By Patrick J. Lynch, medical illustrator - Patrick J. Lynch, medical illustrator, CC BY 2.5, https://commons.wikimedia.org/w/index.php?curid=1498146

1.3.1. Dissection Techniques and Best Practices

Effective learning of gross anatomy is highly reliant on the adoption of proper dissection skills combined with best practices that foster student engagement and comprehension. Although cadaveric dissection is one of the gold standards in anatomy education, its effectiveness is significantly enhanced when combined with emerging approaches such as flipped learning, which increases student motivation and academic performance (Chung et al., 2024).

Moreover, supplementing hands-on dissection with innovative technology like the virtual anatomy dissection table augments the understanding of complex anatomical structures with interactive, three-dimensional visualization beyond two-dimensional images (Martín, 2024). Collectively, these methods foster independent learning, reduce confusion in practice, and support knowledge retention, which are crucial to quality learning experiences in gross anatomy. Adhering to these best practices ensures that students not only learn technical skills but also gain a sense of overall spatial awareness necessary for clinical application.

1.3.2. Imaging Techniques: X-Rays, CT, and MRI

Advances in medical imaging have revolutionized the exploration and understanding of gross anatomy through the capability to see inside the body without resorting to invasive methods. X-rays, among the first imaging technologies, produce two-dimensional images by projecting ionizing radiation through the body, outlining high-density material such as bones. Based on this, CT employs a number of X-ray measurements from different angles to produce cross-sectional images, providing greater anatomical detail and enabling detailed examination of complex spatial relationships between organs. MRI, employing powerful magnetic fields and radio waves, offers greater contrast resolution, especially in soft tissue, thus facilitating extensive examination of muscular, nervous, and vascular systems. These imaging methods play a pivotal role in the research and clinical environments, with current practice integrating refined image registration and fusion methods with the aim of improving diagnosis and therapy planning (Kristy et al., 2017). Moreover, imaging protocols have also been optimized for particular body segments, such as the male lower urinary tract anatomy, emphasizing the importance of appropriate terminology and imaging in clinical practice (Levi et al., 2019).

1.3.3. 3D Modeling and Virtual Anatomy

Technological innovation has played a dramatic role in the way gross anatomy is instructed, from the traditional cadaveric dissection to more recent techniques such as 3D modeling and virtual anatomy. These computer systems provide incredibly detailed and interactive representations of human anatomical structures, allowing students to see and maneuver complex spatial relationships that cannot be done with physical specimens. Integrating virtual reality (VR) in anatomy education has been shown to increase student engagement and understanding of anatomical structures, as well as retention through the delivery of repeatable and interactive learning experiences.

This approach addresses limitations in cadaver availability and ethical concerns, making anatomy more accessible and efficient to learn. The use of computer and virtual models shows a broader trend in pedagogy, augmenting the conventional lecture and dissection with technology-enabled applications supporting diversified learning styles and modern curricula in medicine (Sakshi, 2023; Andrés et al., 2024).

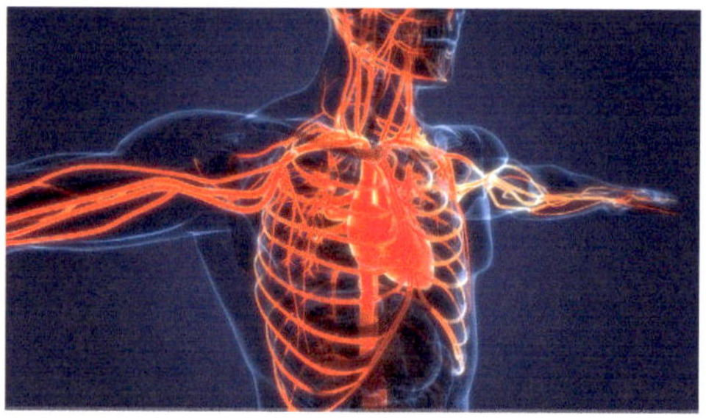

Source:

1.3.4. Cadaveric Studies and their Educational Value

Mastering human anatomy relies on experiential exposure that provides students with the opportunity to engage closely with the intricacies of the human body. In comparison to other pedagogical tools, cadaveric studies remain unrivaled in providing students with a realistic appreciation of spatial relationships and anatomical variations. The unmediated examination of cadavers enables students to relate theoretical learning to tangible structures, encouraging richer understanding and memorability. This activity is highly valued not only by students but also by practicing clinicians who attribute most of their anatomical proficiency to early cadaver exposure. Further, progress has also included integrating technology, such as tablet-based testing, which supplements traditional dissection through immediate feedback and standardized examination, improving learning and overall student outcomes (Polak-Boro et al., 2021). Surveys of healthcare practitioners continue to support the adequacy and suitability of cadaveric experience in anatomy instruction, noting that it plays a critical role in the preparation of clinical practitioners (Giuriato et al., 2020).

1.3.5. Comparative Anatomy: Learning From Other Species

Examination of the anatomical structure of different species provides useful insight into evolutionary biology and functional adaptation. By examining mammalian brain structure, for instance, researchers have revealed conserved scaling relations between neuronal and nonneuronal cells that shed light on the evolution of sophisticated neural systems. Specifically, studies of marsupials and eutherian mammals depict both convergent and divergent trends in brain mass structure and neuron distribution, illustrating evolutionary adaptation and illuminating neurological development (Santos et al., 2017). Similarly, studies in marine mammals such as beaked whales uncover special physiological adaptations to environmental stressors that can only be understood with precise anatomical data. For example, the pathological disorders that acoustic exposure has been found to be related to highlight the significance of anatomical and behavioral studies in such animals (Tara et al., 2023). These comparative anatomy studies not only improve our knowledge of a given species but also enrich the overall system of gross anatomy by giving us knowledge of common characteristics and evolutionary pressure-conditioned differences.

1.3.6. Anatomical Atlases and Resources

Technological innovations have significantly transformed learning gross anatomy by offering new devices that supplement traditional teaching strategies. Anatomy atlases and digital content now offer precise, uniform illustrations that facilitate the understanding of intricate structures and their position in space more profoundly. For instance, advanced software packages allow for automated white matter tractography detail extraction, useful in diverse species, ranging from humans to macaques, hence facilitating comparative neuroanatomy as well as large-scale studies (Warrington et al., 2020). Moreover, the imperative of remote learning, driven by the COVID-19 pandemic, has driven the rapid development and adoption of virtual anatomical interfaces to replicate the haptic and three-dimensional exposure traditionally gained by means of cadaver dissection (Georga et al., 2020). These interfaces overcome the limitations of physical proximity to access, ensuring the guarantee of uninterrupted high-quality learning while enabling academic collaboration and innovative curriculum design. Together, these evolving atlases and resources are a fundamental component of modern gross anatomy education and research (Figure 1.12).

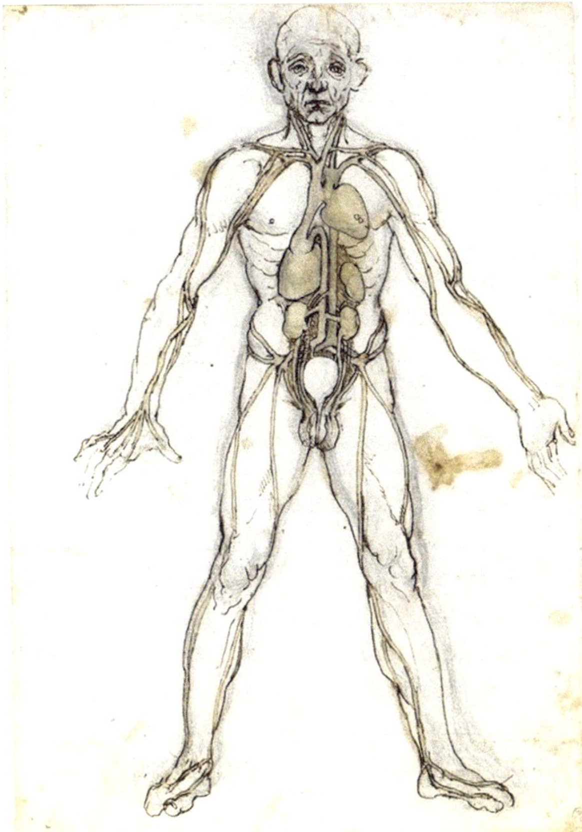

Figure 1.12. Anatomical atlases and resources.

Source: By Leonardo da Vinci - https://www.metmuseum.org/special/Leonardo_Master_Draftsman/tour_gallery4.htm, Public Domain, https://commons.wikimedia.org/w/index.php?curid=1744423

1.3.7. Role of Technology in Modern Anatomy Education

The abrupt transition towards remote learning in times of global disruptions has radically altered anatomy education, compelling institutions to implement technological steps to maintain continuity in teaching. The very nature of anatomy, relying traditionally on cadaveric dissection and manual engagement with three-dimensional structures, poses challenges to virtual conversion that are unique. However, developments in digital materials like interactive software, tutorial videos, and VR sites have become necessary ancillaries to facilitate and, in some contexts, replace hands-on experience. These developments allow for easy access and innovative pedagogic partnerships, but questions remain about their ability to replicate the richness of learning that direct anatomy study offers and their impact on the acquisition of students' clinical competence (Georga et al., 2020). In addition, these platforms should be used thoughtfully and integrated in a manner to bring out optimum interaction of the learners and sustain clinical relevance of the subject to make the resultant health practitioners a thorough anatomist, irrespective of how remote the modality imposes on them (Franchi, 2020).

1.3.8. Challenges in Teaching Gross Anatomy

Despite its foundation in medical education, gross anatomy education has several challenges that make learning and education cumbersome. Traditional application of cadaver dissection is encumbered by logistical problems of increasing numbers of students, fewer cadavers, and heavy maintenance expenses that can restrict experiential learning experiences. Ethical issues and emotional effects on students may also hinder involvement in dissections. Curriculum-wise, integrating anatomy in Competency-Based Medical Education (CBME) curricula necessitates the concurrent development of clinical skills and knowledge but in most cases leaves students with tough content and difficulty in relating theoretical knowledge to practice. Gross anatomy and embryology tend to be targeted as particularly tough topics that further complicate making things easy to teach. To address these challenges, the application of newer visualization tools, such as simulations and virtual dissection tables, has the potential to enhance spatial understanding and engagement alongside modern pedagogical approaches. More student-oriented assessment protocols and embedding clinical relevance in anatomy education are also critical to addressing challenges in learning and improving student performance (Bokil et al., 2025; Veerraju et al., 2025).

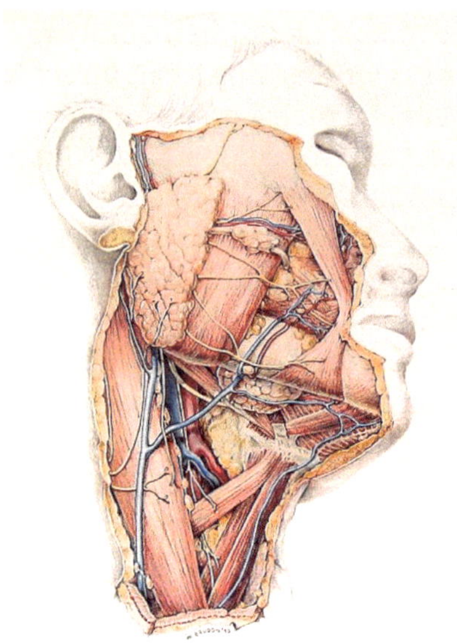

Source: Nicolet College. (2016). *Anatomical Illustration of the Head and Neck Musculature and Vascular Structures.*

1.3.9. Future Trends in Gross Anatomy Research

As technology advances further, science research will go on being revolutionized by technology, and research in gross anatomy will not be left behind. Advances such as three-dimensional imaging, AR, and virtual dissection labs are enhancing visualization and comprehension of complex anatomical structures and consequently educational and clinical uses.

These emerging resources enable precise anatomical mapping and individualized medicine, reducing the utilization of the traditional cadaver dissection technique and expanding access for diverse learners. Besides, interdisciplinary research that unites bioengineering and molecular biology will improve the understanding of anatomical variation and pathologic mechanisms. Still, successful integration of these technologies requires overcoming economic and regulatory challenges, similar to other areas targeting sustainability and modernization (Iwuanyanwu et al., 2024). Paradigms of education also need to evolve with such innovations, creating adaptive curricula that equip future anatomists to handle rapidly changing scientific contexts (Zahroh et al., 2024). Overall, future trends of gross anatomy research indicate towards an active incorporation of technology and pedagogy in shaping both the knowledge and the practice of the discipline.

Test Your Knowledge

1. 1What is the purpose of an anatomical atlas in medical education?
2. What is the advantage of using 3D models in anatomy education?

1.4. Clinical Relevance of Gross Anatomy

Learning Outcome

1. Focus on importance of anatomy in surgical procedures
2. Discuss the anatomy in radiology and imaging
3. Explain the role of anatomy in physical therapy
4. Describe the anatomy in emergency medicine
5. Understand pathology through anatomy
6. Know anatomy in medical education and training
7. Identify case studies highlighting anatomical knowledge
8. Know interdisciplinary approaches to anatomy
9. Learn about future of gross anatomy in healthcare

Awareness of the fundamental structures of the human body is crucial to effective clinical practice, as it informs diagnostic and therapeutic intervention in all medical specialties. While new technologies have introduced new modes of instruction, the kinesthetic experience of cadaveric dissection cannot be replicated by any other means in building a comprehensive spatial awareness and clinical correlation skill required for patient treatment. This hands-on learning not only sharpens anatomical understanding but also cultivates cross-disciplinary skills such as professionalism and empathy, which are essential in healthcare settings. The clinical relevance of gross anatomy education remains unabated even amidst adversity brought about by modern curricular advancements and current disruptions in traditional dissection practice, laying a foundation for safe surgical practice and appropriate clinical judgment. Therefore, the incorporation of dissection alongside adjunct pedagogical techniques ensures that there is well-rounded anatomical training that provides students with hands-on clinical needs, underpinning the argument that gross anatomy is still an integral part of medical education (Ghosh, 2016; Franchi, 2020).

1.4.1. Importance of Anatomy in Surgical Procedures

A thorough understanding of human anatomy is crucial to the success and safety of surgery since it provides the foundation of information upon which to navigate through complex body structures. Surgeons utilize detailed anatomical knowledge to identify landmarks, avoid vital nerves and vessels, and undertake precise interventions. Integrating training in surgical procedures into gross anatomy teaching has also been demonstrated to have significant benefits, with the literature describing enhancement in clinical readiness and student confidence without encroaching on conventional anatomy curricula (Gant et al., 2021). Additionally, advances in medical imaging and segmentation procedures, such as brain MRI, also enhance surgical planning through the accurate visualization of anatomical structures and pathology (Fiaz et al., 2019). They complement anatomical teaching by increasing the surgeon's ability to anticipate difficulty and design interventions on that basis. A refined appreciation of anatomy coupled with newer imaging modalities is thus central to the maximization of surgical outcomes and the further evolution of clinical practice (Figure 1.13).

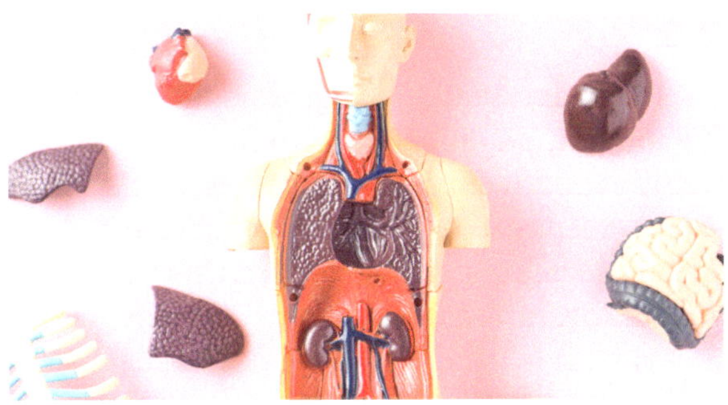

Figure 1.13. Importance of anatomy in surgical procedures.

Source: CIVIS. (n.d.). *Anatomical Model with Detachable Human Organs on Pink Background.*

1.4.2. Anatomy in Radiology and Imaging

Modern radiology and imaging technologies have revolutionized the study and use of gross anatomy by making it possible to visualize internal structures with high accuracy in a painless manner. These advanced imaging technologies, including MRI and CT scans, enable clinicians and anatomists to study anatomical variations, pathological changes, and functional relationships with unprecedented accuracy. MRI, particularly breast imaging MRI, is characterized by exceptional sensitivity in lesion detection and hence enhanced diagnostic accuracy and surgical planning (Ritse et al., 2019). In addition, combining image registration and fusion algorithms allows for precise alignment and comparison of multimodal images, making it easier to provide adaptive treatment strategy and enhance anatomical delineation during radiotherapy (Kristy et al., 2017). This overlap of technology not only facilitates detailed anatomical assessments but also drives individualized medicine by tracking anatomical changes through time. Imaging and radiology are thus critical instruments in the accurate assessment of gross anatomy, bridging traditional cadaveric education with living, dynamic clinical applications.

1.4.3. Role of Anatomy in Physical Therapy

A solid understanding of gross anatomy forms the foundation upon which effective physical therapy is built, enabling clinicians to effectively screen, diagnose, and manage musculoskeletal (MSK) and neurological disorders. Understanding such information helps them identify which anatomical structures are involved in the movement, comprehend their interplay, and gain an understanding of how pathology compromises normal function. For instance, awareness of the intricate arrangement of lymph vessels and nodes informs treatments that steer clear of complications, such as lymphatic blockage following surgery, demonstrating the importance of anatomical precision in treating patients (Ye et al., 2021). Additionally, anatomical awareness of vascular and nervous system development occupies a central role in the treatment of children, as developmental variations affect rehabilitation measures and outcomes (Donna et al., 2019). Hence, gross anatomy not only provides us with a blueprint for human shape but also informs the direct tailoring of physical therapy interventions to the greatest possible patient recovery, through focused evidence-based practice, that respects the complexity of the human body.

1.4.4. Anatomy in Emergency Medicine

A profound understanding of gross anatomy is unavoidable in emergency medicine clinicians, where rapid decision-making often depends on precise knowledge of the human body's structure. In acute settings, for instance, managing aneurysmal subarachnoid hemorrhage, a profound knowledge of topic relevant anatomical regions enhances diagnostic accuracy and guides early interventions, directly impacting patient outcomes (Brian et al., 2023). However, retention of gross anatomy has been shown to decline in the absence of continuing clinical usage, with clinical anatomy retained better due to frequent usage within practice (Brian et al., 2023). This gap indicates the necessity for integrating gross anatomical education with clinical context, especially for emergency medicine physicians dealing with complex, high-stakes cases involving instantaneous understanding of organ systems, vascular structures, and potential trauma pathways. Instructional approaches that support active learning and constant reinforcement can bridge this gap, enabling emergency physicians to apply anatomical principles effectively and, in turn, improve patient care in life-or-death scenarios (Saeed et al., 2025).

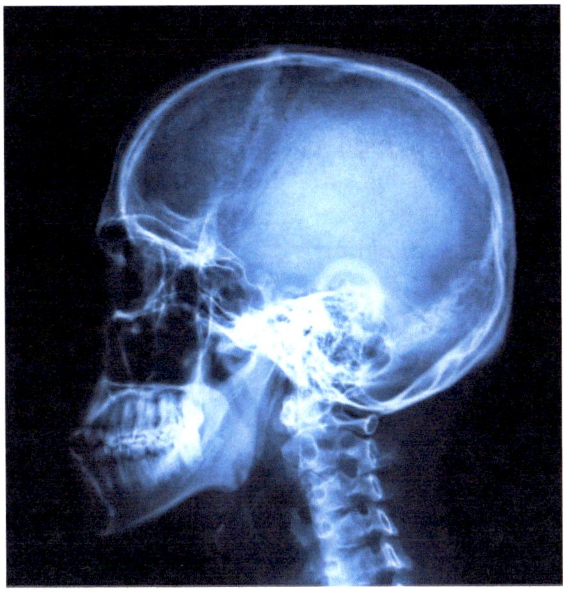

Source: 3D4Medical. (n.d.). *Lateral X-Ray View of Human Skull and Cervical Spine.*

1.4.5. Understanding Pathology Through Anatomy

It is important to have a good knowledge of human anatomy to accurately diagnose and treat disease states, as all disease is expressed within the body's structural framework. Gross anatomy provides a basic foundation by revealing not only the normal arrangement but also the variations and weaknesses present in body structures. For example, recent research identifying the medial meniscal artery enhances meniscal vascularization knowledge, which is crucial for surgical treatment of degenerative meniscus pathologies and surgical planning (Śmigielski et al., 2024). Such detailed anatomical data allow clinicians to better predict how specific pathologies affect function and direct techniques of restoration and preservation. Besides, experiential anatomical learning fosters an appreciation of human complexity and variation, enabling clinicians to anticipate disease presentation variability (Ross et al., 2020). The integrated approach ensures pathology is not addressed alone but rather as a consequence of structural modifications, emphasizing gross anatomy as a vital medical education and clinical practice resource.

1.4.6. Anatomy in Medical Education and Training

Profound knowledge of human anatomy is the keystone for effective medical education, bridging theory and practice. Anatomy has a history that evolved from initial dissection to an essential component of medical curricula across the world, including Korea, where the topic has been cultivated through many pedagogical traditions to serve widening demands for healthcare professionals (In-Kim et al., 2024).

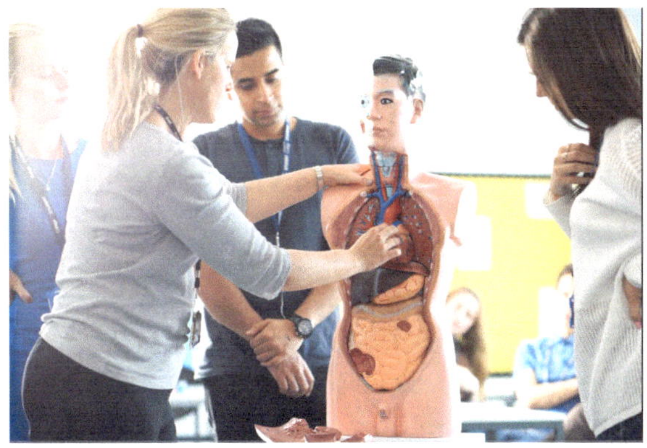

Figure 1.14. Anatomy in medical education and training.

Source: UCLA Extension. (n.d.). *Instructor Demonstrating Human Anatomy Using Torso Model in Classroom.*

Current educational methods blend traditional cadaveric dissection with new multimedia resources such as narrated dissection videos and interactive modules of review to accommodate different learning styles and visualization of complex structures like the nervous system (Matthan et al., 2020). The hybrid approaches address anatomy education issues, such as time limitations for teaching and the occurrence of neurophobia, by promoting independent learning and facilitating anatomical concepts relevant to clinical practice. Hence, integrating traditional and modern teaching techniques is necessary for developing effective physicians who can utilize gross anatomical information in diverse healthcare settings (Matthan et al., 2020; In-Kim et al., 2024) (Figure 1.14).

1.4.7. Case Studies Highlighting Anatomical Knowledge

Clinical case studies are also essential to bridge theoretical anatomical knowledge and application to clinical practice. Tendon transfer procedures, for instance, demand a detailed understanding of muscle anatomy and biomechanics, as supported by a systematic review that outlined essential principles underlying surgical success and trainee education (Ashwood et al., 2023). The incorporation of case discussions within training packages has been shown to significantly enhance trainee anatomical knowledge and surgical confidence, which ultimately leads to improved patient outcomes. Similarly, detailed anatomical research via cadaveric dissection has elucidated the precise course of the first branch of the lateral plantar nerve, yielding reliable landmarks to guide ultrasound interventions for plantar heel pain (Kuechly et al., 2024). These empirical findings underscore the importance of anatomical precision in diagnosis and treatment, illustrating how careful case analysis not only advances educational endeavors but also informs and refines clinical practice. Taken together, these types of case studies demonstrate the immeasurable role of gross anatomy in contributing to medical education and patient care alike.

1.4.8. Interdisciplinary Approaches to Anatomy

The complexity of the human body demands an interdisciplinary effort that transcends traditional field boundaries, promoting collaboration between fields such as biology, engineering, and medical imaging. By a synergistic combination of knowledge from various disciplines, scientists can build more sophisticated models that reveal anatomical structures with greater precision and functional understanding. For example, biomechanical engineering aids in the study of MSK dynamics, while novel imaging technology improves the visualization of internal organs to support both clinical practice and education. Further, interdisciplinary research provides valuable insight into physiological reactions and pathological processes to facilitate innovation in diagnostics and therapy. It is framing the grand challenges of anatomy that necessitate such an interdisciplinary effort, with future breakthroughs promising to transform healthcare and biological science (Guang-Yang et al., 2018). In more specific terms, anatomy and behavioral studies of species affected by environmental change demonstrate the necessity for synergy with physiology, pathology, and ecology, illustrating the extent collaboration can lead to profound understanding (Tara et al., 2023) (Figure 1.15).

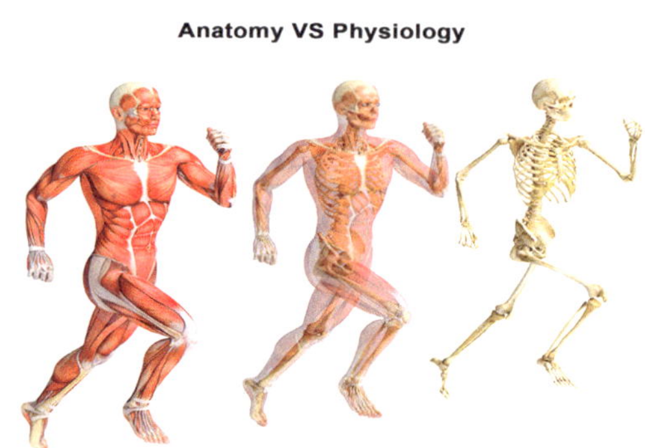

Figure 1.15. The complexity of human anatomy demands an integrative method that transcends traditional disciplinary boundaries.

Source: Knya Med. (2024). *Anatomy vs Physiology – Comparison of Muscular, Internal, and Skeletal Systems.*

1.4.9. The Future of Gross Anatomy in Healthcare

With advances in technology, medical education and practice are going to be revolutionized in ways that optimize learning and clinical utility. Advanced technologies such as AR and VR provide interactive, experiential learning that increases student engagement and retention of complex anatomical information, and encourages critical thinking and collaboration outside the boundaries of traditional dissection labs (Mohammed et al., 2023). Augmenting such developments, three-dimensional printing makes it possible to create patient-specific anatomical models from high-resolution imaging modalities, facilitating individualized preoperative planning and maximizing surgical precision in a broad variety of specialties (José et al., 2022). Such a meeting of technology not only elevates educational methods to a new plan, but also promotes improved patient care by bridging the gap between theoretical learning and actual application. Thus, the future of gross anatomy in medicine will likely center on a multidisciplinary framework that combines digital simulations, physical models, and real-time data to prepare practitioners for the evolving needs of medical science and clinical practice.

Test Your Knowledge

1. What imaging technique provides detailed cross-sectional views of the body?
2. How does anatomy help in identifying pathological changes in organs?

SUMMARY

The challenges faced in gross anatomy teaching, particularly during breakages such as the COVID-19 pandemic, bring into focus the necessity for innovative pedagogical methods that merge traditional and virtual modalities. While the dissection of cadavers remains at the center of learning three-dimensional anatomical associations, teachers have adapted by incorporating web-based components to supplement and even replace practical exercises, with a view to maintaining educational standards despite limitations (Georga et al., 2020). Similarly, the use of multimedia study aids in neuroanatomy illustrates the versatility of different formats like narrated dissection videos and interactive review slides to enhance comprehension and memorization for different learning styles, in effect eliminating the intimidation usually associated with challenging anatomical concepts (Matthew et al., 2020). Together, these breakthroughs mean a balanced gross anatomy curriculum requires an adaptive, multimodal approach to support practical dissection with digital aids, ultimately resulting in greater depth of comprehension and allowing student participation in a dynamic learning community.

Gross anatomy has occupied a prominent place in medical education because it generates the required knowledge for patient management and clinical practice. Emphasizing the need for innovative pedagogic approaches, such as body painting, can enhance understanding of surface anatomy by touch and vision implantation, which has shown to be useful as per current educational research (Gomar et al., 2019). In addition, the emergence of digital resources offers promising tools for students of anatomy but the majority of websites nowadays offer bad content and less effective interactivity, decreasing their learning value. An effective web-based tool for anatomy should be focused on effective content planning that relates to clear learning objectives to facilitate deeper learning than memorization (Kim et al., 2003). These details summarize that gross anatomy education is enriched through both hands-on experiential training and well-designed digital aids, both of which support one another to produce a comprehensive and accessible learning experience.

KEY TERMS FROM THIS CHAPTER

- Anatomical education
- Augmented reality (AR)
- Bibliometric data analysis
- Cardiovascular magnetic resonance (CMR)
- Competency-Based Medical Education (CBME)
- Effective treatment interventions
- Gross anatomical structures
- Gross disease
- Anatomical practice
- Basal ganglia circuits
- Body structures
- Central nervous system (CNS)
- Diagnostic procedures
- Fetal neurosonography
- Gross anatomy
- Health sciences advancement

CRITICAL THINKING QUESTIONS

1. **Which of the following best defines gross anatomy?**
   a. Study of cells and tissues
   b. Study of anatomical structures visible to the naked eye
   c. Study of physiological functions
   d. Study of genetic material
2. **Which plane divides the body into right and left halves?**
   a. Coronal plane
   b. Transverse plane
   c. Sagittal plane
   d. Horizontal plane
3. **Which of the following terms refers to a position closer to the head?**
   a. Inferior
   b. Distal
   c. Proximal
   d. Superior
4. **The study of the structure of organs and organ systems as they relate to the entire body is called:**
   a. Microscopic anatomy
   b. Systemic anatomy
   c. Developmental anatomy
   d. Radiologic anatomy
5. **Which anatomical position describes the body facing forward, with arms at the sides and palms facing outward?**
   a. Lateral
   b. Prone
   c. Anatomical position
   d. Supine

Short Answer Questions

1. What are the main methods used to study gross anatomy?
2. Differentiate between systemic and regional anatomy.
3. What is the anatomical position and why is it important?
4. What is the difference between medial and lateral?
5. Explain the terms proximal and distal with an example.

Answers to Critical Thinking Questions

1. (b) 2. (c) 3. (d) 4. (b) 5. (c)

REFERENCES

1. Ashwood, N. , Hind, J. , Dekker, A. , Elgalli, M. , Alawoya, T. and Mertz, T. (2023) Introducing the Principles of Tendon Transfer for Surgical Trainees to Improve Anatomical Knowledge. *Open Journal of Orthopedics*, **13**, 306-319. doi: 10.4236/ojo.2023.137030.(accessed on 8th May 2025).
2. Albaraa, M., Au, A. L. S., Salah, W., Witting, P. K., & Ahmad, G. (2021). Role for selenium in metabolic homeostasis and human reproduction. *Nutrients, 13*, 3256. https://doi.org/10.3390/nu13093256.
3. AlGerafi, M. A. M., Zhou, Y., Oubibi, M., & Wijaya, T. T. (2023). Unlocking the potential: A comprehensive evaluation of augmented reality and virtual reality in education. *Electronics, 12*, 3953. https://doi.org/10.3390/electronics12183953.
4. Allen, E. A., Damaraju, E., Plis, S. M., Erhardt, E. B., Eichele, T., & Calhoun, V. D. (2012). Tracking whole-brain connectivity dynamics in the resting state. *Cerebral Cortex, 24*, 663–676. https://doi.org/10.1093/cercor/bhs352.
5. Bhattacharjee, S. & Ghosh, S.K. (2023) *The Sun Also Rises*: Tracing the evolution of humanistic values in anatomy pedagogy and research, including cadaveric acquisition practices. *Journal of Anatomy*, 243, 1031–1051. Available from: **https://doi.org/10.1111/joa.13938** (accessed on 8th May 2025).
6. Bianconi, E., Piovesan, A., Facchin, F., Beraudi, A., Casadei, R., Frabetti, F., Vitale, L., et al. (2013). An estimation of the number of cells in the human body. *Annals of Human Biology, 40*, 463–471. https://doi.org/10.3109/03014460.2013.807878.
7. Bolon. (2023). Book review: Toxicologic pathology for non-pathologists. *Toxicologic Pathology, 51*, 87–88. https://www.semanticscholar.org/paper/ce570b29ac1d7ad7ca4f5007500f81c71909781e (accessed on 8th May 2025).
8. Bork, F., Stratmann, L., Enssle, S., Eck, U., Navab, N., Waschke, J., & Kugelmann, D. (2019). The benefits of an augmented reality magic mirror system for integrated radiology teaching in gross anatomy. *Anatomical Sciences Education, 12*, 585–598. https://doi.org/10.1002/ase.1864.
9. Kim, S., Brinkley, J. F., & Rosse, C. (2003). Profile of on-line anatomy information resources: design and instructional implications. *Clinical anatomy (New York, N.Y.), 16*(1), 55–71. https://doi.org/10.1002/ca.10088 (accessed on 8th May 2025).
10. Dawson, L. A., & Jaffray, D. A. (2007). Advances in image-guided radiation therapy. *Journal of Clinical Oncology, 25*, 938–946. https://doi.org/10.1200/jco.2006.09.9515.
11. Fardon, D. F., Williams, A. L., Dohring, E. J., Murtagh, F. R., Rothman, S. L. G., & Sze, G. (2014). Lumbar disc nomenclature: Version 2.0. *The Spine Journal, 14*, 2525–2545. https://doi.org/10.1016/j.spinee.2014.04.022.
12. Faruqi, S., Tseng, C. L., Whyne, C., Alghamdi, M., Wilson, J. R., Myrehaug, S., Soliman, H., et al. (2017). Vertebral compression fracture after spine stereotactic body radiation therapy: A review of the pathophysiology and risk factors. *Neurosurgery, 83*, 314–322. https://doi.org/10.1093/neuros/nyx493.
13. Fleming, K. A., Horton, S., Wilson, M. L., Atun, R., DeStigter, K., Flanigan, J., Sayed, S., et al. (2021). The Lancet Commission on diagnostics: Transforming access to diagnostics. *The Lancet, 398*, 1997–2050. https://doi.org/10.1016/s0140-6736(21)00673-5.

14. Franchi, T. (2020). The impact of the COVID-19 pandemic on current anatomy education and future careers: A student's perspective. *Anatomical Sciences Education, 13*, 312–315. https://doi.org/10.1002/ase.1966.

15. Fratz, S., Chung, T., Greil, G., Samyn, M. M., Taylor, A. M., Valsangiacomo, B. E. R., Yoo, S. J., et al. (2013). Guidelines and protocols for cardiovascular magnetic resonance in children and adults with congenital heart disease: SCMR expert consensus group on congenital heart disease. *Journal of Cardiovascular Magnetic Resonance, 15*, 51. https://doi.org/10.1186/1532-429x-15-51.

16. Gant, T., Chiang, H., Harman, B. D., Axford, D. S., Brisson, P., Brisson, M., & Stephen, D. (2021). Simulating Early Clinical Experiences With Surgical Procedures in the Anatomy Laboratory. *Cureus, 13*(3), e13966. https://doi.org/10.7759/cureus.13966(accessed on 8th May 2025).

17. Giuriato, R., Štrkalj, G., Prvan, T., & Pather, N. (2020). Australian chiropractors' perception of the clinical relevance of anatomical sciences and adequacy of teaching in chiropractic curricula. *Chiropractic & Manual Therapies, 28.* https://doi.org/10.1186/s12998-020-00325-6.

18. Gramfort, A., Luessi, M., Larson, E. D., Engemann, D. A., Strohmeier, D., Brodbeck, C., Goj, R., et al. (2013). MEG and EEG data analysis with MNE-Python. *Frontiers in Neuroscience, 7.* https://doi.org/10.3389/fnins.2013.00267.

19. Grinsell, D., & Keating, C. (2014). Peripheral nerve reconstruction after injury: A review of clinical and experimental therapies. *BioMed Research International, 2014*, 1–13. https://doi.org/10.1155/2014/698256.

20. Harrison, D. J., Geller, D. S., Gill, J., Lewis, V. O., & Görlick, R. (2017). Current and future therapeutic approaches for osteosarcoma. *Expert Review of Anticancer Therapy, 18*, 39–50. https://doi.org/10.1080/14737140.2018.1413939.

21. Inchingolo, F., Santacroce, L., Ballini, A., Topi, S., Dipalma, G., Haxhirexha, K., Bottalico, L., et al. (2020). Oral cancer: A historical review. *International Journal of Environmental Research and Public Health, 17*, 3168. https://doi.org/10.3390/ijerph17093168.

22. Kachlík, V., Musil, A., Blanková, Z., Marvanova, J., Miletin, J., Trachtova, D., Dvořáková, V., et al. (2020). A plea for extension of the anatomical nomenclature: Vessels. *Bosnian Journal of Basic Medical Sciences, 21*, 208–220. https://www.semanticscholar.org/paper/8a869eb301b132fe37da9d44546b00a1519157b5 (accessed on 8th May 2025).

23. Kim, I. B., Joo, K. M., Song, C. H., & Rhyu, I. J. (2024). A brief review of anatomy education in Korea, encompassing its past, present, and future direction. *Journal of Korean Medical Science, 39.* https://doi.org/10.3346/jkms.2024.39.e159.

24. Kok, H. P., Cressman, E. N. K., Ceelen, W., Brace, C. L., Ivkov, R., Grüll, H., Ter Haar, G., et al. (2020). Heating technology for malignant tumors: A review. *International Journal of Hyperthermia, 37*, 711–741. https://doi.org/10.1080/02656736.2020.1779357.

25. Lebow, M., & Chen, A. (2016). Overshadowed by the amygdala: The bed nucleus of the stria terminalis emerges as key to psychiatric disorders. *Molecular Psychiatry, 21*, 450–463. https://doi.org/10.1038/mp.2016.1.

26. Longhurst, G. J., Stone, D., Dulohery, K., Scully, D., Campbell, T., & Smith, C. F. (2020). Strength, weakness, opportunity, threat (SWOT) analysis of the adaptations to anatomical education

in the United Kingdom and Republic of Ireland in response to the COVID-19 pandemic. *Anatomical Sciences Education, 13*, 301–311. https://doi.org/10.1002/ase.1967.

27. Lyall, K., Croen, L., Daniels, J. L., Fallin, M. D., Ladd-Acosta, C., Lee, B. K., Park, B. Y., et al. (2017). The changing epidemiology of autism spectrum disorders. *Annual Review of Public Health, 38*, 81–102. https://doi.org/10.1146/annurev-publhealth-031816-044318.
28. Matthan, J., Cobb, M., McHanwell, S., Moxham, B. J., & Finn, G. M. (2020). The Anatomical Society's core anatomy syllabus for dental undergraduates. *Journal of Anatomy, 236*, 737–751. https://doi.org/10.1111/joa.13133.
29. Montatore, M., Muscatella, G., Eusebi, L., Masino, F., Gifuni, R., Giannubilo, W., Sortino, G., et al. (2023). Current status on new technique and protocol in urinary stone disease. *Current Radiology Reports, 11*, 161–176. https://doi.org/10.1007/s40134-023-00420-5.
30. Mungall, C., Torniai, C., Gkoutos, G. V., Lewis, S., & Haendel, M. (2012). Uberon, an integrative multi-species anatomy ontology. *Genome Biology, 13*. https://doi.org/10.1186/gb-2012-13-1-r5.
31. Nguyen, T. L. A., Vieira-Silva, S., Liston, A., & Raes, J. (2015). How informative is the mouse for human gut microbiota research? *Disease Models & Mechanisms, 8*, 1–16. https://doi.org/10.1242/dmm.017400.
32. Nowak-Sliwinska, P., Alitalo, K., Allen, E., Anisimov, A., Aplin, A. C., Auerbach, R., Augustin, H. G., et al. (2018). Consensus guidelines for the use and interpretation of angiogenesis assays. *Angiogenesis, 21*, 425–532. https://doi.org/10.1007/s10456-018-9613-x.
33. Pescitelli, R. M., Smith, H. F., & Williams, J. M. (2020). Teaching anatomy with dissection in the time of COVID-19 is essential and possible. *Clinical Anatomy (New York, N.Y.), 34*, 1135–1136. https://www.semanticscholar.org/paper/43e0745e5121eafba2338b71b4b355f4753092eb (accessed on 8th May 2025).
34. Pushpa, N. B., Patra, A., Asghar, A., & Ravi, K. S. (2023). Revolutionizing medical education and health care: The crucial role of cross-sectional neuroanatomy. *National Journal of Clinical Anatomy, 12*, 119–120. https://doi.org/10.4103/njca.njca_117_23.
35. Saeed, M., Ahmed, L., AbdAlla, E., Alatawi, Z., Alhowiti, A. M., Elmahdi, T. S. A., Mohammed, S., et al. (2025). Retention of gross and clinical anatomy knowledge among medical graduates in Sudan: A comparative study. *BMC Medical Education, 25*. https://doi.org/10.1186/s12909-025-06832-5.
36. Singh, K., Bharatha, A., Sa, B., Adams, O. P., & Majumder, M. A. A. (2019). Teaching anatomy using an active and engaging learning strategy. *BMC Medical Education, 19*. https://doi.org/10.1186/s12909-019-1590-2.
37. Spaide, R. F., Cheung, C. M. G., Matsumoto, H., Kishi, S., Boon, C. J. F., Van Dijk, E. H. C., Mauget-Faÿsse, M., et al. (2021). Venous overload choroidopathy: A hypothetical framework for central serous chorioretinopathy and allied disorders. *Progress in Retinal and Eye Research, 86*, 100973. https://doi.org/10.1016/j.preteyeres.2021.100973.
38. Xiloyannis, M., Alicea, R., Georgarakis, A. M., Haufe, F. L., Wolf, P., Masia, L., & Riener, R. (2021). Soft robotic suits: State of the art, core technologies, and open challenges. *IEEE Transactions on Robotics, 38*, 1343–1362. https://doi.org/10.1109/tro.2021.3084466.
39. Yabuki, Y. (2020). Twenty-first century radical hysterectomy – Journey from descriptive to practical anatomy. *Gynecologic Oncology Reports, 34*, 100623. https://doi.org/10.1016/j.gore.2020.100623.

UPPER LIMB

2

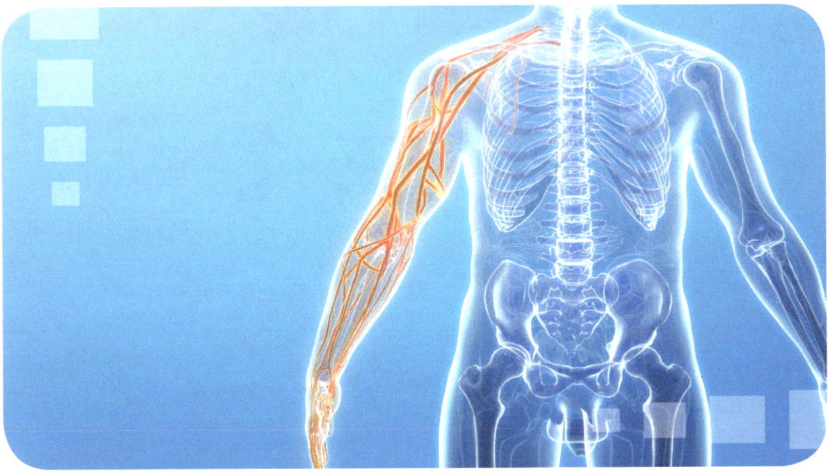

LEARNING OBJECTIVES

After studying this chapter, you will be able to:

1. Discuss the anatomy of the upper limb
2. Focus of bones of the upper limb
3. Explain the muscles of the upper limb
4. Know the joints of the upper limb
5. Focus on neuroanatomy of the upper limb

Introduction

A detailed understanding of the human upper limb is at the core of medical practice and education due to its extremely intricate anatomical structure and functional significance. The extremely complex coordination of bones, muscles, nerves, and vascular systems in the upper limb demands a multifaceted strategy toward learning, using histology, embryology, and anatomy to form a solid base of knowledge. Contemporary educational strategies in medical education, such as case-based learning (CBL), have proved effective in integrating these disciplines, enabling content mastery and facilitating adaptive learning behaviors in medical students during the early years (Merritt et al., 2024). Furthermore, the variability of arterial patterns in the upper limb also highlights the importance of precise anatomical awareness among clinicians and surgeons, as embryological development can result in significant deviations from typical vascular anatomy. Such differences are important for safe surgery and successful diagnostic interventions (Roy et al., 2024). Taken together, these considerations underscore the need for an inclusive introductory framework that connects theoretical foundation and practical application in upper limb research (Figure 2.1).

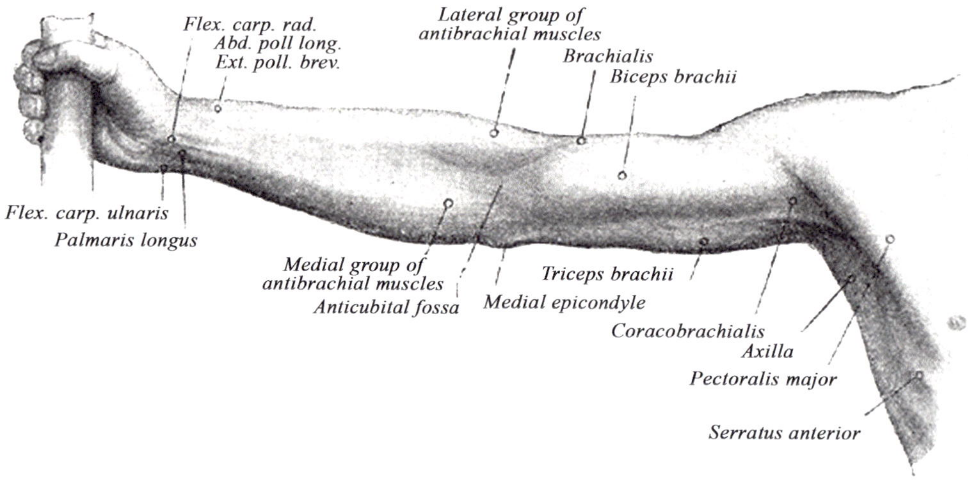

Figure 2.1. The human upper limb.

Source: https://en.wikipedia.org/wiki/File:Gray1231.png

Definition of the Upper Limb

Understanding the anatomy of the human body relies to a large degree upon knowledge of the structure and role of its great parts. The upper limb, a highly complex anatomical region, consists of the shoulder, arm, forearm, and hand, serving as an important conduit between the trunk and the distant limbs. It offers a significant range of movement and manipulations required for daily activities and certain functions. The complexity of this region lies not only in its musculoskeletal (MSK) anatomy but also in its neurovascular architecture, which is of maximum significance to sensory and motor activities. Pedagogical means of acquiring knowledge of the upper limb must keep this multi-planar system in perspective in order to understand better effectively. Latest studies have proved that interactive virtual reality (iVR) technology can supplement classical cadaveric learning in the acquisition of anatomical knowledge, particularly the upper limb, where spatial and touch understanding is critical (Freer et al., 2024). Moreover, clinical practice comes in the form of a vaccine injection, in which exact upper limb anatomy is crucial to prevent complications such as trauma to the shoulder (Mackenzie et al., 2022).

Importance of the Upper Limb in Human Anatomy

Human mobility and dexterity are inseparable and are evolutionary adaptations that have shaped the special anatomy of the upper limb. The upper limb serves to have fundamental functional roles, enabling an enormous variety of movement required for survival and daily living. With the development of the primates, a highly mobile shoulder joint, opposable thumb, and advanced patterns of muscle provided smooth manipulation and advanced tool usage, positioning human beings in contrast to other mammals (Susan, 2018). This adaptability is not merely due to MSK structures but also neurological and vascular systems contained within the limb, which provided its high degree of movement and fine motor capabilities. Besides, the upper limb is also crucial in balance and environmental interaction, with a role in functions ranging from locomotion to communication through gestures. Its importance goes beyond anatomy; it is an evolutionary interface where function and form meet and underscores the need for holistic clinical guidelines in the management of upper limb pathology to preserve its multivalent utility (Baumgartner et al., 2020) (Figure 2.2).

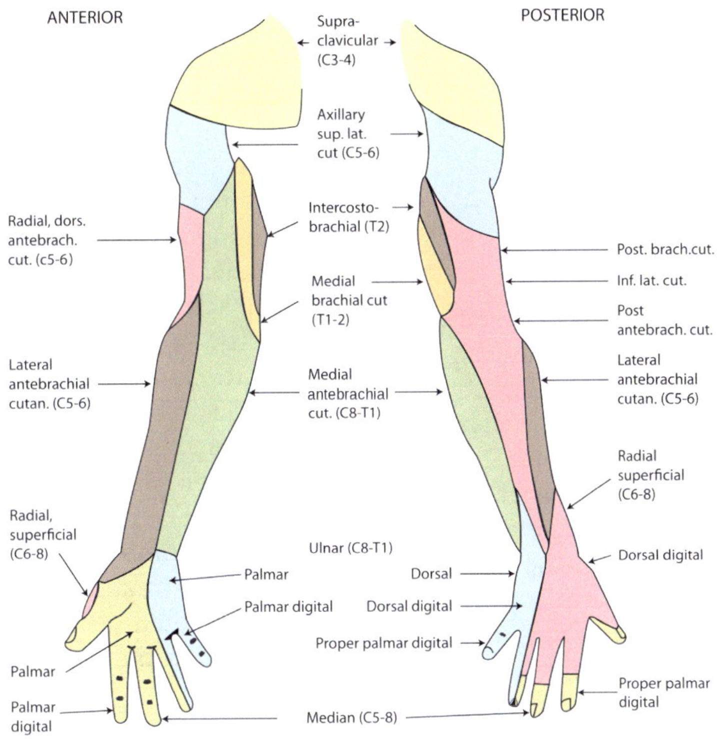

Figure 2.2. The upper limb in human movement.

Source: By Henry Vandyke Carter - Henry Gray (1918) Anatomy of the Human Body (See "Book" section below)Bartleby.com: Gray's Anatomy, Plate 812This is a retouched picture, which means that it has been digitally altered from its original version. Modifications: Vectorised. The original can be viewed here: Gray812and814.PNG: . Modifications made by Fred the Oyster., Public Domain, https://commons.wikimedia.org/w/index.php?curid=9821685

Overview of the Upper Limb's Functions

The sophistication of human movement is based to a large extent on the highly coordinated activity of several anatomical and physiological elements, and the upper limb is a model of such sophistication in its intricate functions. In addition to its fundamental function of enabling reaching, grasping, and manipulation, the upper limb also performs a vital role in sensory perception and fine motor function necessary for activities of daily living. Advances in rehabilitation technology and biomechanical modeling have necessitated the requirement for more accurate estimation of joint kinematics and muscle forces to understand upper limb function, particularly in clinical settings such as stroke rehabilitation. New approaches, such as the use of digital twins and multibody models in conjunction with state observers, allow upper limb mechanics analyses to be more precise with a view to therapeutic treatment and enhanced motor recovery outcomes (Adduci et al., 2024). Moreover, clinical guidelines highlight the imperatives of intensive, tailored rehabilitation to restore upper limb functions, emphasizing its impact on patients' overall quality of life (QoL) and societal participation after neurological defects (Daniel et al., 2024).

Historical Perspective on Upper Limb Studies

The history of upper extremity research reflects astounding advances in anatomical and clinical understanding. Early anatomy studies, frustrated by the lack of means of viewing minuscule and transparent lymphatic vessels, relied heavily upon dissection and mercury perfusion to follow these shadowy paths. While mercury was later abandoned due to toxicity, newer methods like dye injections and radioisotopes made possible the more accurate characterization of the lymphatic system, particularly of the upper extremity. This development underscores the necessity of refining investigation techniques to outsmart anatomical complexity and interindividual differences in lymphatic patterning (Pan et al., 2018). Concurrently, results in symptom-led studies, i.e., chronic cough studies, emphasize a systematic anatomic diagnostic approach that can be applied to musculoskeletal (MSK) and neurovascular exploration of the upper limb. The combining of clinical presentations with anatomical details has made diagnosis more accurate and more effective treatment, illustrating how shifts in methodology over the ages have broadened the depth and breadth of upper limb investigations (Irwin et al., 2001).

Common Injuries and Conditions Affecting the Upper Limb

Upper limb diseases and injuries most often are due to repetitive strain, trauma, or degenerative change, and significantly impair one's functional capacity. The most common conditions include carpal tunnel syndrome, tendinitis, rotator cuff injury, and fracture, each with its own diagnostic and therapeutic complexities. For instance, carpal tunnel syndrome is median nerve compression leading to numbness and weakness, while rotator cuff injury primarily causes pain and loss of motion of the shoulder. Effective treatment plans rely on a profound respect for the upper limb's biomechanical functioning and anatomical complexity, paired with evidence-based clinical recommendations. Clinical acumen is required to be exercised by health professionals in selecting fitting interventions, balancing the requirement for diagnostic precision against individualized care plans to optimize results and restore upper limb function (Baumgartner et al., 2020; Glikson et al., 2021). This approach reaffirms the necessity of combining current knowledge with personalized treatment methods for managing the multifaceted presentations of upper limb pathologies in the clinic.

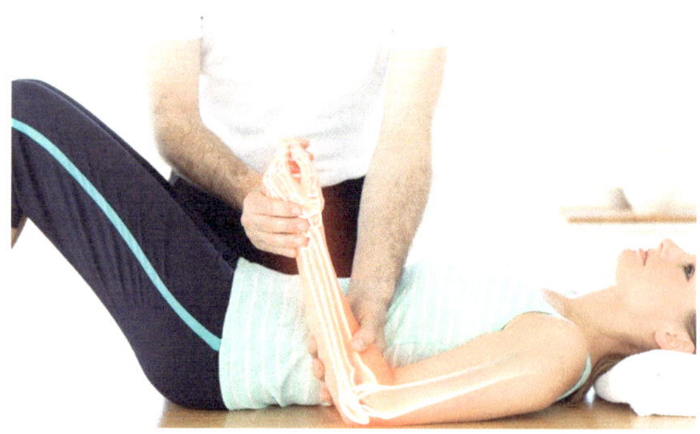

Source: Bradley Physio. (2016). *Upper Limb Physiotherapy Treatment.*

Purpose and Scope of the Essay

Understanding the intricate anatomy and function of the upper limb is a necessary condition for the establishment of clinical practice and biomechanical study. The purpose of this essay is to provide an overview that addresses the skeletal structure, muscles, nerve supply, and blood supply and describes their coordinated functions in movement and dexterity. Through the analysis of these factors, the essay aims to bridge the divide between applied and theoretical knowledge in medical, rehabilitative, and sports contexts. The scope also encompasses the treatment of current controversy and ethical arguments regarding physiological differences and performance improvement in sporting contexts, as evidenced by controversy surrounding inclusion policies (Knox et al., 2019). Although primarily anatomical, the essay is also aware of broader cultural and symbolic applications of limb representation in tradition and art, setting out a multi-faceted method reflecting other complex issues of human embodiment (Maillart-Garg et al., 2019). The scope and aim combined thus try to supply an integrated understanding of the value of the upper limb in both scientific and social contexts.

Brief Outline of the Main Topics

Understanding the upper limb involves exploring several interrelated problems as a whole providing a full image of its anatomy, function, and clinical importance. Initially, the musculoskeletal system is explored to account for bones such as the clavicle, scapula, humerus, radius, and ulna that comprise the structural base for motion. This is followed by an examination of the muscular system, keeping in view important groups of muscles responsible for complex movements like flexion and extension. The neurovascular components then illustrate how nerve impulses and blood supply sustain the limbs' functionality. Besides anatomy, the essay also examines normal treatment and injuries, illustrating case studies in the form of fracture, nerve damage, and soft tissue injury in a demonstration of the depth of trauma care. For instance, complicated trauma necessitates strategic limb salvage versus amputation decision-making that is accentuated by the importance of reconstructive techniques and prevention of infection in planning treatment (Koukos et al., 2025). Furthermore, unique populations such as neonates present with characteristic fracture patterns with typically favorable prognoses that are managed conservatively (Carvalho et al., 2024) (Figure 2.31).

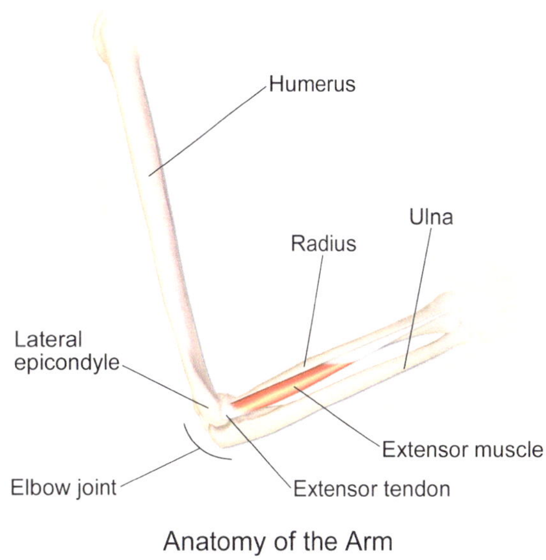

Figure 2.3. The upper limb involves exploring several interconnected topics that collectively provide a comprehensive overview of its anatomy, function, and clinical significance.

Source: By BruceBlaus - Own work, CC BY-SA 4.0, https://commons.wikimedia.org/w/index.php?curid=47008148

Significance of Understanding the Upper Limb

Its intricate anatomy and vital role in everyday life necessitate thorough knowledge of the upper limb to advance both clinical practice and neuroscience research. Mastery of the complex interaction between muscles, nerves, and vasculature must be attained to diagnose and treat upper limb pathology effectively, enhancing patient outcomes through individually tailored therapy. Moreover, knowledge about mechanisms of neural control of the upper limb is at the heart of developing innovative interventions such as non-invasive brain stimulation, which has been shown to have promise in the treatment of neurological disease and motor disability. These advances are increasingly reliant on precise anatomical and physiological knowledge in order to have maximal therapeutic benefits and safe protocols, implying the importance of new clinical guidelines for medical practitioners (Baumgartner et al., 2020; Rossini et al., 2015). Consequently, there is a profound knowledge of the biology of the upper limb, which not only informs surgical and rehabilitative approaches but also generates neuroscientific technology, further indicating its importance across different areas of healthcare and research.

2.1. Anatomy of the Upper Limb

Learning Outcome

1. Give an overview of the skeletal structure
2. How to major bones of the upper limb
3. Explain the joints and their functions
4. Focus on muscles of the upper limb
5. Learn about nerve supply to the upper limb
6. Understand blood supply and circulation
7. How to details connective tissues and fascia
8. Explain the anatomical variations in the upper limb

The anatomy of the upper limb is constrained by its intricate system of bones, muscles, nerves, and vessels that cooperate to allow a myriad of functions from the gross motor through fine dexterity. Anatomical studies recognize the significance of spatial relationships here, particularly as they involve surgical access to significant structures like the brachial plexus and neurovascular bundles. The advances in neuronavigation have shown that familiarity with certain anatomical courses can facilitate safer, less debilitating interventions, improving surgical outcomes without more neurovascular trauma (Signoretti et al., 2025).

Moreover, artificial intelligence (AI) incorporation into anatomy education is transforming how this information is delivered to medical students, where large language models are enhancing the production of clinical cases and test material based on the upper limb. Despite such developments, ongoing improvement is needed to take advantage of AI fully in effectively reflecting the subtle anatomy of the upper limb (Mavrych et al., 2024). Therefore, upper limb anatomy remains a cornerstone of both clinical practice and medical education (Figure 2.4).

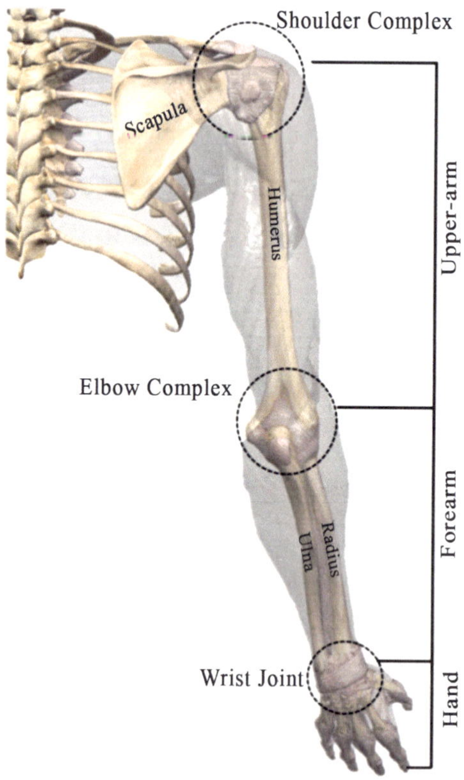

A

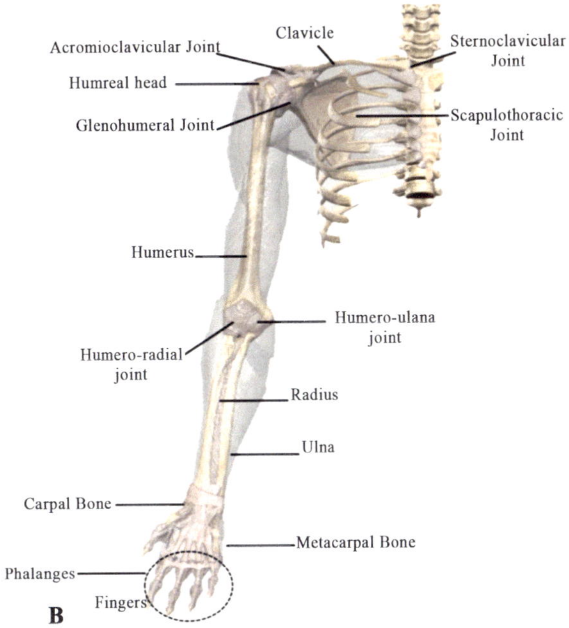

Figure 2.4. Anatomy of the upper limb.

Source: Muhammad, A. G., Shaoping, B., & Thomas B. (2020). *A Review on Design of Upper Limb Exoskeletons.*

2.1.1. Overview of the Skeletal Structure

The fragile architecture of the upper limb is formed by a complex array of bones that provide structural support and allow for a wide range of motion utilized in activities of daily living. Beginning proximally, the scapula and clavicle form the shoulder girdle, suspending the appendage to the axial skeleton while allowing for multidirectional mobility.

The humerus is the only long bone of the arm, joining proximally with the scapula and distally with the radius and ulna at the elbow joint, to enable flexion, extension, and rotation. Distally, the intricate carpal bones constitute the pliable wrist joint, and the metacarpals and phalanges constitute the hand's agile structures for fine manipulation and fine motor skills. Such skeletal structure is biomechanically and functionally maintained by covering soft tissues, whose condition is crucial in the maintenance of musculoskeletal (MSK) system integrity (Caterina et al., 2023).

Advances in therapeutic modalities, such as extracorporeal shockwave therapy, demonstrate evolving clinical techniques for treating concomitant MSK pathologies of the bones of the upper limb (Adam et al., 2022).

2.1.2. Major Bones of the Upper Limb

The upper limb's functional capacity and structural intricacy depend largely on its massive bones, which provide fundamental support while also allowing a huge range of movement. The humerus is the head bone of the arm, and it articulates proximally with the scapula at the shoulder joint and distally with the radius and ulna at the elbow.

The ulna and the radius, in parallel alignment in the forearm, support pronation and supination to enable hand orientation and dexterity. The intricate structure of the carpal bones in the wrist supports both flexibility and stability necessary for delicate motor skills. Not only do these bones bear mechanical loads, but they also serve as an attachment site for movement-coordinating muscles and ligaments that supply strength.

Debilitating injuries to these bones, such as fractures or oncologic resections, are challenges to their management, reflective of their central importance to maintaining limb function, justifying the urgency of new reconstruction and rehabilitation approaches to facilitate upper limb use (Codazza et al., 2024; Mascia et al., 2024) (Figure 2.5).

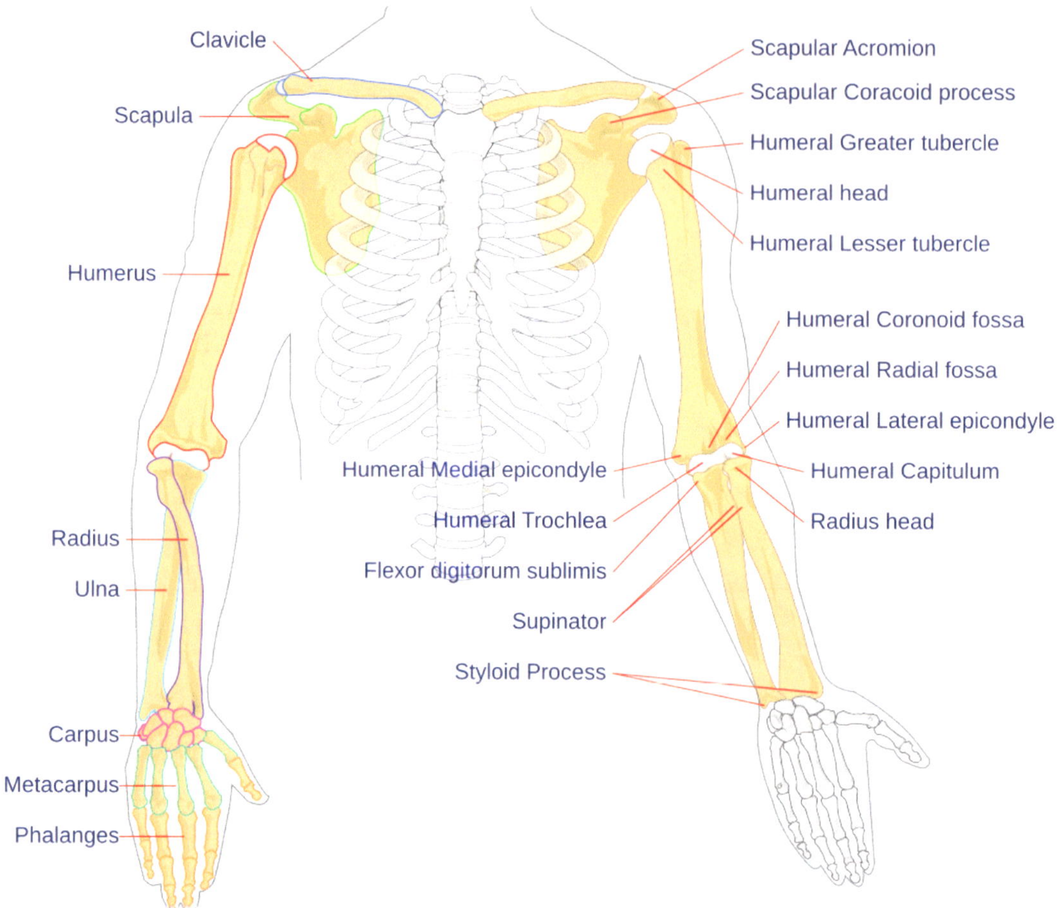

Figure 2.5. Major bones of the upper limb.

Source: By LadyofHats Mariana Ruiz Villarreal - Some of my sources: [1], Gray's Anatomy "Williams & Warwick", Atlas der anatomie des menschen "Sobotta", Anatomia del cuerpo humano "Yokochi, Rhoen, weinreb", and a lamina printed by "rüdiger-anatomie GmbH"- LadyofHats, Public Domain, https://commons.wikimedia.org/w/index.php?curid=1522438

2.1.3. Joints and their Functions

The intricate arm structure relies primarily on the dynamic interaction of its joints, enabling extensive movement required for daily activities. Joints such as the glenohumeral, elbow, and wrist work synergistically to provide stability alongside mobility. Specifically, the shoulder joint demonstrates this balance through its complex anatomy, often likened to an industrial crane, where the base, axial tower, and clavicular structures collaborate with a suspensory cascade that stabilizes and mobilizes the arm in space. The rotator cuff muscles and ligaments envelop the humeral head, providing both support and delicate control with movement. Furthermore, the coracoid also acts as a pulley system that provides fine control in force transmission, demonstrating the sophisticated biomechanical design of the upper limb (Gregory et al., 2019). Such coordination between joints and muscles forms the foundation for effective motor control that can be maximally improved through rehabilitative devices that replicate the intrinsic synergies of joints, demonstrating the central importance of joint function in facilitating limb utility restoration (He et al., 2021).

2.1.4. Muscles of the Upper Limb

The intricate function of the upper limb relies on the cooperative action of numerous muscles, which allow for a coordinated range of movements required for normal functions along with complex motor skills. Compartments of muscle are organized into groups based on where and what they are doing, such as the limb's anterior flexors and posterior extensors, each of which is involved in precise articulation at the shoulder, elbow, wrist, and fingers. Advances in biomedical engineering, based on accurate anatomical and biomechanical modeling of such muscles and their tendinous attachments, have enabled the development of highly effective wearable exoskeleton robots that can rehabilitate or assist disabled limb function (Li et al., 2017). Furthermore, advances in bioelectronic interfaces enhance the selectivity of targeting upper limb muscles to be activated with neuromodulation, allowing unprecedented accuracy in intervention treatments through modeling endogenous patterns of muscle activation (Schiavone et al., 2020). Such cross-departmental methods accentuate the sophistication and potential for rehabilitating upper limb muscular function after illness or injury (Figure 2.6).

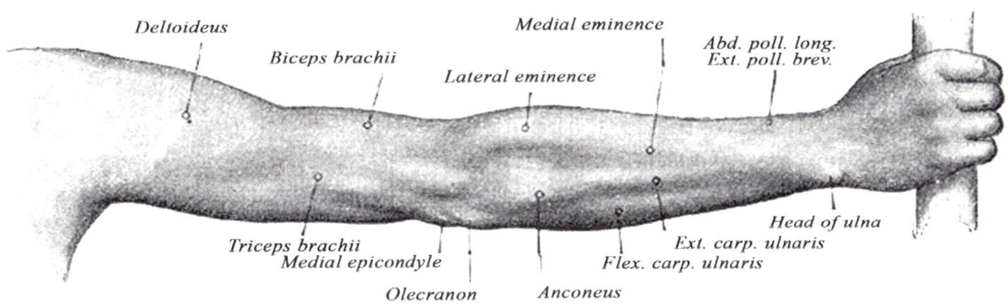

Figure 2.6. The intricate functionality of the upper limb.

Source: By Henry Vandyke Carter - Henry Gray (1918) Anatomy of the Human Body (See "Book" section below)Bartleby.com: Gray's Anatomy, Plate 1232, Public Domain, https://commons.wikimedia.org/w/index.php?curid=564846

2.1.5. Nerve Supply to the Upper Limb

Functional complexity of the upper limb, in return, depends largely on its intricate nerve supply, enabling fine motor control and sensory function. This plexus is derived primarily from the brachial plexus, which is a complex of cervical and upper thoracic spinal nerves' nerve roots, dividing widely to innervate the arm, forearm, and hand muscles and skin. Certain forearm muscles, such as the flexor carpi ulnaris and pronator teres, have distinct neuromuscular compartments, each supplied by specific nerve branches, which show a very high degree of organization that enables fine motor coordination and control and compartmentalized muscle action. Detailed anatomical studies through techniques like modified Sihler's staining have substantiated the nerve innervation in the compartments, which is of critical relevance in surgical operations like tendon transfer procedures for limb restoration (Liu et al., 2014). This intricate nerve topology should be comprehended by clinicians while formulating treatment plans to ensure proper diagnosis and therapy (Bharadwaj et al., 2024).

2.1.6. Blood Supply and Circulation

The intricate relationship between tissue temperature and blood flow accounts for the significance of local heating in perfusion control of the upper limb. Local heating of single muscle groups has been found to cause a localized increase in tissue temperature, which locally enhances blood flow precisely in the heated region without the participation of adjacent areas. This hyperemia is crucial for the maintenance of optimal oxygen delivery and exchange of nutrients in tissues, favoring efficient metabolic processes and repair (Esteves et al., 2024).

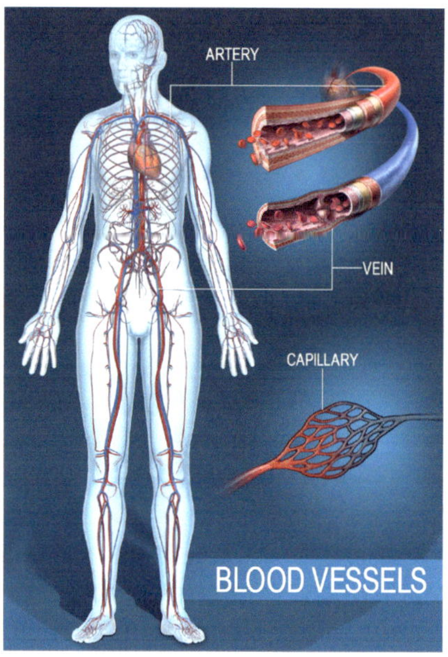

Figure 2.7. Blood supply and circulation.

Source: Visible Body. (n.d.). *Blood Vessels: Arteries, Veins, and Capillaries*.

In the case of trauma or composite injury to the upper limb, maintenance of an adequate and competent blood supply takes on importance. Adequate assessment of peripheral circulation by palpation of pulses, skin color, warmth, and capillary refill is central to determining limb viability. Prompt multidisciplinary management with a bias towards limb salvage is very much dependent upon the maintenance of this vascular integrity, which dictates both functional outcome and amputation/reconstruction decisions (Bharadwaj et al., 2024) (Figure 2.7).

2.1.7. Connective Tissues and Fascia

The complex relationship between fascia and connective tissues is crucial for the upper limb's functional integrity and mobility. The tissues exist as a continuum that ensheaths muscles, vessels, and nerves, thereby facilitating coordinated movement and force transmission. Fascial layers compartmentalize muscles but also permit gliding between the different tissue planes, which reduces friction during joint articulation and limb manipulation. In addition, fascial dynamism reacts to mechanical stresses, contributing to proprioception and injury prevention. An understanding of fascial mechanical properties and anatomy in the upper limb is important for clinical approaches to MSK injury and surgical intervention. This wider perspective aligns with evolving perceptions that emphasize fascia's dynamism rather than a static barrier notion, a concept of relevance to both rehabilitation and treatment interventions (Wong et al., 2015). Moreover, advances in imaging and regional anesthesia techniques have highlighted the contribution of connective tissues to guiding safe and effective nerve block procedures in limbs (Tran et al., 2019).

2.1.8. Anatomical Variations in the Upper Limb

The upper limb anatomy is typically complex and presents variations of which clinical significance is significant. Variations in the brachial plexus, such as variations of origin and patterns of nerve branching, are not uncommon and impact sensory and motor function, particularly after injury or surgery. For instance, studies have seen a noticeable disparity between the right and left upper limbs in musculocutaneous nerve branching, with a higher frequency of variations on the right side (Omuga et al., 2023). Similarly, arterial upper limb variations are relatively frequent and can cause diagnostic challenges. Research on cadaveric specimens revealed that about 10% of the upper limbs have abnormal arterial paths or courses, and it may complicate the diagnosis, surgery, and radiological examination (Kannappan et al., 2022). Anatomical variations like these should be made known by medical practitioners to prevent errors and improve patient care, emphasizing the necessity for detailed anatomical knowledge for both instruction and clinical practice.

Test Your Knowledge

1. Which major nerve innervates the flexor muscles of the forearm?
2. Why is it important for clinicians to be aware of anatomical variations?

2.2. Bones of the Upper Limb

Learning Outcome

1. Give an overview of the skeletal structure
2. Discuss the clavicle: anatomy and function
3. Explain the scapula: anatomy and function
4. Understand humerus: anatomy and function
5. Focus on radius: anatomy and function
6. Know ulna: anatomy and function
7. Identify carpal bones: types and arrangement
8. Discuss metacarpals: structure and significance
9. Explain the phalanges: types and roles

A detailed understanding of the bones of the upper limbs is required to ascertain how function and mobility are influenced by structural design. The bony anatomy consists of the clavicle, scapula, humerus, radius, and ulna, each contributing in a specialized way to the overall function of the limbs. Not only do these bones provide support and stability, but they also create a highly mobile system that allows a wide range of motion necessary for daily use and complex tasks. Fascinatingly, as significantly as the length and strength of bones like the humerus and radius help contribute to body function, their coordination with surrounding soft tissues like muscles and tendons is equally significant in maximizing mobility and strength.

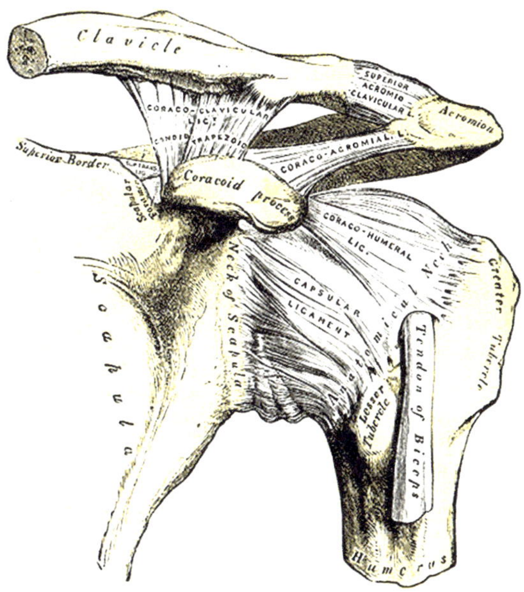

Figure 2.8. Bones of the upper limb.

Source: By Henry Vandyke Carter - Henry Gray (1918) Anatomy of the Human Body (See "Book" section below)Bartleby.com: Gray's Anatomy, Plate 326, Public Domain, https://commons.wikimedia.org/w/index.php?curid=85420

It is now understood that upper limb MSK networks exhibit significant integration and complexity, substantiating the fact that functional anatomy is more an issue of not bone structure by itself, but how these structures work in unison to generate efficient movement (Goswami et al., 2015). Such a multifaceted interplay underscores the importance of maintaining bone health along with anatomical variations in upper limb functionality (Figure 2.8).

2.2.1. Overview of the Skeletal Structure

The skeletal system is at the core of the overall upper extremity function and biomechanics. As a composite structure of bones, cartilage, and ligaments, the skeleton not only facilitates motion but also provides essential support and protection for vital structures. The modularity of the skeletal elements allows motion to be diverse while providing stability, a balance that is critical for both normal and pathologic conditions. For instance, Anatomical Network Analysis studies give valuable details of the MSK organization, showing that upper limb skeletal networks differ greatly from those of the lower limb, particularly their proximal regions (Goswami et al., 2015). Furthermore, conditions such as Morquio A syndrome highlight the difficulty of limb skeletal deformities, referring to the need for personalized management strategies that address both dysfunction and quality of life (QoL) (Bache et al., 2014). Clarifying such dynamics is important in enhancing clinical outcomes and functional performance in patients.

2.2.2. Clavicle: Anatomy and Function

The collarbone, or clavicle, plays a significant role in shoulder movement and upper limb mobility, serving as a vital anatomical link between the upper limb and the trunk. Its S-shaped, single structure is favorable to both strength and flexibility, allowing it to bear loads and withstand numerous stresses during movement. Since it is a part of the shoulder girdle, the clavicle stabilizes the scapula to enable a multitude of motions, e.g., lifting and reaching (Bache et al., 2014). Further, its articulation with the sternum and the acromion of the scapula offers critical points of muscular attachment to enable effective propulsion in upper limb function. This connection not only enhances the overall biomechanical efficiency of the upper limb but also minimizes the risk of damage by distributing forces across the shoulder area. Thus, the understanding of the clavicle's anatomy and function is essential to appreciate the sophisticated mechanics of the upper limb as a unity (Figure 2.9).

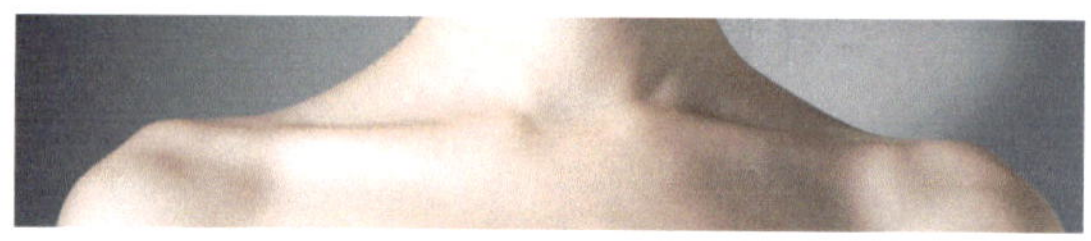

Figure 2.9. Clavicle: anatomy and function.

Source: By Exey Panteleev - This image has been extracted from another file, CC BY 2.5, https://commons.wikimedia.org/w/index.php?curid=78504238

2.2.3. Scapula: Anatomy and Function

The scapula or shoulder blade plays a key role in upper limb movement by offering a wide range of arm movements. Located behind the rib cage, its triangular shape enables a convergence of muscular attachments that offer functional mobility and stability. This arrangement allows mechanisms like glenohumeral joint movements that are crucial in activities involving elevation and rotation of the arm. In addition, the scapula is also a site where muscular force is produced, and muscles acting around the shoulder joint display typical leverage and joint mobility. For instance, an analysis revealed that muscle actions are largely influenced by limb posture, which means that scapular anatomy evolution has a close correlation with locomotor adaptations in different archosaurian lineages (Otero et al., 2017).

Besides, an understanding of the modularity and integration of scapular skeletal musculature gives insight into its wide-ranging functions, highlighting that structure-function relationships are essential for the effective functions of the upper limb (Goswami et al., 2015).

2.2.4. Humerus: Anatomy and Function

The humerus is a vital component of the upper limb whose anatomical form and functional capacity directly rely on it. It is the bone connecting the shoulder to the elbow, not only providing structural support but also facilitating extensive movement in numerous ways required for daily activities. Its anatomy, characterized by head features, greater and lesser tubercles, and deltoid tuberosity, has a crucial role in joint mobility and muscle attachment.

Muscles that move the shoulder joint, like those responsible for rotation and elevation, are largely under the control of the morphology of the humerus. For instance, modifications in muscle leverage and joint mobility have extensive implications, as noted by studies of limb postures in limb evolution, where the development of a more erect posture among sauropodomorphs is associated with greater locomotor efficiency (Otero et al., 2017).

Understanding the specialized humerus biomechanics enhances knowledge of locomotor behavior in a variety of animals, with significance of its evolutionary implications (Maidment et al., 2012) (Figure 2.10).

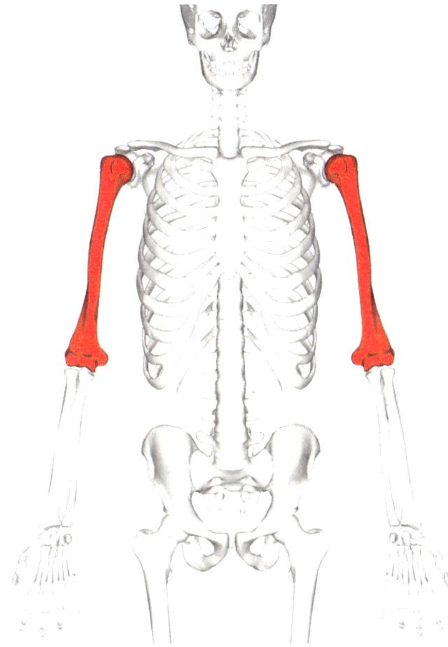

Figure 2.10. Humerus: anatomy and function.

Source: By Anatomography - en:Anatomography (setting page of this image), CC BY-SA 2.1 jp, https://commons.wikimedia.org/w/index.php?curid=23389521

2.2.5. Radius: Anatomy and Function

The radius is an essential part of the upper limb's functional anatomy, particularly in loading and movement. As one of the two long bones in the forearm, it not only adds strength to the arm's framework but also functions as the primary bone for wrist joint articulation and rotation. Its anatomical design offers a unique range of motions like pronation and supination that are crucial for fine motor functions needed in everyday life. The relationship of the ulna with the radius is crucial, and the interosseous membrane connecting the bones assists in the distribution of forces along the forearm in various movements. This interaction is consistent with findings of anatomical research, demonstrating how forelimb posture correlates with muscle leverage and joint mobility, enhancing total limb function (Otero et al., 2017). The radius is thus pivotal not only for movement but also for the complex interplay of muscle actions involved in successful upper limb function (Goswami et al., 2015).

2.2.6. Ulna: Anatomy and Function

The ulna, which is one of the two long forearm bones, plays a critical role in the functional anatomy of the upper limb. It lies on the medial side and extends from the elbow to the wrist and serves as a stabilizing anchor for arm motion. Its unique morphology, which includes a trochlear notch that engages the humerus, accommodates a wide range of motion, particularly in flexion and extension at the elbow joint. This degree of freedom is required for many activities of daily living, such as lifting and reaching. In addition, the ulna's functional significance is emphasized when locomotor transitions in terrestrial vertebrates are considered. As revealed by Otero et al. (2017), limb posture and muscle leverage are important to each other. In this, the ulna is responsible for providing optimal alignment, as well as optimal distribution of forces, thereby contributing to the efficiency of upper limbs function. Through its structure, the ulna not only helps with numerous movements but also stabilizes via tasks (Figure 2.11).

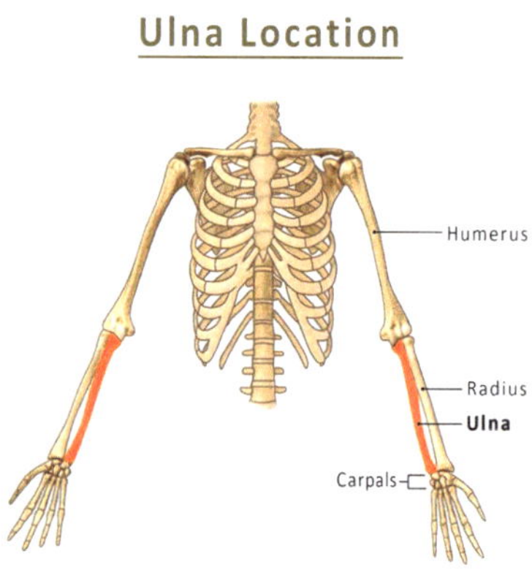

Figure 2.11. Ulna: anatomy and function.

Source: The Skeletal System. (2018). *Ulna Location in the Human Skeleton*.

2.2.7. Carpal Bones: Types and Arrangement

The division and arrangement of the carpal bones are critical to the function and mechanics of the entire upper limb. The eight carpal bones are type of short bones arranged into two rows: the proximal and distal rows. The proximal row consists of the lunate, triquetrum, scaphoid, and pisiform, and the distal row consists of the capitate, hamate, trapezoid, and trapezium. This unique arrangement provides a variety of complex movements, and it facilitates the grip and manipulation ability required for activities ranging from everyday activities to complex biomechanical activities. As studies on biomechanics reveal, coordination of these bones helps in effective hand movements, which are essential in activities with the requirement for fine motor activities (Harris et al., 2012). Additionally, studies have shown that the pattern and coherence of the carpal bones within other primate lineages are not the same, presumably affecting functional adaptations within areas like thumb mobility (Diogo et al., 2017). These bone dynamics are important to recognize within anatomical research as well as clinical practice under MSK injury.

2.2.8. Metacarpals: Structure and Significance

The five long bones located in the middle part of the hand are responsible for the functionality and mobility of the hand. The bones connect the carpals of the wrist to the proximal phalanges of the fingers, forming a flexible system which allows different movements needed for the activities of daily life. Their particular anatomy, consisting of base, shaft, and head, provides for several levels of grip strength and precision. The metacarpals also contribute to forearm biomechanics, and changes in their integrity—such as those caused by trauma or disease—result in compromised function. This is indicative of the importance of their anatomy, as evidenced by studies of the interaction of forces delivered through the forearm and subsequent surgical procedures, such as in radial head arthroplasty, that could mimic native biomechanics (Lanting et al., 2014). This careful examination of the metacarpals thus demonstrates the essential role played by them in the efficiency and adaptability of the upper limbs (Figure 2.12).

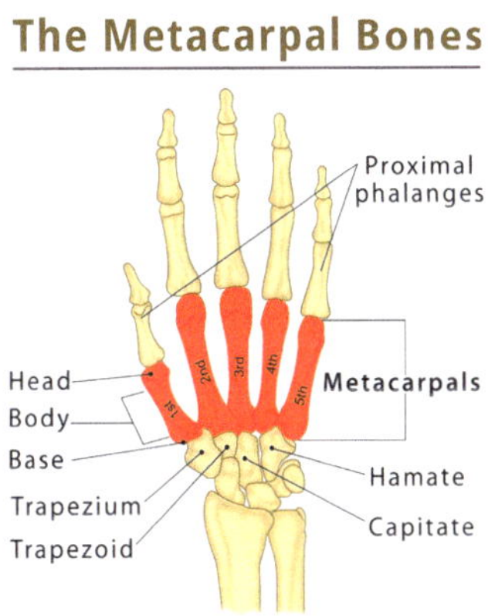

Figure 2.12. Metacarpals: structure and significance.

Source: The Skeletal System. (2018). *The Metacarpal Bones of the Hand.*

2.2.9. Phalanges: Types and Roles

The phalanges are 14 distinct bones found in each hand and are categorized into three different types: proximal, middle, and distal. The three types of phalanges have different functions in the provision of complex movement and gripping mechanisms. The proximal phalanges are connected to the metacarpals that are essential support for the hands' architecture, while the middle phalanges serve additional leverage to the fingers that increase the dexterity of the hands. The distal phalanges are the most distal bones of upper limb and carry the essence of fine motor activities with precision and sensitivity. The evolutionary developments of modern human hands put in the limelight a trade-off with these structures, balancing locomotion and manipulation (Tracy et al., 2022). Further, the functionality of phalanges is directly connected to the central nervous system (CNS) because the ability to execute multifunctional grasping and holding functions is the outcome of neural pathways that regulate such movements (Zhengrun et al., 2022). The knowledge of phalanges' types and functions helps in understanding the overall functionality of the hands and their evolutionary significance.

Test Your Knowledge

1. Give an overview of the skeletal structure
2. Discuss the clavicle: anatomy and function
3. Explain the scapula: anatomy and function

2.3. Muscles of the Upper Limb

Learning Outcome

1. Give an overview of muscle groups
2. Discuss the shoulder muscles: rotator cuff and others
3. Explain the arm muscles: anterior and posterior compartments
4. Focus on forearm muscles: flexors and extensors
5. Describe the hand muscles: intrinsic vs. extrinsic
6. Know muscle innervation and blood supply
7. Understand functional roles of major muscle groups
8. Focus on muscle actions during movement
9. Discuss the common injuries and conditions

The complex design of the upper limb is not only for purposeful use but also for protection, as observed in the organization of its anatomical and muscular components. The elaborate analysis of muscles in the upper limb reveals a highly sophisticated interaction designed to guard vital components, especially against external trauma. Based on dissection class anatomy studies, protective architecture design emphasizes arterial integrity at the expense of muscle and nerve integrity, and this suggests a life-protecting system (Francesco et al., 2022).

The design emphasizes the fact that even with trauma, upper limb musculature is designed to preserve maximum function at the expense of compromising as little as possible on important structures. Also, the upper limb muscles from the shoulder to the fingers afford great motion range and dexterity, both being important for normal functions. Last but not least, an understanding of this complex interaction contributes to knowledge about evolutionary alterations in human anatomy.

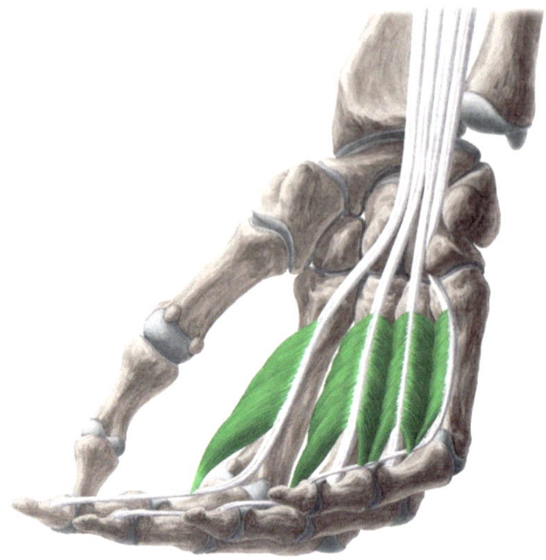

Source: Gordana S. (2023). *Lumbrical Muscles of the Hand.*

2.3.1. Overview of Muscle Groups

Upper limb muscle groups play a fundamental role in facilitating diverse movements and maintaining structural stability. The muscle groups can be described as flexors, extensors, abductors, and adductors that act together to facilitate the general function of the arm and hand. For instance, the flexor muscles, such as the biceps brachii, facilitate bending at the elbow joint, while the extensor muscles, such as the triceps brachii, facilitate straightening actions. It is this complex coordination of muscle activity that underpins the capacity for performing everyday tasks, ranging from lifting to precision manipulations. Furthermore, the modularity and integration of these muscle groups also reflect their evolutionary functions in adapting to various locomotor demands, thereby optimizing survival at no expense of functional potential, as expressed in both normalcy and pathology (Goswami et al., 2015). Thus, the understanding of these muscle groups is essential for movement science and rehabilitation professionals to implement specific interventions to facilitate motor recovery (Altarocca et al., 2019).

2.3.2. Shoulder Muscles: Rotator Cuff and Others

The shoulder function is, nonetheless, complex because of the complex interaction between all the multiple groups of muscles, most importantly the rotator cuff, which consists of several large muscles: the supraspinatus, infraspinatus, teres minor, and subscapularis. They work synergistically to stabilize the glenohumeral joint but enable a tremendous amount of arm movement. Outside the rotator cuff, several other muscles help move the shoulder, including the deltoid, pectoralis major, and latissimus dorsi, all of which play significant roles in the strength and stability of movement with exercise.

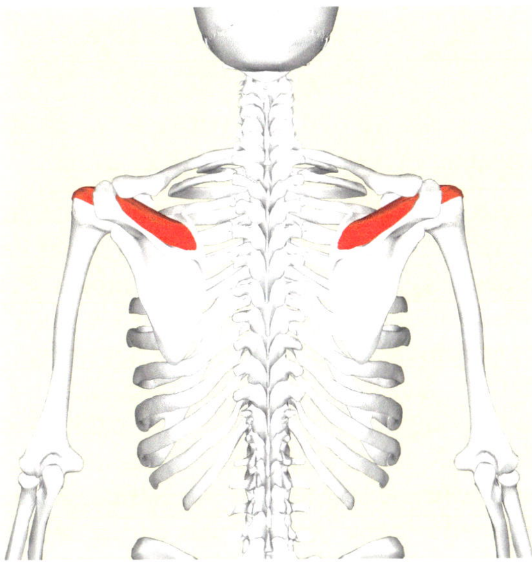

Figure 2.13. Shoulder muscles: rotator cuff and others.

Source: By Anatomography - en:Anatomography (setting page of this image), CC BY-SA 2.1 jp, https://commons.wikimedia.org/w/index.php?curid=22813514

Rehabilitation of injury to the shoulder, especially to these muscles, needs an appreciation of the mechanics involved. For example, Ellenbecker & Cools (2010) stress the intervention of individual factors for pain, scapular dysfunction, and muscle strength to improve patient outcomes. In addition, studies using models illustrate how structural damage compromises shoulder stability, which shows that rehabilitative strategies based on anatomical differences are needed (Klemt, 2018). As such, comprehensive knowledge of the musculature of the shoulder is needed for proper intervention and rehabilitation (Figure 2.13).

2.3.3. Arm Muscles: Anterior and Posterior Compartments

The arm contains separate anterior and posterior compartments with specific muscular roles important for the stability and mobility of the upper limb. The anterior compartment consists primarily of flexor muscles including the biceps brachii and brachialis, responsible for flexion of the elbow and lifting objects. On the other hand, the extensor muscles such as triceps brachii form the posterior compartment, employed in extending the arm and aiding in a wide range of functions. Importantly, information about the anatomy of structures and innervation patterns of these muscles is important in applications towards functional electrical stimulation, as reported through research on motor points of muscles in the forearm. This research brings to the fore the significance of proper electrode placement for optimal muscle function because most of the forearm muscles have multiple motor points with focal areas on the proximal third of the muscle (Safwat & Abdel-Meguid, 2007). The segmental innervation of the deltoid muscle, for instance, reflects the complex intersensory interrelations within the muscle groups that control coordinated movement (Krasucki et al., 2014).

2.3.4. Forearm Muscles: Flexors and Extensors

The fine balance between the flexor and extensor muscles of the forearm is essential to effective movement and functional capacity of the upper limb. Flexors, placed anteriorly within the forearm, produce actions such as gripping and wrist flexion, while extensors, placed posteriorly, perform wrist and finger extension. This division not only facilitates large motion (i.e., movement within a lot of space) but also plays an important role in everyday activities involving power and fine motor. Dysfunction or fatigue of these muscle groups can significantly impair performance; e.g., muscle fatigue is a frequent complaint of patients with neuro-muscular disease, leading to impaired motor control and sensorimotor integration (Mugnosso, 2020). These impairments are reflected in challenges to doing simple tasks; hence, maintaining healthy flexor and extensor muscles is of paramount importance to maximize upper limb function (Goswami et al., 2015). Thus, knowledge about these muscle dynamics becomes crucial for rehabilitation and prevention of injury (Figure 2.14).

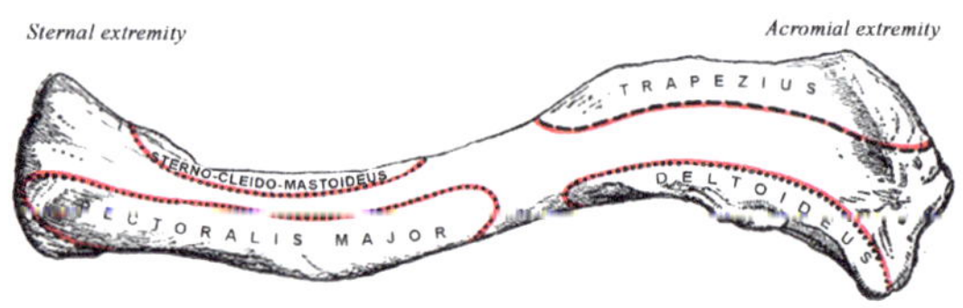

Figure 2.14. Forearm muscles: flexors and extensors.

Source: By Henry Vandyke Carter - Henry Gray (1918) Anatomy of the Human Body (See "Book" section below)Bartleby.com: Gray's Anatomy, Plate 200, Public Domain, https://commons.wikimedia.org/w/index.php?curid=792173

2.3.5. Hand Muscles: Intrinsic vs. Extrinsic

Among the components of hand anatomy, there is a fundamental distinction between intrinsic and extrinsic muscles, both of which play significant roles in hand function. The intrinsic muscles, intrinsic to the hand, are chiefly responsible for fine movement and precision of action, such as writing and object manipulation. These muscles, particularly noted for greater atrophy in older people, contribute significantly to hand dexterity, which is essential for the performance of activities of daily living (ADL) (Hsu, 2009). Extrinsic muscles, however, originate in the forearm and extend into the hand, permitting stronger movements like gripping or throwing. Aging alterations that include reductions in both the dimensions and strength of these muscles establish a correlation between these muscles and overall hand dexterity, evidencing the interdependence of strength-fine motor (Hsu, 2009). Identification of this dissociation not only demarcates functional dynamics of the upper limb but also the imperative of targeted rehabilitation to guarantee the functionality of the hand, most notably in aged adults.

2.3.6. Muscle Innervation and Blood Supply

The complex relationship between innervation of the muscles and blood supply to the upper limb is crucial in order to maintain both mobility and function. Innervation of each group of muscles comes from individual peripheral nerves, which not only facilitate voluntary movement but also provide sensory feedback for balance and coordination. For instance, the brachial plexus is a significant provider of nerve fibers, which divide into large nerves such as the median, ulnar, and radial, each targeting unique areas of muscles. Coupled with this neural system is the blood system in which arteries such as the brachial and radial are of utmost significance in supplying oxygen-rich blood for energizing muscle contractions. Adequate blood supply ensures that muscles can function optimally with activation from light motor tasks to increased weights. Alteration of either blood supply or innervation may lead to impaired function, thus emphasizing the importance of identifying these interdependencies for effective clinical intervention and the rehabilitation strategy (Figure 2.15).

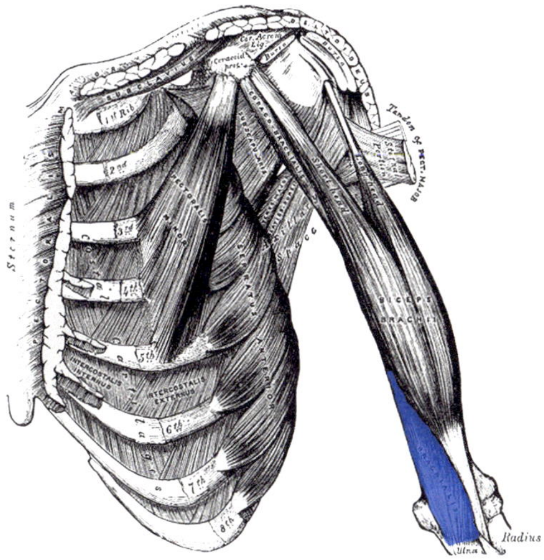

Figure 2.15. Muscle innervation and blood supply.

Source: By Me - I created this from Gray's Anatomy plate 411 using Gimp, Public Domain, https://commons.wikimedia.org/w/index.php?curid=1672637

2.3.7. Functional Roles of Major Muscle Groups

Muscle groups of the upper limb perform several significant functional roles allowing for a variety of movement and action. The deltoid, for example, plays a vital role in shoulder abduction, while rotator cuff muscles help control and stabilize arm movement. This complex combination allows for both subtle motor skill and heavy lifting, demonstrating the importance of muscle structure in movement proficiency.

In addition, muscles such as the triceps brachii and biceps brachii perform reciprocal roles in flexion and extension at the elbow, highlighting their functional collaboration with everyday activities. Furthermore, the research on other limb musculature shows that architecture specializations influence function; for instance, the muscle architecture's proximo-distal gradient is responsible for locomotive stability and efficiency in quadrupedal animals (Cappellari et al., 2016). This is a key concept to recognize, as it identifies how evolutionary changes within musculature in humans can lend to both strength and dexterity within upper limb function. Scaling of musculature also, such as in felids, emphasizes the need for muscle groups to contribute proportionate strength relative to body size (Adams et al., 2016). The understanding of these functional roles helps to further identify the biomechanical foundation needed for both athletic and daily functioning.

2.3.8. Muscle Actions During Movement

Upper limb motor function is founded to a great degree on the highly organized activity of heterogeneous groups of muscles, each adapted to fulfill specific functional demands. For instance, the complex muscular architecture allows fine control and broad versatility of motion necessary for functions such as reaching, grasping, and fine motor tasks.

A recent study highlighted the importance of muscle actions by demonstrating how the mobility of the forelimb in different species is correlated with their locomotor adaptations; for example, the contrasting muscle mechanics of Crocodylus and Mussaurus demonstrate the adaptation of muscle action to environmental pressures and postural changes (Otero et al., 2017). Similarly, when muscles of the mouse hindlimb are taken into account, specific adaptations can be seen, allowing for exact functions like force generation and stability during locomotion (Cappellari et al., 2016). Clarification of these kinds of muscle functions not only enhances knowledge regarding functional anatomy but also offers therapeutic justification for pathologies and injuries of the upper limb (Figure 2.16).

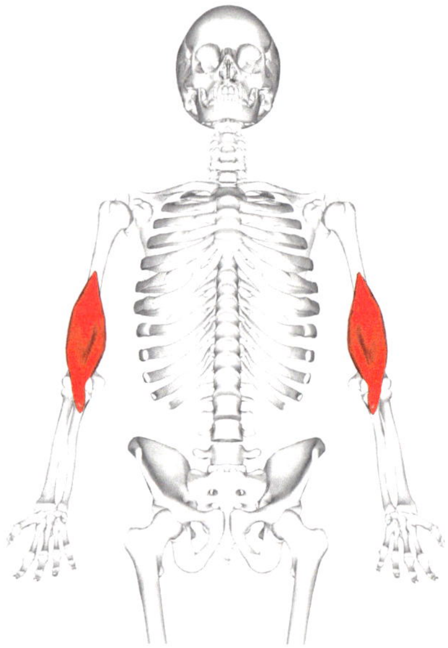

Figure 2.16. Muscle actions during movement.

Source: By Anatomography - en:Anatomography (setting page of this image), CC BY-SA 2.1 jp, https://commons.wikimedia.org/w/index.php?curid=27463169

2.3.9. Common Injuries and Conditions

Injuries and illnesses of the upper limb can potentially minimize function severely and impact everyday living. Rotator cuff injury, fractures, and nerve injury are some of the most prevalent conditions. These normally arise due to repetitive strain, trauma, or long-standing degenerative changes. For instance, tears of the rotator cuff may restrict arm movement and lead to major pain and can occur in both athletes and the general population. Nerve injury, particularly of the brachial plexus, can lead to phantom perception or sensation, which impairs the rehabilitation process (Pazzaglia et al., 2019). Despite the advent of prosthetic limbs, amputees can still be plagued by problems related to their prosthetic limbs, which lag behind user satisfaction because of the issue of functionality and control (Aszmann et al., 2016). Knowledge of these prevalent injuries and their consequences is important for the creation of effective rehabilitation and treatment strategies, ultimately improving QoL.

Test Your Knowledge

1. What is the difference between agonist and antagonist muscles?
2. Define concentric and eccentric muscle contractions with examples.

2.4. Joints of the Upper Limb

Learning Outcome

1. Give an overview of joint types
2. Explain the shoulder joint: structure and movement
3. Focus on elbow joint: structure and movement
4. Discuss wrist joint: structure and movement
5. Know finger joints: types and movements
6. Understand range of motion in upper limb joints
7. Discuss the joint stability and mobility
8. Focus on common joint disorders
9. Understand rehabilitation of joint injuries

The joints of the upper limb are all-critical connections between the skeleton and various muscles that allow extensive movements. The articulations, e.g., glenohumeral (shoulder), elbow, and wrist joint, allow flexure and stability most suitable for complex action. The ball-and-socket glenohumeral joint maintains extensive mobility while accommodating a series of movements including flexion, extension, and rotation. But this liberty is at the expense of joint stability, with the need for synchronized action from surrounding muscles to be able to provide integrity during dynamic movements. To comprehend the biomechanics of such joints, one can refer to comparisons drawn with locomotor adaptations in other animals; for instance, research points out the disparity in muscle function and joint mobility between sprawling and erect postures in archosaurs (Otero et al., 2017). These analyses point out that the mutual design of the human upper limb optimizes fine motor control required for everyday tasks (Figure 2.17).

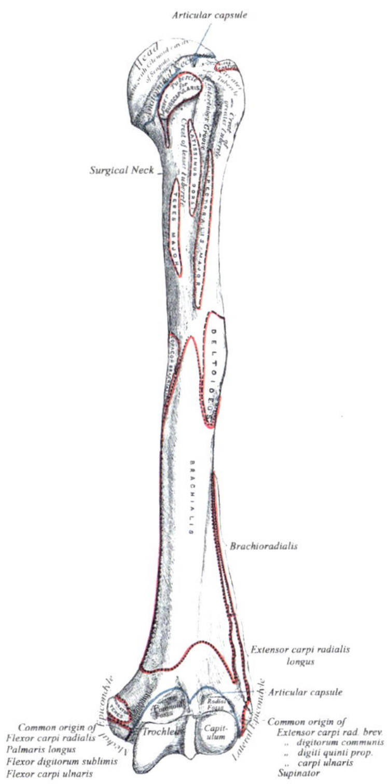

Figure 2.17. Joints of the upper limb.

Source: By Henry Vandyke Carter - Henry Gray (1918) Anatomy of the Human Body (See "Book" section below)Bartleby.com: Gray's Anatomy, Plate 207, Public Domain, https://commons.wikimedia.org/w/index.php?curid=327856

2.4.1. Overview of Joint Types

Joints are significant connections in the skeletal system, enabling a variety of movements essential for everyday activity. The primary joints are hinge joints, ball-and-socket joints, pivot joints, and gliding joints, each allowing a variety of motion suited to its anatomical location. For instance, hinge joints, like the elbow, permit flexion and extension, while ball-and-socket joints, like the shoulder, provide multidirectional movement and rotation, with a high level of freedom of movement. These variations in joint types are at the core of the function of the upper limbs, shaping everything from simple tasks to more complex maneuvers. Complex prosthetic limbs, as discussed in recent reviews of upper limb prosthetics, are heavily dependent on comprehension of these joint mechanics to effectively and precisely replicate natural movement (Aszmann et al., 2016). As such, an appreciation of the wide variety of joint types is relevant to both anatomical knowledge and innovative prosthetic joint design and demonstrates their relevance for restorative and rehabilitative applications (Rust et al., 2009).

2.4.2. Shoulder Joint: Structure and Movement

The fantastic range of motion of the shoulder joint is structured to support a variety of motions required for the function of the upper limbs. It is a ball-and-socket joint formed through the articulation of the humerus and the shallow glenoid cavity of the scapula to form flexibility of rotation, elevation, and reaching. The anatomy and its potential to offer a gigantic range of motion are at the expense of inconvenience in stability. The muscles surrounding the shoulder, i.e., the rotator cuff, play crucial roles in stabilizing the joint as well as facilitating its movement. Biomechanical study reveals gigantic variations in the function of muscles at the shoulder joint, especially between sprawling ones like Crocodylus and more upright postures displayed by Mussaurus, proving that the placement of the scapula makes the leverage of the muscles (Otero et al., 2017). Therefore, understanding the interaction between motion and structure at the shoulder is critical to address clinical conditions as well as enhancing rehabilitation techniques in biomechanics (Harris et al., 2012) (Figure 2.18).

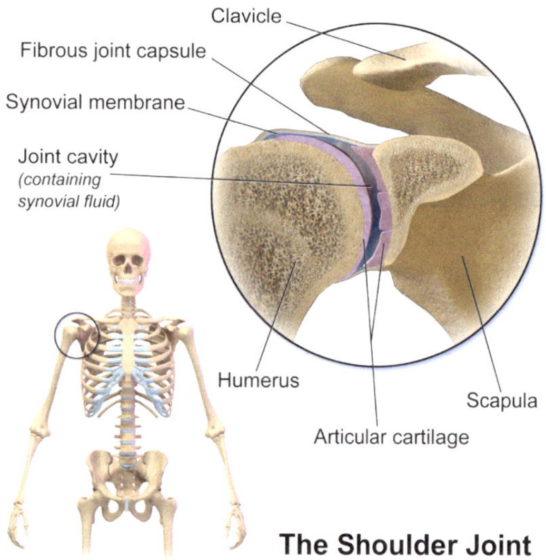

Figure 2.18. Shoulder joint: structure and movement.

Source: By BruceBlaus. When using this image in external sources it can be cited as:Blausen.com staff (2014). "Medical gallery of Blausen Medical 2014". WikiJournal of Medicine 1 (2). DOI:10.15347/wjm/2014.010. ISSN 2002-4436. - Own work, CC BY 3.0, https://commons.wikimedia.org/w/index.php?curid=27796970

2.4.3. Elbow Joint: Structure and Movement

The elbow joint, the medial hinge of the arm, allows for an awe-inspiring range of motions required for daily tasks. Structurally, the elbow is made up of three individual bones: the humerus, radius, and ulna, which are formed together in a manner that would allow them to flex and extend as well as accommodate some rotating motion at the forearm. Its formation is also supported by its ligaments, which provide stability but allow for mobility. In evolutionary limb history, the ability of the elbow joints can be contrasted with the more sprawling forms in other archosaurs, such as Crocodylus, whose joint mobility is limited by their anatomy (Otero et al., 2017). These adaptations highlight the biomechanical importance of the efficiency of the human elbow since it can facilitate the type of precise and coordinated motion involved in various activities. Ultimately, familiarity with these structural elements is crucial to comprehend the functional intricacies of the upper limb.

2.4.4. Wrist Joint: Structure and Movement

Positioned at the distal end of the forearm, the wrist joint serves as a critical pivot point that allows for a wide variety of movements essential to the functioning of the hand. The wrist joint is composed of eight carpal bones organized in two rows and accommodates flexion, extension, and rotation movements, which are essential to activities that require precision and dexterity. The interaction of these bones with the ulna and radius creates a complex structure with multidirectional motion, which is vital in everyday life. Wrist mobility deficiencies, however, can significantly impede hand function as indicated by studies that demonstrate that inadequate actively controllable movements in prosthetics lead to user abandonment (Boccardo et al., 2023). With further enhancement of wrist prosthetic mobility, i.e., active flexion-extension and pronation-supination, the designers aim to bridge the existing gap between natural and artificial limb performance and thus improve amputees' outcomes (Boccardo et al., 2023). Ultimately, appreciation of the intricacy of the wrist's structure and motion will be crucial for advancing the application of both prosthetic and rehabilitation technology in upper limb anatomy.

2.4.5. Finger Joints: Types and Movements

The complexity of finger joints is a fundamental aspect of upper limb function, providing a high range of fine motion necessary for activities of daily life. There are three large groups of finger joints: hinge joints, such as the interphalangeal joints, that allow flexion and extension; saddle joints, such as the carpometacarpal joint of the thumb, allowing oppositional movement; and ellipsoid joints, which are two of the metacarpophalangeal joints, and these allow both flexion/extension and abduction/adduction. They all combine to perform fine activities, ranging from typing to playing music. Understanding the mechanism of such joints is crucial, as their interaction between physical structure and mechanical needs reveals how neuromuscular adaptation influences movement efficiency (Santello et al., 2017; Pereira, 2022). With sustained observation of these kinds of joints and their movements, we are better able to understand the evolutionary structure behind the human hand and its dexterity in grasping and manipulation.

2.4.6. Range of Motion in Upper Limb Joints

The testing of range of motion in upper limb joints suggests tremendous complexity, primarily controlled by anatomical factors as well as biomechanical considerations. To be precise, the shoulder joint possesses the largest range of motion among all upper limb joints with the capacity to perform various motions such as flexion, extension, abduction, and rotation. This diversity plays a critical role in various functional movements, ranging from reaching up to throwing. However, as seen in Otero et al. (2017), the different joint mobilities for sprawling and erect postures may have effects on the functional capacity of the shoulder and elbow in different animals, including humans. Furthermore, the importance of muscle leverage in the movement of joints further highlights this complexity; particular muscle activity around the shoulder and elbow is important for maximal movement economy and prevention of injury, as illustrated in Harris et al. (2012). Finally, grasping these dynamics is most important to applications in rehabilitation and sports training, where joint range maximization and injury risk minimization are primary concerns.

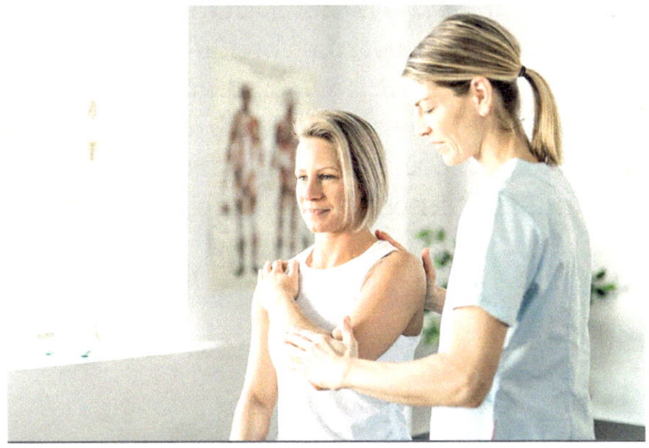

Source: National Academy of Sports Medicine (NASM). (n.d.). *Range of Motion Assessment for Upper Extremities.*

2.4.7. Joint Stability and Mobility

The precarious balance between joint stability and mobility is critical for the functional anatomy of the upper limb. Stability, in general, takes precedence to allow the efficacy and safety of movement to take place, precluding injury with dynamic motion. Stability is mainly a function of the cooperation among the various anatomical elements such as ligaments, tendons, and muscles, all working together to allow the maintenance of the joints. For instance, as biomechanics research suggests, advanced biomechanical model methods can reveal anatomical differences leading to joint stability within different species, including extinct ones like the sthenurine kangaroos, to be balanced and supported during motion (Harris et al., 2012). In contrast, mobility provides a range of movement for an active daily life and specialized function, with direct effects on the functional implications of upper limb mechanics. Lastly, stability/mobility balance is an essential prerequisite for optimal performance and prevents dysfunction of the upper limb.

2.4.8. Common Joint Disorders

Arthropathies are prevalent diseases that can significantly impact an individual's mobility and general QoL. The most common of these conditions are osteoarthritis, rheumatoid arthritis, and bursitis, which tend to affect the functioning of the upper limb. Osteoarthritis is due to the breakdown of cartilage leading to pain and stiffness of joints bearing weight.

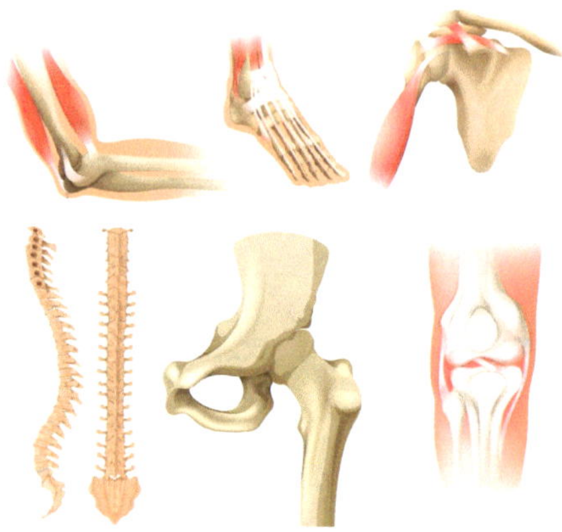

Source: Unknown. (n.d.). *Illustration of Various Joints and Skeletal Structures.*

In contrast, rheumatoid arthritis is an autoimmune disorder causing inflammatory damage to joints that gradually impairs their function. Bursitis due to inflammation of the bursae also causes pain in the shoulder and elbow, further making daily activities difficult. Early intervention and management approaches are necessary for coping with these disorders. As recognized in recent studies, understanding the anatomical and functional consequences of such conditions enhances clinical approaches to prevent complications and improve patient outcomes among affected groups, including those with Morquio A syndrome (Bache et al., 2014) and broiler chickens (Paxton et al., 2014).

2.4.9. Rehabilitation of Joint Injuries

Successful rehabilitation of joint injuries requires a thorough understanding of the specific anatomical and functional characteristics of the joint involved. A meticulous clinical evaluation is necessary, allowing clinicians to establish the precise structures involved and the mechanisms of pain or dysfunction. This detailed examination mandates a tailored rehabilitation program that not only alleviates immediate symptoms but also addresses underlying issues such as muscle strength deficiencies and aberrant movement patterns. As highlighted in the current literature, such as the necessity to treat scapular dysfunction and rotator cuff weakness in patients with glenohumeral impingement, rehabilitation must be multifaceted, incorporating both specific exercise and manual therapy to facilitate healing and restore function (Ellenbecker & Cools, 2010). Also, technological and methodological advances enable clinicians to utilize multi-objective measures in tracking patient progress so that interventions are not just evidence-based but also effective (Aszmann et al., 2016). Lastly, having a systematic approach enables patients to recover full function and restart activities of daily living with confidence.

Test Your Knowledge

1. What is the normal range of motion for shoulder abduction?
2. Which joint movements are possible at the elbow joint?
3. Why is pain management important in joint injury rehabilitation?

2.5. Neuroanatomy of the Upper Limb

Learning Outcome

1. Give an overview of the nervous system's role
2. Explain the brachial plexus: structure and function
3. Focus on major nerves: median, ulnar, radial
4. Discuss sensory innervation of the upper limb
5. Understand motor innervation of the upper limb
6. Explain the reflexes involving the upper limb
7. Know neurological conditions affecting the upper limb
8. Discuss how to impact of nerve injuries on function
9. Focus on rehabilitation strategies for nerve injuries

The complex neuroanatomy of the upper limb lies at the heart of determining its functional capacity and the impact of neurological disease. Motor control of the upper limbs is founded upon the complex inter-relationship between many neural structures, including the primary motor cortex, the corticospinal tract, and peripheral nerves, which all interact to facilitate voluntary movement. Dysfunctions or deteriorations in these neural tracts can lead to severe motor impairment. For instance, injuries to the spinal cord can interfere with such circuits, causing loss of independence and dysfunctional ADLs (Mittal, 2021). Besides, neuroimaging studies prove that conditions such as Alzheimer's disease not only can affect cognition but also the integrity of white matter pathways responsible for motor control, further demonstrating the importance of knowing the upper limb neuroanatomy both for rehabilitation and treatment of neurodegenerative diseases (Alves et al., 2012). Each element in this neuroanatomical structure plays a critical part in setting up the mechanisms of the functional upper limb (Figure 2.19).

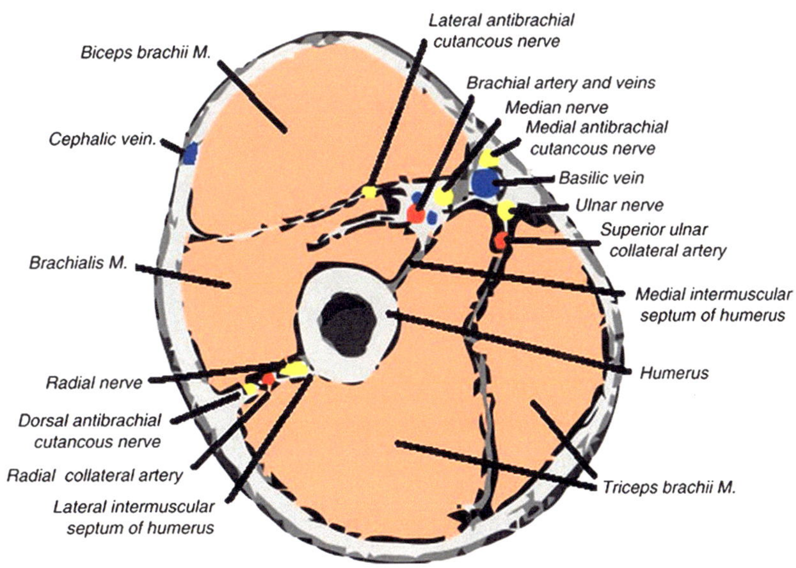

Figure 2.19. Neuroanatomy of the upper limb.

Source: By Henry Vandyke Carter - Henry Gray (1918) Anatomy of the Human Body (See "Book" section below)Bartleby.com: Gray's Anatomy, Plate 413, Public Domain, https://commons.wikimedia.org/w/index.php?curid=3270164

2.5.1. Overview of the Nervous System's Role

The complex function of the nervous system forms the foundation for the overall function of the upper limb, combining sensory feedback and motor response to facilitate movement. The system not only reads information from the environment but also enables an individual to act on their environment appropriately. For example, when a brachial plexus injury or anesthesia is experienced, as realized by recent studies, phantom sensations that are produced reflect the complex interaction between body consciousness and sensory feedback (Pazzaglia et al., 2019). The neuromechanical hypothesis suggests that behavior is the result of physical structure and neural control interacting, which illustrates the way both biological and engineered robotic analogs try similar mechanical tasks even as they have different origins (Santello et al., 2017). It is important to grasp this dynamic since it is what leads to the rehabilitation of individuals with limb loss and increases our knowledge of motor function under health and pathology. Last, the nervous system is the chief intermediary of movement and sensation of the upper limb.

2.5.2. Brachial Plexus: Structure and Function

The brachial plexus is a vital collection of nerves emerging from the spinal cord to innervate the upper limb for both motor and sensory purposes. Its complex nature originates from the spinal nerve anterior rami C5 to T1, which join together to give five roots that blend to form trunks, divisions, cords, and terminal branches. All of these components play a critical role in signaling back and forth to and from the arm and hand for coordinated motion and sensory feedback. Notably, damage to the brachial plexus can lead to extreme impairment, indicated by phantom sensations following injury. These events highlight its importance in perception and motor control and illustrate the collaboration between peripheral and central mechanisms in neural processing (Pazzaglia et al., 2019). Furthermore, advances in imaging technology have enhanced our understanding of the anatomical subtleties of this plexus for use in guiding surgical applications and facilitating orthopedic therapeutic planning (Audenaert et al., 2010).

2.5.3. Major Nerves: Median, Ulnar, Radial

The complex plexus of peripheral nerves of the upper limb are part of both motor and sensory function, and the median, ulnar, and radial nerves are particularly significant.

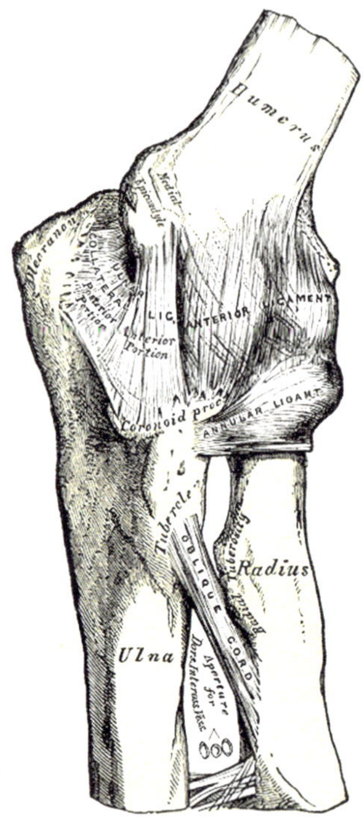

Figure 2.20. Major nerves: median, ulnar, radial.

Source: By Henry Vandyke Carter - Henry Gray (1918) Anatomy of the Human Body (See "Book" section below)Bartleby.com: Gray's Anatomy, Plate 329, Public Domain, https://commons.wikimedia.org/w/index.php?curid=792114

Each of these three nerves has a separate course through the upper limb, influencing different groups of muscles and sensory distributions. The median nerve, whose chief role is the innervation of the forearm flexors and some intrinsic hand muscles, is essential for precision grip and thumb opposition. In comparison, the ulnar nerve controls hand muscles that are vital to fine motor function and grip, often in jeopardy of injury or compression. The radial nerve, however, controls the extensor muscles that allow wrist and finger extension. Understanding these nerves' spatial relationship to the axillary artery and their anatomical variations, as highlighted in studies, is relevant for clinical application, particularly with anesthetic techniques for regional blocks (Ates et al., 2018; Francesco et al., 2022) (Figure 2.20).

2.5.4. Sensory Innervation of the Upper Limb

The complexity of sensory innervation of the upper limb is essential to its functional anatomy. Nerves such as the median, ulnar, and radial nerves are responsible for the transmission of touch, pain, and temperature sensations from the skin to the CNS to give an integrated response to the environment. This pathway not only protects the limb from harm but also fine-tunes the fine motor control required for day-to-day life. Damage to these nerve pathways can result in phenomena like phantom sensations that ironically demonstrate the brain's ongoing representation of the body with no sensory information (Pazzaglia et al., 2019). Moreover, the interface of peripheral mechanisms and central processing explains how brachial plexus disorders can alter sensory function, impacting overall limb performance and rehabilitation techniques (Cozart et al., 2017). Lastly, this knowledge is crucial in building useful treatments for sensory impairment in the upper limb.

2.5.5. Motor Innervation of the Upper Limb

The upper limb's complex motor innervation is of utmost significance for smooth motion and function, as it involves an complex network of nerves originating from the brachial plexus. This neural element is responsible for transmitting motor commands to various groups of muscles, conveying a superior range of motion and dexterity required for daily activities. The organization of the brachial plexus reflects evolutionary adaptations that replicate the locomotive pressures on the arm and shoulder. Notably, studies reveal certain differences in the brachial plexus across primate lineages, with lineages showing excessive locomotor modifications tending to show rapid evolution in their patterns of nerves, with a focus on the direct correlation between locomotion and neural adaptation (Shearer, 2019). Understanding these pathways is crucial to the functional anatomy of the upper limb since motor innervation directly influences both the mechanics of movement and the ability to execute skilled movements. Collectively, the dissection of the complexities of the innervation of the upper limb illustrates the basic interaction between anatomy, function, and evolution.

2.5.6. Reflexes Involving the Upper Limb

Reflexes play a significant role in the functional anatomy of the upper limb, facilitating rapid responses essential for survival. Reflexes such as the flexor withdrawal reflex and the stretch reflex enable the body to respond instantly to stimuli, avoiding injury and maintaining it in a stable condition while in motion. Such upper limb reflexes are closely associated with motor pathways with structures such as the striatum and motor cortices. For instance, the impairment of righting reflexes in basal ganglia illnesses points to the importance of such neural circuits, particularly maintaining coordination and control (Bakheit et al., 1990). Moreover, integrating sensory inputs and ensuing motor responses show how reflexes help execute complex actions such as writing or playing a musical instrument. This complex interplay between motor output and sensory input enhances the upper limbs flexibility, controlled by reflex mechanisms to allow voluntary and involuntary movements during daily activities (Figure 2.21).

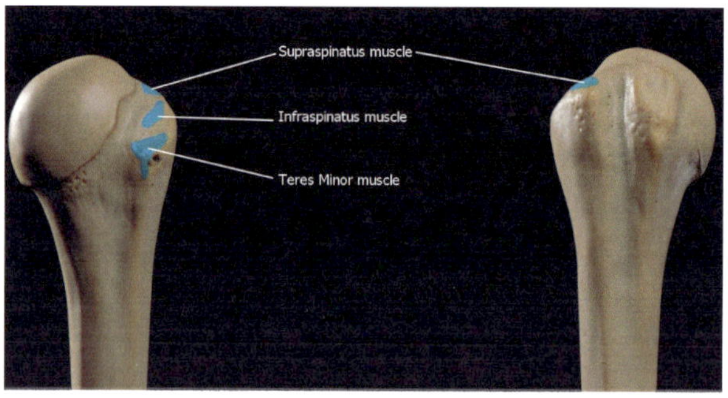

Figure 2.21. Reflexes involving the upper limb.

Source: By Doctor Jana - https://docjana.com/Humerus-3d-Anatomy/, CC BY-SA 4.0, https://commons.wikimedia.org/w/index.php?curid=77075723

2.5.7. Neurological Conditions Affecting the Upper Limb

Neurological diseases can extensively impair the functioning of the upper limb, leading to difficulty in carrying out activities of daily living and QoL. For example, patients after total shoulder arthroplasty (TSA) or reverse shoulder arthroplasty (RSA) may have deranged kinematics in reaching movements, which has a direct influence on the performance of tasks. These procedures are usually performed to address disabling shoulder pathologies; however, the postoperative changes in proprioception may disrupt motor coordination and fluidity of motion (Carbone et al., 2015). Further, treatments like guided motor imagery and cross education are explored to regain upper limb function impaired by neurological disorders, by stimulating neural circuits that cause movement without actual physical exertion (Bouchard, 2014). As research continues, integrating such therapeutic interventions may enhance recovery outcomes, and this identifies the importance of establishing the neurological underpinnings of upper limb biomechanics in rehabilitation.

2.5.8. Impact of Nerve Injuries on Function

Nerve damage can significantly impact the upper limb's function, disrupting sensory perception along with motor control. After the brachial plexus has been injured or blocked, as documented in recent studies, patients also begin to experience phantom sensations, which demonstrate the complexity of body representation in the brain (Pazzaglia et al., 2019). This division not only affects the physical possibility of movement but also harms the sensory feedback necessary for interaction with the environment, resulting in a range of social and psychological consequences. Further, innovations in prosthetic devices have attempted to minimize these consequences. Traditional devices often did not have this, and because of this, high abandonment rates were seen as a result of limitations in functionality and control for the user (Aszmann et al., 2016). However, the union of improved robotics and enhanced interfacing techniques is hopeful of returning more normal motion and sensation, and, eventually, enhancing the QoL in victims of nerve trauma.

2.5.9. Rehabilitation Strategies for Nerve Injuries

Effective rehabilitation procedures for nerve damage have a key function in the restoration of function and improvement of the QoL of such individuals. In a protocol, operative procedures such as nerve transfer or microneural reconstruction are implemented to facilitate regeneration via the damaged involved nerve tract, which adds to the restoration of function. For example, procedures like lower subscapular nerve transfer can prove to be extremely beneficial, enabling the restoration of shoulder movement in brachial plexus injury (Baj et al., 2023). Rehabilitation also includes rigorous non-surgical interventions like physical therapy, which enhances the range of motion and strengthens surrounding muscles, ultimately enabling the restoration of dexterity and coordination. Moreover, integrating new technologies, like advanced prosthetics, enhances the capacity of patients to perform daily activities, validating the role of a multidisciplinary approach. Lastly, the tailored rehabilitation program combining surgical and therapeutic modalities is the optimal means of maximizing nerve injury recovery (Figure 2.22).

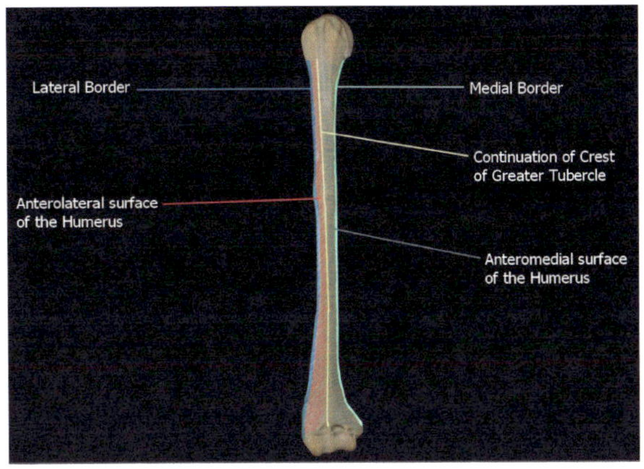

Figure 2.22. Knowledge of upper limb anatomy.

Source: By Doctor Jana - https://docjana.com/Humerus-3d-Anatomy/, CC BY-SA 4.0, https://commons.wikimedia.org/w/index.php?curid=77075724

Test Your Knowledge

1. What are common symptoms of peripheral nerve injuries?
2. What is the role of physiotherapy in nerve injury recovery?
3. How can occupational therapy help restore daily function after a nerve injury?

SUMMARY

With the anatomy of the upper limb, the complex relationships of bone, muscle, and nerve become apparent, demonstrating that these relationships not only provide for a high amount of motion but also serve critical biomechanical functions. The arrangement and construction of the parts enable sophisticated movements required for normal living, reinforcing their importance in the healthy state as well as in the rehabilitation state. For example, just as those limitations that were evident in the sthenurine kangaroos which were specialized for locomotion are likewise applied today to any dysfunction in the functional anatomy of the upper limb as causing considerable dysfunction in movement patterns and overall functionality, emphasis on research indicates that sthenurines adaptations provide insight into the emergence of mobility and how structural differences can affect functionality, that knowing these principles is essential for effective therapeutic intervention. In summary, reinforcement of our knowledge of upper limb anatomy and mechanics can guide superior clinical practice and optimize recovery outcomes for those facing MSK challenges (Jones et al., 2016).

The functional anatomy of the upper limb comprises a highly developed interaction among bones, muscles, and connective tissues, which in total facilitate a wide range of movements and functions required in daily activities. The major characteristic of this system is the unique modularity and coordination of various anatomical structures, particularly when comparing upper limb versus lower limb structures. Research involving Anatomical Network Analysis (AnNA) highlights this distinction, showing that there exist dramatic differences between the bone networks of the upper and lower limbs when muscle involvement is taken into consideration, defying the classic belief that such limbs are serial homologs (Goswami et al., 2015). Additionally, the evolution of such specialized anatomy suggests adaptive mechanisms to enhance the survivability and functionality of humans in various environments. Understanding these facts is achievable only through a greater appreciation of how our upper limb supports both fine manipulation and gross motor function and how they express their critical status in human behavior and physiology (Ricci et al., 2022).

KEY TERMS FROM THIS CHAPTER

Archosaurian lineages
Case-based learning (CBL)
Embryological development
Human movement
Multidirectional mobility
Biomechanical study
Clavicular structures
Gross motor
Lymphatic patterning
Multivalent utility
Carpal tunnel syndrome
Elbow joint
Human mobility
Mercury perfusion

CRITICAL THINKING QUESTIONS

1. **Which bone articulates with the scapula at the shoulder joint?**
   a. Radius
   b. Humerus
   c. Ulna
   d. Clavicle
2. **Which nerve supplies the muscles in the anterior compartment of the arm?**
   a. Radial nerve
   b. Ulnar nerve
   c. Musculocutaneous nerve
   d. Median nerve
3. **What is the main artery of the upper arm?**
   a. Subclavian artery
   b. Axillary artery
   c. Brachial artery
   d. Radial artery
4. **Which carpal bone is most commonly fractured?**
   a. Scaphoid
   b. Lunate
   c. Triquetrum
   d. Pisiform
5. **Which structure passes through the carpal tunnel?**
   a. Ulnar nerve
   b. Brachial artery
   c. Median nerve
   d. Radial nerve

Short Answer Questions

1. What are the main joints present in the upper limb?
2. Describe the boundaries and contents of the axilla.
3. Define the brachial plexus and its role in the upper limb.
4. What is the brachial plexus and what is its function?
5. Which arteries supply blood to the upper limb?
6. Describe the anatomical snuffbox and its clinical importance.

Answers to Critical Thinking Questions

1. (b) 2. (c) 3. (c) 4. (a) 5. (c)

REFERENCES

1. Safwat, M. D., & Abdel-Meguid, E. M. (2007). Distribution of terminal nerve entry points to the flexor and extensor groups of forearm muscles: an anatomical study. *Folia morphologica*, *66*(2), 83–93. (accessed on 8th May 2025).
2. Allen, V., Hutchinson, J. R., Otero, A., & Pol, D. (2017). Forelimb muscle and joint actions in Archosauria: Insights from *Crocodylus johnstoni* (Pseudosuchia) and *Mussaurus patagonicus* (Sauropodomorpha). *PeerJ*. https://core.ac.uk/download/141887609.pdf Otero A, Allen V, Pol D, Hutchinson JR. 2017. Forelimb muscle and joint actions in Archosauria: insights from Crocodylus johnstoni (Pseudosuchia) and Mussaurus patagonicus (Sauropodomorpha) PeerJ 5:e3976 https://doi.org/10.7717/peerj.3976 (accessed on 8th May 2025).
3. Altarocca, A., Altieri, M., Camerota, F., Celletti, C., Di Piero, V., Giuliani, G., Jannini, T. B., Maestrini, I., Mastria, G., Ruggiero, M., Toscano, M., Vicenzini, E., & Vigano, A. (2019). *Short-Term Effects of Focal Muscle Vibration on Motor Recovery After Acute Stroke: A Pilot Randomized Sham-Controlled Study.* Frontiers Media SA. https://core.ac.uk/download/231747785.pdf (accessed on 8th May 2025).
4. Aszmann, O. C., Farina, D., & Vujaklija, I. (2016). *New Developments in Prosthetic Arm Systems.* Dove Medical Press Ltd. https://core.ac.uk/download/78075208.pdf (accessed on 8th May 2025).
5. Baj, J., Korga, M., Kowalczyk, A., Małyska, J., Sikora, K., Tokarzewska, A., & Tybulczuk, B. (2023). *Current Strategies of the Brachial Plexus Palsy Management.* Nicolaus Copernicus University, Toruń, Poland. https://core.ac.uk/download/587246448.pdf (accessed on 8th May 2025).
6. Bakheit, A. M. O. (1990). *The Basal Ganglia as a Gate Control Mechanism for Postural Set.* [ProQuest Dissertations & Theses. https://core.ac.uk/download/286351427.pdf (accessed on 8th May 2025).
7. Jones, P. S., Pomeroy, V. M., Wang, J., Schlaug, G., Tulasi Marrapu, S., Geva, S., Rowe, P. J., Chandler, E., Kerr, A., Baron, J. C., & SWIFT-Cast investigators (2016). Does stroke location predict walk speed response to gait rehabilitation?. *Human brain mapping*, *37*(2), 689–703. https://doi.org/10.1002/hbm.23059 (accessed on 8th May 2025).
8. Maidment SCR, Linton DH, Upchurch P, Barrett PM (2012) Limb-Bone Scaling Indicates Diverse Stance and Gait in Quadrupedal Ornithischian Dinosaurs. PLoS ONE 7(5): e36904. https://doi.org/10.1371/journal.pone.0036904 (accessed on 8th May 2025).
9. Bonilla-Yacelga, K. A., Guzmán-Moreno, K. I., Iñiguez-Jimenez, S. O., Llumiquinga-Panchi, E. D., & Maldonado-Cornejo, J. G. (2024). *Physiotherapeutic Assessment in Oncological Post-Mastectomy Patients.* Uphills Publishers LLC, United States. https://core.ac.uk/download/616974475.pdf (accessed on 8th May 2025).
10. Bouchard, Emily, "Integrating Guided Motor Imagery and Cross Education into Rehabilitation: Scientific Review and Clinical Application" (2014). Honors College Capstone Experience/Thesis Projects. Paper 448. http://digitalcommons.wku.edu/stu_hon_theses/448 (accessed on 8th May 2025).
11. Reinkensmeyer, D.J., Burdet, E., Casadio, M. *et al.* Computational neurorehabilitation: modeling plasticity and learning to predict recovery. *J NeuroEngineering Rehabil* **13**, 42 (2016). https://doi.org/10.1186/s12984-016-0148-3(accessed on 8th May 2025).

12. Cappellari, O., Charles, J. P., Hutchinson, J. R., Spence, A. J., & Wells, D. J. (2016). *Musculoskeletal Geometry, Muscle Architecture and Functional Specializations of the Mouse Hindlimb.* Public Library of Science (PLoS). https://core.ac.uk/download/45467680.pdf (accessed on 8th May 2025).

13. Paxton, H., Tickle, P. G., Rankin, J. W., Codd, J. R., & Hutchinson, J. R. (2014). Anatomical and biomechanical traits of broiler chickens across ontogeny. Part II. Body segment inertial properties and muscle architecture of the pelvic Ellenbecker, T. S., & Cools, A. (2010). Rehabilitation of shoulder impingement syndrome and rotator cuff injuries: an evidence-based review. *British journal of sports medicine*, *44*(5), 319–327. https://doi.org/10.1136/bjsm.2009.058875 (accessed on 8th May 2025).

14. Ricci, G., Marzella, L. ., De Vitis, R., Gravina, P., & De Francesco, F. (2021). Upper Limb Structural Anatomic Mechanisms of Protection (SAMPs). *Organisms. Journal of Biological Sciences*, 1–10. https://doi.org/10.13133/2532-5876/17506 (accessed on 8th May 2025).

15. Gao, Z., Pang, Z., Chen, Y. M., Lei, G., Zhu, S., Li, G., Shen, Y., & Xu, W. (2022). Restoring after central nervous system injuries: Neural mechanisms and translational applications of motor recovery. *Neuroscience Bulletin, 38*, 1569–1587. https://doi.org/10.1007/s12264-022-00959-x.

16. Pazzaglia, M., Leemhuis, E., Giannini, A. M., & Haggard, P. (2019). The Homuncular Jigsaw: Investigations of Phantom Limb and Body Awareness Following Brachial Plexus Block or Avulsion. *Journal of clinical medicine*, *8*(2), 182. https://doi.org/10.3390/jcm8020182(accessed on 8th May 2025).

17. Vargesson, N., & Hootnick, D. R. (2017). Arterial dysgenesis and limb defects: Clinical and experimental examples. *Reproductive toxicology (Elmsford, N.Y.)*, *70*, 21–29. https://doi.org/10.1016/j.reprotox.2016.10.005 (accessed on 8th May 2025).

18. Hsu, J. (2009). *Aging Related Differences in Hand Intrinsic and Extrinsic Muscles for Hand Dexterity: An MRI Investigation.* http://hdl.handle.net/1903/9988

19. https://core.ac.uk/download/56106559.pdf (accessed on 8th May 2025).

20. Kivell, T. L., Baraki, N., Lockwood, V. A., Williams-Hatala, E. M., & Wood, B. (2022). Form, function and evolution of the human hand. *American Journal of Biological Anthropology, 181*, 6–57. https://doi.org/10.1002/ajpa.24667.

21. Klemt, C. (2018). *Musculoskeletal Shoulder Modelling for Clinical Applications.* Doctoral dissertation, Imperial College London. Bioengineering, Imperial College London. https://core.ac.uk/download/266987656.pdf (accessed on 8th May 2025).

22. Lanting, B. A. (2014). *The Development and Application of a Forearm Simulator to Investigate Radial Head Biomechanics.* Master's thesis, Western University. *Scholarship@Western.* https://core.ac.uk/download/61644598.pdf (accessed on 8th May 2025).

23. Latey, P. (2018). *Measuring and Managing Foot Muscle Weakness.* Master's thesis, University of Sarajevo Faculty of Health Sciences. https://core.ac.uk/download/212695406.pdf (accessed on 8th May 2025).

24. Legleiter, K. (2023). Occupational therapy graduate students,' recent graduates,' and educators' perceptions of the value of anatomy knowledge. *Journal of Occupational Therapy Education*, v7 n2 Article 10 2023 https://core.ac.uk/download/572737989.pdf (accessed on 8th May 2025).

25. Levin, M. (2022). Technological approach to mind everywhere: An experimentally-grounded framework for understanding diverse bodies and minds. *Frontiers in Systems Neuroscience, 16*. https://doi.org/10.3389/fnsys.2022.768201.

26. Rosse, C., Mejino, J.L.V. (2008). The Foundational Model of Anatomy Ontology. In: Burger, A., Davidson, D., Baldock, R. (eds) Anatomy Ontologies for Bioinformatics. Computational Biology, vol 6. Springer, London. https://doi.org/10.1007/978-1-84628-885-2_4 (accessed on 8th May 2025).

27. Mittal, N. (2021). *Intermittent Theta Burst Stimulation: Application to Spinal Cord Injury Rehabilitation and Computational Modeling*. VCU Scholars Compass. https://core.ac.uk/download/489493638.pdf (accessed on 8th May 2025).

28. Mugnosso, M. (2020). *Coupling Robot-Aided Assessment and Surface Electromyography to Evaluate Wrist and Forearm Muscles Activity, Muscle Fatigue and its Effect on Proprioception*. Master's thesis, Università degli Studi di Genova. https://core.ac.uk/download/286529306.pdf (accessed on 8th May 2025).

29. Nichols, R. (2019). *UGA Laboratory Manual for Functional Human Anatomy. GALILEO Open Learning Materials*. https://core.ac.uk/download/287027371.pdf (accessed on 8th May 2025).

30. Pereira, M. S. (2022). *Numerical-Experimental Characterization of a Hand Prosthesis: Pilot Project Built by Additive Manufacturing*. Master's Dissertation Integrated Masters in Biomedical Engineering Biomaterials, Rehabilitation and Biomechanics. https://core.ac.uk/download/553665950.pdf (accessed on 8th May 2025).

31. Reinkensmeyer, D. J. (2019). *JNER at 15 Years: Analysis of the State of Neuroengineering and rehabilitation*. eScholarship, University of California. https://core.ac.uk/download/286362777.pdf (accessed on 8th May 2025).

32. Rust, C., Whiteley, G., & Wilson, A. (2000). Experimental Making in Multidisciplinary Research. *The Design Journal, 3*(3), 16–25. https://doi.org/10.2752/146069200789390088(accessed on 8th May 2025).

33. Shearer, B. M. (2019). *The Morphology and Evolution of the Primate Brachial Plexus*. Doctoral dissertation, City University of New York. CUNY Academic Works. https://academicworks.cuny.edu/cgi/viewcontent.cgi?article=4113&context=gc_etds (accessed on 8th May 2025).

LOWER LIMB

3

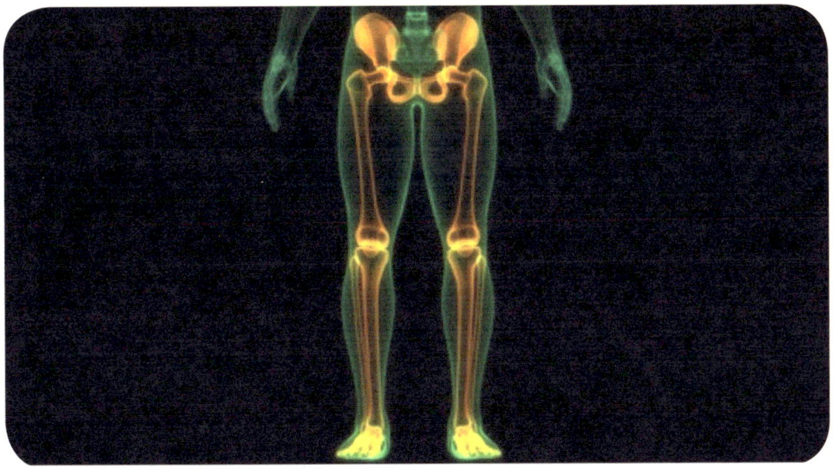

Introduction

The lower limb, which is a great anatomical structure, plays a key role in mobility and stability in human beings. It is the complex interworking of bones, muscles, ligaments, tendons, and joints, each contributing a synergistic degree of motion to enable walking, running, and other movements. Awareness of lower limb functional anatomy not only demonstrates the importance of its components but also describes how these structures function together to support load and facilitate motion. This study of the lower limb anatomy is particularly relevant in fields such as medicine, physical therapy, and sports science, in which anatomical relationship information can aid in the diagnosis and treatment of injuries. Lastly, an in-depth review of the lower limb functional anatomy reveals complex biological designs, which show how important these structures are in maintaining overall human health and function.

LEARNING OBJECTIVES

After studying this chapter, you will be able to:

1. Explain the anatomy of the lower limb
2. Explain the bone structure of the lower limb
3. Identify the muscular system of the lower limb
4. Learn about joints and ligaments of the lower limb
5. Give an overview of the nervous system in the lower limb

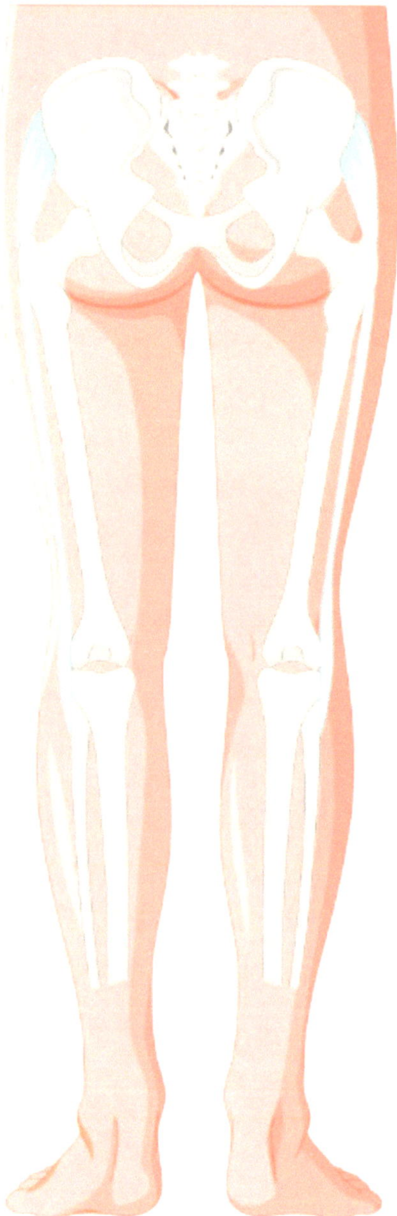

Source: Freepik. (n.d.). *Human Leg and Pelvis Anatomy (Posterior View).*

Definition of the Lower Limb

The human body relies on complex anatomical structures to enable movement and stability with each component having a specific role in the musculoskeletal (MSK) system. Of these, the lower limb is a critical region that encompasses all regions from the hip to the foot to enable locomotion and weight-bearing functions that are necessary for daily activities. It is made up of the thigh, leg, ankle, and foot, and comprises bones, muscles, tendons, ligaments, blood vessels, and nerves that work synergistically to enhance balance and mobility. Proper functioning of this area is not only crucial for ordinary activities such as walking and running but also for postural stabilization in various situations. Understanding the definition of the lower limb and its internal structures is fundamental to clinical evaluation and management of related pathologies and, as such, the value of evidence-based practice and methods in medical guidelines and interventions (Jean-Ricco et al., 2017; Paul et al., 2017).

Importance of the Lower Limb in Human Movement

The anatomical configuration of the lower limb has a significant influence on human movement complexities, performing crucial functional roles. The lower limbs stabilize, support, and push in the execution of numerous everyday activities, such as walking, running, and jumping, illustrating the importance of sports and everyday life. Bone, muscle, tendon, and joint connectivity in the lower limbs offers an impressive range of motion and dynamic balance. This interaction allows individuals to perform complex movements in an effective way, and this is valuable to athletes, as seen on platforms like the EuroSciCon Sports Science Summit, which discusses progress and results regarding performance enhancement through greater understanding of biomechanics (Chawla et al., 2015). Also, limb design in prosthetics, as researched at Sheffield Hallam University, reflects the importance of anatomical accuracy in the facilitation of movement and the improvement of Calidad de Vida, demonstrating how the application of innovation can optimize function through an understanding of the human anatomy (Rust et al., 1999) (Figure 3.1).

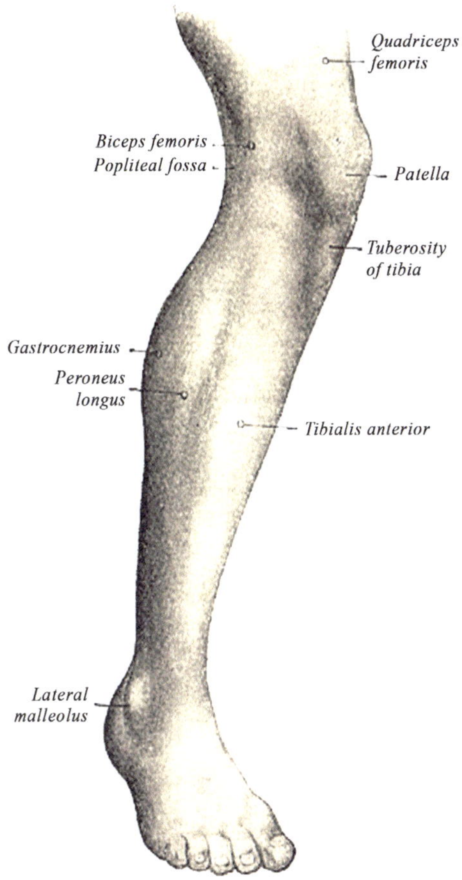

Figure 3.1. The lower limb in human movement.

Source: https://en.wikipedia.org/wiki/File:Gray1240.png

Overview of the Lower Limb Structure

The lower limb is a highly developed machine that is crucial for stability and movement. Composed of several vital parts—involving the pelvic girdle, thigh, leg, and foot—the lower limb is designed to support the body weight and enable an individual to walk, run, or jump. Each segment consists of a unique arrangement of bones, muscles, ligaments, and tendons, all of which work together to enable movement. For instance, the hip joint connecting the femur to the pelvis is a ball-and-socket joint that allows a wide range of motion, and the knee joint is a crucial hinge that gets subjected to very high loads while performing many activities. Furthermore, 3D anatomical modeling development has widened knowledge of lower limbs anatomical and functional correlations to provide greater clinical applications in areas of rehabilitation and biomechanics (Magnenat-Thalmann et al., 2010; Standring, 2015). From these studies, it can be seen that all structural elements of the lower limbs are related in a very correlated manner with its functional capabilities.

Brief History of Lower Limb Anatomy Studies

Beginning from ancient history, the physiology of the lower limbs has evolved significantly, punctuated by sequential cultural and scientific advances. The early anatomical knowledge, predicated largely on dissections, laid the ground for the understanding of bone and muscle morphology. The formative period was dominated by limited access to human cadavers and reliance on animal anatomy, which forestalled an adequate human physiology understanding. The Renaissance kindled interest again and more systematic investigations were carried out that included observational techniques as well as anatomical drawings. As the subject evolved, the advent of modern methodologies like Anatomical Network Analysis (AnNA) has transformed our understanding of lower limb dynamics. For instance, AnNA has given valuable insights into the functional integration of muscles and skeletal networks in primates, illuminating the differences between proximal and distal limb structures in primates (Diogo et al., 2017). This evolution is in line with an overall trend in anatomy from descriptive to integrative complex analysis, ultimately enhancing the understanding of lower limb function under both health and disease (Goswami et al., 2015) (Figure 3.2).

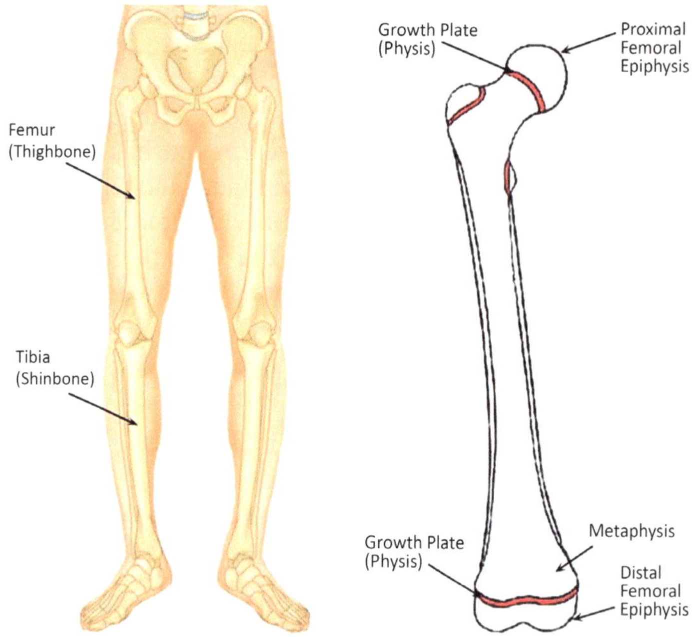

Figure 3.2. Brief history of lower limb anatomy studies.

Source: American Academy of Orthopedic Surgeons (AAOS). (n.d.). *Growth Plate Anatomy of the Femur and Tibia.*

Significance of Studying the Lower Limb

Careful understanding of the lower limb is essential in both surgical and clinical scenarios due to its complex anatomy and frequent lower limb involvement in disease and trauma. Variations in neural and vascular anatomy significantly impact surgical success and therapeutic treatment success. For instance, knowledge about arterial anomalies such as the upper limb superficial brachial artery emphasizes the recognition of anomalous vessels so that they are not accidentally damaged while performing an operation, a stipulation that may be extended to the arteries of the lower limb as well (Prabhakar et al., 2024). Similarly, the sciatic nerve, which is the main neural anatomy of the lower limb, shows anatomical variations like high division, which have far-reaching implications on intramuscular injection, nerve blocks, and effective injury management (Shah et al., 2023). Knowledge of such variations enhances the precision of medical interventions, reduces complications, and fosters personalized treatment approaches, reflecting the crucial role of lower limb anatomy in medicine.

3.1. Anatomy of the Lower Limb

Learning Outcome

1. Give an overview of the skeletal structure
2. Discuss the major bones of the lower limb
3. Focus on joints in the lower limb
4. Define muscles associated with the lower limb
5. Explain the nerves supplying the lower limb
6. Understand blood supply to the lower limb
7. Describe the fascia and connective tissues in the lower limb
8. Focus on variations in lower limb anatomy
9. Explain the developmental aspects of the lower limb

It is required to comprehend the complex anatomy of the lower limb to enhance both clinical intervention and biomechanical engineering applications. The lower limb has major joints such as the hip, knee, and ankle, which are all involved in generating complex movements like walking and standing up from a sitting position. Exoskeleton designs with different levels of freedom replicate these joint motions to assist individuals with lower limb motor dysfunction, showing the importance of aligning assistive technology with normal human anatomy and gait mechanics (Chen et al., 2024). The designing of prosthetic devices to fulfill personalized anatomical and functional needs is also highly reliant on detailed anatomical information. Integrating CAD design and strength analyses, based on ISO standards, ensures that not only do prostheses meet anatomical requirements, but they also withstand real-world mechanical stresses, with enhanced safety and efficacy for users (Siwek, 2023). This intersection of anatomy, engineering, and materials science underscores the complexity of designing lower limb support systems that are synchronized with human motion (Figure 3.3).

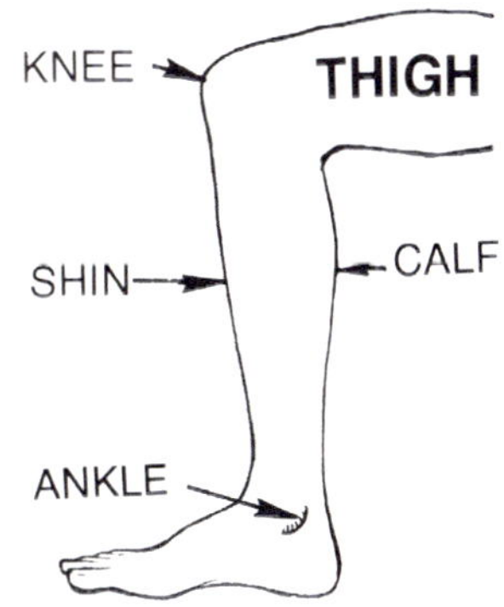

Figure 3.3. The anatomy of the lower limb.

Source: By Pearson Scott Foresman - This image has been extracted from another file, Public Domain, https://commons.wikimedia.org/w/index.php?curid=87549104

3.1.1. Overview of the Skeletal Structure

The complex pattern of the lower limbs' skeletal system serves as the central foundation for mobility and stability. Composed of the femur, tibia, fibula, and the bones of the foot, this structure provides effective weight-bearing and mobility. The femur, which is the longest and strongest bone, plays the central role in force distribution during movement, while structural support and balance are provided by the tibia and fibula. Moreover, the relationship between muscle and bone, as determined by fiber content such as in the soleus and rectus femoris muscles, directly influences functional performance and endurance (Nair et al., 2023). Biomechanical engineering advances, such as improvements in exoskeleton actuators, rely heavily on exact knowledge of this skeletal framework to develop rehabilitation technology. For instance, series elastic–damping actuators are specifically designed with the mechanical properties and dynamics of lower limb joints to facilitate improved human-machine interaction in assistive devices (Zhao et al., 2024). This convergence of anatomical structure and technology applied works to emphasize the importance of both the skeletal system in biological terms and the skeletal system in clinical terms.

3.1.2. Major Bones of the Lower Limb

Support and function of the structural integrity of the lower limb are offered by a complex arrangement of major bones that permit mobility and weight-bearing. The basic component of this system is the femur, the longest and strongest bone, which articulates the hip to the knee, permitting ambulation and support. The tibia and fibula, distally, provide the necessary support for weight transfer while permitting ankle flexibility. These bones, along with the patella, play very essential roles in locomotion and shock absorption. The foot skeleton composed of tarsals, metatarsals, and phalanges supports balance and propulsion when walking. Evolutionary differences in these bones present primates' diverse locomotor behavior and reveal the function of the lower limb in various means of mobility from arboreal locomotion to terrestrial bipedalism (Susan, 2018). Ultrasound imaging techniques have provided information regarding complex fetal bone formation during early pregnancy, which underscores the importance of skeletal assessment for the identification of anomalies and appropriate musculoskeletal (MSK) growth (Caterina et al., 2023).

3.1.3. Joints in the Lower Limb

Lower limb structural integrity and function are primarily reliant upon the delicate cooperation of its joints, which provide support for mobility and bearing functions essential to human movement. Of all such joints, the hip, knee, and ankle joints are of greatest importance, each possessing unique anatomical characteristics suited to specific biomechanical demands. The sacroiliac joint, which joins the lower limb to the axial skeleton, is of particular significance, but its involvement in pathological processes such as sacroiliitis can critically interfere with lower limb function, such as in situations demonstrating pain and neurological presentation following pregnancy or surgery (Kandanuri et al., 2025). While the majority of the literature focuses on upper limb pseudarthrosis and surgery (Puseva et al., 2021), the principles of joint stability, osteosynthesis, and restoration of anatomy are also relevant, emphasizing the importance of proper diagnosis and targeted treatment in lower limb joint disorder management. Understanding the anatomy and pathology of these joints is crucial in advancing therapeutic methods in lower limb treatment.

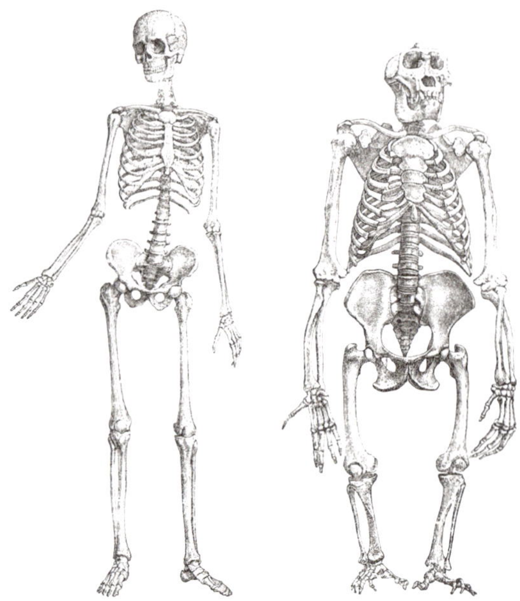

Source: By Unknown author - Brehms Tierleben, Small Edition 1927, Public Domain, https://commons.wikimedia.org/w/index.php?curid=32184

3.1.4. Muscles Associated with the Lower Limb

The complex coordination of the muscles surrounding the lower limb plays a central role in locomotion and joint stability, in particular the hip and the knee joints. The deep muscles like the iliopsoas, which includes the iliacus, psoas major, and psoas minor, are primary hip flexors significant in activities ranging from normal walking to sports, and their compromise can significantly impact mobility (Lifshitz et al., 2020). In addition to static anatomy, dynamic forces arising from muscle activity play a large part in joint loading; for instance, co-contraction of the gastrocnemii and quadriceps muscles has been demonstrated to substantially increase tibio-femoral contact forces to nearly two bodyweights during stair negotiation, also adding to wear in osteoarthritic or prosthetic joints (Trepczynski et al., 2018). Hence, awareness of the anatomy and biomechanical functions of lower limb muscles is not only essential for pathology diagnosis but also for the development of rehabilitative interventions that optimize muscle function to protect joint integrity and enhance patient mobility (Trepczynski et al., 2018; Lifshitz et al., 2020).

3.1.5. Nerves Supplying the Lower Limb

Effective motor control and sensory perception of the lower limb rely on an elaborate network of peripheral nerves that arise primarily from the lumbar and sacral plexuses. The plexuses give rise to main nerves such as the femoral, obturator, sciatic, tibial, and common peroneal nerves that supply certain groups of muscles and regions of skin. The evolution of ultrasound-guided regional anesthesia has enhanced clinical understanding of these neural channels, allowing for accurate nerve blocks for enhanced surgical outcome and pain control with minimal complications. These developments emphasize the need for careful anatomical knowledge while managing lower limb disorders using medical as well as imaging modalities. Besides, the coordination of neural supply and vascular tissues is vital for limb function, predicting the need for thorough diagnostic methods in case of neurovascular pathology (Tran et al., 2019; Yadav et al., 2019). This holistic knowledge enables targeted interventions, proving the significance of nerves for the functional integrity of the lower limb.

3.1.6. Blood Supply to the Lower Limb

The complex vascular network supplying the lower limb is a reflection of the intricacy and functionality required for ambulation and weight-bearing. Originating primarily from the femoral artery, blood supply meanders through different branches such as the profunda femoris and popliteal arteries to supply sufficient perfusion to skin, bones, and muscles.

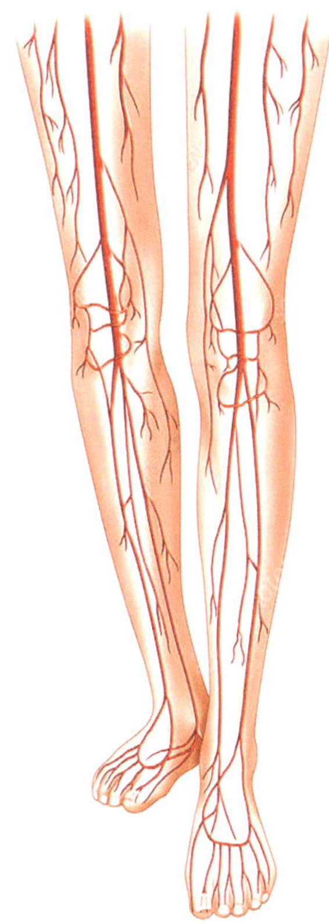

Source: Science Photo Library. (n.d.). *Arteries of the Legs*.

Collateral circulation guarantees adequate supply of blood in the case of limb movement or if the main vessels undergo blockage. It is important to have an in-depth understanding of this vascular anatomy for surgery and circulatory pathology diagnosis. Modern anatomical education, complemented by multimodal learning strategies like the dissection of a cadaver, helps further develop this understanding so that medical students have an improved comprehension of the spatial and functional relationship in the lower limb (Albanese et al., 2018). In addition, integrating such detailed anatomical ontologies like the Foundational Model of Anatomy (FMA) enables not only the clinical application but also the enablement of computational analysis of vascular anatomy, thus improving both education and research regarding lower limb vasculature (Rosse & Mejino, 2008).

3.1.7. Fascia and Connective Tissues in the Lower Limb

The complex network of fascial and connective tissue of the lower limb both stabilizes structure and facilitates function and has a critical role in force transmission and joint stabilization. They not only surround muscle and bone but also contribute to proprioception and load transfer during movement. Technological advances, such as ultrasound and computational modeling, have in recent times enabled a better understanding of their mechanical properties *in vivo* so that a more accurate measurement of elasticity and tissue strain is possible that approximates near-natural physiological conditions (Patel et al., 2014). Alterations in these connective structures can have important effects on function in the lower limbs and are involved in pain or reduced flexibility conditions. Therapeutic interventions for the treatment of fascia, such as unique self-care, were found to be capable of reviving tissue thickness, improving viscoelastic functions, and easing pain, reinforcing the functional aspect of connective tissue health towards maintaining lower limb biomechanics and general mobility (Sanjana et al., 2016).

3.1.8. Variations in Lower Limb Anatomy

Anatomical variation in the lower limb is of great clinical relevance, often dictating surgical approaches and results.

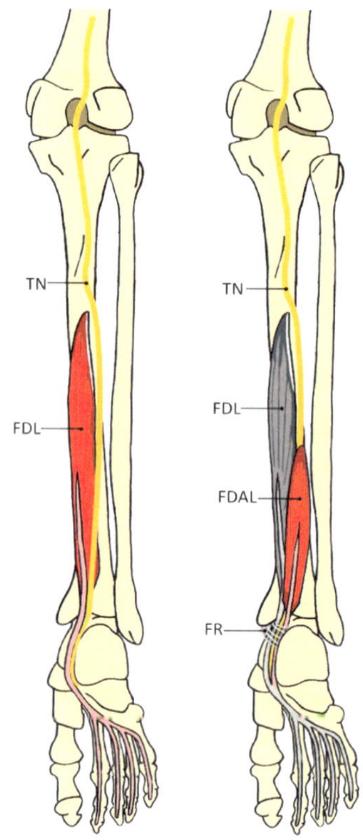

Source: Valenzuela-Fuenzalida JJ, Inostroza-Wegner A, Osorio-Muñoz F, Milos-Brandenberg D, Santana-Machuca A, Nova Baeza P, Donoso MO, Bruna-Mejias A, Iwanaga J, Sanchis-Gimeno J, et al. The Association between Anatomical Variants of Musculoskeletal Structures and Nerve Compressions of the Lower Limb: A Systematic Review and Meta-Analysis. Diagnostics. 2024; 14(7):695. https://doi.org/10.3390/diagnostics14070695

The great saphenous vein (GSV), for example, exhibits variable branching and diameter variability that is linked to the complexity of its tributaries, with a marked influence on the development and management of chronic venous disease. Increased GSV diameter is also accompanied by more complex anatomical arrangements, emphasizing the need for precise preoperative assessment in venous reflux surgery (Munteanu et al., 2024). Similarly, arterial vessels such as the femoral artery also show considerable variation in their origin and branching. While the femoral artery typically arises from the middle inguinal region, variations including branches of the superficial epigastric and external pudendal arteries have been documented, with implications for both surgical technique and image interpretation. Understanding such variations not only assists in reducing intraoperative complications but also in enhancing the success of reconstructive and interventional procedures of the lower extremities (Sagari et al., 2021).

3.1.9. Developmental Aspects of the Lower Limb

Formation of the lower limb is a complex process of coordinated genetic, cellular, and molecular processes that guide its morphogenesis from the early embryonic stage. Limb buds develop as outgrowths of the lateral plate mesoderm, and proximal-distal, cranial-caudal, and dorsal-ventral patterning necessary for normal limb development are regulated by complex signaling pathways. Disruption in these pathways results in congenital deformities of the limb that change its structure and function. Recent advances in genetic research have expanded our understanding of these developmental processes, clarifying the role of specific genes and signaling molecules responsible for tissue growth and differentiation. The application of newer genomic techniques has improved the diagnosis of developmental disorders of lower limb malformations, enabling more precise diagnostic and therapeutic approaches. Although tremendous strides have been made, ongoing research with animal models and stem cell technologies continues to delineate developmental pathways that can inform future clinical interventions and improve patient outcomes (Peter et al., 2016; Pierpont et al., 2018).

Test Your Knowledge

1. What is a common vascular variation found in the lower limb?
2. How does the rotation of the lower limb during development affect adult anatomy?

3.2. Bone Structure of the Lower Limb

Learning Outcome

1. Give an overview of lower limb bones
2. Explain the anatomy of the femur
3. Describe the structure of the patella
4. Understand anatomy of the tibia
5. Know anatomy of the fibula
6. Define structure of the tarsal bones
7. Know anatomy of the metatarsals
8. Describe the structure of the phalanges
9. Explain the role of bones in lower limb function

Its complex bone structure is required for stability and flexibility and is facilitated by its structural characteristics. Composed primarily of the femur, tibia, fibula, and several tarsal, metatarsal, and phalangeal bones, each part plays a significant role in supporting body weight and facilitating movement. The femur, being both the longest and strongest, is designed to withstand major forces with walking and running. Furthermore, the tibia and fibula also confer a dynamic structure that facilitates proper motion and weight bearing, essential for agility and balance. The articulatory connections between these bones, especially within the knee and ankle areas, provide evidence of the significance of bony structure in safeguarding sensitive structures like ligaments and tendons that work together to ensure optimal performance in everyday activity and athletics (Appolinaire et al., 2021). Such morphological harmonization between bone structures is evidence of an evolutionary adaptation to biped locomotion, witness to the functionally conditioned significance of anatomical form (Figure 3.4).

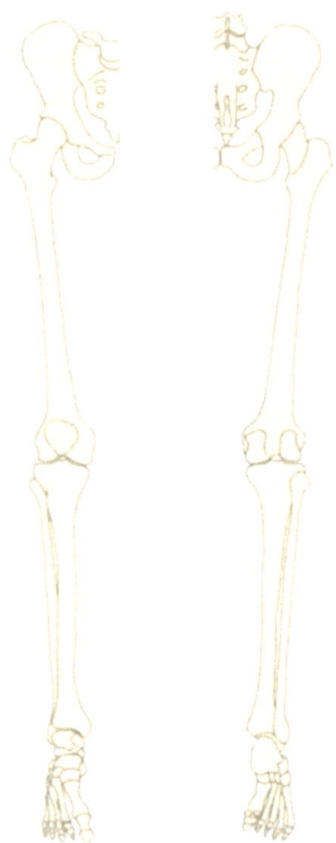

Figure 3.4. The architecture of the lower limb bones.

Source: MAIOS. (n.d.). *Bones of the Lower Limb – Anterior View.*

3.2.1. Overview of Lower Limb Bones

The lower limb holds several major bones which work together to offer mobility and support structure. Being its base, the femur is the strongest and longest bone joining the hip and the knee and bears significant weight during running and walking. The knee is formed by the femur, the tibia, and the patella, of which the tibia is the primary weight-bearing lower leg bone. The fibula, not a primary weight-bearing but contributing to ankle fixation and points of muscle attachment, is also involved. Anatomical complexity of the lower limbs further involves the formation of tarsal bones in the foot, upon which there is complex movement as well as mobility to allow for varied terrains. Understanding this skeletal structure is central to uses such as biomechanics and rehabilitation, where maximizing mobility and treating lower limb function-related pathologies take precedence, as shown in studies of MSK modeling (Magnenat-Thalmann et al., 2010) and analysis of motor control systems (Ferrand, 2000).

3.2.2. Anatomy of the Femur

The femur, which is the longest, largest and strongest of the bones in the human body, plays a major role in mobility, as it supports bearing weights. The bone is anatomically divided into many important regions, such as the head, neck, greater and lesser trochanters, and the shaft, which all contribute to the formation of the bone's function. Specifically, the femoral neck angle of about 125 degrees influences hip joint mechanics to offer a functional range of motion essential for walking and running functions. The relationship between the femur and structures like muscles and ligaments is of prime significance in maintaining stability and function. Surgical interventions of femoral fractures, particularly predisposed to complications or non-union, validate the importance of familiarity with femoral anatomy in clinical practice, as evidenced by research demonstrating the benefits of dual implantation techniques (Chanda et al., 2022). Furthermore, the advent of customized endoprosthetic options, including the Kyocera Modular Limb Salvage System, highlights the dynamic development of femoral reconstruction according to anatomical considerations (Rubio et al., 2020).

3.2.3. Structure of the Patella

At the intersection of biomechanics and evolution through adaptation is the patella anatomy, an essential component of the knee joint. Utilized to enhance the leverage of the extensor muscles to make the economy of knee extension in walking more efficient, this sesamoid bone is an essential adaptation for the species.

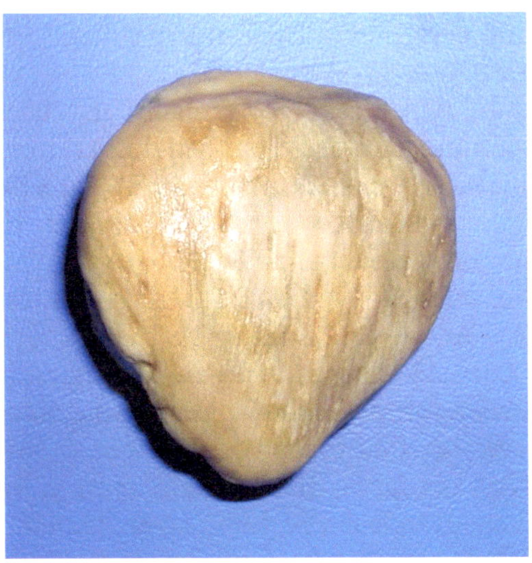

Source: Public Domain, https://commons.wikimedia.org/w/index.php?curid=65520

The unique anatomical characteristics of the patella, which may differ between species, are an evolutionary trend toward optimal function. For instance, while the adult ostrich contains two patellae, which is a characteristic unique to ratites, its functional component is a fascinating comparison to lizards, in which the occurrence of patella is not as consistent. Up-to-date studies have revealed that various species of lizards possess mineralized patellae, and this proves there is a degree of polymorphism in this structure (Benjamin et al., 2016). Such differences highlight the adaptive utility of the patella in taxa, testifying to the functional anatomy of the lower limb. Enjoying such variations has further insight into the mechanical constraints placed upon the knee joint and illuminates the evolutionary pathways that shape anatomical form.

3.2.4. Anatomy of the Tibia

The tibia, also known as the shinbone, is an important part of the structural and functional component of the lower limb. It is the larger and stronger of the two bones in the lower leg and supports the weight of most of the body when in motion. The tibia anatomy is segmented into several areas: the tibial plateau, shaft, and the medial malleolus. The tibial plateau, which is at the proximal end, is the primary weight-carrying surface, uniting the femur at the knee joint to provide a wide range of motion that enables walking and running. The importance of the tibia is its function in case of injuries such as tibial plateau fractures, where mobility and quality of life (QoL) can be severely affected in middle-aged and old people (Dushyant et al., 2020). A precise understanding of the anatomy of the tibia opens doors to better therapeutic interventions, like rehabilitation, where the results can be significantly enhanced and recovery enhanced in lower limb disability patients.

3.2.5. Anatomy of the Fibula

Located alongside the tibia, the fibula is a slender bone that significantly contributes to stabilizing the ankle and lower leg. Its anatomy comprises the head, shaft, and lateral malleolus, which play a crucial role in maintaining the integrity of the ankle joint. The incisura fibularis, on the tibia, is an essential region of articulation for the fibula, which helps stabilize the tibiofibular syndesmosis. Interestingly, the variation in the fibula's shape, specifically the depth and the incisura fibularis's angle, has been linked to susceptibility to ankle injury, as discussed in elaborate studies (Ruben et al., 2023). The recognition of such variations in the fibula's anatomy is paramount for medical practitioners, particularly during the diagnosis and treatment of lower limb injury. This information assists in creating rehabilitation programs with specific regard for osseous and ligamentous factors that influence ankle stability as well as overall lower limb function.

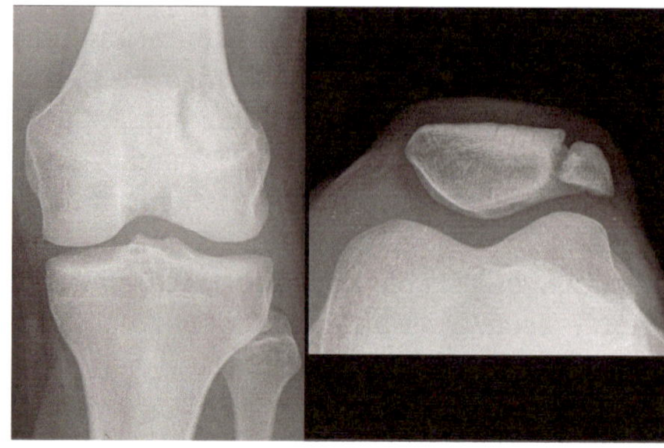

Source: By Hellerhoff - Own work, CC BY-SA 3.0, https://commons.wikimedia.org/w/index.php?curid=9462329

3.2.6. Structure of the Tarsal Bones

The tarsal bones play a key role in providing shape and stability to the foot and thus significantly influencing its overall mobility and function. The tarsals, which are composed of seven distinct bones, i.e., the talus, calcaneus, cuboid, navicularand the cuneiforms (medial, intermediate and lateral cuneiforms), form a compound structure that supports weight-bearing and motion.

The design structure allows for a wide range of motions, which is so critical in daily activities such as walking, running, and jumping. Furthermore, the sophisticated geometry of these bones is accompanied by variations in mechanical and density properties, as revealed by studies on bone composition. For instance, the analysis of morphological and mechanical properties of bird species reveals how variations in tarsal bone morphology influence locomotion and biomechanical response to stress (Marcin et al., 2021). Understanding the anatomical nuances of the tarsal bones plays a vital role in the determination of injury mechanisms and optimizing athletic performance, hence making them significant in the lower limb functional anatomy.

3.2.7. Anatomy of the Metatarsals

The metatarsals are of crucial significance to the function of the foot. They serve as anchors for the toes, support the arch, and permit movement. They are five long bones, constructed to withstand a great deal of mechanical stress, particularly in running and jumping. Interestingly, metatarsal stress fractures account for a significant percentage of sports injuries, which highlights their vulnerability under situations of overloading, as evidenced in many research studies (Francesca, 2024). An understanding of the trabecular and cortical structure of the metatarsals is essential for assessing their biomechanical features, as this discrimination could have a bearing on force distribution upon weight-bearing exercises. Besides, advancements in modeling techniques, such as Finite Element Analysis, have made it possible for researchers to simulate stress patterns in these bones and therefore gain insights on avoiding injury and developing treatment interventions, which is particularly relevant for individuals with mobility impairments.

3.2.8. Structure of the Phalanges

The phalanges are the constitutive parts of the skeletal structure of lower limbs, particularly during movement and balance. Comprising 14 bones, the phalanges in each foot are classified into three types: proximal, middle, and distal except the hallux which has only proximal and distal. Each of the types is unique from the others structurally, supporting various functions like walking, running, and gripping while climbing or descending. The complex system of tendons and muscles that connect these bones enables fine motor and stability in locomotion, testifying to their survival advantage in the context of functional pressures placed on the feet (Diogo et al., 2017). Moreover, observation of phalangeal architecture reveals that morphological differences in length and width in bones play significant roles within their biomechanical function across varying primate orders, inferring phalange structure isn't structurally significant, but also functionally significant for entire limb function (Rosse et al., 2000). Hence, knowledge regarding the structure of the phalanges increases our awareness regarding lower limb form and function.

3.2.9. Role of Bones in Lower Limb Function

The lower limb bones have significant roles to play in the supply of structure, support, and mobility required for a variety of functional movements such as walking, running, and jumping. In copying the dynamics of biological systems, the lower limb femur, tibia, and fibula bones create a structure that not only is competent enough to support weight but also optimal as far as movement patterns are concerned. This position is also accentuated by how the skeletal structure interlocks with surrounding ligaments and muscles, allowing for well-coordinated action that is pivotal in locomotion. As stated, the lower limb anatomy facilitates accurate control and flexibility in movement, a factor that is particularly important during sports or when walking over rough terrain (Appolinaire et al., 2021). In addition, how bone strength and mobility interact underlines the importance of skeletal strength and, therefore the bones function in locomotion and overall lower limb fuction (Guillermo et al., 2020).

Test Your Knowledge

1. What is the functional significance of the first metatarsal bone?
2. Why are the bones of the lower limb adapted for stability and locomotion?

3.3. Muscular System of the Lower Limb

Learning Outcome

1. Describe the major muscle groups in the lower limb
2. Focus on anatomy of the quadriceps
3. Explain the anatomy of the hamstrings
4. Understand anatomy of the calf muscles
5. Explain the role of gluteal muscles
6. Know intrinsic muscles of the foot
7. Explain the muscle actions during locomotion
8. Evaluate muscle innervation and blood supply
9. Identify importance of muscle strength and flexibility

The lower limb muscular system plays a vital role in facilitating movement, stability, and weight-bearing functions required for optimal function. The system may be segregated into several major groups of muscles with specific functions like locomotion, balance, and posture. Some of the primary muscles involving the quadriceps, hamstrings, and calf muscles synergistically work to facilitate activities like walking, running, and jumping. Furthermore, the relationship of these muscles to the skeleton supports the effective passage of forces for locomotion. For instance, the hamstrings facilitate the strength required in hip extension and knee flexion crucial in bending and straightening movement of the leg. Further study reveals that extensive knowledge of this musculature is essential for occupational therapy professionals, as it has widespread implications in joint movement and functional mobility examinations (Ottero et al., 2017). Through a thorough examination of these groups of muscles, it can be appreciated how the interface between the function and anatomy of the lower limb comes together (Ottero et al., 2017) (Figure 3.5).

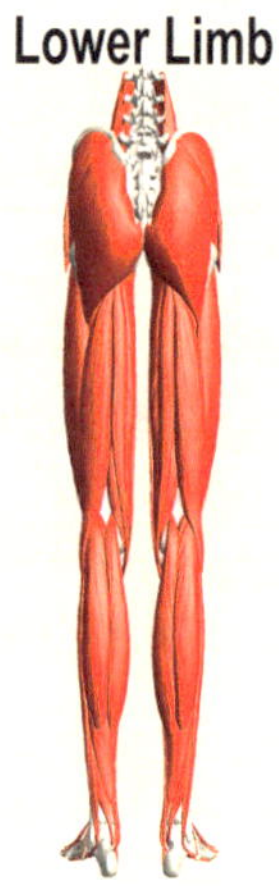

Figure 3.5. The muscular system of lower limb.

Source: Muscle Atlas. (n.d.). *Lower Limb Muscles – Posterior View.*

3.3.1. Major Muscle Groups in the Lower Limb

The structure of the lower limbs has some significant groups of muscles that are involved in a range of movements required for locomotion and stability. Quadriceps in the front are crucial in straightening the knee and are vital in running and jumping. Conversely, the hamstrings along the back are crucial in the bending of the knee and straightening of the hip, providing balance and power in walking and other dynamic movements. Also, calf muscles such as gastrocnemius and soleus are important in propelling the body ahead during walking and running and also assist in balance and support during standing. Hip flexors such as iliopsoas facilitate hip flexion, required during activities like climbing stairs or cycling. Hence, coordination among such groups of muscles is necessary for the functional anatomy of the lower limb in a manner that promotes effective movement as well as round-the-clock agility (Ottero et al., 2017).

3.3.2. Anatomy of the Quadriceps

Understanding the anatomy of the quadriceps femoris is essential to appreciate its functional role within the lower limb. The quadriceps is a powerful anterior thigh muscle that consists of four discrete heads, namely the rectus femoris, vastus lateralis, vastus medialis, and vastus intermedius. Knee extension is contributed to by all four heads, and the quadriceps is hence essential for activities such as walking, running, and jumping.

Research highlights that protocol focal vibrations, combined with muscle contractions, can be applied to effectively enhance quadriceps strength and overall athletic performance, echoing the responsiveness of muscles to training stimuli (Max et al., 2024). Furthermore, anatomical investigations of different species, such as domestic dogs and shalaykas, reveal variations in muscle attachment points and their functional importance (Shirokova et al., 2023). From these considerations, one can gain an appreciation of the quadriceps' essential role in both mechanics and the subtleties of adaptation to the different forms of locomotion.

3.3.3. Anatomy of the Hamstrings

Hamstrings play a great role in movement as well as in stabilizing the lower limb, particularly in movements such as walking, running, and jumping. The muscles located at the posterior part of the thigh are composed of three main components namely the biceps femoris, semitendinosus, and semimembranosus. They are fixed to the ischial tuberosity of the pelvis and inserted at several locations on the tibia and fibula, thus allowing them to generate flexion at the knee and extension at the hip. Remarkably, their purpose extends beyond locomotion; they assist in maintaining posture, stabilizing the body during dynamic movement, and shock absorption on landing.

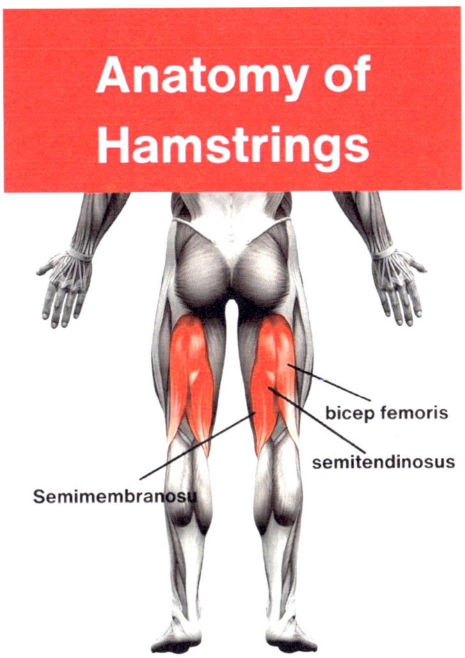

Figure 3.6. Anatomy of the hamstrings.

Source: Pinterest. (n.d.). *Anatomy of Hamstrings – Posterior View Highlighting Semimembranosus, Semitendinosus, and Biceps Femoris.*

In addition, the functional interplay of the hamstrings with other muscles, such as the quadriceps, optimizes functional movement while reducing the chances of injury. Understanding the hamstring anatomy lies at the core of rehabilitation strategies in addition to training program formulation designed to optimize lower limb function (Adam et al., 2022; César et al., 2020) (Figure 3.6).

3.3.4. Anatomy of the Calf Muscles

The calf muscles, composed primarily of the gastrocnemius and soleus, play an important role in lower limb function to allow activities such as walking, running, and jumping. The two-headed gastrocnemius is primarily located at the back of the lower leg and is the muscle that plantarflexes the foot at the ankle joint as well as contributes to knee bending. Conversely, the soleus is underneath the gastrocnemius and plays a crucial role in posture and stability when standing and moving. Coordination and strength in these muscles are important indicators of lower limb function as a whole, and deficiencies can lead to injury, including knee-related injuries like ACL injuries, where excessive frontal plane movement can place undue stress on the knee (see Shephard et al., 2013). Understanding the anatomy and mechanics of the calf muscles is vital in developing efficient rehabilitation and prevention techniques for injury, particularly among athletes predisposed to developing mobility and stability complications like foot-drop.

3.3.5. Role of Gluteal Muscles

The gluteal muscles have a function beyond cosmetic appeal, with a critical role in general lower limb mobility and stability. The gluteus maximus and Medius, specifically, are required for proper pelvic alignment and dynamic movement in physical activity. Gluteal muscle strengthening or neuromuscular control impairments may lead to biomechanical dysfunction, which has the potential to lead to injury, e.g., Achilles tendinopathy, when low hip muscle strength is correlated with increased ankle strain (Julien, 2023). Moreover, evidence indicates that gluteus maximus activity can be enhanced by spinal manipulation, indicating a neurophysiological interaction that augments the gluteal muscles' contribution to lower limb mechanics (Ottero et al., 2017). Therefore, a thorough understanding of the gluteal muscles is necessary not only for rehabilitation but also for preventing injury, underscoring their role in maintaining functional integrity throughout the kinetic chain.

3.3.6. Intrinsic Muscles of the Foot

The intrinsic muscles of the foot, that is, the small muscles in the foot, are important in ensuring stability, ease of movement, and overall foot function. Lying deep within the foot, the muscles assist in the regulation of toe movements and serve to build the integrity of the arch, which is important for balance and thrust during activities such as walking and running.

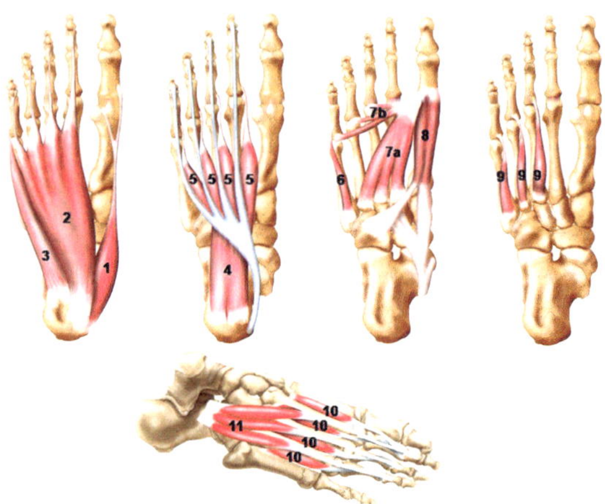

Figure 3.7. The foot's intrinsic muscles, comprising the small muscles within the foot.

Source: Fraser, J. (2016). *Intrinsic Muscles of the Foot (Plantar View, Multiple Layers).*

Interestingly, studies have shown that individuals with flatfoot deformity may exhibit variations in intrinsic muscle function compared to people with neutral foot posture, highlighting the importance of these muscles for ensuring foot well-being and preventing damage (Maarten et al., 2023). In addition, intrinsic foot muscles have been said to be strengthened through dedicated exercises and might even prevent over-pronation and lower limb injury (Maarten et al., 2023; Raf et al., 2023). It is through the understanding of their functional anatomy that we are able to grasp their role in sporting activity and rehabilitation (Figure 3.7).

3.3.7. Muscle Actions During Locomotion

Muscle operation and locomotion interaction illustrate deep adaptations that allow for the maximal economy of movement among birds, notably emus and ostriches. Although they are growing up, the birds' force-production capacity from the muscles as a fraction of the body weight gets enhanced, and this is something that allows them to persist in locomotion without regard to fast growth (Abourachid et al., 2014). The adaptation allows them to maintain efficient forms of movement against the change that comes with their anatomy. In ostriches, a biomechanical computer model shows that muscle moment arms and joint angles do not optimize these parameters with locomotion, suggesting that other factors, such as muscle and tendon dynamics, may be more crucial in locomotor efficiency (Hutchinson et al., 2015). Recognition of these complex interactions provides us with an appreciation of the machinery of muscle action in locomotion, illustrating how evolutionary pressures shape the functional anatomy of the lower limb in bird species.

3.3.8. Muscle Innervation and Blood Supply

The relationship between muscle innervation and blood supply is crucial to maintaining function of the lower limb. Nerves not only enable motor control but also sensory feedback and reflex. The peripheral nervous system (PNS), through numerous spinal nerves such as the sciatic and femoral nerves, innervates muscles to provide for the fine movements required in walking and running. Concurrently, the arterial supply, primarily through the popliteal and femoral arteries, enables the muscles to receive the oxygen and nutrients needed for metabolism and energy generation. Any disruption of this equilibrium is bound to lead to pathologies like vascular dysfunction, which has been found to be present alongside cardiovascular disease symptoms, probably impairing function and performance in the lower limb (Rachel, 2023). Hence, the synchronization of vascular supply and innervation is to be understood in the clinical assessment and rehabilitation treatment of lower limb-disabled patients.

3.3.9. Importance of Muscle Strength and Flexibility

Muscle strength and flexibility are important components of functional movement that directly impact total physical health as well as performance. Strong muscles provide joint stability, reduce the possibility of injury, and enhance athletic performance, which is especially important in activities that vary from daily chores to competitive sports. Flexibility, however, allows for a greater range of motion, which aids in proper posture and reduces the risk of strain and sprain. These properties alone not only allow for fluid motion but also play a critical role in rehabilitating injuries. For instance, advancements in functional electrical stimulation illustrate the importance of muscle strength in rehabilitation because the technologies aim at re-establishing movement and function after paralysis (César et al., 2020). At the same time, the role of flexible interfaces in rehabilitation demonstrates how enhanced muscle performance and flexibility can impact patients' outcomes, confirming that investment in muscle strength and flexibility is essential to maintaining mobility and QoL (Wenzheng et al., 2021).

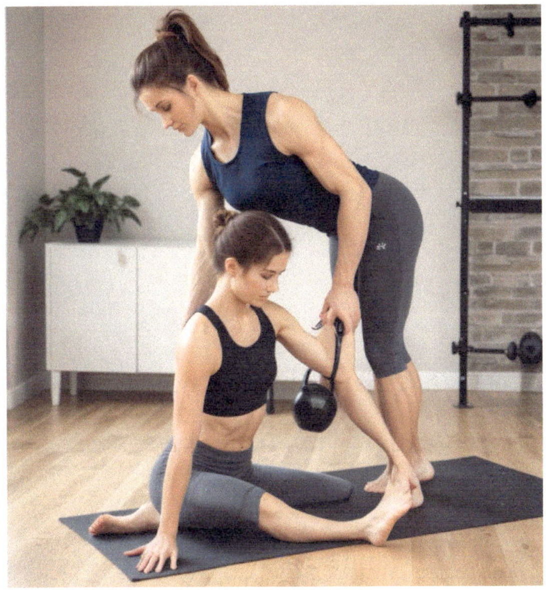

Source: Lanatomie. (n.d.). *Personal Training Session: Assisted Kettlebell Exercise.*

3.4. Joints and Ligaments of the Lower Limb

The complex joint and ligament alignment of the lower limb is especially crucial in facilitating movement, stability, and weight transfer. The knee joint itself is a great representation of this intricacy and has multiple ligaments that support it, but in addition, facilitates dynamic movements like running and walking. As a case in point, the two-bundle anterior cruciate ligament (ACL) is central to stabilizing the knee during running and walking. Specifically, studies indicate that customized anatomical characteristics exert significant effects on *in vivo* ligament forces, subject-specific models being superior to scaled-generic models as predictors of ACL forces during exercise, and individualized analysis is prioritized in the understanding of joint mechanics (Ottero et al., 2017). Additionally, advances in prosthetic technology and bio-inspired joint systems point toward continued efforts to replicate the intrinsic functions of such biological structures for enhancing rehabilitation technologies and functional mobility in individuals with lower limb deficiency (Appolinaire et al., 2021) (Figure 3.8).

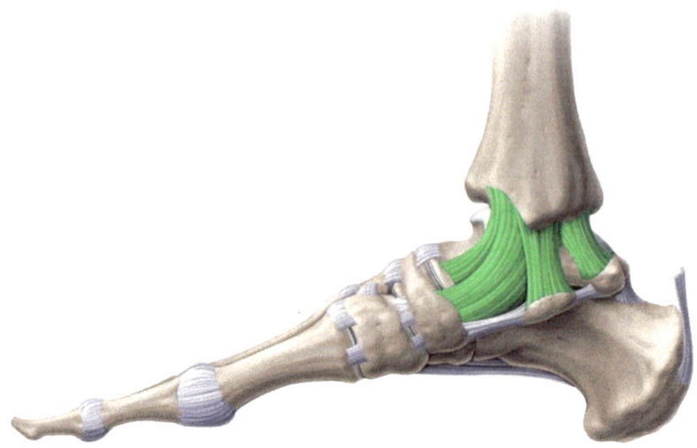

Figure 3.8. Joints and ligaments of the lower limb.

Source: Kenhub. (n.d.). *Deltoid Ligament of the Ankle (Medial View).*

Test Your Knowledge

1. Which artery commonly supplies blood to the quadriceps muscle group?
2. How can regular exercise improve both muscle strength and flexibility?
3. Discuss the joints and ligaments of the lower limb

3.5. Overview of Lower Limb Joints

Learning Outcome

1. Discuss the anatomy of the hip joint
2. Focus on anatomy of the knee joint
3. Explain the anatomy of the ankle joint
4. Discuss the role of ligaments in joint stability
5. Define the common injuries to lower limb joints
6. Focus on joint movements and their significance
7. Understand relationship between joints and muscle function
8. Explain the rehabilitation of joint injuries
9. Learn about neurovascular supply of the lower limb

The lower limb is made up of a complex series of joints that bear weight and facilitate movement. The principal joints, for the most part, are the hip, the knee, and the ankle, and each of these has a unique function in mobility and balance. The hip joint is a ball-and-socket joint that allows for a wide range of motion required for activities like walking and running. Conversely, the knee joint is a hinge joint, which is most famous for playing a crucial role in flexion and extension, in addition to permitting rotational movements to some extent. Lastly, the ankle joint, which is made up of the tibia, fibula, and talus, promotes stability and flexibility, enabling various forms of locomotion. Knowing the complicated anatomy and function is vital due to the fact that issues such as joint injuries may result in serious impairment of mobility. Also, inflammation or edema of surrounding structures like the pericruciate fat pad (PCFP) may complicate the functioning of the knee, as seen in studies on its anatomy and vascularization (Michał et al., 2023). Moreover, anatomical studies highlight vasculature and joint health relations with a focus on structures like the middle genicular artery in operations (Oliinyk et al., 2021).

3.5.1. Anatomy of the Hip Joint

The hip joint is a key part of the functional anatomy of the lower limb, permitting a wide range of movements as well as being strong enough to bear body weight. Structurally, it is a ball-and-socket joint formed by the acetabulum of the pelvis and the head of the femur articulating together. This type of construction enables one to flex, extend, abduct, adduct, and internally and externally rotate, which are necessary for walking and balance. The surrounding musculature, such as the large muscle groups of gluteals and iliopsoas, contributes significantly to the stability and efficiency of movement of the joint, illustrating the interdependence of the muscular and skeletal apparatus. Furthermore, as observed in emus, muscle mass and physiological cross-sectional area show positive allometry with growth, suggesting an increase in force-generating capacity relative to body weight (Abourachid et al., 2014). Thus, the anatomical configuration of the hip joint is essential to both mobility and stability, underscoring its importance in the overall functional dynamics of the lower extremity.

3.5.2. Anatomy of the Knee Joint

The structure of the knee joint is complex, with multiple different parts that work in concert to provide movement and support the weight of the body. The primary structure of the knee is two types of cartilage: articular cartilage, which lines the ends of the femur and the summit of the tibia, and menisci, semicircular cartilage pads that absorb shock and add stability. Ligaments are vital in maintaining the integrity of the knee, with the ACL and posterior cruciate ligament (PCL) controlling forward and backward movement, respectively. The collateral ligaments also provide side-to-side stability, and the joint capsule encloses the entire structure, producing synovial fluid to minimize friction in the joint. Successful functioning of these structures is required for activities ranging from walking to jumping, and familiarity with their anatomy is instrumental in diagnosing and treating knee injuries (Gordon et al., 2013) (Figure 3.9).

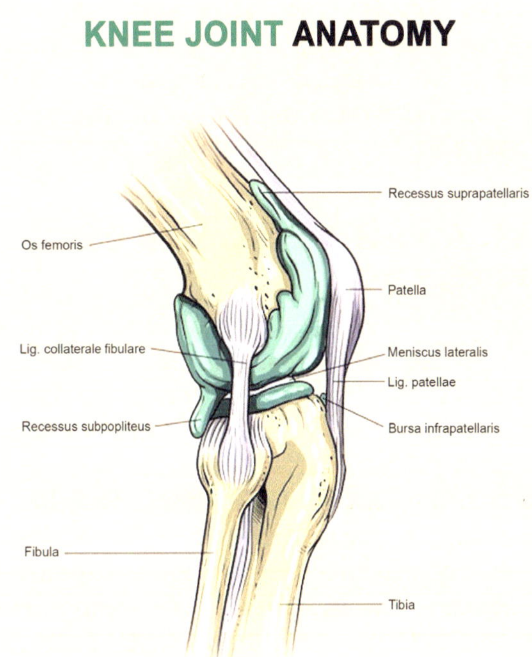

Figure 3.9. Anatomy of the knee joint.

Source: Freepik. (n.d.). *Illustration of Knee joint Anatomy Diagram*.

3.5.3. Anatomy of the Ankle Joint

The ankle joint, a multi-articular complex that enables mobility and stability, consists primarily of the tibia, fibula, and talus bones. It is a hinge joint that enables dorsiflexion and plantarflexion, essential for walking, running, and jumping. It is stabilized by various ligaments that provide stability to its anatomical framework, including the lateral ligaments and medial deltoid ligament. The complicated ligamentous system limits hypermobility, which protects the joint from overuse injuries that are so inextricably associated with physical exercise and sport. Furthermore, the interaction among the ankle joint and the muscles and tendons nearby dictates successful function in locomotion. That is, in modeling with simulation software like OpenSim, knowledge of biomechanics within the ankle helps replicate the adaptive kinematics through different activities and conditions (Ottero et al., 2017). As a result, anatomical integrity at the ankle joint is vital to both the function of the ankle and lower limb mechanics as a whole.

3.5.4. Role of Ligaments in Joint Stability

Ligaments are an intrinsic component of the MSK system responsible for a significant amount of joint stability. Ligaments are fibrous connective tissues that bind bones to other bones at joints, providing structural support and limiting excessive movement. Stability is important in preventing injury; for example, the ACL of the knee plays a significant role in maintaining the integrity of the joint during dynamic activities, such as sports (Siddhi et al., 2024). When compromised, say in sprains, the joint is rendered unstable and alters the pattern of movement as well as increased vulnerability to re-injury. Also, proper diagnosis and understanding of the function of ligaments are crucial to effective therapy, as the assessment of knee injury (Roșu et al., 2022) exemplifies. Hence, the functional state of ligaments has a direct effect on functional activity and the overall health state of lower limb joints.

3.5.5. Common Injuries to Lower Limb Joints

Lower limb joints are particularly prone to a range of injuries due to the critical functions they undertake in locomotion and weight-bearing. Ligament sprain, particularly in the knee and ankle, where changes of direction or force are excessive, resulting in impaired joint stability, is a frequent injury.

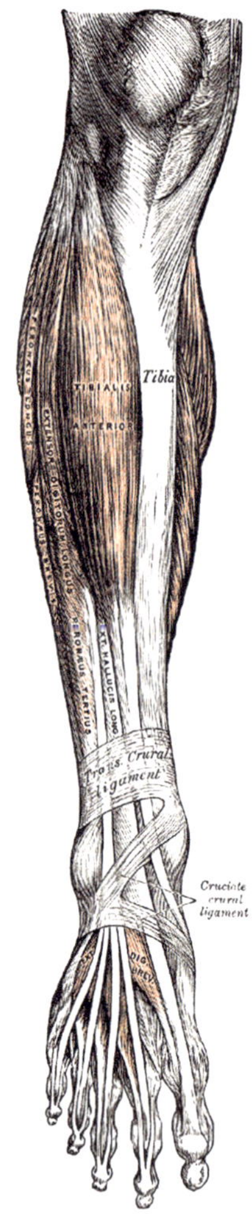

Source: By Henry Vandyke Carter - Henry Gray (1918) Anatomy of the Human Body (See "Book" section below)Bartleby.com: Gray's Anatomy, Plate 437, Public Domain, https://commons.wikimedia.org/w/index.php?curid=527206

Tendonitis, however, is extremely prevalent among athletes, due to overuse and repetitive strain, involving the knee, ankle, and hip joints. Degenerative joint disease in the form of osteoarthritis is also significant, typically caused by the additive wear and tear that joints sustain over a lifetime. Developments in prosthetics over recent years, such as those described in Aszmann et al. (2016), have been placing increasing emphasis on restoring the joint to a state of normal function, and thus further underlining the need to understand these common injuries. Advanced designs for prosthetic limbs aim to reverse the disability caused by lower limb joint injuries, which underscores the broader consequences of joint health for mobility and QoL.

3.4.6. Joint Movements and their Significance

Articular movement is focal to the functional capability and function of the lower limb and constitutes the dynamic connection between muscular function and skeletal structure. The complexity of these motions, including flexion, extension, abduction, and adduction, allows the broad range of walking, running, and jumping that requires sensitive coordination between a wide variety of joint mechanisms and groups of muscle. An exhaustive anatomical description explains that the architecture of mouse hindlimb muscles exhibits drastic adaptations to support joint control, particularly in hip extensors and adductors, which explains that these adaptations are significant for the achievement of stability and economy of locomotion (Cappellari et al., 2016). Moreover, morphological integration analysis reveals contrasting patterns in the chimpanzee forelimb and hindlimb to humans, highlighting how diverse evolutionary pressures have evolved joint movements to meet different functional demands (Esteve-Altava et al., 2018). This is required for developing interventions in sports medicine and rehabilitation.

3.4.7. Relationship Between Joints and Muscle Function

Joints play an important role in determining muscle function in terms of the range of motion and mechanical advantage at which the muscles operate. For instance, joint positions directly influence moment arms, which play a significant role in optimizing the application of muscle force when walking. In studies of avian locomotion, it was found that ostriches fail to align limb orientations to maximize moment-generating abilities or muscle moment arms, and thus it is possible that dynamic muscle properties may be a leading cause of locomotor efficiency (Hutchinson et al., 2015). Similarly, the morphological transformations of sauropodomorph dinosaurs suggest that a shift from sprawling to erect limb posture deeply alters patterns of muscle action, which increase leverage during locomotion (Otero et al., 2017). Thus, the interdependence of joint mechanics and the functioning of muscles, far from showing the importance of structural anatomy, suggests evolutionary changes that allow effective movement modes in various species.

3.5.8. Rehabilitation of Joint Injuries

Effective rehabilitation of joint injuries is crucial for the restoration of function and preservation of mobility after trauma. Rehabilitation typically involves a combination of physical therapy, strengthening, and in some cases, surgery, particularly in the event of severe injury. For instance, the use of a vascularized fibular graft, as mentioned in Vinay et al. (2018), is a valuable surgical alternative when dealing with extensive bony defects following tumor resections in the lower limb. This method can allow early ambulation and reduce morbidity, making rehabilitation easier. Additionally, advances in simulation platforms, such as those provided by OpenSim, make possible precise modeling of joint mechanics and muscle dynamics.

Rehabilitation practitioners can now use these sophisticated tools to provide deeper insights into the person's biomechanical profiles and modify intervention approaches accordingly. In general, an organized rehabilitation program, combining novel surgical methods with computational modeling, greatly improves the outcomes of recovery and functional mobility in patients suffering from joint injury.

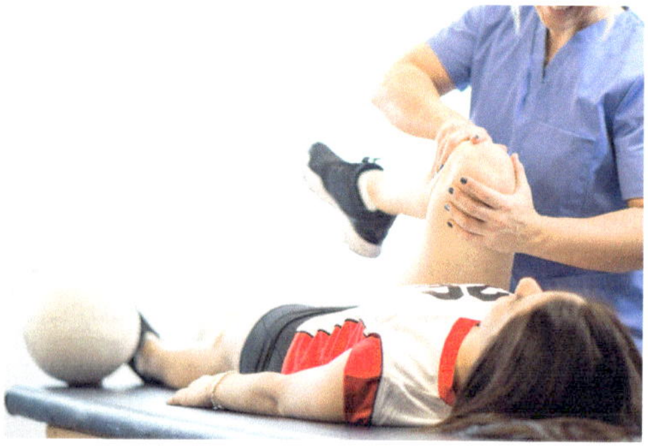

Source: Orange County Physical Therapy Clinic. (2021). *Female Volleyball Player Receiving Rehabilitation for Sports Injury.*

3.5.9. Neurovascular Supply of the Lower Limb

The neurovascular supply of the lower limb is significant in motor activity and sensory perception, basically governing the limb's function altogether. The complex network begins with the lumbar and sacral plexuses, extending into major nerves such as the femoral, sciatic, and tibial nerves, supplying innervation to muscles and sensation to various regions of the limb. There is this neural supply that comes with copious vascular supply; the femoral artery provides the popliteal artery, which divides into anterior and posterior tibial arteries to supply suffused blood required for metabolic needs and wound healing. As emphasized in the ongoing work to enhance regional anesthesia education, familiarity with this vascular and neural anatomy is key to optimizing interventions aimed at pain relief and surgical results (De Tran et al., 2019). Furthermore, conditions arising within this region, such as osteosarcoma, emphasize the need for precise knowledge of the neural and vascular anatomy to prevent complications during treatment (Amirhossein et al., 2018) (Figure 3.10).

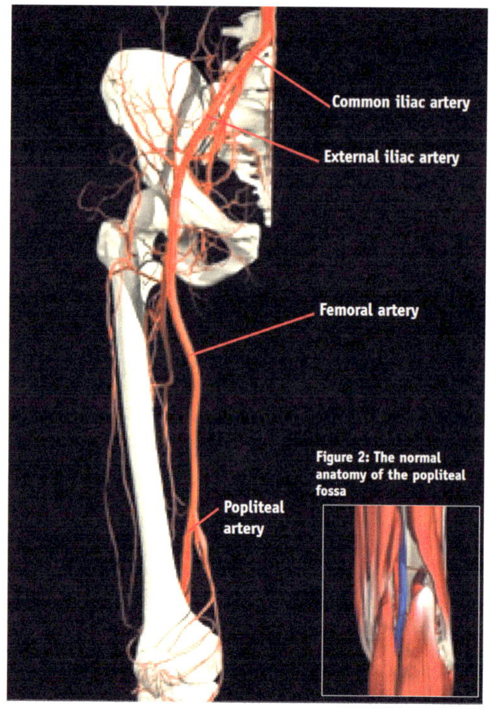

Figure 3.10. Neurovascular supply of the lower limb.

Source: Taylor, A. (n.d.). *Arteries of the Lower Limb.*

Test Your Knowledge

1. How does physiotherapy assist in restoring joint function?
2. How does the neurovascular supply affect lower limb movement and sensation?

3.6. Overview of the Nervous System in the Lower Limb

Learning Outcome

1. Discuss the major nerves of the lower limb
2. Explain the blood supply to the lower limb
3. Describe the role of the sciatic nerve
4. Understand function of the femoral artery
5. Focus on importance of venous return
6. How to impact of nerve injuries on function
7. Understand vascular diseases affecting the lower limb
8. Focus on neurovascular considerations in surgery

The lower limb nervous system is the focal point of movement, sensation, and balance, in association with the MSK anatomy of the leg. Constructed by a series of peripheral nerves, the lower limb is primarily supplied by the lumbar and sacral plexuses, which are derived from spinal nerves L2-S5. These plexuses form massive nerves, including the femoral, sciatic, and tibial nerves, which provide motor innervation to locomotory muscles and sensory input from the joints and skin. Such sensory input is required for the coordination of complex movements and postural stability. In addition, an understanding of the interplay between the nervous system and sleep and cognition is essential in the management of lower limb injury, which demonstrates that mobility impairments can affect overall neurological function and outcome (Adam et al., 2017). Thus, an understanding of the functional anatomy of the nervous system of the lower limb is essential to the diagnosis and management of related movement disorders.

3.6.1. Major Nerves of the Lower Limb

In understanding the functional anatomy of the lower limb, the major nerves play a crucial role in motor as well as sensory function. The body's largest nerve, the sciatic nerve, branches into the tibial and common peroneal nerves, which innervate the posterior compartment muscles and the anterior and lateral leg compartments, respectively. This complex network enables coordinated motion and balance on walking or running. Moreover, the femoral nerve also supplies the muscles in the front thigh to facilitate activities such as knee extension, an important movement activity in actions like stairs climbing or rising from sitting. Pathologies requiring reconstructive surgeries, such as in the case of complicated wound cases where the Achilles tendon is exposed, also point out the importance of preserving nerve integrity during rehabilitation (Chou et al., 2013). Thus, the identification of these significant nerves not only indicates their overt role in movement but also their significance in the clinical scenarios of the lower limb, which reinforces the significance of accurate anatomical information.

3.6.2. Blood Supply to the Lower Limb

The complex system of vessels that provides the lower extremities is vital in maintaining its function in place and its general health. The femoral artery mostly goes downward into the thigh, dividing into the popliteal artery behind the knee, and the popliteal artery splits into the anterior and posterior tibial arteries. They supply oxygenated blood to the muscles and tissues to support movement and survival. The anterior tibial artery supplies the anterior compartment of the leg, while the posterior tibial artery predominantly supplies the posterior compartment and the plantar surface of the foot. Interestingly, compromised blood supply can lead to severe implications, ranging from ischemia or necrosis, as seen in a case of a large wound with an exposed Achilles tendon requiring reconstruction via a free anterolateral thigh flap (Chou et al., 2013). The implications for vascular health are diverse, emphasizing the need for adequate blood supply to permit efficient locomotion and prevent potential damage (Vargesson & Hootnick, 2017) (Figure 3.11).

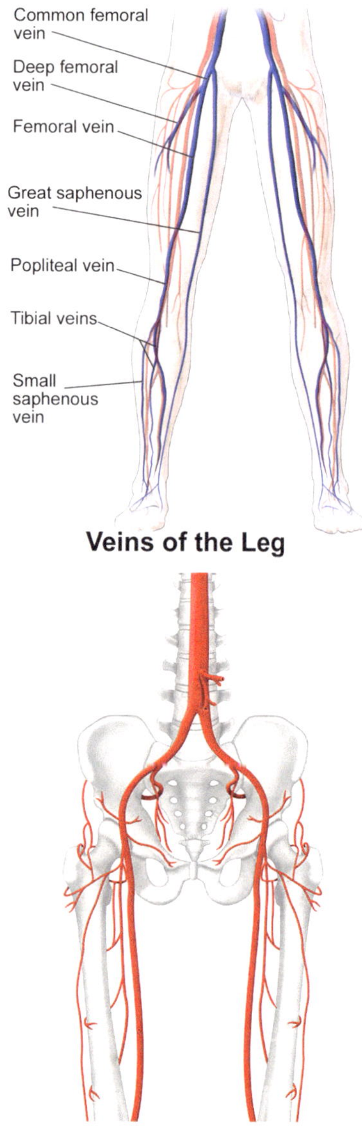

Figure 3.11. Blood supply to the lower limb.

Source: By BruceBlaus. When using this image in external sources it can be cited as:Blausen.com staff (2014). "Medical gallery of Blausen Medical 2014". WikiJournal of Medicine 1 (2). DOI:10.15347/wjm/2014.010. ISSN 2002-4436. - Own work, CC BY 3.0, https://commons.wikimedia.org/w/index.php?curid=30634279

3.6.3. Role of the Sciatic Nerve

In the context of the functional anatomy of the lower limb, the sciatic nerve is a key figure in somatic motor control and sensory perception in the posterior thigh and lower leg. It is the largest peripheral nerve of the body, originating in the lumbosacral plexus and extending down through the hip and into the thigh. It provides different muscles utilized in movements such as walking, running, and jumping, specifically targeting the hamstring group, the role of which is crucial for hip extension and knee flexion.Further, branching into the tibial and common peroneal nerves indicates its importance in providing sensation to the lower leg and to the foot and facilitating movement. It is crucial to realize the anatomical structure and physiology of sciatic nerves, particularly concerning conditions like deep vein thrombosis that may arise from its anatomical variations and impacts on venous return and movement (Ayub et al., 2024).

3.6.4. Function of the Femoral Artery

The femoral artery is a critical one to supply oxygenated blood to the lower limb and is a big vascular route of the human body. It branches off from the external iliac artery and runs along the thigh, branching out into multiple routes to nourish the muscles, skin, and tissues. By continuing as the popliteal artery at the posterior surface of the knee, the femoral artery suffices during exercise-stimulating activities such as walking and running. Potential interruption of this vascular chain may lead to severe complications, including ischemia or necrosis of tissue, particularly in damaged or infected areas, such as with severe injuries like a large posterior leg wound with Achilles tendon exposure (Chou et al., 2013). Thus, the integrity and functionality of the femoral artery are very crucial to the overall health and functionality of the lower limbs (Vargesson & Hootnick 2017).

3.6.5. Importance of Venous Return

Proper venous return is necessary to have optimal circulatory dynamics within the body, particularly in the lower limbs. The venous circulatory system is responsible for returning blood that has become deoxygenated to the heart, a process that is critical in preventing pooling and potentially serious conditions such as varicose veins, which Ayurveda categorizes as Siraj granthi and Siragat Vata (Samiksha et al., 2024). The function of venous valves serves a pivotal role in this respect in that it prevents backward flow of blood, enabling it to flow smoothly against gravity, especially during exercise. Incompetence of venous return can lead to venous reflux and associated complications like transient vestibular symptoms and exertional headaches (Takahiro, 2024). Through understanding the importance of venous return and its influence on overall vascular health, we can have a sense of appreciation for the complex design of the venous system and its critical contribution to the physiological demands placed on the lower extremities.

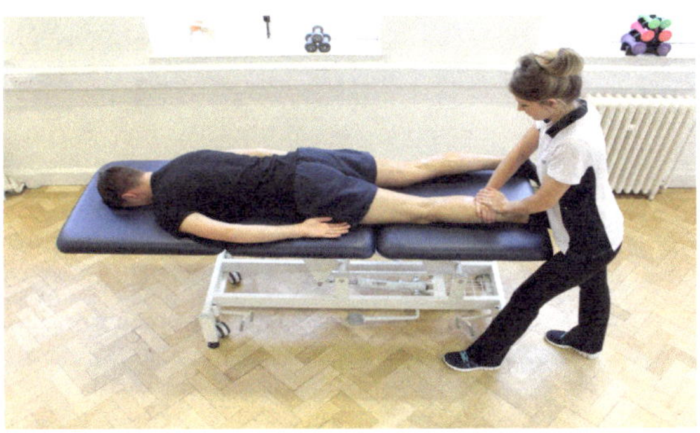

Source: Physio.co.uk. (n.d.). *Physiotherapist Performing Leg Massage to Increase Venous Return.*

3.6.6. Impact of Nerve Injuries on Function

Nerve injury can severely hinder the functional capacities of the lower limb, leading to extensive motor and sensory deficits. The synergy between nerve repair methods and recovery outcomes emphasizes the requirement for effective interventions. For instance, in sciatic nerve injury patients, the application of spinal cord electrical stimulation with standard therapy was shown to substantially improve motor nerve conduction velocity and lower extremity function (Shi et al., 2024). These findings reflect the encouraging possibility for improved rehabilitation in nerve injury cases. Furthermore, water therapy exercise has been shown to considerably improve lower limb function in stroke survivors by enhancing balance, walking ability, and coordination, which play a fundamental role in everyday functioning (Ning et al., 2023). These illustrations demonstrate the significant function that sensory and motor nervous systems have in maintaining function and QoL, affirming that effective therapeutic measures can counteract the adverse effects of nerve injury.

3.6.7. Vascular Diseases Affecting the Lower Limb

Decreased blood flow to the legs can lead to a range of vascular conditions, significantly impairing mobility and quality of life. Peripheral artery disease (PAD) is one of the most prevalent, resulting from atherosclerosis that narrows the arteries and reduces leg blood flow. Symptoms typically consist of pain in the legs during walking, or claudication, significantly limiting mobility and QoL. In addition, chronic venous insufficiency can occur when veins do not return blood to the heart, leading to swelling, varicose veins, and ulceration. These conditions indicate the relationship between vascular diseases and lower limb function. Lifestyle interventions such as diet, exercise, and smoking cessation can decrease risk factors associated with these diseases and improve patient outcomes. It is important to understand these vascular diseases to prevent complications and encourage interventions that support healthy lower limb function and overall health (Márquez-Chin & Popović, 2020) (Figure 3.12).

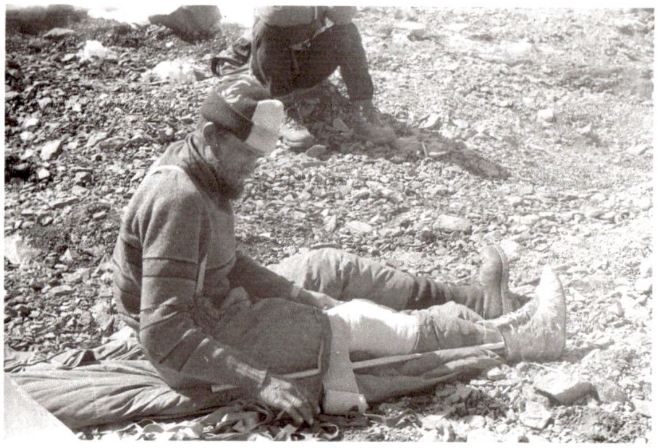

Figure 3.12. Vascular diseases affecting the lower limb.

Source: By Jaan Künnap - Jaan Künnap, CC BY-SA 4.0, https://commons.wikimedia.org/w/index.php?curid=39687909

3.6.8. Neurovascular Considerations in Surgery

Surgical procedures on the lower limb require complete awareness of neurovascular anatomy and the complications that may occur during surgery. An impeccable understanding of the delicate proximity between nerves and arteries is important for minimizing the risks of neuropathy or ischemia. For instance, precise dissection in the proximity of the femoral nerve can prevent unnoticed damage that causes sensory and motor deficits. Furthermore, investigation into regional anesthetic techniques, such as the erector spinae plane (ESP) block, can improve postoperative pain management by targeting relevant neural pathways. Investigation has indicated that the primary mechanism of the ESP block is through direct local anesthetic diffusion to neural structures within fascial planes, which can ensure quicker recovery and reduce opioid use (Márquez-Chin & Popović, 2020). Lastly, the inclusion of neurovascular data in surgical planning gives more successful operations and safer outcomes for patients undergoing lower limb surgery.

Test Your Knowledge

1. What is peripheral artery disease (PAD) and how does it affect the lower limb?
2. How does knowledge of anatomical variations assist in safer surgical procedures?

SUMMARY

The elegant structure of the lower limb, particularly its bony and ligamentous components, highlights the complexity of the process of maintaining stability and function in walking. Findings from recent anatomical studies highlight the critical role of the interrelated ligaments, including the newly named lateral Lisfranc ligament, which extends from the second to fifth metatarsal, providing crucial support to the transverse and longitudinal arch of the foot. This ligamentous framework can explain lateral stability's longevity in the face of midfoot trauma, pointing to the importance of preserving such structures in practice (Mason et al., 2019). Furthermore, clinical guidelines serve as a reminder to clinicians regarding the importance of integrating evolving anatomical understanding with evidence-based care to optimize patient outcomes, underscoring an individualized strategy that respects distinct health status and current regulatory expectations (Cosentino et al., 2019). Lastly, an overall understanding of lower limb anatomy and biomechanics is needed to make appropriate diagnosis, treatment, and rehabilitation protocols.

The discussion of the lower limb illustrates its complex anatomy, biomechanical function, and clinical relevance to mobility and stability. Central to this discussion is the critical structural components, including bones, muscles, nerves, and vascular supply, which interact synergistically to allow locomotion and balance. The understanding of the extensive interaction among these factors explains the mechanisms of common injuries and pathologies, which normally result from trauma or degenerative processes. Additionally, technological advances in diagnostic methods and treatment options highlight the significance of evidence-based clinical care, affirming the influence of individualized therapeutic interventions to achieve enhanced patient outcomes. Clinical professionals have to incorporate these findings while applying clinical judgment to treat conditions effectively, constantly adapting to changing guidelines and ethical obligations. Thus, extensive knowledge of the anatomy and physiology of the lower limb is not only crucial for prevention but also for management of lower limb diseases in the broader healthcare context (Márquez-Chin & Popović, 2020).

KEY TERMS FROM THIS CHAPTER

- Anatomical accuracy
- Assistive technology
- Axial skeleton
- Ball-and-socket joint
- Biomechanical engineering
- Biomechanics
- Clinical intervention
- Distal limb structures
- Dorsal-ventral patterning
- Exoskeleton designs
- Facilitate motion
- Gluteal muscle strengthening
- Great saphenous vein (GSV)

CRITICAL THINKING QUESTIONS

1. **Which bone is the longest and strongest in the human body?**
   a. Tibia
   b. Femur
   c. Fibula
   d. Humerus
2. **Which artery is the main blood supply to the lower limb?**
   a. Subclavian artery
   b. Radial artery
   c. Femoral artery
   d. Brachial artery
3. **Which nerve is the largest in the lower limb?**
   a. Obturator nerve
   b. Tibial nerve
   c. Femoral nerve
   d. Sciatic nerve
4. **What type of joint is the knee joint?**
   a. Hinge joint
   b. Ball and socket joint
   c. Pivot joint
   d. Saddle joint
5. **Which of the following muscles is NOT part of the quadriceps femoris group?**
   a. Rectus femoris
   b. Vastus lateralis
   c. Vastus medialis
   d. Biceps femoris

Short Answer Questions

1. Describe the anatomical location and function of the patella.
2. Which nerve supplies the anterior compartment of the thigh?
3. Explain the role of the iliotibial tract.
4. What is the significance of the femoral triangle?
5. How does the sciatic nerve divide in the lower limb?
6. What is the role of the tibia in weight-bearing?

Answers to Critical Thinking Questions

1. (b) 2. (c) 3. (d) 4. (a) 5. (d)

REFERENCES

1. Aerts, P., Ayuso, M., Prims, S., Van Cruchten, S., Van Ginneken, C., & Vanden, H. C. (2019). Does intrauterine crowding affect the force generating capacity and muscle composition of the piglet front limb? *Public Library of Science (PLoS).* https://core.ac.uk/download/287940318.pdf (accessed on 8th May 2025).
2. Otero A, Allen V, Pol D, Hutchinson JR. 2017. Forelimb muscle and joint actions in Archosauria: insights from Crocodylus johnstoni (Pseudosuchia) and Mussaurus patagonicus (Sauropodomorpha) PeerJ 5:e3976 https://doi.org/10.7717/peerj.3976 (accessed on 8th May 2025).
3. Arditi, F. (2024). *Comparative Analysis of FEM Models with Homogeneous and Structured Bone in the Foot-Ankle Complex for the Study of Stress Fractures in the First Metatarsal.* Master's thesis, University of Padua. https://thesis.unipd.it/retrieve/2504a759-6034-43c0-a8ac-e47fd5029a70/Arditi_Francesca.pdf (accessed on 8th May 2025).
4. Aszmann, O. C., Farina, D., & Vujaklija, I. (2016). *New Developments in Prosthetic Arm Systems.* Dove Medical Press Ltd. https://core.ac.uk/download/78075208.pdf (accessed on 8th May 2025).
5. Ayub, K., Lemashon, M., Nurani, K., & Wambua, B. (2024). *Beyond the Ordinary: A Case of a Unilateral Persistent Sciatic Vein.* Vol 5 No 1 (2024): https://doi.org/10.61797/ijcsav.v5i1.309(accessed on 8th May 2025).
6. Bartels, E. M., Juhl, C. B., Christensen, R., Hagen, K. B., Danneskiold-Samsøe, B., Dagfinrud, H., & Lund, H. (2016). Aquatic exercise for the treatment of knee and hip osteoarthritis. *Cochrane Database of Systematic Reviews, 2016.* https://doi.org/10.1002/14651858.cd005523.pub3.
7. Bei, N., Long, D., Bei, Z., Chen, Y., Chen, Z., & Xing, Z. (2023). Effect of water exercise therapy on lower limb function rehabilitation in hemiplegic patients with the first stroke. *Alternative Therapies in Health and Medicine, 29*(7), 429–433. http://www.alternative-therapies.com/oa/pdf/8228.pdf (accessed on 8th May 2025).
8. Cappellari, O., Charles, J. P., Hutchinson, J. R., Spence, A. J., & Wells, D. J. (2016). Musculoskeletal geometry, muscle architecture and functional specializations of the mouse hindlimb. *PLoS One 11*(4), e0147669. Public Library of Science (PLoS). https://core.ac.uk/download/45467680.pdf (accessed on 8th May 2025).
9. Chawla, A., & McGregor, A. (2015). Highlights from day three of the EuroSciCon 2015 Sports science summit. *Future Sci. OA, 1*(3), FSO14. Future Science Ltd. https://core.ac.uk/download/77021863.pdf (accessed on 8th May 2025).
10. Chin, K. J., & El-Boghdadly, K. (2021). Mechanisms of action of the erector spinae plane (ESP) block: A narrative review. *Canadian Journal of Anesthesia, 68,* 387–408. https://doi.org/10.1007/s12630-020-01875-2.
11. Hutchinson, J. R., Rankin, J. W., Rubenson, J., Rosenbluth, K. H., Siston, R. A., & Delp, S. L. (2015). Musculoskeletal modelling of an ostrich (Struthio camelus) pelvic limb: influence of limb orientation on muscular capacity during locomotion. *PeerJ, 3,* e1001. https://doi.org/10.7717/peerj.1001 (accessed on 8th May 2025).
12. Evans, F. G. (2023). *Rehabilitation Plan and Process to Treat a Patient with Chronic Lower Back Pain* Master's thesis, Masaryk University. https://is.muni.cz/th/zsyfb/Francesca_Evans_Thesis_Final_IS_System.pdf (accessed on 8th May 2025).

13. Ferrand, C. (2000). *Speech Science: An Integrated Approach to Theory and Clinical Practice.* Ear and Hearing 22(6):549. DOI:10.1097/00003446-200112000-00011(accessed on 8th May 2025).
14. Pazzaglia, M., Leemhuis, E., Giannini, A. M., & Haggard, P. (2019). The Homuncular Jigsaw: Investigations of Phantom Limb and Body Awareness Following Brachial Plexus Block or Avulsion. *Journal of clinical medicine, 8*(2), 182. https://doi.org/10.3390/jcm8020182 (accessed on 8th May 2025).
15. Heng, W., Solomon, S. A., & Gao, W. (2021). Flexible electronics and devices as human–machine interfaces for medical robotics. *Advanced Materials, 34.* https://doi.org/10.1002/adma.202107902.
16. Vargesson, N., & Hootnick, D. R. (2017). Arterial dysgenesis and limb defects: Clinical and experimental examples. *Reproductive toxicology (Elmsford, N.Y.), 70*, 21–29. https://doi.org/10.1016/j.reprotox.2016.10.005(accessed on 8th May 2025).
17. Liu, Y., Pharr, M., & Salvatore, G. A. (2017). Lab-on-skin: A review of flexible and stretchable electronics for wearable health monitoring. *ACS Nano, 11*, 9614–9635. https://doi.org/10.1021/acsnano.7b04898.
18. Márquez-Chin, C., & Popović, M. R. (2020). Functional electrical stimulation therapy for restoration of motor function after spinal cord injury and stroke: A review. *BioMedical Engineering OnLine, 19.* https://doi.org/10.1186/s12938-020-00773-4.
19. Misaghi, A., Goldin, A. N., Awad, M., & Kulidjian, A. A. (2018). Osteosarcoma: A comprehensive review. *SICOT-J, 4*, 12. https://doi.org/10.1051/sicotj/2017028.
20. Oliver, G., Kipnis, J., Randolph, G. J., & Harvey, N. L. (2020). The lymphatic vasculature in the 21st century: Novel functional roles in homeostasis and disease. *Cell, 182*, 270–296. https://doi.org/10.1016/j.cell.2020.06.039.
21. Parab, S., & Kumar, N. (2024). Effect of low-moderate plyometric exercise in post anterior cruciate ligament reconstruction: A case study. *International Journal of Physical Education, Sports and Health, 11*(2), 293–297. https://doi.org/10.22271/kheljournal.2024.v11.i2e.3298.
22. Rosse, C. (2000). *Terminologia Anatomica; Considered from the Perspective of Next-Generation Knowledge Sources.* https://core.ac.uk/download/pdf/9412243.pdf (accessed on 8th May 2025).
23. Rust, C., Whiteley, G., & Wilson, A. (1999). *First Make Something – Principled, Creative Design as a Tool for Multi-Disciplinary Research in Clinical Engineering.* https://core.ac.uk/download/100292.pdf (accessed on 8th May 2025).
24. Shcherbakov, M. S., Svetlitsky, A. O., Chernavsky, A. V., & Matvieishyna, T. M. (2024). Human anatomy: Central and peripheral part of nervous system. *Sense Organs* (p. 128). Zaporizhzhia State Medical and Pharmaceutical University. https://dspace.mphu.edu.ua/bitstream/123456789/21156/1/MSQ%20NS%2BOS.pdf (accessed on 8th May 2025).
25. Standring, S. (2015). *Gray's Anatomy: The Anatomical Basis of Clinical Practice.* https://www.semanticscholar.org/paper/2aac5fe3844cd46ee28cad2a4b307c7d436f18c1 (accessed on 8th May 2025).

THORAX REGION

4

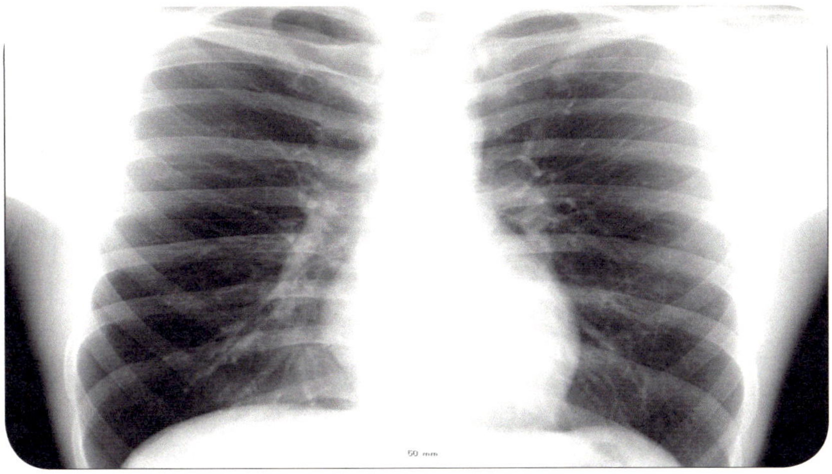

LEARNING OBJECTIVES

After studying this chapter, you will be able to:

1. Talk about thorax anatomy
2. Explain the anatomy of thoracic organs
3. Emphasize thoracic pathologies
4. Apply thorax to clinical practice

Introduction

The thorax is a basic crossroad in the anatomical and functional structure of the human organism. This region hosting vital organs such as the heart and lungs plays a primary role in both respiratory and circulatory functions. Composed of the thoracic vertebrae, ribs, and sternum, the thorax is not only an armored cage but also a flexible system that accommodates the essential movements of breathing. The anatomy of this area is key to an understanding of the highly interrelated character of various systems of the body. Moreover, studying the thorax also provides information on numerous clinical conditions that can result, demonstrating the significance of this region in both health and disease. As we examine the complex structures and functions of the thorax, we will discover its relevance in ensuring overall physiological homeostasis and resolving possible medical implications.

Definition of the Thorax Region

Lying between the neck and the abdomen, the thorax region is a significantly important anatomical compartment that houses essential organs like the heart and lungs. Its superior boundary begins at the thoracic inlet, extending to the diaphragm, which forms its inferior boundary.

Medical professionals need to be aware of the precise demarcation of the thorax, particularly in imaging and radiation therapy. For example, the development of automatic anatomical recognition systems, as highlighted in various studies, calls for clearly defined body regions like the thorax to enhance precision in medical interventions, such as contouring in radiation therapy (Vibhu et al., 2020). Not only is the respiratory and circulatory system a priority area in this region, but it is also a priority area of study for automatic anatomy recognition to enable improved treatment planning and patient prognosis (Xingyu et al., 2019). Therefore, accurate segmentation of the thorax is most significant for both diagnosis and therapy developments (Figure 4.1).

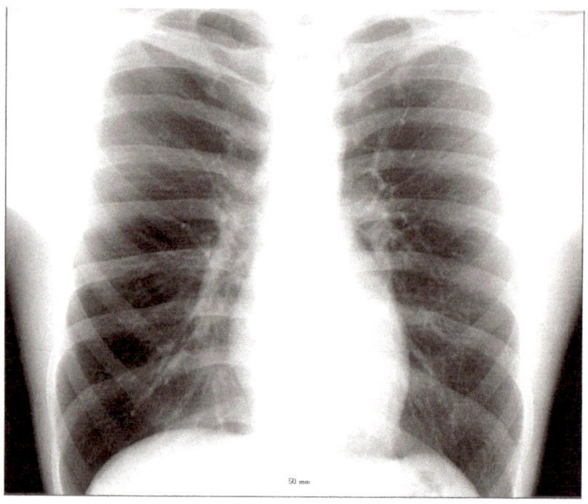

Figure 4.1. Thorax anatomical region.

Source: CC BY-SA 3.0, https://commons.wikimedia.org/w/index.php?curid=817752

Importance of the Thorax in Human Anatomy

The thorax is a significant component of the human anatomy, harboring essential organs and structures required for existence. Not only does this region protect the heart and lungs, but it also plays a critical role in the act of respiration and circulation as well. The thoracic cavity is housed within the rib cage, providing protection while allowing for inflation and deflation of the lungs during the act of breathing. This function is critical since it provides for the exchange of gases during cellular metabolism. In addition, the thorax contains important vascular organs such as the aorta and superior vena cava that are components of the circulatory system of the body. Besides, the importance of accurate anatomical knowledge to the understanding of the thorax is also underscored further by studies that promote the benefits of innovative pedagogies, such as the employment of the body painting method to comprehend surface anatomy, to enhance the medical students' knowledge of this vital region (Almorza et al., 2019). Knowledge about the thorax is therefore the foundation for effective medical practice and broad human physiology knowledge (Ayeni et al., 2019).

Overview of Thoracic Structures

The thorax is a protective space with essential organs of the body, the heart and lungs, that are involved in considerable physiological activity. It is bordered by the rib cage and consists of a bony cavity created by the ribs, sternum, and thoracic vertebrae and serves as protection, support, and also as support to mechanics of respiration. All closely linked with many body structures, the thorax consists of various significant systems such as the cardiovascular, respiratory, and lymphatic systems, all of which play a significant role in the maintenance of homeostasis. Research on thoracic structures has been made more accessible through technological advancements, enabling extensive understanding of spatial and symbolic anatomy (Bradley et al., 1997). Moreover, learning materials have been created to complement learning, i.e., laboratory manuals dealing with anatomies such as the cardiovascular and respiratory systems that properly fill in loopholes of traditional learning methods (Georgakopoulos & Lasrado, 2022). Overall, the thorax is a sophisticated but streamlined region central to processes that support life (Figure 4.2).

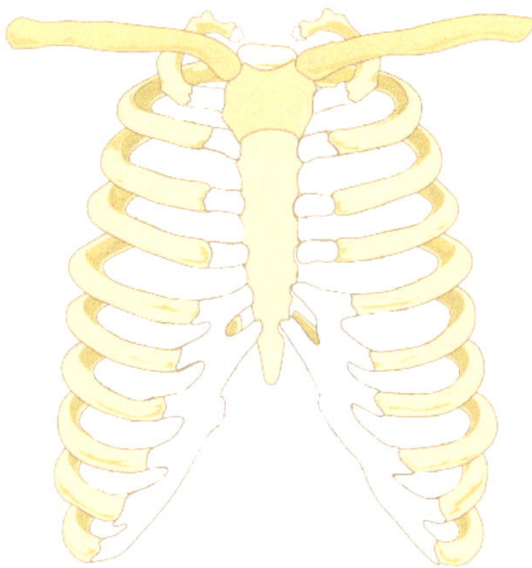

Figure 4.2. Overview of thoracic structures.

Source: By Mikael Häggström - Image:Human_skeleton_front.svg (Public domain license), Public Domain, https://commons.wikimedia.org/w/index.php?curid=6111860

Functions of the Thorax

The thorax is an essential protective and functional area in the human body that houses vital organs such as the heart and lungs. The primary role of the thorax is respiration and circulation since the design of the rib cages allows for expansion and contraction during breathing. The thorax also serves as a protective covering for these organs, minimizing damage from external forces. The intercostal muscles, which are between the ribs, play an essential role in the mechanics of breathing as they assist in raising and lowering the rib cage. Also, the area is utilized as a passage for nerves and blood vessels that aid in the body's overall functioning. This body configuration highlights the significance of the thorax not merely as a compartment but as an active contributor to homeostasis by its complex relations with surrounding systems, demonstrating the sophistication of human physiology as a whole (Figure 4.3).

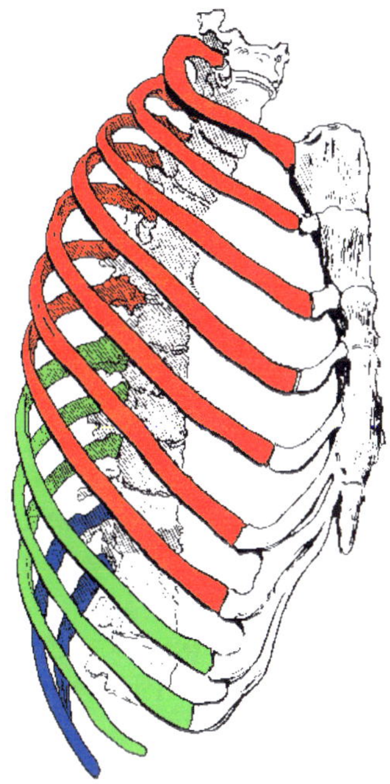

Figure 4.3. Thorax and its functions.

Source: By Cristobal carrasco - Own work, Public Domain, https://commons.wikimedia.org/w/index.php?curid=8922104

Historical Perspective on Thoracic Studies

The past of thoracic research can be traced back through significant milestones in the area of medical science and technology, which greatly influenced treatment and diagnostic protocols. Initial comprehension of the thoracic cavity derived from observations that were predominantly anatomical in their scope, as practitioners tried to understand the nuances within the rib cage and corresponding organs.

Initially reliant on rudimentary techniques, such as palpation and auscultation, the field progressed with innovations like radiography, which emerged in the late 19th century, allowing for unprecedented insights into thoracic structures. This shift was paralleled in other areas of medicine, where detailed data collection became essential for identifying conditions like lung cancer. Surveys across 37 European countries revealed the discrepancy in mechanisms for gathering lung cancer data, paving the way for improved-designed datasets and benchmarks within thoracic research (Alfageme et al., 2018). Enhanced research techniques and technology have continued to enable a greater understanding of the thorax, which in itself has led to enhanced patient outcomes and a cohesive understanding of thoracic health.

Relevance in Medical Fields

Within the areas of therapy and imaging in medicine, accuracy in dose calculation algorithms is not just important but also essential when treating thoracic regions. The Anisotropic Analytical Algorithm is quite precise when it comes to photon doses with 2% agreement in uniform media and 2.5% in complex cases containing inhomogeneities such as bone and lung tissues (Ahnesjö et al., 2006). This precision is significant as it directly impacts the success of radiation therapy as a tool for curing thoracic disease, such as lung cancer. Furthermore, studies like the Automatic Annotation Task in medical imaging highlight the importance of classification systems in the diagnosis and management of thoracic diseases (González et al., 2005). By applying precise calculations and advanced imaging techniques, clinicians are able to tailor treatment programs more effectively, enhancing patient outcome in this serious area of medicine. The employment of exact computations and automated mechanisms emphasizes the complementary nature of technology and clinical practice, ushering in improved treatment strategies.

Methodology of Research

In examining the thorax region, a solid methodology is required to gain reliable and pertinent data. The research primarily involves advanced imaging techniques, such as computed tomography (CT) scans, which provide quantitative information on the structural and mechanical properties of thoracic bones, especially in children. For instance, studies on Hounsfield Units of children's ribs demonstrate the potential to link imaging data with mechanical property measurements to enable enhanced understanding of growth patterns and bone density variations (Propper & Rigg, 2006). In addition, medical image analysis with artificial intelligence (AI) has increased in importance. Designing deep neural networks that can automatically segment and annotate regions of interest in X-ray images is a significant achievement. By integrating textual reports with visual data, researchers can enhance diagnostic accuracy, thereby improving results in thoracic-related conditions (Guo et al., 2018). Overall, a comprehensive and multidisciplinary research methodology is crucial in advancing knowledge in the thorax field.

4.1. Anatomy of the Thorax

Learning Outcome

1. Give an Overview of Thoracic Cavity
2. Focus on Rib Cage Structure and Function
3. Explain the Thoracic Vertebrae Characteristics
4. Discuss the Sternum Anatomy
5. Understand Intercostal Muscles and their Role
6. Know Diaphragm Structure and Function
7. Describe the Mediastinum and its Subdivisions
8. Know Thoracic Inlet and Outlet
9. Evaluate Vascular and Nervous Supply of the Thorax

To explore the structural complexity of the thorax is to discover a remarkable arrangement of bones, muscles, and organs that serve vital roles in the human body. The region, bordered by the rib cage, holds the lungs and heart, central to breathing and circulation functions. Appreciation of thorax anatomy arises from cutting-edge technologies that allow close imaging and dissection studies. For instance, the use of 3-D atlases has revolutionized the visualization of thoracic anatomy into an interactive means of spatial arrangement navigation between structures. Additionally, access to these resources across the globe has implied a great demand for anatomical training (Bradley et al., 1997). With a foundation of knowledge in thoracic anatomy established, it is apparent that specialized knowledge not only supports clinical practices but also augments higher-level research efforts, hence further promoting appreciation of the complexity of human physiology (Casagrande-Jaloretto et al., 2013).

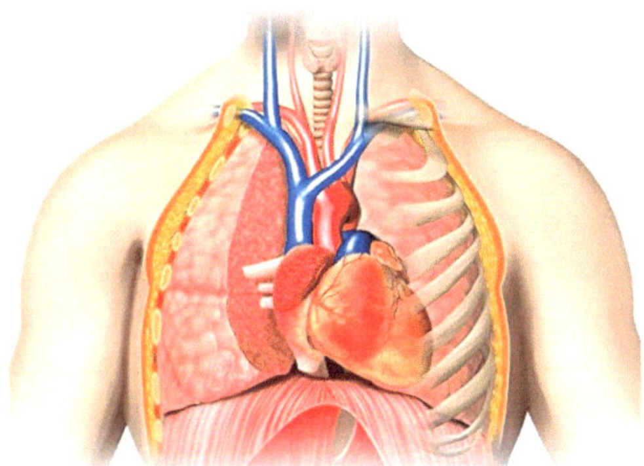

Source: Amazon. (n.d.). *Human Thoracic Cavity Anatomy*.

4.1.1. Overview of Thoracic Cavity

The thoracic cavity, as an essential part of the human body, is in charge of holding essential organs and supporting essential physiological functions. The thoracic cavity is covered by the ribs, vertebral column, and sternum to provide a protected compartment for the lungs and heart. Within this compartment lies the mediastinum, home to the heart, great vessels, and trachea, and around every lung lie the pleural cavities responsible for creating a lubricated interface that reduces friction during breathing. It is valuable to be familiar with the complex anatomy of the thoracic cavity, especially its function in various medical conditions and imaging techniques. For instance, advanced imaging methods such as SPECT/CT have been employed to image the biodistribution of drug delivery systems based on nanoparticles, providing information on their interaction with thoracic organs, such as the heart and lungs, *in vivo* (Prashant et al., 2018). This convergent information puts the thoracic cavity in the limelight as far as anatomy and clinical interventions are concerned (Figure 4.4).

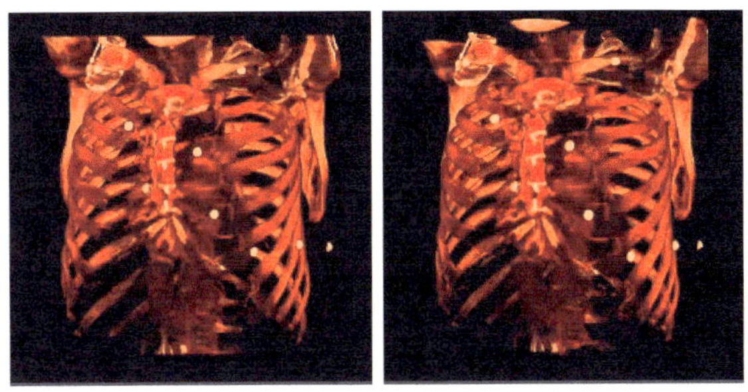

Figure 4.4. The thoracic cavity is the superior cavity in the ventral body cavity.

Source: By KieranMaher at English Wikibooks - Transferred from en.wikibooks to Commons by Adrignola using CommonsHelper., Public Domain, https://commons.wikimedia.org/w/index.php?curid=8750249

4.1.2. Rib Cage Structure and Function

The rib cage is important in respiratory mechanics as it acts as an enclosure that safeguards vital organs during the process of breathing, yet makes breathing efficient. Its special design, made up of ribs, costal cartilage, and sternum, promotes rigidity as well as flexibility. During inspiration and expiration of humans, the rib cage undergoes significant morphological change; during maximum forced inspiration, the superior part expands in antero-posterior dimensions while the inferior part undergoes medio-lateral expansion (Agostini et al., 2017). The dynamic movement highlights compartmentalization of the thoracic cavity with the pulmonary and diaphragmatic region having a differential contribution to respiration. Furthermore, the developmental trends of the rib cage in children show that the costal cartilage forms a high proportion of rib length, illustrating the structural development over the years in a child (Propper & Rigg, 2006). This complicated design not only optimizes respiratory function but also develops throughout development, illustrating the rib cage's essential role in human physiology (Figure 4.5).

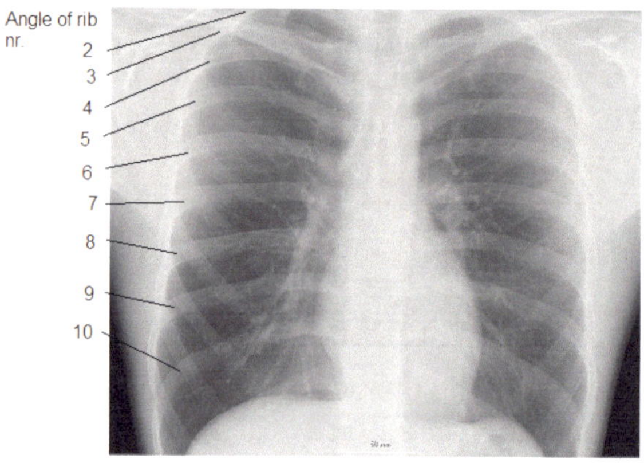

Figure 4.5. Rib cage diagram.

Source: By Mikael Häggström (User:Mikael Häggström) - Image:Chest.png, CC BY-SA 3.0, https://commons.wikimedia.org/w/index.php?curid=3415318

4.1.3. Thoracic Vertebrae Characteristics

Thoracic vertebrae, which are noted for their uniqueness, play a significant role in protecting the spinal cord and structurally supporting the upper part of the body. Comprised of 12 vertebrae (T1-T12), the vertebrae incorporate facets for rib attachment, hence facilitating articulation of the rib cage, imparting stability and mobility to the thoracic cavity. Kyphotic curvature of the thoracic spine is one aspect of its distinct shape, facilitating load distribution in activities. In addition, the alignment of thoracic vertebrae facilitates the execution of paraspinal nerve blocks, which are essential in controlling pain when undertaking thoracic operations. Research has shown that blocks like paravertebral and erector spinae plane (ESP) block target anatomy relevant to thoracic surgery with varying degrees of success in pain alleviation (Kim, 2022). Hence, the structural characteristics and functional importance of thoracic vertebrae should be known for anatomical studies as well as a medical practice.

4.1.4. Sternum Anatomy

Located at the center of the chest is a plate-like bone that is a part of thoracic anatomy and acts as an anchor point for the ribs and as a critical protector of the heart and lungs. Its composition consists of three broad sections: manubrium, body, and xiphoid process, all of which contribute to the overall function and stability of the ribcage. Studies have indicated that sternum morphology varies considerably with age and demonstrates robust reliance on growth, with its volume disclosing appreciable change in children (Propper & Rigg, 2006). Significantly, the sternal structure has an effect on respiratory mechanics since its particular shape makes room for the attachment of the ribs, critical for effective ventilation. Also, the analysis of thoracic shape in primates reveals that the more extensive sternum configuration in hominoids has a close relationship with their locomotor specializations, emphasizing the interactive relationship between skeletal anatomy and functional evolution (Chan et al., 2014).

4.1.5. Intercostal Muscles and their Role

The complex interplay among the intercostal muscles plays a key function in the respiration process. The muscles between the ribs play an important role in the accommodation of inhalation as well as exhalation. During inhalation, the external intercostal muscles contract and consequently elevate the rib cage, as well as the widening of the thoracic cavity, through which air flows into the lungs. Conversely, during exhalation, the muscles of the internal intercostal contract to decrease the rib cage and expel air. Not only does this coordinated effort ease breathing, but it also serves to maintain intrathoracic pressure. It is noteworthy to learn about the anatomy and physiology of these muscles because they are also directly involved in the overall efficiency of the respiratory system further emphasized by studies on *Caiman crocodilus* muscular structure (Mariluce et al., 2023). Thus, precise information about intercostal muscles gives insight into the dynamics of the thoracic area along with its impact on respiratory health as well as disease avoidance (Figure 4.6).

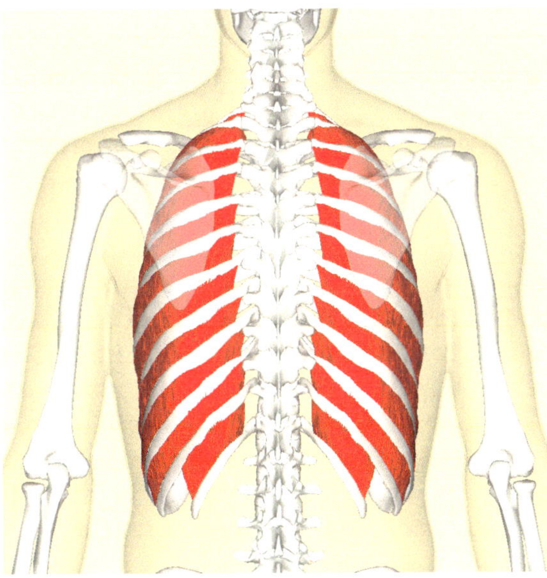

Figure 4.6. Intercostal muscles and their role.

Source: By Anatomography - en:Anatomography (setting page of this image), CC BY-SA 2.1 jp, https://commons.wikimedia.org/w/index.php?curid=22754501

4.1.6. Diaphragm Structure and Function

The diaphragm plays a vital role in breathing and is one of the primary thoracic anatomical structures. Physiologically, the diaphragm is a dome-shaped sheet of muscle that separates the thoracic and abdominal cavities and is made largely of skeletal muscle and connective tissue. When the diaphragm contracts to breathe in, it causes the volume of the thoracic cavity to increase such that pressure is reduced and therefore allows air into the lungs. Secondarily, the role of the diaphragm is supported by its attachment with bordering structures, i.e., the esophageal hiatus, which is formed by the right crus of the diaphragm (Ghahremani et al., 2020). This is for a proper lower esophageal sphincter to prevent gastroesophageal reflux. Therefore, understanding the diaphragm structure and function is critical to an understanding of its function in breathing, as well as the maintenance of thoracic and abdominal pressure integrity. Such analysis puts diaphragm importance to respiratory mechanics and thoracic health into perspective.

4.1.7. Mediastinum and its Subdivisions

Between the lungs lies the thoracic mediastinum, a crucial compartment of the thoracic cavity, between the thoracic inlet and the diaphragm. The space, without any physical divides, is classically divided into four sections: superior, anterior, middle, and posterior mediastinum. The subdivisions harbor important anatomical structures essential to numerous body functions. For instance, the middle mediastinum contains the great vessels and heart, which are critical to the circulatory system, and the posterior mediastinum contains important nerves and the thoracic aorta. As discussed in similar literature, the mediastinum houses many important structures like the heart, great vessels, trachea, and important nerves (Mete & Akbudak, 2018).

An understanding of these subregions is not only important for anatomical understanding but also for the diagnosis of pathologies that may arise in this complex region, emphasizing its clinical importance in both health and disease.

4.1.8. Thoracic Inlet and Outlet

Located at the superior border of the thoracic cavity, the thoracic inlet is a vital opening through which structures that are entering and exiting the chest pass. The anatomy of this location includes vital elements such as the trachea, esophagus, great vessels, and nerves, all of which travel between the thorax and neck.

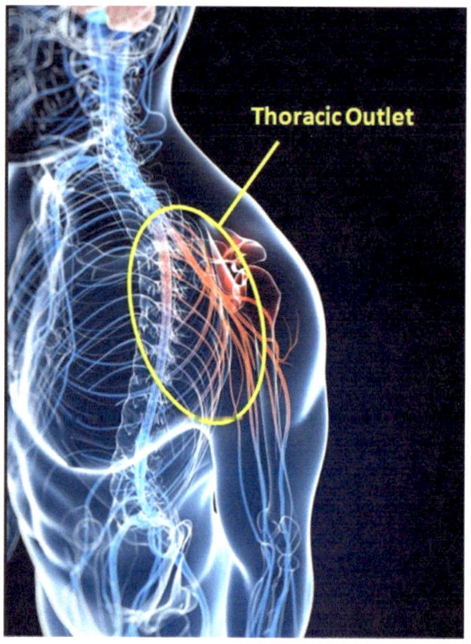

Figure 4.7. Thoracic inlet and outlet.

Source: Beaumaris Physiotherapy. (n.d.). *Thoracic Outlet Syndrome (TOS).*

The arrangement of the inlets has a close correlation with the thoracic outlet function, located at the upper surface of the diaphragm and containing similar structures on their exit directed into the upper limb and abdomen. Specifically, the inter-scalene triangle, which is delineated by the anterior and middle scalene muscles, is significant in the position of the brachial plexus, determining the role of thoracic inlets in the function of the upper limb (Mete & Akbudak, 2018). Syndromes or abnormalities along these pathways, such as thoracic outlet syndrome (TOS), carry significant health implications for a person, underpinning the critical role of the thorax in respiratory and circulatory systems (Mete & Akbudak, 2018) (Figure 4.7).

4.1.9. Vascular and Nervous Supply of the Thorax

The thorax is provided in a complicated way by both vascular and nervous components that are crucial for normal physiological activity. The vascular supply primarily comes from the aorta and includes branches such as the subclavian and intercostal arteries, which give adequate blood supply to essential structures in the thorax . In addition, venous drainage is provided by a rich network of veins centered on the superior and inferior vena cavae. Importantly, the thoracic cavity also houses critical parts of the nervous system, namely the autonomic fibers for involuntary control of the heart and lungs, and sensory and motor pathways with priority given to upper limb sensation and movement. This complex supply chain enables the thorax to effectively fulfill both structural role and dynamic physiological processes, highlighting its pivotal role in overall human function.

Test Your Knowledge

1. Which veins drain the thoracic wall into the superior vena cava?
2. What is the role of the intercostal nerves in thoracic function?

4.2. Thoracic Organs

Learning Outcome

1. Discuss the Lungs: Structure and Function
2. Explain the Heart: Anatomy and Physiology
3. Focus on Esophagus and Its Role in Digestion
4. Explain the Trachea and Bronchial Tree
5. Describe the Thymus Gland and its Significance
6. Understand Major Blood Vessels in the Thorax
7. Know Lymphatic System in the Thoracic Region
8. Give details Pleura and Pleural Cavity
9. Thoracic Organs in Relation to Respiratory Health

The thorax is a significant hub of different organ systems, especially in insects like the honey bee (*Apis mellifera*) and the armored ground cricket (*Acanthoplus speiseri*). In this region, the thoracic musculature facilitates significant movements, including flight, walking, and some adaptations to their environments.

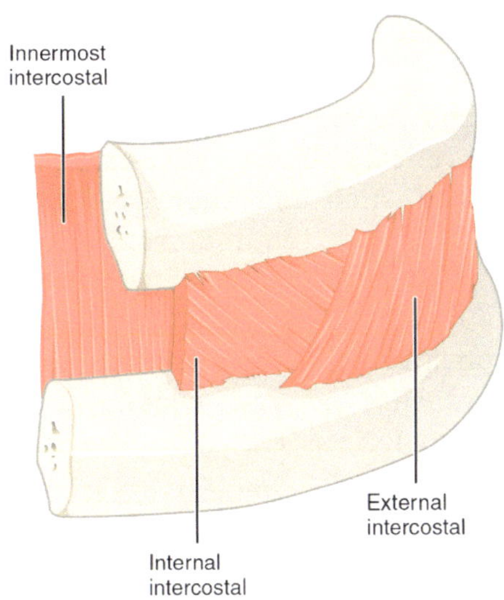

Figure 4.8. The thorax serves as a critical hub for various organ systems.

Source: By CFCF - Own work, CC BY-SA 4.0, https://commons.wikimedia.org/w/index.php?curid=44308826

It has been noted in research on *A. speiseri* that the musculature of this species exhibits sexual differences due to divergent functions, such as the presence of modified tegmina among males that are accountable for stridulation (Mbata et al., 1985). Besides, the thoracic chamber features vital respiratory and circulatory features accountable for efficient gas exchange and blood flow required in maintaining homeostasis. The complex arrangement of thoracic organs not only enables survival but also adds to the versatility of these insects, illustrating the evolutionary significance of thoracic morphology in the range of ecological niches. Thus, the thorax becomes a functionally variable region central to the organism's overall physiology and behavior (Figure 4.8).

4.2.1. Lungs: Structure and Function

The human lungs are amazing organs that support the process of gas exchange by which life is maintained. Their very sophisticated structure comprising millions of alveoli ensures the maximum surface area to allow oxygen into the blood and carbon dioxide out. Lungs not only cover respiration but also aid in physiological processes like maintaining blood pH levels stable and removing toxic compounds. Recent advances in medical technology, for instance, thoracic electrical impedance tomography (EIT), have enhanced our understanding of lung function through the capability of real-time imaging of ventilation distribution with mechanical ventilation (Mete & Akbudak, 2018). Moreover, animal model studies have elucidated radiation exposure impact on lung integrity and identified it to have detrimental roles like pulmonary vascular resistance and loss of microvascular density, which accumulate under radiation pneumonitis conditions (Mete & Akbudak, 2018). Overall, these observations attest to the lungs complex functions and susceptibility to environmental stress (Figure 4.9).

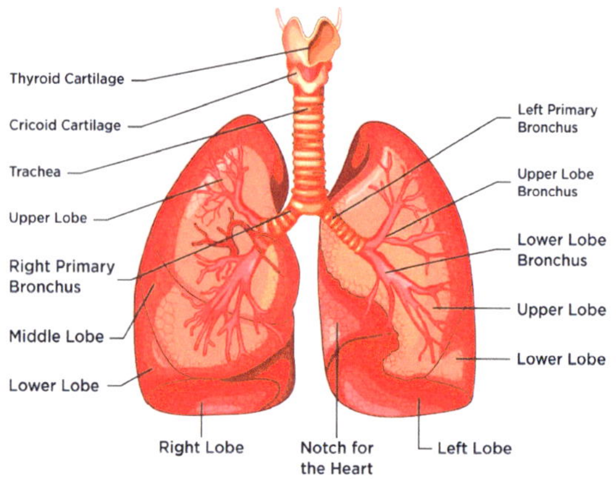

Figure 4.9. Structure of lung.

Source: Biology Notes Online. (n.d.). *Lung Structure, Location, Functions, and Diseases.*

4.2.2. Heart: Anatomy and Physiology

The heart, a muscular organ located in the thorax cavity, plays a vital role in the circulatory system by pumping blood throughout the body. Composed of four chambers—the right atrium, right ventricle, left atrium, and left ventricle—it operates on a synchronized contraction cycle, powered by electrical impulses generated by the sinoatrial (SA) node, also referred to as the heart's natural pacemaker. This complex anatomy facilitates the heart to effectively separate oxygenated and deoxygenated blood flow in order for tissues to receive oxygen and nutrients and remove carbon dioxide. The structure-function interrelation of the heart is even more pronounced when one considers its extremely complex valve system, which prevents backflow and permits unidirectional blood flow. Overall, the heart represents an exemplary model of complex coordination of anatomy and physiology, a requirement for life and an indicator of general health dynamics within the thoracic cavity (Mete & Akbudak, 2018).

4.2.3. Esophagus and Its Role in Digestion

It is situated within the thoracic cavity, and the esophagus is a vital food transport tube that links the stomach to the mouth. The muscle tube not only moves ingested material by rhythmic contraction or peristalsis, but it also highlights the role of anatomy within the process of digestion. Translocation of the food from the pharynx to the esophagus occurs in an impressive orderly fashion, as higher airway structures, i.e., the larynx and pharynx, are key to swallowing (Akbudak et al., 2018). Reaching the level of the esophagus, food is driven downwards by being propelled by esophageal sphincters preventing reflux, delivering single-way movement of material. Without such efficient mechanisms, digestion would be severely compromised, illustrating the esophagus's vital role as an advanced buffer in the complex system of human digestion and overall thoracic function.

4.2.4. Trachea and Bronchial Tree

Being part of the respiratory apparatus, the trachea and its bronchial tree dividing into a chain of bronchi and bronchioles are important for air conduction and filtering. The trachea, a flexible tube extending from the larynx, divides into the right and left main bronchi, which further divide into smaller bronchi and bronchioles inside the lungs to form a highly branched network enabling maximum surface area for gas exchange. The branching anatomy of the bronchial tree not only ensures optimal flow of air but also plays a vital role in humidifying and warming the air before it enters the sensitive alveoli. Of prime importance is the fact that the bronchial arteries supply oxygenated blood to the lungs' tissues, a lung anatomical feature is essential in ensuring healthy respiratory function (Mete & Akbudak, 2018). This complex system within the thoracic cavity underscores the importance of respiratory anatomy knowledge because other pathologies may arise, affecting airflow and the effectiveness of gas exchange (Mete & Akbudak, 2018) (Figure 4.10).

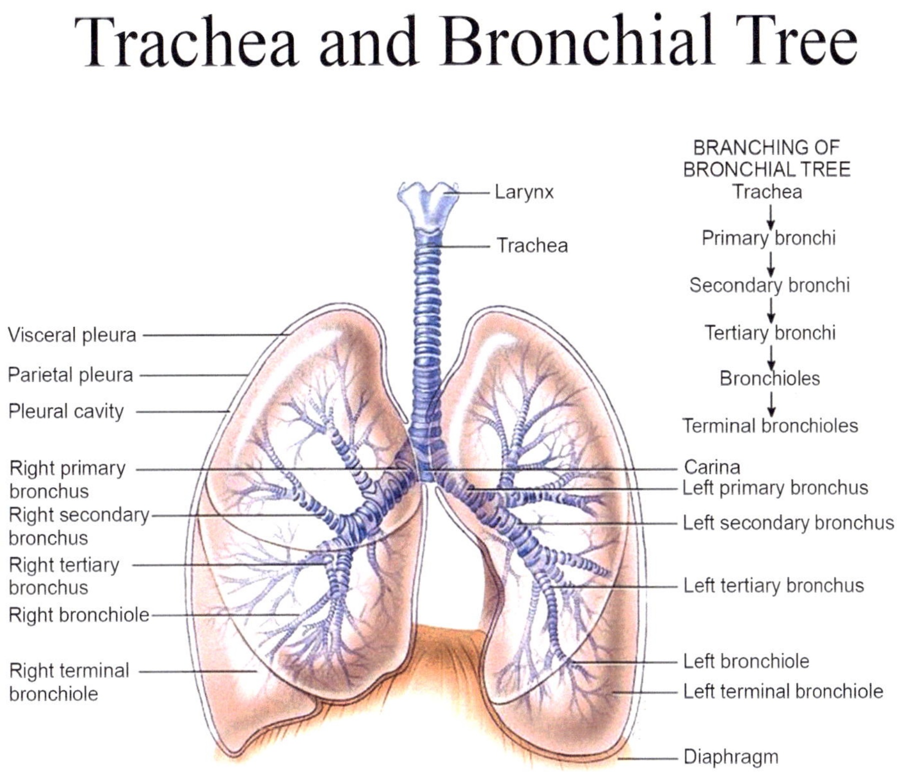

Figure 4.10. Trachea and bronchial tree.

Source: SlidePlayer. (n.d.). *Trachea and Bronchial Tree.*

4.2.5. Thymus Gland and its Significance

In the upper anterior part of the thoracic cavity, the thymus gland is tasked with helping the immune system, particularly in the process of T lymphocyte development, which is essential in adaptive immunity. Being a principal primary lymphoid organ, the thymus provides space for T cell maturation so that they may be able to identify and combat pathogens effectively. The thymus is of most vital concern during childhood and adolescence, when it is in its most active state; effectiveness wanes with age, resulting in a disruption of immune response efficiency. The disruption can result in an increase in susceptibility to infection and autoimmune diseases in older age. Also, the process of learning the thymus's function and how it has relationship with the thorax area suggests that it plays an important role in overall health and well-being. The study of this gland underscores the need for more research on its function and potential therapeutic applications in immunologically related diseases (Gray et al., 1933) (Figure 4.11).

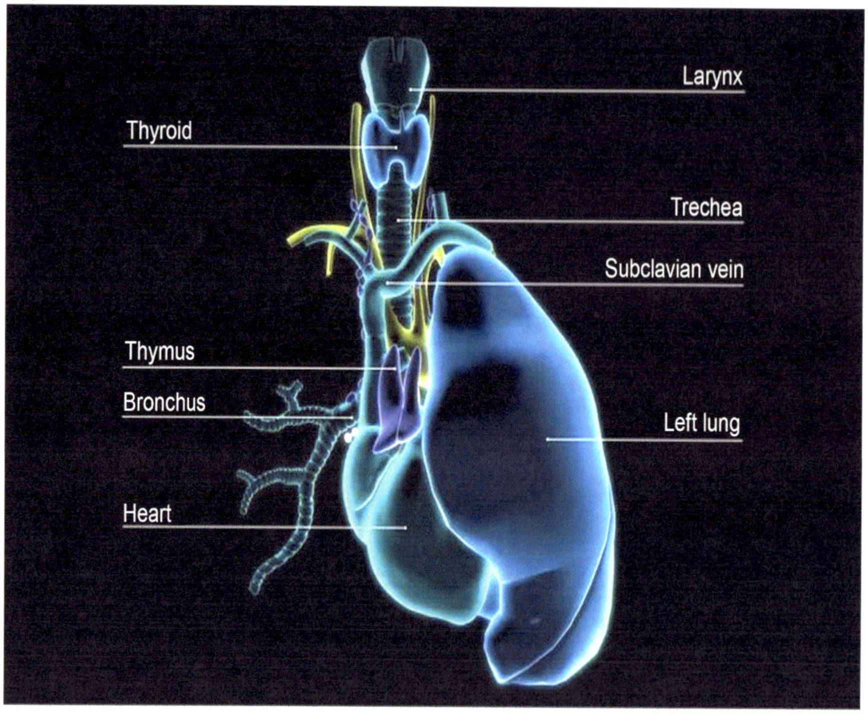

Figure 4.11. Thymus anatomy.

Source: https://www.thoughtco.com/thymus-anatomy-373250.

4.2.6. Major Blood Vessels in the Thorax

The thoracic cavity is important to both the respiratory and circulatory systems, offering large blood vessels that enable the vital processes of the body. The aorta is the primary artery here, arising from the left ventricle of heart and distributing oxygenated blood to the body. Aortic branches include the brachiocephalic trunk, left common carotid artery, and left subclavian artery, which all supply blood to critical areas such as the head and arms. The superior and inferior vena cavae also play critical roles by returning deoxygenated blood from the body to the right atrium of the heart. The system of pulmonary veins and pulmonary arteries is also responsible for efficient gas exchange within the lungs, taking in oxygen to body tissues and bringing in carbon dioxide for exhalation, respectively. These vascular networks allow the thorax to maintain homeostasis, linking respiratory and circulatory processes that keep life in this body center alive (Georgakopoulos & Lasrado, 2022).

4.2.7. Lymphatic System in the Thoracic Region

Housed within the thoracic region is the lymphatic system that maintains fluid and immune levels in the body to ensure smooth function. An assemblage of vessels and nodes transports the body fluid comprising immune cells named lymph throughout the thorax as well as elsewhere within the body. The thoracic duct, the largest of the lymph vessels, drains lymph from most of the body back into the venous system, underscoring its important function in returning fluid from the interstitium back to the circulation. Its malfunction may lead to severe complications such as protein-losing enteropathy and plastic bronchitis, particularly observed in patients with conditions like the Fontan circulation (Viktor et al., 2021). In addition, the pig model has proven useful as a valuable tool for investigation, yielding an understanding of lymphatic physiology and pathology, and the manner by which specific treatments may mitigate lymphatic disease in large animal models (Reinhard, 2020). Elucidating such mechanisms informs effective treatment as well as optimized patient outcomes.

4.2.8. Pleura and Pleural Cavity

The thorax holds key structures enveloped and organized by the pleura and pleural cavity, which play significant roles in respiratory mechanics. The pleura is two thin membranes, the visceral and parietal pleura, that envelop the lungs and line the thoracic cavity, respectively. This structure creates the pleural cavity, a potential space filled with pleural fluid that permits lung expansion and contraction during breathing. Pressure gradients across the cavity are important in maintaining the lungs to the thoracic wall to allow ventilation to be effective. Disruption of pleural fluid balance can lead to complications such as pneumothorax or pleural effusion, which can catastrophically interfere with respiratory function. Understanding the anatomy and physiological function of the pleura and pleural cavity highlights their function in the thorax area and interdependence of thoracic structures maintaining important body processes (Figure 4.12).

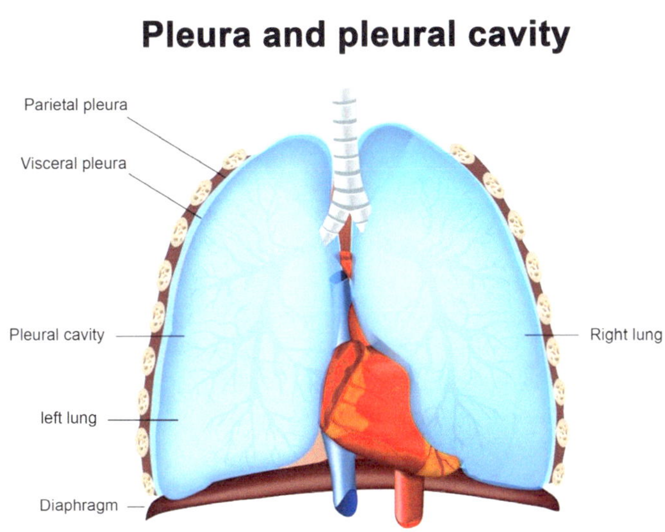

Figure 4.12. Pleura and pleural cavity.

Source: Alamy. (n.d.). *Lung, Pleura, and Pleural Cavity – Medical Vector Illustration*.

4.2.9. Thoracic Organs in Relation to Respiratory Health

The thoracic cavity harbors vital organs that are tasked with guaranteeing respiratory well-being. At the center of the system is the lungs, which are tasked with gas exchange where oxygen is drawn in and carbon dioxide is expelled. The pleurae, which encase the lungs, create a protective sheath that guarantees smooth movement during respiration. The diaphragm, a large muscle that is situated under the lungs, is crucial in regulating airflow through contracting and relaxing. Any interference with these thoracic organs may lead to severe respiratory complications, such as those experienced with pneumonia or lung cancer. Also, infections of contiguous structures, like deep spaces of the neck, can extend into thoracic cavities, triggering potentially fatal conditions such as mediastinitis or septic shock (Mete & Akbudak, 2018). Therefore, it is important to know and preserve thoracic organ integrity for upholding optimal respiratory capacity and overall health.

Test Your Knowledge

1. What is the pleural cavity and why is it important for lung function?
2. How do the lungs and diaphragm work together during respiration?

4.3. Thoracic Pathologies

Learning Outcome

1. Discuss the Common Thoracic Diseases
2. Explain the Thoracic Trauma and Injuries
3. Understand Respiratory Disorders (e.g., Asthma, COPD)
4. Focus on Cardiovascular Diseases Affecting the Thorax
5. Know Tumors and Cancers in the Thoracic Region
6. Evaluate Infections (e.g., Pneumonia, Tuberculosis)
7. Focus on Congenital Anomalies of the Thorax
8. Describe the Diagnostic Imaging Techniques
9. Know Treatment Options for Thoracic Conditions

The thoracic region is of vital importance in the understanding of various clinical conditions, particularly trauma and muscle function. Of the significant issues are pectoralis minor muscle-related injuries, which may lead to altered scapular alignment and arm movement dysfunction. This adaptive shortening may be the cause of shoulder movement-related disability frequently seen in patients with shoulder disorders (Mete & Akbudak, 2018). Furthermore, the diagnostic evaluation of thoracic pathologies is crucial to effective patient management, particularly in trauma. Current studies confirm that low-dose CT significantly enhances the detection of thoracic injuries compared to traditional X-ray imaging with greater sensitivity and specificity (Alpaslan et al., 2013). All these observations characterize the complex nature of thoracic pathologies and emphasize the importance of effective diagnostics and rehabilitation interventions in managing these conditions.

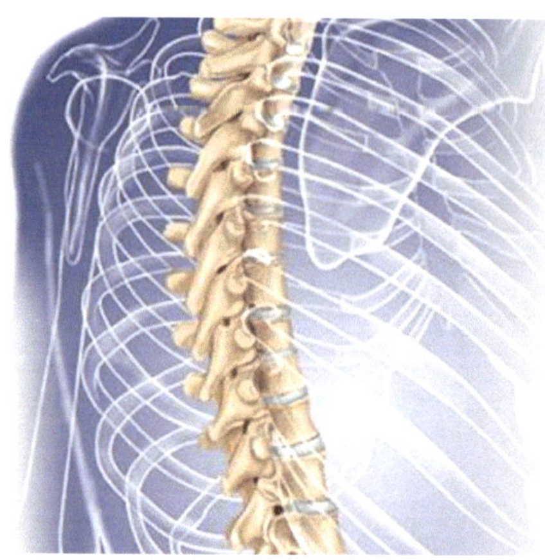

Source: Centre du Dos Genève. (2019). *Colonne Thoracique*.

4.3.1. Common Thoracic Diseases

The thoracic region is susceptible to many diseases that can have a major impact on respiratory and cardiovascular functions. Pneumonia, chronic obstructive pulmonary disease (COPD), and congestive heart failure

(CHF) are some of the frequent diseases that, if left untreated, can lead to serious complications. Pneumonia, which is often caused by infection, can lead to inflammation of lung tissue, leading to high morbidity in the affected population. Chronic conditions like COPD not only compromise lung function but also incur greater rates of hospitalization and economic burden to healthcare systems (Liang et al., 2023). In addition, the integration of advanced diagnostic tools, such as deep learning models, has promoted thoracic disease classification and prognosis. For instance, ThoraX-PriorNet utilizes anatomical prior distributions in CNN models for the enhancement of chest X-ray-based disease detection, pointing to the necessity of accurate diagnostics in addressing common thoracic disease (Iqbal et al., 2022). Thus, an understanding and treatment of these diseases are crucial for improving patient outcomes in the thoracic region (Figure 4.13).

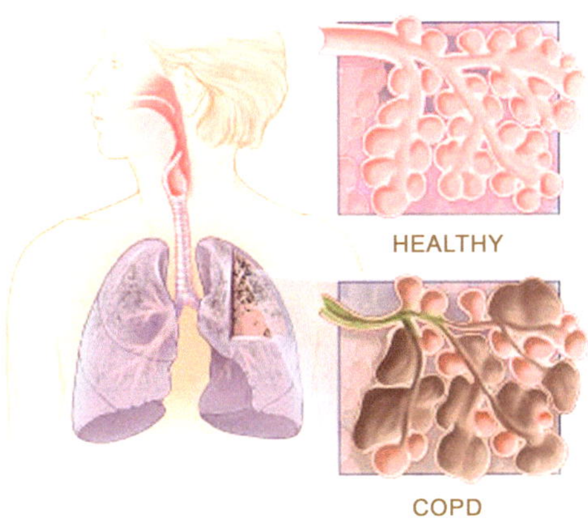

Figure 4.13. Chronic obstructive lung disease (COLD).

Source: By Original source: http://www.nhlbi.nih.gov/health/public/lung/copd/campaign-materials/html/copd-patient.htm, Public Domain, https://commons.wikimedia.org/w/index.php?curid=14853266

4.3.2. Thoracic Trauma and Injuries

Thoracic trauma is particularly dangerous due to its potential for instant death and severe complications. Trauma analysis shows that nearly 45% of the patients with significant trauma develop thoracic injury, and overall mortality for such an injury was 9.3% (Helsloot et al., 2023). Particularly, the early post-injury time is critical, with approximately 25% of fatalities in this scenario occurring during the first hour of admission, highlighting the necessity of appropriate intervention within this therapeutic window. Further, the concomitance of blunt thoracic aortic injury and blunt abdominal trauma comes with unique challenges; patients requiring thoracic endovascular aortic replacement (TEVAR) have a heightened risk of intra-abdominal hemorrhage post-procedure (Yu-Chieh et al., 2022). These findings underscore the importance of quick and professional intervention protocols since early intervention would mitigate avoidable deaths from thoracic injuries. This is critical in maximizing outcomes in trauma care.

4.3.3. Respiratory Disorders (e.g., Asthma, COPD)

Chronic respiratory diseases, such as COPD and asthma, have a notable impact on the thoracic region and overall respiratory function. These conditions most often develop due to complex interaction among lifestyle, environmental, and genetic determinants that lead to structural remodeling and airway inflammation. Asthma, with hyperreactivity of airways and inflammation, typically occurs as a result of allergen and irritant exposures and leads to bronchoconstriction, wheezing, and shortness of breath (Kenneth et al., 2020). COPD, by contrast, is due to chronic noxious particulate exposure, i.e., cigarette smoking, leading to chronic airway obstruction and dyspnea. Anatomy and physiology of the lung also change with age, which entails reduced regenerative capacity, rendering older people more vulnerable to such diseases (Soo et al., 2019). Understanding the risk factors and the pathophysiological processes underlying such respiratory diseases is pivotal in ensuring effective control and intervention in their management.

4.3.4. Cardiovascular Diseases Affecting the Thorax

The thorax is a region harboring vital structures of the heart and lungs and is therefore most susceptible to most of cardiovascular diseases. These usually manifest as chest pain, dyspnea, or palpitations, indicative of underlying pathology that must be addressed urgently.

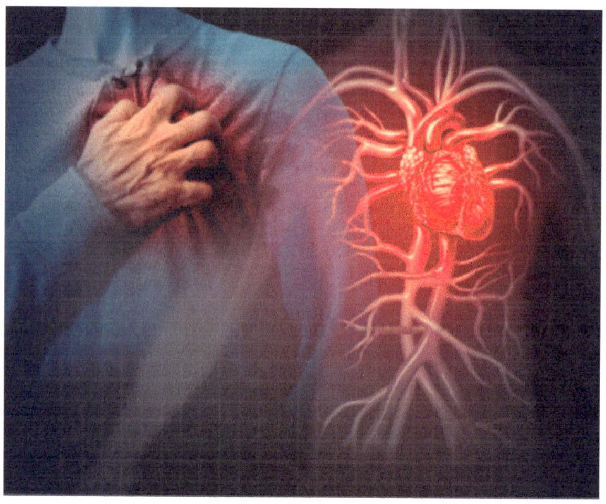

Source: Healthily. (n.d.). *Cardiovascular Disease Illustration.*

An important characteristic of cardiovascular diseases of this region is that they can exacerbate underlying respiratory disease, particularly in the case of COPD patients. Scientific research has also indicated that COPD exacerbations are most prevalent during winter months, suggesting environmental factors, i.e., increased viral infections during cold weather, play a prominent part in their development (Donaldson et al., 2014). Random findings like heart murmurs can also frequently remain stealthy until they coincide with other thoracic symptoms, highlighting the importance of proper cardiovascular exams in animals as well (Abbott et al., 2015). Understanding these factors in total is important for successful prevention and control.

4.3.5. Tumors and Cancers in the Thoracic Region

Within the thoracic cavity, tumors and cancers pose some of the most challenging health conditions, with the lungs and surrounding tissues most implicated. Such cancers are often aggressive and may arise in various forms, necessitating precise diagnostic tools to inform treatment. Recent advances in imaging studies, such as positron emission tomography (PET) and contrast-enhanced computed tomography (CE CT), enhance our ability to assess tumor characteristics and staging. For instance, the creation of PET images using multi-channel generative adversarial networks (M-GAN) greatly improves the visualization of high-uptake regions, which aids in tumor detection, especially in patients with lung cancer (Mete & Akbudak, 2018). In addition, fractal analysis of time sequence CE CT images has also been demonstrated as a promising method for differentiating between aggressive and nonaggressive lung tumors with as much as 83.3% accuracy of predictions based on vascular patterns (Mete & Akbudak, 2018). These advances not only assist in staging but also in planning personalized treatment strategies, reflecting the indispensable role of technological innovation in oncology.

4.3.6. Infections (e.g., Pneumonia, Tuberculosis)

The prevalence of such infections like pneumonia and tuberculosis significantly affects health outcomes, particularly in the region of the thorax. Hospitalization and a high mortality rate often result from community-acquired pneumonia (CAP), which is a significant public health issue in sub-Saharan Africa, particularly causing hospitalization and high mortality among young adults as a result of the high prevalence of HIV infection and associated comorbidities (Mete & Akbudak, 2018). Patients usually report presenting with combined conditions that are complicating for diagnosis and treatment paths, requiring adequate medical facilities and skills that may not be available at all times. Further, consequences of early life exposure to risk factors such as respiratory infections persist in adult life and predispose individuals to chronic respiratory disease (Mete & Akbudak, 2018). This connection emphasizes the need for broad-based public health interventions that address both the shorter-term problems of infectious disease and the longer-term determinants of lung function, ultimately enhancing overall health impacts in vulnerable populations.

4.3.7. Congenital Anomalies of the Thorax

Congenital thoracic anomalies present a daunting challenge to pediatric medicine, encompassing a range of structural abnormalities that can impact respiratory and cardiac function. These anomalies, such as congenital diaphragmatic hernia and thoracic scoliosis, result from abnormal development during embryogenesis and are associated with lethal complications. The etiology is however never always known, but environmental exposures, genetic predispositions, and prenatal exposures play crucial roles in their causation. Importantly, the occurrence of individual congenital anomalies is associated with geographic clusters and therefore suggests that local environmental factors may be implicated in the prevalence of disorders like congenital diaphragmatic hernia (Mete & Akbudak, 2018). Secondly, advances in prenatal imaging and diagnosis have increased the detection rate of such anomalies, presenting opportunities for early intervention and management. It is essential to comprehend these congenital diseases to develop specific treatments and interventions, ultimately improving the lives of those afflicted (Figure 4.14).

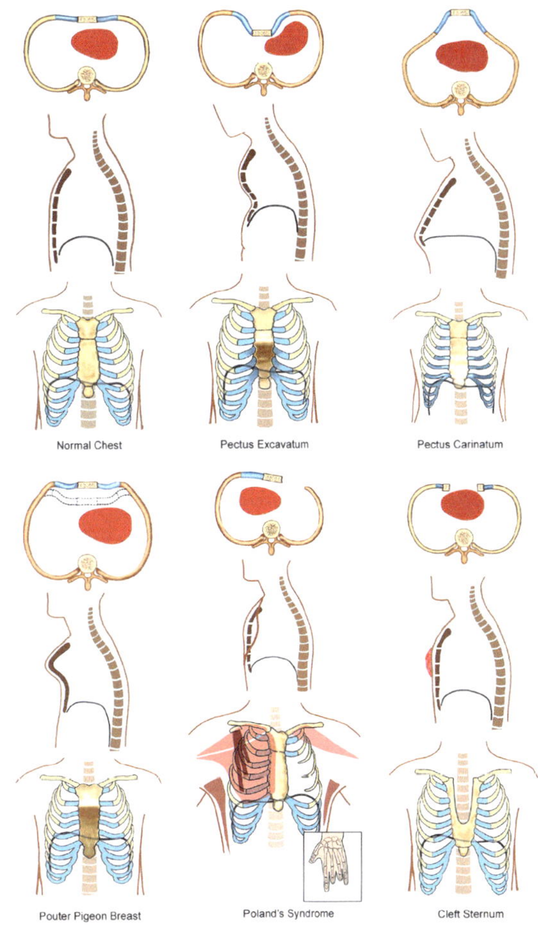

Figure 4.14. Congenital anomalies of the thorax represent a significant challenge in pediatric medicine.

Source: Alexander A. F., Nury M. S., William A. A., Karen, E. A. (2009). Anatomical, histologic, and genetic characteristics of congenital chest wall deformities. *Surgical Repair of Anterior Chest Wall Deformities: The Past, the Present, the Future*, *21*(1), 44–57.

4.3.8. Diagnostic Imaging Techniques

In the diagnostic medical area, imaging modalities play a very crucial role in evaluating various regions of the body, including the thorax. Of these sophisticated modalities, magnetic resonance imaging (MRI) and computed tomography (CT) have the ability to produce detailed cross-sectional images. As an illustration, the study validates the usefulness of CT to image carotid body tumors, for instance, in the case of one Labrador Retriever where useful imaging was utilized in staging before treatment (De Cock et al., 2012). As part of the comparative analysis of imaging techniques, priority in optimizing methodologies highlights the protection from radiation and with particular relevance the breast among other sensitive areas against radiation when imaging with CT. Research confirms that advanced protocols can reduce doses significantly without sacrificing image quality, such as the application of 80 kV techniques and consequent breast and lung dose reduction (Mete & Akbudak, 2018). These advancements are significant in enhancing diagnostic efficacy with respect to patient safety.

4.3.9. Treatment Options for Thoracic Conditions

Effective management of thoracic disease in most instances is a multidisciplinary approach with consideration of short-term symptom relief and long-term health benefits. Interventions may vary from pharmacologic, such as bronchodilators for conditions like COPD, to surgical management for more advanced anatomical malformations or malignancies. For instance, in patients with lung cancer and concurrent complications of COPD, coordination of care among specialists is critical. These experts can develop personalized treatment plans that address both the malignancy and the primary pulmonary condition, offering holistic care. In addition, conditions like Morquio A syndrome demonstrate the necessity of multidisciplinary strategies. As this syndrome involves several thoracic symptoms and complications, coordinated efforts between specializations like pulmonology, cardiology, and orthopedics can optimize treatment efficacy while enhancing patients' quality of life (QoL) (Berger et al., 2014). Finally, the holistic approach to thoracic management will yield improved outcomes and comprehensive treatment of patients.

Test Your Knowledge

1. What is pectus excavatum and how does it affect thoracic anatomy?
2. What role does minimally invasive surgery play in thoracic treatment today?

4.4. Thorax in Clinical Practice

Learning Outcome

1. Discuss the importance of thoracic examination
2. Explain the techniques for auscultation
3. Discuss the role of thoracic surgery
4. Understand interventional procedures in the thorax
5. Focus on rehabilitation for thoracic patients
6. Know thoracic anatomy in medical education
7. How to research advancements in thoracic medicine
8. Understand multidisciplinary approach to thoracic care
9. Learn about future trends in thoracic health

In modern clinical practice, understanding the thorax's complexities is crucial in proper diagnosis and management. The thorax is involved in the cardiovascular and respiratory mechanisms, and advances in monitoring techniques, such as thoracic EIT, have led to dramatically enhanced patient care. EIT offers a noninvasive method of lung function measurement by reconstructing a cross-sectional image of conductivity within the thoracic cavity, thus providing ventilation distribution information during mechanical ventilation (Mete & Akbudak, 2018). These new techniques are invaluable, particularly for patients with conditions like acute lung injury, where monitoring and responsive treatment can be the difference between huge outcomes. In addition, evidence from studies on cutaneous melanoma emphasizes the interplay between thoracic anatomy and lymphatic drainage, emphasizing the importance of thorough evaluation in regional lymph node areas for the detection of metastases effectively (Blum et al., 2006). Hence, a comprehensive understanding of the thorax is important in optimizing clinical practice and patient care (Figure 4.15).

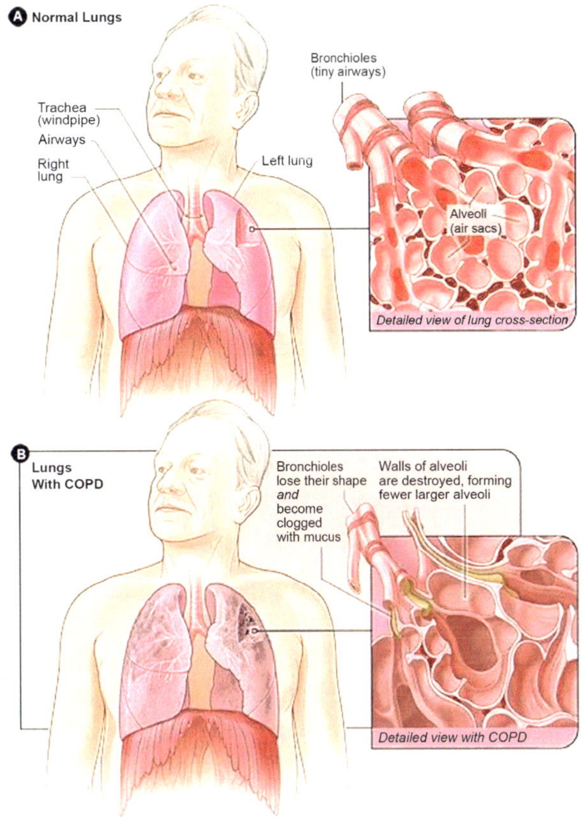

Figure 4.15. Thorax in clinical practice.

Source: By National Heart Lung and Blood Institute - National Heart Lung and Blood Institute, Public Domain, https://commons.wikimedia.org/w/index.php?curid=29583200

4.4.1. Importance of Thoracic Examination

A correct investigation of the thoracic cavity is of utmost significance for the prompt diagnosis and therapy of various medical conditions, having a strong impact on the prognosis in patients. Situated at the center of the respiratory and circulatory systems, the thorax contains the vital organs such as the lungs, heart, and great vessels. The importance of this examination is underscored by advancements in imaging techniques like MRI, which can reveal abnormalities not visible through standard assessments. For instance, coronal images have proven valuable in detecting extra-spinal lesions that may affect thoracic anatomy, highlighting the necessity of comprehensive imaging for accurate diagnoses (Ahmed et al., 2010). Furthermore, sophisticated optical measurement systems provide non-invasive methods for assessing complex thoracic wall deformities with guaranteed precision, allowing for accurate assessment of anatomical disparities and aiding surgical decision-making. In conclusion, accurate thoracic evaluation is vital in the early diagnosis of conditions, facilitating maximally optimized treatment regimens, and advancing world patient care.

4.4.2. Techniques for Auscultation

Within the clinical environment, auscultation is a core skill in thoracic sound evaluation and allows practitioners to adequately assess cardiac and respiratory function. Familiarity with the normal auscultation points is essential, particularly in musculoskeletal (MSK) environments where concurrent complications will be identifiable as abnormal findings upon examination. For instance, the application of MSK ultrasound can complement the application of auscultation techniques by the application of visual feedback on the anatomical structures and conditions, such as inflammation and instability of the tissues (Mete & Akbudak, 2018). With harmonization with dynamic MSK examination, diagnostic accuracy could be enhanced concurrently while practitioners have improved pathology awareness. This three-dimensional route to assessing thoracic health not only improves patient outcomes but also validates the need for auscultation in conjunction with advanced imaging techniques, illustrating its enduring relevance in clinical practice.

4.4.3. Role of Thoracic Surgery

The complexity of the thorax necessitates specialized surgical care, particularly in the treatment of lung diseases and conditions such as COPD and lung cancer. Thoracic surgery is critical in the treatment of these conditions by enabling precise diagnostic and therapeutic maneuvers that significantly improve patient outcomes.

For instance, patients with COPD have a high risk of lung cancer, which is often accompanied by pathologies such as chronic inflammation and oxidative stress. Lobectomies and resections are among the surgical procedures that can effectively remove cancerous tissue while addressing the comorbid pulmonary condition, thus aligning treatment modalities with the comorbid condition of the patients. Moreover, new imaging technologies such as SPECT/micro-CT provide important information regarding anatomical and functional alterations in the lungs, with improved surgical planning and surveillance (Tschanz & Lombardo, 2024). Through interprofessional strategies, thoracic surgery not only addresses immediate issues concerning health but also contributes to the whole-care services within the region of the thorax (Figure 4.16).

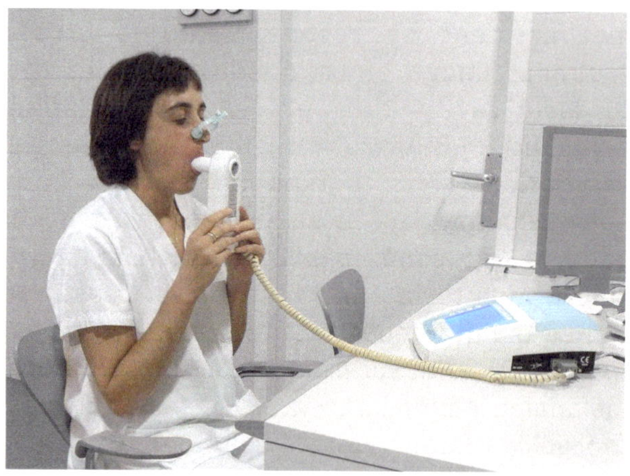

Figure 4.16. A surgeon performs thoracic (chest) surgery.

Source: By Jmarchn - Own work, CC BY-SA 3.0, https://commons.wikimedia.org/w/index.php?curid=26590234

4.4.4. Interventional Procedures in the Thorax

The thorax is a very complicated region that often requires to be addressed by an array of interventional techniques to diagnose and manage many conditions. These interventions, like chest drain placements, are also crucial in the management of complications like pleural effusions, which can occur post-operatively or secondary to many diseases. In a study comparing over 590 liver transplant recipients, it was noted that nearly 61% required chest drains within the first 10 days post-surgery, indicating the prevalence of this complication in high-risk patients (Tschanz & Lombardo, 2024). In addition, thoracic interventional radiology entails more than drainage placement; it entails modalities like CT scanning, which has shown an increase in patient utilization among cystic fibrosis patients, and this has prompted issues with cumulative radiation exposure (Mete & Akbudak, 2018). Thus, the growing demand for these interventional procedures necessitates ongoing evaluation of their efficacy and accompanying risks, particularly among vulnerable populations.

4.4.5. Rehabilitation for Thoracic Patients

Effective thoracic patient rehabilitation is of the highest priority in improving their overall QoL, as well as functional mobility. Such rehabilitation is usually holistic, involving multidisciplinary treatment that can be tailored to the specific condition of the patient, such as spinal deformity or neuromuscular diseases. For instance, in idiopathic scoliosis, current guidelines suggest the conjunction of bracing and physiotherapeutic scoliosis-specific exercises (PSSE) to avoid growth progress and to promote postural alignment, with emphasis on evidence-based concepts in therapy (Stefano et al., 2018). Furthermore, in spinal muscular atrophy (SMA) patients, providing a standard of care with orthopedic management and respiratory function is essential to optimize recovery and maintain respiratory health (Mete & Akbudak, 2018). Ultimately, a comprehensive rehabilitation program with physical therapy and patient education can contribute significantly to achieving long-term health and enhancing functional abilities in thoracic patients.

4.4.6. Thoracic Anatomy in Medical Education

Understandings of thoracic anatomy are critical aspects of medical studies because they provide the foundation upon which various conditions in the thoracic cavity are diagnosed and managed. Mastery of this subject allows students to understand the functional relationships between structures such as the lungs, heart, and great vessels, which supports enhanced clinical skills assessment.

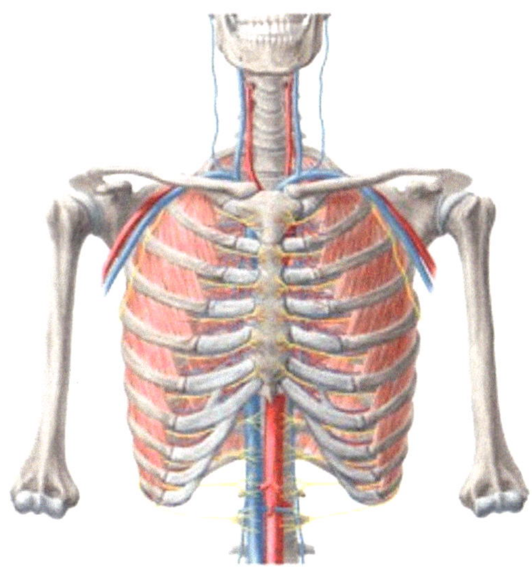

Source: Kenhub. (n.d.). *Muscles, Bones, And Vessels of the Thorax.*

For instance, the anatomy of the thoracic cavity, its musculature, and also its relation to respiratory mechanics are all important when handling respiratory pathologies. In addition, imaging modalities in medicine like X-rays and CT scans are very useful tools in the evaluation of thoracic anatomy. More specifically, newer imaging methods can reveal subtle findings that are not evident on standard examinations (Volckaert et al., 2016). As established by existing studies, the implication of thoracic anatomy extends beyond mere structure to influence locomotion and respiratory performance, thereby indicating its significance in an all-encompassing medical curriculum (Mete & Akbudak, 2018). Appropriate training in this area is important for the next generation of healthcare professionals.

4.4.7. Research Advancements in Thoracic Medicine

Significant breakthroughs in thoracic medicine have arisen from ongoing research that examines both the genetic etiology and surgical techniques associated with thoracic disease. For instance, a greater understanding of the inherited causes of asthma has played an important role in the establishment of treatment strategies focused on afflicted populations, particularly in regions like Pakistan, where asthma is unreasonably widespread. Literature has indicated that over 334 million individuals are afflicted with this condition globally, and genetic vulnerabilities are augmenting the environmental risks of city life (Tschanz & Lombardo, 2024). Also, the study of traumatic diaphragmatic hernias in veterinary medicine indicates that there are advantages to thoracic research as a multidisciplinary field of research. Surgical techniques like repair of diaphragmatic hernia enhance patient outcomes and highlight the demand for continued innovation in intervention approaches. Together, these studies demonstrate how collaborative research activities in thoracic medicine are unlocking the doors to more advanced diagnostic and therapeutic options, ultimately converting into better patient outcomes in diverse settings (Mete & Akbudak, 2018).

4.4.8. Multidisciplinary Approach to Thoracic Care

Effective thoracic care relies heavily on a multidisciplinary team, unifying various specialties in addressing the complexities of lung disease patients. This not only enhances diagnostic accuracy but also treatment outcomes, as specialists collaborate to create tailored treatment plans. For instance, in interstitial lung diseases (ILDs), the role of multidisciplinary conferences becomes evident. As noted, a study found that 71% of patients brought to multidisciplinary discussion received an absolute diagnosis, which indicates the level to which such collaborative care can render dramatic improvement in patient care (Khalifa et al., 2022). Additionally, conditions like Morquio A syndrome highlight the significance of involving multiple healthcare practitioners, e.g., pulmonologists and geneticists, to properly address both skeletal and non-skeletal presentations (Berger et al., 2014). Ultimately, the role of a variety of professionals allows healthcare professionals to deliver complete and holistic care to thoracic patients with complex conditions.

4.4.9. Future Trends in Thoracic Health

Advances in medical technology and science can potentially transform the landscape of thoracic health over the next few years. Perhaps most significantly, the integration of artificial intelligence (AI) into diagnostic imaging has the potential to enhance the accuracy and efficiency of thoracic diseases identification, most significantly in infections like COVID-19, where early detection can have a dramatic effect on outcomes. For instance, it has emerged in recent studies that computer-based image analysis of chest CT could identify pneumonia that indicates severe respiratory infections accurately (Tschanz & Lombardo, 2024). Further, the increasing interest in preventive healthcare, like screening tests to diagnose lung conditions early on, will become more regimented. This is indicated through fresh evidence illustrating extended viral shedding in respiratory illnesses (Chen et al., 2020). Ultimately, the integration of advanced technology and innovation in medicine will usher in a new era for thoracic well-being, equipped with improved patient care and consequent improved clinical outcomes.

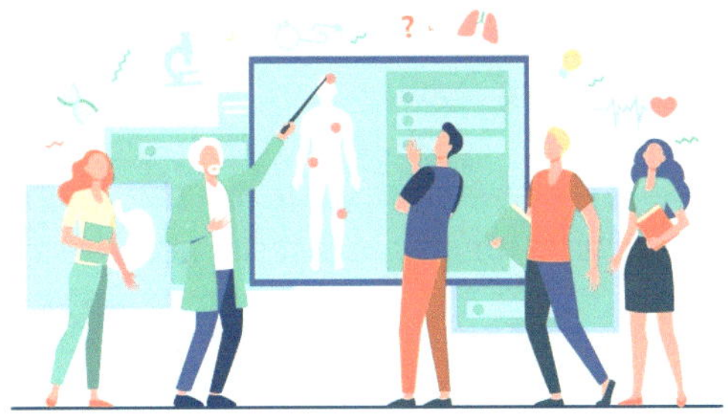

Source: Healthray. (2024). *The Future of Healthcare: Innovations in Hospital Management System Software.*

Test Your Knowledge

1.

SUMMARY

The assessment of the thoracic region shows its complexity and that it is a vital area in various medical conditions. The knowledge of lymphatic drainage from cutaneous melanoma, as discussed byMete & Akbudak (2018), shows the necessity of stringent follow-up treatment, particularly in high-risk patients. This is also a demonstration of the power of metastases to occur beyond expected anatomical areas, thus the necessity to have a systematic approach in follow-up after surgery patients. Besides, the results of infections of the deep neck spaces as described by Tschanz & Lombardo (2024)) illustrate the complicated interaction between the different anatomical sites and the need for multidisciplinary management. In conclusion, the thorax region is a significant site in oncology and infection control management, requiring constant research and clinical focus to improve patient outcomes and minimize complications. Its diversified associated structures and conditions identification are important for clinical treatment and patient education.

Thorax is an indispensable component of the function and health of insects and humans alike and embodies the delicate ballet of form and function. In insects, particularly dipteran flies, the thorax architecture attains a dramatic flight capability by the precise adjustments of their power and steering muscles. Research has confirmed that these flight steering muscles, which constitute fewer than 3% of the total flight muscle mass, utilize nonlinear mechanisms to enhance maneuverability in flight, with the thorax's role in maximizing movement and aerodynamics (Wisser et al., 2014). In humans, however, the thorax plays a critical role in respiratory and cardiovascular health, with its intactness being directly correlated to overall health. The resultant health effect of air quality, for instance, higher mortality caused by PM2.5, demonstrates the importance of a healthy thoracic environment in human beings (Mete & Akbudak, 2018). The thorax region's significance, thus, is not specific to species, emphasizing its universal role of movement, health, and adaptation.

KEY TERMS FROM THIS CHAPTER

- Anatomical recognition systems
- Antero-posterior dimensions
- Cellular metabolism
- Community-acquired pneumonia (CAP)
- Congenital diaphragmatic hernia
- Congestive heart failure (CHF)
- Anisotropic Analytical Algorithm
- Automatic anatomy recognition
- Chronic obstructive pulmonary disease (COPD)
- Computed tomography (CT)
- Congenital thoracic anomalies
- Connective tissue

CRITICAL THINKING QUESTIONS

1. **Which structure encloses and protects the heart and lungs?**
   a. Pelvic girdle
   b. Thoracic cage
   c. Abdominal wall
   d. Vertebral column
2. **Which of the following is NOT a part of the sternum?**
   a. Manubrium
   b. Body
   c. Xiphoid process
   d. Clavicle
3. **How many pairs of ribs are there in the human body?**
   a. 10
   b. 11
   c. 12
   d. 14
4. **Which muscle is the primary muscle of respiration?**
   a. External oblique
   b. Diaphragm
   c. Rectus abdominis
   d. Latissimus dorsi
5. **Which rib is considered the first true rib?**
   a. 7th
   b. 6th
   c. 1st
   d. 12th

Short Answer Questions

1. Describe the anatomical position and function of the diaphragm.
2. What is the mediastinum and what structures does it contain?
3. Which muscle is primarily responsible for inspiration?
4. Describe the position and function of the sternum.
5. What is the role of intercostal muscles during respiration?

Answers to Critical Thinking Questions

1. (b) 2. (d) 3. (c) 4. (b) 5. (c)

REFERENCES

1. Abbott, J. A., Cote, E., Edwards, N. J., Ettinger, S. J., Fuentes, V. L., MacDonald, K. A., Scansen, B. A., & Sisson, D. D. (2015). Management of incidentally detected heart murmurs in dogs and cats. *Journal of Veterinary Cardiology, 17*, 245e261. Elsevier BV. https://core.ac.uk/download/36779155.pdf (accessed on 8th May 2025).
2. Agrawal, V., Udupa, J. K., Tong, Y., & Torigian, D. A. (2020). BRR-Net: A tandem architectural CNN–RNN for automatic body region localization in CT images. *Medical Physics, 47*, 5020–5031. https://doi.org/10.1002/mp.14439.
3. Mete, A., & Akbudak, İ. H. (2018). Functional Anatomy and Physiology of Airway. InTech. doi: 10.5772/intechopen.77037 (accessed on 8th May 2025).
4. Al-Kadi, O. S., & Watson, D. (2008). *Texture Analysis of Aggressive and Nonaggressive Lung Tumor CE CT Images*. Institute of Electrical and Electronics Engineers (IEEE). https://core.ac.uk/download/2709596.pdf (accessed on 8th May 2025).
5. Aston, R. J., & Rylance, J. (2016). *Community-Acquired Pneumonia in Sub-Saharan Africa*. Georg Thieme Verlag KG. https://core.ac.uk/download/74363962.pdf (accessed on 8th May 2025).
6. Ayeni, O. A., Baeyens, A., Kotzen, J. A., Minnaar, C. A., & Vangu, M. D. T. (2019). *Defining Characteristics of Nodal Disease on PET/CT Scans in Patients with HIV-Positive and -Negative Locally Advanced Cervical Cancer in South Africa*. Grapho, LLC. https://core.ac.uk/download/322827598.pdf (accessed on 8th May 2025).
7. Banda, N. P. K., Masekela, R., Mortimer, K., & Rylance, S. (2020). Determinants of lung health across the life course in sub-Saharan Africa. *International Union Against Tuberculosis and Lung Disease, 24*(9). https://core.ac.uk/download/338225918.pdf (accessed on 8th May 2025).
8. Barbero, P., Bidondo, M. P., Gili, J. A., Gimenez, L. G., Groisman, B., Liascovich, R., López Camelo, J. S., & Poletta, F. A. (2016). Geographic clusters of congenital anomalies in Argentina. *J. Community Genet., 8*, 1–7. Springer Science and Business Media LLC. https://core.ac.uk/download/159291453.pdf (accessed on 8th May 2025).
9. Bilardo, C. M., Chaoui, R., Hyett, J., Kagan, K. O., Karim, J., Papageorghiou, A. T., Poon, L. C., Salomon, L., Syngelaki, A., & Nicolaides, K. H. (2023). ISUOG practice guidelines (updated): Performance of 11–14-week ultrasound scan. *Ultrasound in Obstetrics & Gynecology, 61*, 127–143. https://doi.org/10.1002/uog.26106.
10. Canoy, D., Elliott, P., Harju, T., Hartikainen, A. L., Järvelin, M. R., Laitinen, J., Little, M. P., Patel, S. P., Pekkanen, J., Pouta, A., & Rodriguez, A. (2011). Associations between pre-pregnancy obesity and asthma symptoms in adolescents. *BMJ*. https://core.ac.uk/download/371468.pdf (accessed on 8th May 2025).
11. Che, S., Guy, C. L., Jan, N., Rosu-Bubulac, M., Weiss, E., & Zhao, S. (2018). *Evaluation of Image Registration Accuracy for Tumor and Organs at Risk in the Thorax for Compliance with TG 132 Recommendations*. VCU Scholars Compass. https://core.ac.uk/download/232207267.pdf (accessed on 8th May 2025).
12. Ciosi, M., Gitau, J., Masiga, D., Mugasa, C. M., Ndungu, N., & Villinger, J. (2018). Morphological re-description and molecular identification of *Tabanidae* (Diptera) in East Africa. *ZooKeys, 769*, 117–144. Pensoft Publishers. https://core.ac.uk/download/201756320.pdf (accessed on 8th May 2025).

13. Morais, N., & Cruz, J. (2016). The pectoralis minor muscle and shoulder movement-related impairments and pain: Rationale, assessment and management. *Physical therapy in sport : official journal of the Association of Chartered Physiotherapists in Sports Medicine, 17*, 1–13. https://doi.org/10.1016/j.ptsp.2015.10.003(accessed on 8th May 2025).

14. Czymmek, K., Hossler, F., Pauwels, E., Van Hoorebeke, L., Van Loo, D., & Wagner, R. (2010). *High-Resolution Imaging of Kidney Vascular Corrosion Casts with Nano-CT.* Cambridge University Press (CUP). https://core.ac.uk/download/55755127.pdf (accessed on 8th May 2025).

15. Volckaert, E. Vandermeulen, S. Daminet, J.H. Saunders, K. Peremans (2016). *Hyperthyroidism in Cats, Part I: Anatomy, Physiology, Pathophysiology, Diagnosis and Imaging.* Vlaams Diergeneeskundig Tijdschrift, 2016, 85.(accessed on 8th May 2025).

16. De Cock, H., Gielen, I., Kromhout, K., Van Bree, H., & Van Dyck, K. (2012). *Magnetic Resonance and Computed Tomography Imaging of a Carotid Body Tumor in a Dog.* Springer Science and Business Media LLC. https://core.ac.uk/download/55853440.pdf (accessed on 8th May 2025).

17. Dogra, P., Adolphi, N. L., Wang, Z., et al. (2018). Establishing the effects of mesoporous silica nanoparticle properties on *in vivo* disposition using imaging-based pharmacokinetics. *Nature Communications, 9.* https://doi.org/10.1038/s41467-018-06730-z (accessed on 8th May 2025).

18. Donaldson, G., & Wedzicha, J. (2014). *The Causes and Consequences of Seasonal Variation in COPD Exacerbations.* Dove Medical Press Ltd. https://core.ac.uk/download/77003007.pdf (accessed on 8th May 2025).

19. Dorsher, P. The Neuroanatomic Basis of the Acupuncture Principal Meridians. *Nat Prec* (2009). https://doi.org/10.1038/npre.2009.3795.1(accessed on 8th May 2025).

20. Esteva, A., Gholipour, A., Hoh, C. K., et al. (2017). Synthesis of positron emission tomography (PET) images via multi-channel generative adversarial networks (GANs). *Computer Vision and Pattern Recognition.* http://arxiv.org/abs/1707.09747 (accessed on 8th May 2025).

21. Eustace, J. A., Maher, M. M., McGarrigle, A. M., McWilliams, S. R., Mullane, D., O'Connell, O. J., O'Connor, O. J., Plant, B. J., & Shanahan, F. (2012). *Radiologic Imaging in Cystic Fibrosis: Cumulative Effective Dose and Changing Trends Over 2 Decades.* American College of Chest Physicians. https://core.ac.uk/download/160477137.pdf (accessed on 8th May 2025).

22. F Freer, G Ail, T Chan, M Jones, J Broad, G P Canale, P Elston, J Leeney, P Vickerton, 1017 Out With the Old, in With the New? Virtual Reality vs. Cadaveric Based Teaching Materials for Anatomy Education, British Journal of Surgery, Volume 111, Issue Supplement_6, July 2024, znae163.315, https://doi.org/10.1093/bjs/znae163.315 (accessed on 8th May 2025).

23. Georgakopoulos B, Lasrado S. Anatomy, Head and Neck: Inter-scalene Triangle. [Updated 2022 Nov 9]. In: StatPearls [Internet]. Treasure Island (FL): StatPearls Publishing; 2025 Jan-. Available from: https://www.ncbi.nlm.nih.gov/books/NBK544222/ (accessed on 8th May 2025).

24. Ghahremani, G., Horgan, S., Kumar, D., Kunkel, D. C., Mittal, R. K., & Zifan, A. (2020). *Morphology of the Esophageal Hiatus: Is it Different in 3 Types of Hiatus Hernias?* eScholarship, University of California. https://core.ac.uk/download/323065805.pdf (accessed on 8th May 2025).

25. González, C. J. C., Goñi, M. J. M., Martínez, F. J. L., & Villena Román, J. (2005). *MIRACLE's Naive Approach to Medical Images Annotation.* E.T.S.I. Telecomunicación (UPM). http://oa.upm.es/4696/ (accessed on 8th May 2025).

26. Guo, Y., Gur, Y., Madani, A., Moradi, M., & Syeda-Mahmood, T. (2018). *Bimodal Network Architectures for Automatic Generation of Image Annotation from Text.* http://arxiv.org/abs/1809.01610 (accessed on 8th May 2025).

27. Hernández-Dávila, E. R., Torres-García, E., Aranda-Lara, L., Roldán-Valadez, E., Isaac-Olivé, K., & Flores-Reyes, M. (2024). CNN application for automated determination of the patient's size to obtain the size-specific dose estimated in CT. *Scientific Reports, 10.* https://www.semanticscholar.org/paper/1046f95012290d225162a7a632f5fa0c48ebdba4 (accessed on 8th May 2025).

28. Hough, K. P., Curtiss, M. L., Blain, T. J., Liu, R. M., Trevor, J., Deshane, J. S., & Thannickal, V. J. (2020). Airway remodeling in asthma. *Frontiers in Medicine, 7.* https://doi.org/10.3389/fmed.2020.00191.

29. Hraška, V., Hjortdal, V. E., Dori, Y., & Kreutzer, C. (2021). Innominate vein turn-down procedure: Killing two birds with one stone. *JTCVS Techniques, 7,* 253–260. https://doi.org/10.1016/j.xjtc.2021.01.045.

30. Iman, B. N. (2024). *Studi Kasus Perbaikan Traumatic Diaphragmatic Hernia Pada Kucing di Pet First Veterinary Centre, Kuala Lumpur, Malaysia.* Undergraduate thesis, IPB University. https://core.ac.uk/download/622354986.pdf (accessed on 8th May 2025).

31. Jacobs, E. R., Krenz, G. S., Medhora, M., Molthen, R. C., Moulder, J. E., & Wu, Q. (2009). *Imaging Radiation Pneumonitis in a Rat Model of a Radiological Terrorism Incident*. e-Publications@Marquette. https://core.ac.uk/download/213084486.pdf (accessed on 8th May 2025).

32. Kamm, M. (1930). *The Structure, Function, and Pathology of the Thyroid Gland.* Master's thesis, Boston University. https://open.bu.edu/bitstream/2144/7484/1/thestructurefunc00kamm.pdf (accessed on 8th May 2025).

33. Khalifa, A. (2022). *Diagnostic Ability of Multidisciplinary Discussion in Interstitial Lung Diseases and Rare Lung Diseases.* Doctoral dissertation, Christian-Albrechts-Universität Zu Kiel. https://core.ac.uk/download/599598608.pdf (accessed on 8th May 2025).

34. Kim, S. (2022). Anatomical classification and clinical application of thoracic paraspinal blocks. *Korean Journal of Anesthesiology, 75,* 295–306. https://www.semanticscholar.org/paper/89f83857689fabaf81ff8938d4940e3adff9788f (accessed on 8th May 2025).

35. Laurent, G., & Richard, D. (1986). *The Organization and Role During Locomotion of the Proximal Musculature of the Cricket Foreleg: I. Anatomy and Innervation.* The Company of Biologists. https://core.ac.uk/download/4879155.pdf (accessed on 8th May 2025).

36. Litjens, G., Kooi, T., Ehteshami, B. B., Setio, A. A. A., Ciompi, F., Ghafoorian, M., Van Der Laak, J., Van Ginneken, B., & Sánchez, C. I. (2017). A survey on deep learning in medical image analysis. *Medical Image Analysis, 42,* 60–88. https://doi.org/10.1016/j.media.2017.07.005.

37. Lu, Y. C., Yu, S., Fu, C. Y., Bajani, F., Bokhari, M., Mis, J., Poulakidas, S., & Bokhari, F. (2022). Increased intra-abdominal hemorrhage after thoracic endovascular aortic replacement in patients with concomitant blunt aortic injuries and abdominal trauma: A National Trauma Data Bank analysis. *Eur. J. Cardiothorac. Surg., 62*(6), ezac494. https://www.semanticscholar.org/paper/1b3dd64aa055e27f88e42410c09a8611622ec76a.

38. Mayo, P. H., Copetti, R., Feller-Kopman, D., Mathis, G., Maury, É., Mongodi, S., Mojoli, F., Volpicelli, G., & Zanobetti, M. (2019). Thoracic ultrasonography: A narrative review. *Intensive Care Medicine, 45,* 1200–1211. https://doi.org/10.1007/s00134-019-05725-8.

39. Pabst, R. (2020). The pig as a model for immunology research. *Cell and Tissue Research, 380,* 287–304. https://doi.org/10.1007/s00441-020-03206-9.

40. Carol Propper & John A. Rigg, 2006. "**Understanding socio-economic inequalities in childhood respiratory health**," CASE Papers case109, Centre for Analysis of Social Exclusion, LSE. (accessed on 8th May 2025).

41. Rohmann, E. (2008). *Identification of the Molecular Basis of the Lacrimo-Auriculo-Dento-Digital (LADD) Syndrome.* Doctoral dissertation. https://core.ac.uk/download/12010069.pdf (accessed on 8th May 2025).

42. Shome, R., Elbardan, H., & Yazdifar, H. (2023). *Banking Research in the GCC Region and Agenda for Future Research – A Bibliometric Examination.* https://www.semanticscholar.org/paper/97b242d1de00bb19e20f9aaaec932b7d995445a9 (accessed on 8th May 2025).

43. Tschanz, D., & Lombardo, P. (2024). The Ultrasound Analysis of the Most Important Musculoskeletal Issues: Visual presentation of common standard ultrasound imaging techniques in the Musculoskeletal area. (2024). *Swiss Journal of Radiology and Nuclear Medicine, 9*(2), 1-76. https://doi.org/10.59667/sjoranm.v9i2.12(accessed on 8th May 2025).

THORACIC WALL AND BREAST

5

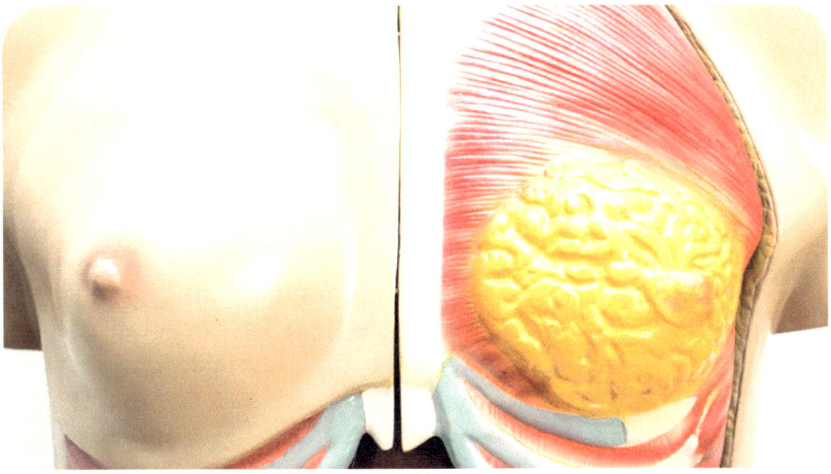

LEARNING OBJECTIVES

After studying this chapter, you will be able to:

1. Discuss the anatomy of the thoracic wall
2. Focus on blood supply to the thoracic wall
3. Explain the innervation of the thoracic wall
4. Know the anatomy of the breast
5. Understand blood supply and innervation of the breast
6. Focus on clinical considerations

Introduction

The human thoracic wall is a complex anatomic structure that protects vital organs such as the heart and lungs, enables respiratory movement, and provides structural support for the upper body. The region is comprised of bone, muscle, cartilage, and connective tissue and plays a fundamental role in physiological stability. Its complex structure enables it to maintain a balance between rigidity and flexibility in a way that it resists any external forces while creating space for the expansion and contraction of the lungs during respiration. The thoracic wall also provides an attachment for muscles involved in upper limb movement and respiration. Understanding the detailed anatomy and function of the thoracic wall is required to appreciate many clinical procedures, including surgical interventions and anesthetic techniques, that are frequently undertaken in this area. The breast, which lies over the anterior thoracic wall, possesses unique anatomical and physiological characteristics that dictate both its function and its liability to disease. Structurally, the breast tissue is made up of glandular tissue, fat tissue, and connective tissue, all of which co-exist within the supportive framework of the breast, the superficial fascia of the thoracic wall. This not only allows for lactation but also integrates with the lymphatic and vascular systems necessary for tissue viability and immune function. The anatomy of the breast in relation to the underlying thoracic wall is also important for both diagnostic and therapeutic interventions, such as imaging and reconstructive surgery. The advancement of ultrasound-guided interventions has improved clinical access to structures in immediate proximity to the thoracic wall, allowing greater accuracy and safety in interventions such as nerve blocks and tumor resections (Luyet et al., 2017).

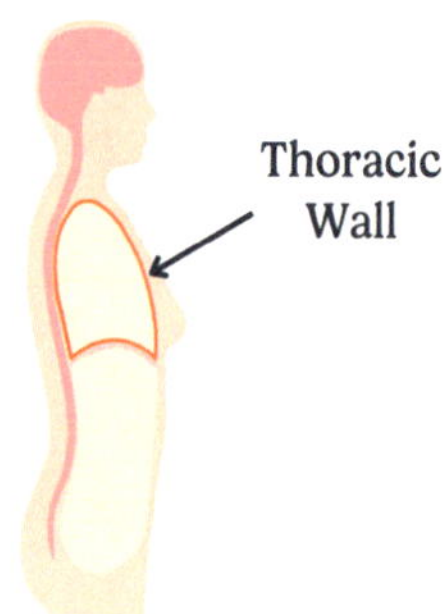

Figure 5.1. The human thoracic wall serves as a complex anatomical framework that protects vital organs.

Source: The Lactation Collection. (2024). *Thoracic Wall Illustration*.

Thoracic wall and breast pathologic disorders may significantly impact patient quality of life (QoL), requiring innovative approaches to management and treatment. Congenital thoracic wall deformities, such as pectus carinatum, highlight the importance of synchronized anatomical and biomechanical considerations. This deformity of abnormal sternum and rib protrusion highlights the challenge of developing a balance between aesthetic and functional outcomes in treatment. Modern interventions, such as orthotics designed especially for women patients, show promise for individualized treatments that honor anatomical distinction and enhance patient satisfaction with corrective results (Mompart et al., 2024). With continued research and technology, the relationship between the integrity of the thoracic wall and breast health continues to be a priority area for the advancement of clinical treatment (Figure 5.1).

Definition of the Thoracic Wall

Its complexity is based on its anatomically layered composition, which besides padding vital thoracic organs acts as a supporting structure to the breast. Basically, the thoracic wall comprises skin, subcutaneous tissue, muscles, bones such as the ribs and the sternum, and fasciae, all working synergistically for mechanical support as well as for the potential to expand during respiration. Fascial layers, i.e., Campers and Scarpa's fasciae have significant roles in determining boundary and internal compartmentalization of chest structures. The breast, lying superficial to the thoracic wall, is anatomically supported by these fascial layers, which envelop mammary glands and fatty pads, creating a discrete breast pocket that maintains breast shape and position over the underlying thorax. An understanding of this functional anatomy is important, particularly in the context of surgical operations, as the composition of the thoracic wall directly affects operations on the breast and accompanying structures (Hall et al., 2024). Apart from offering structural definitions, the anatomical features of the thoracic wall hold considerable clinical importance, primarily in studying the pathology and treatment follow-up of the breast operation. Breast surgical procedures are intimately related to thoracic wall layers, and great caution should be exercised in not compromising the integrity of the chest wall. Emerging evidence indicates that radiotherapy after breast-conserving surgery can pose hazards for very rare but serious complications such as thoracic soft tissue sarcomas. These findings underscore the mechanisms by which treatments on or near the thoracic wall influence secondary cancer risk, underscoring the significance of both the thoracic wall and breast anatomy to post-treatment monitoring and long-term patient care. Such correlations underscore the significance of an accurate anatomical understanding of the thoracic wall in managing and preventing these significant outcomes (Whelan et al., 2023). Embryologically, the wall of the thorax and its accessories, like the breast, come to be due to complex interaction between the mesenchymal and epithelial layers. The mammary glands arise as epidermal invaginations that grow backwards into the fascial matrix of the thoracic wall, i.e., in the fat pads of Campers fascia. This glandular tissue is overlaid by membranous Scarpa's fascia to form anterior and posterior lamellae, which are very important in suspensory support required for anchoring the breast against the thoracic wall. This circummammary ligament formed by Scarpa's fascia is a significant anatomical feature that ensures the mechanical position and functional balance of the breast with respect to the chest. Knowledge of these embryological and anatomical connections is central to the understanding of normal breast form as well as breast illness pathophysiology (Hall et al., 2024).

Importance of the Thoracic Wall in Human Anatomy

Thoracic wall is a vital structural barrier that protects significant organs in the thoracic cavity, including the heart, lungs, and main blood vessels. The mechanical protection provided by this bony and muscular support is complemented by assistance with respiratory function through the facilitation of lung inflation and deflation during breathing. In addition, the thoracic wall also provides points of attachment for muscles involved in upper limb movements and respiration, further emphasizing its multifaceted function. Its intimate association with the breast tissue further delineates its clinical and anatomical importance, as thoracic wall pathology directly influences breast shape and function. Knowledge of the thoracic wall's integrity and biomechanics is therefore essential for healthcare providers to make diagnoses and manage diseases of both thoracic organs and the breast tissue itself (Halvorsen et al., 2022). Clinically, the structures within the thoracic wall , that is, ribs, sternum, and intercostal muscles , bear direct implications for therapeutic and diagnostic treatments of the breast. For example, breast imaging and breast surgical interventions must consider the underlying thoracic anatomy to avoid damage to important structures and to optimize outcomes. Progress in ultrasound technology, such as that proposed by recent multidisciplinary committees, has optimized the ability to assess not just the breast tissue but also the integrity of the thoracic wall, to improve clinical accuracy. These new imaging modalities emphasize the importance of a sound understanding of thoracic anatomy in breast health to distinguish between superficial breast pathology and deeper thoracic abnormalities (Hall et al., 2024). This integration of thoracic and breast imaging is a wonderful example of how anatomy drives effective patient care. Moreover, the biomechanical characteristics of the thoracic wall influence breast morphology and susceptibility to trauma. The rigidity and elasticity of the ribs and their associated muscles create a dynamic platform upon which breast tissue resides and determines its position and form. Any trauma or deformity of the thoracic wall can impact the appearance or function of the breast and have both aesthetic and physiological implications. Additionally, since the thoracic wall contains important neurovascular structures that supply the breast, the integrity of this wall directly affects breast viability and sensitivity. Therefore, the importance of the thoracic wall is not just its protective function; it is vital background support for the anatomy and health of breasts, which emphasizes their interdependence on each other in clinical as well as anatomical contexts (Halvorsen et al., 2022; Hall et al., 2024) (Figure 5.2).

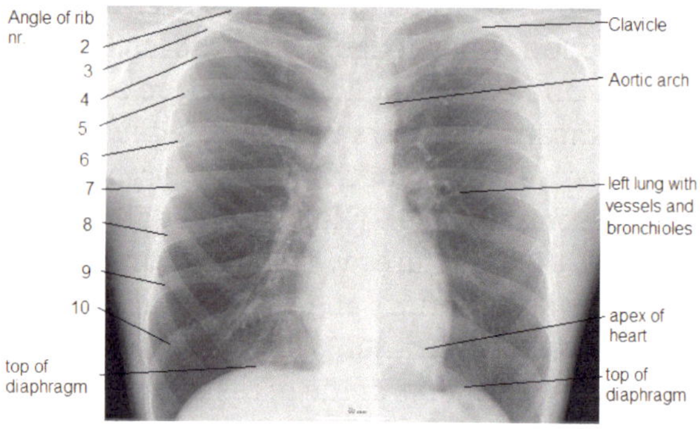

Figure 5.2. The thoracic wall in human anatomy.

Source: By Chikumaya and Mikael Häggström (User:Mikael Häggström) - Image:Chest.png and Essential Clinical Anatomy. K.L. Moore & A.M. Agur. Lippincott, 2 ed. 2002. Page 92, CC BY-SA 3.0, https://commons.wikimedia.org/w/index.php?curid=3415343

Overview of the Breast Structure and Function

Superficial to the pectoral muscles, the breast lies as a preponderance of glandular, fibrous, and fatty tissues closely interrelated to serve its structural and functional purposes. Mammary glands, the essence of breast physiology, are organized in lobes composed of minute lobules in which milk secretion occurs. The lobules are linked via a branching system of ducts that open close to the nipple to facilitate optimum delivery of milk during lactation. Circumjacent connective tissue and fat are used to support and mold, differing greatly from one person to another. Innervation allows for sensory perception and vascular and lymphatic patterns deliver necessary nutrients and offer immunity defense. Multidimensional anatomy is what gives the double role of the breast: as an endocrine-responsive organ and as a special exocrine gland essential for neonatal nutrition. Understanding of this organization is crucial regarding the breast's integration with the thoracic wall and its physiological function (Standring, 2015). The organismic ability of the breast includes more than milk production, dynamically altering in response to hormonal influences that govern tissue morphology and activity. The growth and cyclical alteration of the mammary glands are regulated by estrogen and progesterone, preparing them for potential pregnancy and lactation. During pregnancy, the proliferation of the ducts and proliferation of the alveoli occurs to augment milk production and release, followed by secretion of colostrum during postpartum. Myoepithelial cells around the alveoli operate to contract on oxytocin exposure, allowing the ejection of milk through the ductal system. This functional maturity is complemented by the breast's rich innervation and lymphatic drainage, also providing sensory input and immune surveillance, respectively. The breast thus constitutes a choreographed interaction of cellular, hormonal, and neural components critical to its reproductive function in the broad context of thoracic anatomy (Standring, 2015). The supportive structure of the breast is ensured by specialized connective tissue components in the form of Cooper's ligaments, which suspend the glandular tissue above the dermis and underlying fascia. These fibrous septa contribute to shaping the breast and the mechanical support and adjust volume and tension changes with physiological conditions such as puberty, pregnancy, and senescence. The location of the breast atop the thoracic wall, draping primarily over the pectoralis major muscle and fascia, emphasizes the contribution of musculoskeletal (MSK) support to maintaining form and function. Also, the original blood supply of the breasts mainly via the internal thoracic, lateral thoracic, and intercostal arteries reiterates the breast reliance on the thoracic wall for perfusion. The intimate anatomical relationship underscores the compound nature of the breast as an extension of the chest wall structure, both structural and functional (Standring, 2015).

5.1. Anatomy of the Thoracic Wall

Learning Outcome

1. Discuss the components of the thoracic wall
2. Explain the muscles associated with the thoracic wall
3. Describe the role of the thoracic wall in respiration

It requires an appreciation of the complex interaction between the muscular and skeletal components of the upper torso to have an understanding of thoracic mechanics and their clinical importance. The thoracic wall contains a protective shield over essential organs as well as a foundation for respiratory motion. It is composed primarily of the sternum anteriorly, the 12 sets of ribs anterolaterally, and the thoracic vertebra posteriorly. Muscles such as intercostals, serratus anterior, and pectoralis major overlie these bony elements to facilitate protection and mobility. This multi-layered configuration not only supports respiratory function but also provides an anatomical basis for breast tissue positioning that is superficial to the rib and thoracic wall muscles. This relationship brings to prominence the importance of thoracic wall anatomy in diagnostic imaging and surgery for breast pathology in order to ensure structural integrity under clinical maneuvers (Agnihotri et al., 2016). Beneath superficial skin and muscle, the complex vascular and nervous components are responsible for the functional competence of the thoracic wall and adjacent structures. The intercostal spaces house the neurovascular bundles of arteries, veins, and nerves, which travel just beneath each rib. These bundles provide innervation to the thoracic wall muscles and overlying skin, as well as to the breast tissue, with marked overlap in anatomical territories. Besides, the brachial plexus, an important cluster of nerves emanating from the cervical region, passes through the thoracic outlet, closely related to the upper thoracic wall and shoulder girdle. Advances in imaging and three-dimensional reconstruction techniques have enabled more precise delineation of these nerve tracts, allowing better surgical planning and minimizing iatrogenic injury in thoracic walls and breast procedures (Audenaert et al., 2008). The dynamic nature of the thoracic wall is further highlighted by its involvement in respiratory mechanics and movement of the upper limb, with a direct impact on breast physiology and clinical assessment. The ribs' flexibility, facilitated by costal cartilages and intervertebral joints, accommodates expansion during inspiration and mechanical loads from upper limb motion.

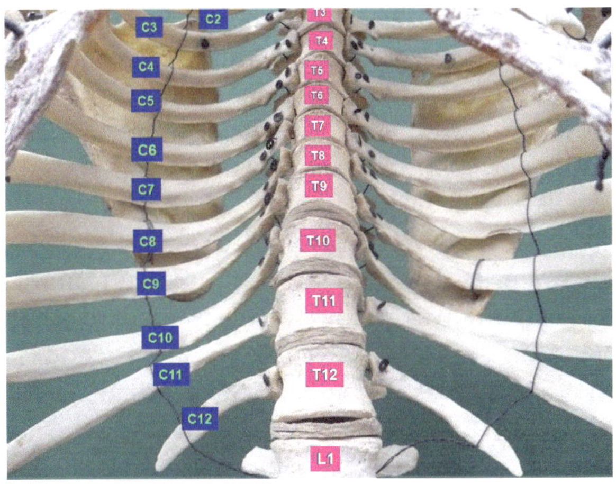

Figure 5.3. Anatomy of the thoracic wall.

Source: By Anatomist90 - Own work, CC BY-SA 4.0, https://commons.wikimedia.org/w/index.php?curid=35277552

This biomechanical interaction influences the position and tension of muscular and nervous structures of the thoracic wall, potentially influencing breast mobility and sensory innervation. Understanding these functional relationships is essential to predict post-surgical outcomes, such as after breast reconstruction or thoracic surgery where nerve preservation must take place to avoid the complications of chronic pain or sensory loss. Thus, synergy between in-depth anatomical knowledge and practice enhances patient management for thoracic and breast disorders (Audenaert et al., 2008; Agnihotri et al., 2016) (Figure 5.3).

5.1.1. Components of the Thoracic Wall

The thoracic wall also serves as a critical protective and structural element of the organs within the thorax consisting of both bony and soft tissue elements that offer support and flexibility. The skeletal framework consists of the thoracic vertebrae in the posterior, the ribs in the lateral, and the sternum anteriorly surrounding a cage-like structure that safeguards vital organs such as the heart and lungs. Intercostal muscles fill the intercostal spaces between ribs to facilitate respiratory movements required in ventilation. Connective tissues and fascia also provide stability and integrity to the thoracic wall. This kind of composite arrangement allows the dynamic increase and decrease of the thoracic cavity with protection guaranteed. An understanding of the minute anatomy of the thoracic wall is important, especially when planning surgical interventions or procedures on related structures such as the brachial plexus, which are affected by positional changes during surgery (Audenaert et al., 2008). Beneath the bony component, the thoracic wall has many layers of muscles that play not only a role in respiratory physiology but also in breast and chest contour and movement. The outer, inner, and innermost intercostal muscles act in a coordinated manner in expanding and depressing the ribs for inspiration and expiration. These are supplemented by the accessory muscles, including the serratus anterior and pectoralis major and minor, which serve to assist with movements of the upper limbs along with stabilizing the shoulder girdle. The neurovascular and vascular components of the thoracic wall, including intercostal veins, arteries, and nerves, run along the ribs within the neurovascular bundles, with an adequate blood supply and sensory innervation. Such a complex relationship among muscular and neurovascular elements is of primary importance in clinical contexts, like regional anesthesia and radiotherapy positioning, where precise anatomical knowledge prevents complications and maximizes therapeutic efficiency (Audenaert et al., 2008). The anterior part of the thoracic wall is particularly significant since it houses the breast, which drapes over the musculature and upper ribs. It consists of several layers: skin, a subcutaneous tissue replete with fat, glandular breast tissue, and deep fascia over the pectoralis major muscle.

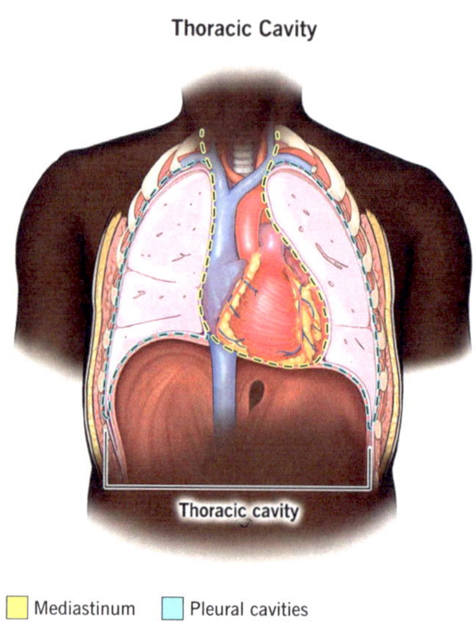

Figure 5.4. Components of the thoracic wall.

Source: Cleveland Clinic. (n.d.). *Thoracic cavity: Illustration of Mediastinum and Pleural Cavities.*

The complex vascularization of the breast is caused principally by branches of the internal thoracic artery and lateral thoracic artery, and lymphatic drainage proceeds in a predictable pattern fundamental to the understanding of metastasis in breast carcinoma. Structural support from the thoracic cage and muscular investment maintains the breast tissue in optimal position for functional and cosmetic considerations. Therapeutic positioning technologies, such as prone and crawl positions with specialized expertise during irradiation, take advantage of the anatomical characteristics of the thoracic walls to improve treatment results with reduced exposure to organs at risk without compromising target coverage (Figure 5.4).

5.1.2. Muscles Associated with the Thoracic Wall

Thoracic wall structural strength and movement basically depend on a complex system of muscles that work together to allow breathing and protect thoracic organs. Under the skin and superficial fascia, intercostal muscles course through the intervals between the ribs and play a central role in the mechanics of breathing. These are three-layered muscles: external, internal, and innermost intercostals, all with specific orientations of fibers that take part in the elevation or depression of the ribs in inspiration and expiration. The external intercostal muscles play a primary role in elevating the ribs to expand the thoracic cavity, while the internal and innermost ones contribute to rib depression to aid in forced expiration. In addition, accessory muscles such as the serratus anterior and subclavius provide stability and movement to the thoracic cage. One should appreciate the dynamic function of these muscles when taking into consideration the respiratory function of the thoracic wall and its interaction with adjacent anatomical structures, including the breast (Georgakopoulos & Lasrado, 2022). Furthermore, the muscular support of the thoracic wall is enhanced by the pectoral muscles, which not only play a role in the movement of the upper limb but also influence thoracic mechanics. The pectoralis major muscle is a large fan-shaped muscle that originates on the clavicle, sternum, and ribs and attaches to the humerus to facilitate movements such as arm flexion, adduction, and medial rotation. Deep to it lies the pectoralis minor, which stabilizes the third to fifth ribs to the scapula's coracoid process, and assists in scapular stabilization and minor rise of the ribs in deep breathing. These muscles are intimately associated with the anterior thoracic wall and overlie important neurovascular elements supplying the breast.

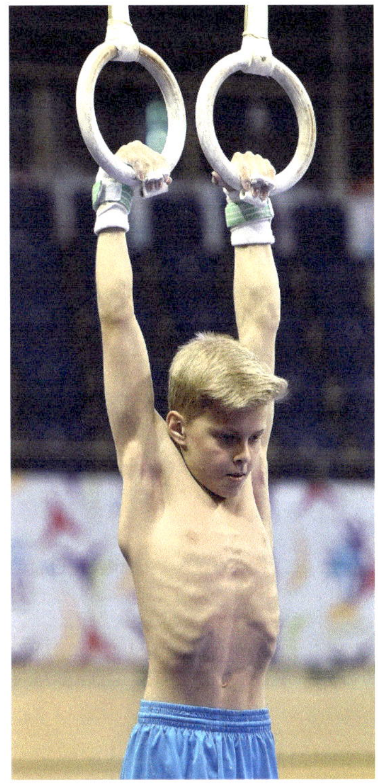

Figure 5.5. Muscles associated with the thoracic wall.

Source: By Martin Rulsch, Wikimedia Commons, CC BY-SA 4.0, CC BY-SA 4.0, https://commons.wikimedia.org/w/index.php?curid=62725717

Their close anatomical proximity and functional connection to each other point towards the complexity of the thoracic wall musculature, engaging them in chest and breast wall surgery and clinical pathology (Iqbal & Harahap, 2021). Other muscles such as the subcostal, transversus thoracis, and serratus posterior muscles have definite roles within the muscular complex of the thoracic wall. The subcostal muscles, on the inside of the lower ribs, facilitate the depression of the ribs during expiration, while the transversus thoracis muscles, which are placed in the front wall of the thorax, facilitate reducing the volume of the thoracic cavity by pulling the ribs downward. Serratus posterior muscles, made up of both superior and inferior parts, assist respectively in raising and depressing the ribs and thus contribute respectively to the period of inspiration and expiration. These muscles, though less prominent in respiration than the intercostals or pectoral muscles, contribute individually as well as collectively to the fine control of thoracic expansion, the protected innervation of internal organs, and provide a critical basis for the support of breast tissue as well as surgical landmarks (Iqbal et al., 2021; Georgakopoulos & Lasrado, 2022) (Figure 5.5).

5.1.3. Role of the Thoracic Wall in Respiration

The complex structure of the thoracic wall contributes to the respiratory mechanics by providing a rigid, albeit pliable, enclosure containing essential organs and making space for the expansion of the lungs. The rib cage, intercostal muscles, and associated connective tissues form the thoracic wall and are jointly responsible for producing the dynamic alterations in the thoracic volume required for respiration. On inspiration, the external intercostal muscles contract, elevating the ribs and expanding the thoracic cavity, thereby decreasing intrathoracic pressure and allowing air to flow into the lungs. The coordinated motion emphasizes the role of the biomechanical characteristics of the thoracic wall in breathing, allowing for efficient ventilation without sacrificing protection for the breasts and underlying structures (Georgakopoulos & Lasrado, 2022). Of equal importance is the structural relationship between the breast and the thoracic wall, with the wall acting as a supportive base essential for both physiological and mechanical functions. Anatomical research highlights that the rigidity and elasticity of the thoracic wall directly affect not only respiratory efficiency but also the positioning and mobility of the breast. The relationship between the thoracic muscles and the breast tissue that overlies them can impact respiratory dynamics, as the changing volume of the thorax during breathing subtly shifts the breast contour and tension. The relationship gives insight into the reason for such detailed knowledge of thoracic anatomy being necessary for medical education, as evidenced by ongoing efforts to internationalize core anatomical knowledge for clinical relevance (Loukas et al., 2020). Moreover, the structural integrity of the thoracic wall is critical in maintaining optimum respiratory mechanics, particularly in pathologic conditions that compromise its structure. Trauma, congenital deformities, or thoracic wall surgery may disrupt the synchronized movement of the ribs and adjacent muscles and thereby interfere with efficient ventilation. This bargain not only risks pulmonary function but also compromises the aesthetic and biomechanical support of the breast, demonstrating the interconnectedness of these anatomical spaces. Detailed anatomical education and clinical awareness are necessary to manage both respiratory and breast pathology, emphasizing the thoracic wall's dual role of protection and function within the human body (Loukas et al., 2020; Georgakopoulos & Lasrado, 2022).

Test Your Knowledge

1. What are the main structural components of the thoracic wall?
2. How does the thoracic wall contribute to the process of respiration?

5.2. Blood Supply to the Thoracic Wall

Learning Outcome

1. Discuss Major Arteries Supplying the Thoracic Wall
2. Understand Venous Drainage of the Thoracic Wall
3. Explain Importance of Blood Supply in Surgical Procedures

The complex vascular supply to the thoracic wall is essential to the function and integrity of the thorax and the breast tissue. The intercostal arteries, which are branches of the internal thoracic arteries and thoracic aorta , supply the thoracic wall with blood . These arteries run parallel to the ribs and supply blood to the skin and muscles. The anterior perforating branches, as they arise from the internal thoracic artery, are of utmost significance in the cutaneous vascularization of the breast skin. It is particularly important to maintain these branches during surgical intervention of the breast and thoracic wall because injury to them may cause necrosis of the tissue. For example, the significance of preservation of anterior perforating branches is noted in nipple-sparing mastectomy to limit postoperative necrosis as well as to yield the best possible surgical outcome (Amanti et al., 2015). The knowledge of arterial supply of the thoracic wall is fundamental with special consideration given to plastic or reconstructive breast surgeries. Anatomical studies have determined that there are more arterial perforators in specific regions of the thoracic wall, with direct surgical planning implications. Notably, the internal mammary perforator arteries, the most frequent location being the second intercostal space, provide a considerable source of blood supply to the upper inner quadrant of the breast. Data indicate that nearly half of the perforators of the arteries are located in this quadrant, with overall lower quadrats as a whole having the greatest vascular supply. Such accurate topography emphasizes the individualization of surgical techniques to maintain robust circulatory flow and avoid vascular pedicle compromise (López-de-Celis et al., 2024). The surgical importance of the vascular anatomy of the thoracic walls extends beyond mastectomy to a wide range of thoracic and breast surgery.

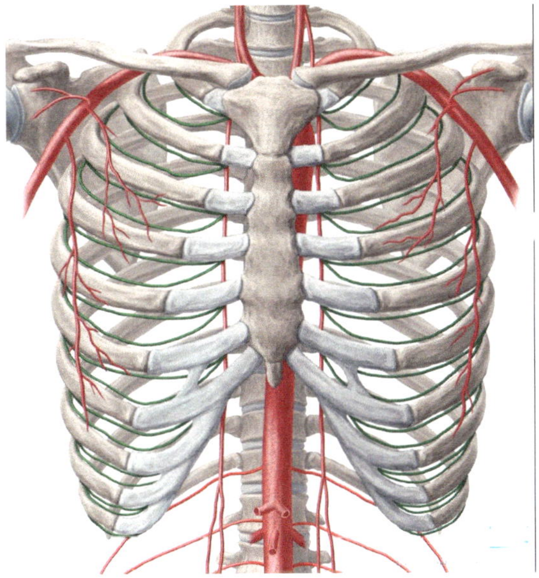

Figure 5.6. Blood supply to the thoracic wall.

Source: Kenhub. (n.d.). *Intercostal Arteries and Veins.*

Regardless of performing reduction mammoplasty or reconstructive surgeries, surgeons must be careful with the vascular territories to ensure tissue viability and prevent ischemic complications. Preservation of the nipple-areola complex (NAC) vascularization, based mainly on the anterior perforating branches and the internal mammary perforators, is very critical. It has been demonstrated that careful preoperative planning of the operation, e.g., localization of the incision in the inframammary fold or periareolar areas, can reduce total or segmental NAC necrosis rates. Thus, well-established knowledge of the thoracic wall vascular supply not only enhances the results of the operation but also provides a ground for minimizing postoperative complications of vascular insufficiency (Amanti et al., 2015; López-de-Celis et al., 2024) (Figure 5.6).

5.2.1. Major Arteries Supplying the Thoracic Wall

The thoracic wall is supplied with blood, which serves an important function in physiological processes and surgical procedures, especially during breast surgery. Blood is supplied to the thoracic wall from cervical and intercostal arteries, and their primary function is to maintain oxygenation and delivery of nutrients to the skin, muscles, and interior tissues. Of all the vessels, the internal thoracic artery plays a central role in the sense that it courses with the sternum and gives rise to anterior intercostal branches that supply the anterior chest wall. Preservation of these branches in oncologic procedures such as nipple-sparing mastectomies is important since they contribute to the vascularization of the skin and NAC as well. Involvement of these arteries can lead to such complications as necrosis, attesting to the delicate balance that needs to be reached by surgeons between tumor extirpation and preservation of functional blood supply (Amanti et al., 2015). Except for the internal thoracic artery, the intercostal and lateral thoracic arteries contribute significantly to the arterial blood supply of the thoracic wall. The lateral thoracic artery, which is a branch of the axillary artery, courses along the lateral chest, supplying the serratus anterior muscle and overlying tissues. Intercostal arteries, which originate from the thoracic aorta, course through the intercostal spaces and are the arteries which vascularize the intercostal muscles and overlying tissue with branches to the breast in females. This extensive supply network highlights the complexity of thoracic wall vasculature and its relevance to clinical interventions, including breast reconstruction and image-guided procedures aimed at assessing vascular structures (Jesinger et al., 2014). It is necessary to understand the spatial distribution and anatomical variability of these arteries to achieve successful surgical outcomes and minimize postoperative complications. Imaging modalities such as contrast-enhanced MRI allow detailed visualization of the arterial supply, assisting in planning interventions that preserve critical blood supply. Intercommunication between the intercostal arteries, lateral thoracic artery, and internal thoracic artery allows a good anastomotic plexus that can take over in regional interruption but must also have the correct surgical technique to avoid ischemic injury. This vascular network also supports both the thoracic musculature and the delicate breast tissue pattern, underlining the importance of knowing specific anatomy to carry out both reconstructive and oncological breast surgery (Jesinger et al., 2014; Amanti et al., 2015).

5.2.2. Venous Drainage of the Thoracic Wall

The circulatory system within the thoracic cavity is well-organized to facilitate structural and functional requirements, where venous return plays a key role in the maintenance of tissue homeostasis. Venous return from the thoracic wall occurs primarily through a network of superficial and deep veins that replicate the course of the arteries to accommodate efficient blood return into the heart. This venous network includes the anterior and posterior intercostal veins, which are significant channels for draining blood from the intercostal spaces. The anterior intercostal veins empty into the internal thoracic vein, while the posterior intercostal veins empty into the azygos venous system. This arrangement supports collateral circulation, which is able to adapt to variations in venous pressure and flow. Their structural connection to surrounding tissue is significant in the context of the thoracic wall general physiology and the resulting implications for breast vascularization and procedures (Agnihotri et al., 2016).

Deep venous pathways of the thoracic wall communicate with greater vessels essential to cardiovascular wellness, connecting thoracic venous networks to the superior vena cava system. The azygos venous system, including the accessory hemiazygos and hemiazygos veins, is specifically important to posterior thoracic wall drainage, providing an ancient embryologic and anatomical route for the return of blood. Venous drainage along the anterior surface of the thorax is secondarily aided significantly by the internal thoracic vein, in tandem with the internal thoracic artery. This vein also receives tributaries from the venous plexus of the breast and thoracic wall, showing the interdependence of venous drainage between the two regions. Familiarity with this venous anatomy is important in operative planning, especially in thoracic wall and breast surgeries, where incidental injury to these veins can result in severe complications or compromise blood supply (Agnihotri et al., 2016). Because of the reciprocal anatomic adjacency and interconnected vascular pathways, the venous drainage of the thoracic wall is clinically directly relevant to breast disease and treatment. The venous drainage of the breast typically parallels its arterial supply and lymphatic drainage, with venous paths coursing deep into the thoracic wall veins to facilitate efficient outflow of blood. Varying communication between superficial and deep venous channels in this region demands careful consideration during diagnostic imaging and surgery. Imaging techniques like contrast-enhanced MRI and nuclear medicine lymphoscintigraphy rely on a strong understanding of this venous anatomy to avoid misinterpretation and to guide effective, safe treatment planning. Because the vascular anatomy of the breast is intimately associated with thoracic wall veins, venous compromise will influence tissue perfusion and surgical success in oncologic resections or breast reconstruction (Jesinger et al., 2014).

5.2.3. Importance of Blood Supply in Surgical Procedures

Successful surgical results in the thoracic wall and breast region significantly depend on the meticulous preservation and optimization of blood supply. The integrity of the vasculature is crucial in ensuring tissue viability, particularly when reconstructive techniques like chest wall perforator flaps are employed. The flaps rely on large perforators from arteries like the lateral thoracic, anterior intercostal, and lateral intercostal arteries to supply nutrition to grafted segments of tissue. The significance of this vascular supply cannot be overstated, as poor perfusion can lead to flap necrosis, delayed healing, and infection. In addition, the strategic incorporation of several perforators in the design of flaps increases perfusion and flap survival, demonstrating the versatility of surgical planning to patient-specific vascular anatomy. This technique has been validated in recent clinical studies, which underscore low complication rates and excellent patient satisfaction when large perforators are adequately preserved in oncoplastic breast-conserving surgery (Xie et al., 2025). Other than the viability of a flap, blood supply quality influences postoperative recovery and aesthetic outcomes in breast surgery. Accurate perfusion facilitates aggressive wound healing, reducing the incidence of fibrosis and capsular contracture, which are common complications affecting both function and aesthetics. For instance, fat grafting procedures, which are widely used to restore deformities and tighten the skin in breast and thoracic wall surgeries, are dependent on recipient site vascularization to ensure graft survival and integration. An inefficient blood supply jeopardizes the regenerative potential of fat tissue, leading to fat resorption and suboptimal cosmetic results. Operative planning must thus include steps aimed at maintaining or enhancing regional blood supply, e.g., postoperative interventions such as physiotherapy that facilitate tissue healing by regulating inflammation and stimulating circulation (Alves et al., 2024). Such a holistic vision of blood supply maximizes functional and aesthetic results. Furthermore, awareness and application of the vascular anatomy of the thoracic region are oncologic assurance and surgical precision. Adequate blood flow around the NAC and areas of resection allow surgeons to achieve negative margins while preserving tissue viability. This is a critical equilibrium for tumor management and reconstruction, as illustrated by operations that spare the NAC using well-vascularized flaps for breast conservation. Integrating intraoperative diagnostics, such as frozen section results, with anatomic data of perforator location optimizes margins and minimizes ischemic complications. The innovation is an indicator of the shift in the relevance of blood supply concerns in advancements in surgery to limit morbidity and improve survival and cosmetic outcomes in patients with thoracic and breast operations (Xie et al., 2025).

Test Your Knowledge

1. Which veins are primarily involved in the venous drainage of the thoracic wall?
2. Why is knowledge of thoracic wall blood supply important in surgical procedures like mastectomy or thoracotomy?

5.3. Innervation of the Thoracic Wall

Learning Outcome

1. Discuss the Nerves Involved in the Thoracic Wall
2. Explain the Sensory and Motor Functions of Thoracic Nerves
3. Focus on Clinical Significance of Thoracic Nerve Damage

The complexity of innervation of the thoracic wall is an integral part of understanding its sensory and motor functions, which are essential for respiration as well as defense of the organs beneath. The primary innervation is provided by the intercostal nerves, which are the anterior rami of the thoracic spinal nerves T1 to T11. These nerves run in the costal groove of every rib, innervating motor to the intercostal muscles and sensory branches to the superficial skin and parietal pleura. The subcostal nerve, which originates from T12, also provides the innervation to the lower thoracic and upper abdominal walls. This complex network of neurons offers coordinated muscular function for respiration and transmits sensory information necessary for pain, temperature, and touch perceptions. The joint function of these nerves is particularly crucial in surgery of the thoracic wall and breast, where unintended nerve damage can lead to complications. Besides the intercostal nerves, the thoracic wall is also innervated with autonomic innervation that further refines the regulation of vascular tone and sweat glands to contribute to the homeostasis of the skin and musculature. Sympathetic fibers accompany the intercostal nerves and have vasomotor and sudomotor functions to control skin temperature and wetness. Parasympathetic inputs, though not so prominent, are indirectly activated via the vagus nerve and influence thoracic organ activity regulation. Dermatomal spread of intercostal nerves is clinically significant in determining the pattern of sensory loss or pain following thoracic injury or surgery. Accurate understanding of this pattern provides support to clinicians for diagnosing referred pain or impairment of nerve conditions, particularly in thoracic wall reconstruction and breast surgery (Raikos et al., 2011). The nervous system of the thorax, thus, is a delicate interaction between the somatic and autonomic components vital for the functional integrity of the area. The clinical application of thoracic innervation of the wall goes as far as complications management and postoperative recovery, particularly in breast surgery such as mastectomy. Disruption or damage to an intercostal nerve during surgical dissection can result in chronic pain syndromes or loss of sensation, which significantly affect patient QoL. Effective postoperative management methods, such as the utilization of continuous suction drainage, have been discovered to reduce complications such as seroma production and flap necrosis, indirectly maintaining nerve function through tissue integrity and healing (Hall et al., 2024). Therefore, accurate knowledge of thoracic wall innervation forms the basis of surgical intervention to preserve nerve integrity to provide a balance between oncologic control and preservation of function and avoid nerve damage in favor of optimal outcome (Figure 5.7). This intersection of anatomy and clinic highlights nerve preservation in ensuring the quality of recovery and preventing morbidity of surgery in thoracic wall and breast interventions.

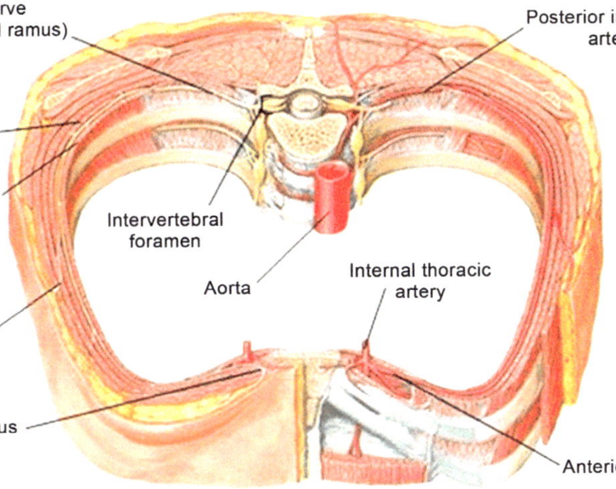

Figure 5.7. Innervation of the thoracic wall.

Source: Thoracickey. (2016). *Intercostal Space Anatomy – Transverse Section*.

5.3.1. Nerves Involved in the Thoracic Wall

The complex anatomy of the thoracic wall requires a complete understanding of its neural elements, which are central to sensory as well as motor functions. Peripheral nerves that arise from the brachial plexus and intercostal nerves supply the thoracic wall, controlling the contraction of muscles and conveying cutaneous sensations. The brachial plexus, with its complex cluster of nerve fibers, has been well investigated by employing sophisticated three-dimensional reconstruction methods to examine its morphology and mechanical properties. Such investigations demonstrate that nerve orientation and stretching, particularly in the lateral and medial roots, have a considerable impact on thoracic nerve function affecting movement and sensation. Such detailed anatomical mapping provides better clinical intervention, including anesthetic blocks and surgeries that involve precise knowledge of nerve courses along the thoracic region (Audenaert et al., 2008). Such information becomes critical while designing interventions involving the breast and thoracic wall to avoid unnecessary nerve damage. Thoracic wall motor innervation is provided primarily by intercostal nerves, which have their origin in the anterior rami of thoracic spinal nerves. They serve a dual purpose: motor supply to the intercostal muscles, which are necessary for respiratory mechanics, and sensory innervation to the overlying skin and the parietal pleura. Every intercostal nerve travels within the costal groove of the rib, providing segmental innervation that is responsible for the thoracic walls' functional integrity and protective sensory input. Taking their anatomy course into consideration, these nerves are vulnerable during surgeries such as mastectomy or thoracic wall reconstruction, where care must be taken during dissection to prevent nerve damage. Damage to these nerves may result in postoperative morbidity in the form of pain, sensory impairment, or impaired respiratory movements and underscores the need to appreciate their function in clinical practice. The clinical relevance of thoracic wall nerve preservation is emphasized in breast surgery, where postoperative morbidity such as seroma formation and flap necrosis is influenced by surgical technique and nerve management. Advanced drainage techniques intended to prevent fluid accumulation and injury to tissues have improved the outcomes of recovery, but such treatments must be weighed against the need for thoracic nerve preservation, particularly intercostobrachial nerve preservation, which is sacrificed when lymph nodes are dissected. Preservation of the nerves during surgeries not only decreases sensory deficits but also enhances QoL during the postoperative period. Understanding the correlation between surgical technique and nerve anatomy enables individualized techniques that minimize complications while enabling oncological clearance (Hall et al., 2024). Thus, integrating anatomical data concerning thoracic wall nerves into clinical strategies remains imperative in a bid to achieve maximum functional and therapeutic outcomes in breast surgery.

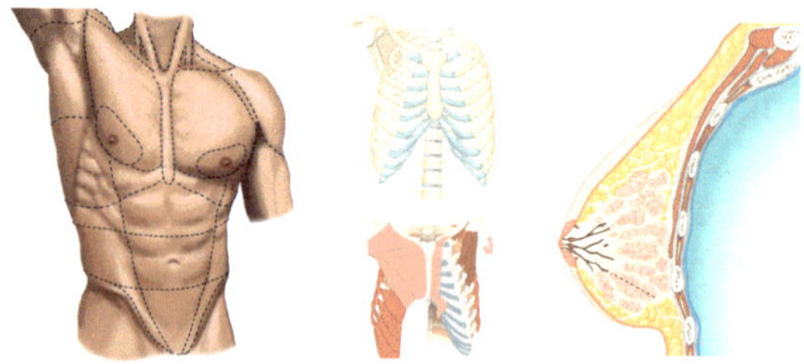

Source: IMAIOS. (n.d.). *Thoracic Wall and Breast Anatomy Illustration.*

5.3.2. Sensory and Motor Functions of Thoracic Nerves

Thoracic nerves are accountable for integrating sensory and motor functions within the thoracic wall and breast that underpin protective and functional mechanisms. Thoracic nerves originate from the spinal cord, dividing into dorsal and ventral rami, and the ventral rami form the intercostal nerves. Each intercostal nerve provides a specific thoracic dermatome with cutaneous sensation to the thoracic wall and skin of the breast. In addition to their sensory role, they have motor fibers that innervate the intercostal muscles responsible for respiration. The sensory carries pain, temperature, and light touch information, which is critical for the appreciation of injury or pathological processes in the thoracic organs. Therefore, the cooperative sensory and motor function of thoracic nerves is the foundation for the sophisticated interaction between movement and sensation in the sophisticated processes that provide respiratory efficiency and protective reflexes in the thoracic cavity. Thoracic motor innervation is essential to the maintenance of the mechanical integrity of the thoracic wall through the modulation of intercostal musculature and associated musculature with precise control. These motor fibers induce muscle contraction that contributes to rib cage expansion with inspiration and to effective ventilation directly. The thoracic nerves also innervate accessory muscles employed in forceful breathing, thereby facilitating adaptive responses to physiological stress. In the breast, motor innervation is not so prominent; however, the nerves are involved in the autonomic regulation of the smooth muscle fibers in the nipple and areolar region, which is critical for reflex actions such as nipple erection in response to stimulus. These motor roles emphasize the double function of thoracic nerves both in voluntary as well as in involuntary muscle control, indicating their increased role in the thoracic wall and breast physiology. Sensory modalities carried on thoracic nerves extend beyond simple touch, and an active function in visceral and somatic mechanisms of communication have an impact on gastrointestinal and systemic homeostasis. Recent data demonstrate that thoracic sensory pathway neurotransmitters and neuromodulators, such as glutamate, play a central role in mediating sensory transmission affecting local tissue as well as central neuroimmune transactions across the microbiota-gut-brain axis. This two-way communication pathway indicates the clinical importance of thoracic nerve sensory function in modulating nearby thoracic structures and controlling systemic responses to gut and brain health (Baj et al., 2019). The understanding of these complex sensory networks extends the knowledge base of thoracic nerve involvement in pathophysiological disease and provides potential targeted therapeutic opportunities that utilize neuroactive molecules for sensory dysfunction of thoracic region-related disorders (Alessandro et al., 2015).

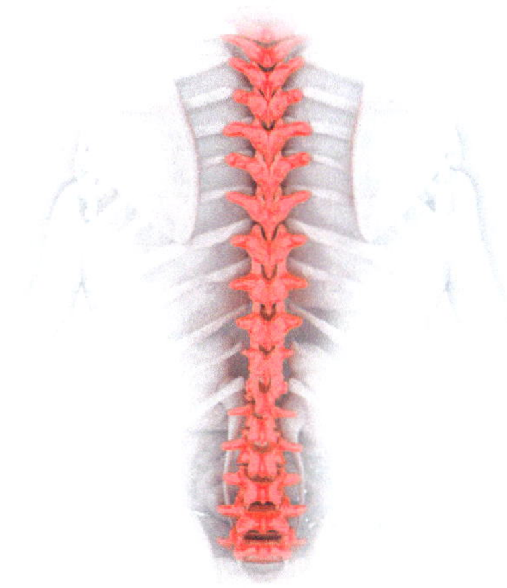

Source: iStock. (n.d.). *3D Illustration of Human Spine Isolated.*

5.3.3. Clinical Significance of Thoracic Nerve Damage

The complex anatomy of the breast and thoracic wall involves a complex interaction of nerves responsible for sensory sensation as well as motor function. Damage to these thoracic nerves, particularly during surgeries such as mastectomy or thoracic surgery, can have severe clinical implications. Preservation and identification of these nerves is one of the key difficulties in thoracic surgery to prevent postoperative complications. The intercostobrachial nerve, for example, plays a critical role in innervation of the chest and arm. Its iatrogenic injury during surgery for mastectomy later results in sensory loss, chronic pain, or neuropathic syndromes. Knowledge of the detailed anatomy and identification of variance between these branches of nerves are therefore essential to surgeons since they have a direct influence on patient QoL as well as postoperative recovery (Smith et al., 2015). Post-mastectomy pain syndrome (PMPS) provides a dramatic illustration of the clinical implications of thoracic nerve injury. PMPS is a chronic neuropathic pain disorder that frequently occurs in women undergoing breast cancer surgery and is extremely linked to intercostobrachial nerve injury. Recent clinical studies emphasize that preserving this nerve during surgery significantly reduces the incidence and severity of PMPS. Patients with intact intercostobrachial nerve function are less painful and have fewer sensory deficits compared to patients with transected nerves. Additionally, knowledge of anatomical variations of this nerve is crucial, as it directs the surgical procedure and nerve-sparing techniques, enhancing postoperative outcomes and reducing long-term morbidity (Chayampurath et al., 2017). Besides sensory defects, thoracic nerve damage can result in motor function and structural integrity defects of the breast and thoracic wall. Thoracic nerve damage can result in paralysis or weakness of muscles, impairing respiratory mechanics and upper limb motion. These functional defects not only affect physiological processes but also have psychological as well as rehabilitative consequences for the patient. Therefore, sound integration of the anatomy of thoracic nerves and clinical significance is vital in patient counseling and surgical planning. Integration of anatomical detail with clinical experience helps to ensure the facilitation of reduction in nerve injury and overall better results in thoracic and breast surgeries (Smith et al., 2015; Chayampurath et al., 2017).

Test Your Knowledge

1. Which nerves are primarily responsible for innervating the thoracic wall?
2. What are the sensory and motor functions of the intercostal nerves in the thoracic region?
3. What clinical issues can arise from damage to thoracic nerves, such as intercostal nerve injury?

5.4. Anatomy of the Breast

Learning Outcome

1. Describe the Structure of Breast Tissue
2. Explain the Location and Significance of Mammary Glands
3. Understand Role of Connective Tissue in Breast Support

Understanding the complex organization of the anatomical layers in the anterior thoracic wall is necessary to understand the structural intricacy of the breasts. The breast is superficially placed over the thoracic wall, and superficial fatty tissue and membranous layers such as Campers fascia and Scarpas fascia play a crucial role. These fasciae develop from the anterior body wall and assist in defining the boundaries and internal architecture of the breast. Specifically, the glandular tissue of the mammary, or corpus mammae in an operative sense, is enclosed by a membrane-lined structure and is not diffused throughout the breast. This bank of glandular tissue is ensconced in the mammary fat pad, which itself is more than likely derived from Campers fascia, and Scarpas fascia covers this pad and forms demarcated anterior and posterior laminae. This two-layering permits not only the aesthetic contour but also functional compartmentalization of the breast against the thoracic wall, so that structural support and mobility are provided relative to underlying muscles (Hall et al., 2024). The relationship of the breast to its suspensory mechanism further demonstrates the coordination of connective tissues in sustaining breast position. Suspensory ligaments have been classically defined as direct cutaneous attachments but may be better defined as retinaculae cutis spanning the deep fascial planes. These fibrous bands run from the anterior and posterior lamellae of Scarpas fascia, suspending the breast from the chest wall but not attached to the overlying skin. This arrangement allows for dainty movement of the breast in relation to the chest while giving mechanical support that resists gravity. This anatomical precision highlights the subtle relationship between superficial fascia and connective tissue in disease and health, e.g., breast ptosis or during surgical interventions. The knowledge of these fascial inputs is essential during surgical planning and understanding breast biomechanics (Hall et al., 2024).

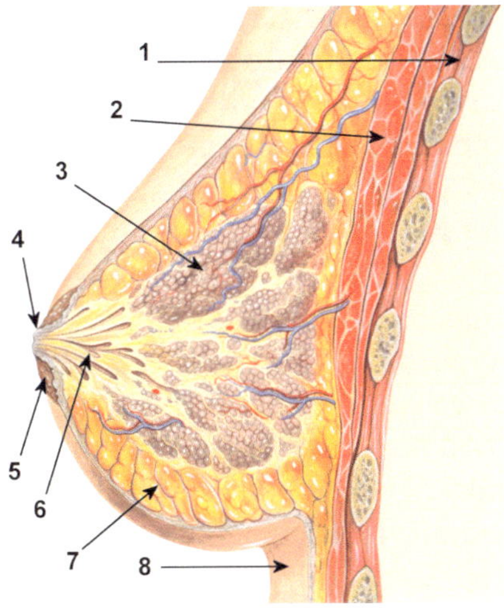

Figure 5.8. Anatomy of the breast.

Source: By Original author: Patrick J. Lynch. Reworked by Morgoth666 to add numbered legend arrows. - Patrick J. Lynch, medical illustrator, CC BY 3.0, https://commons.wikimedia.org/w/index.php?curid=2676813

The vascular anatomy of the breast and its positional relevance to thoracic structures are strongly interconnected for both physiological and clinical reasons. Though outside the breast proper, thoracic arterial branch abnormalities can influence local anatomy and surgical technique. Such anomalies of vascular structures as a retroesophageal right subclavian artery demonstrate the variability and complexity of arteries traversing the thoracic wall. These artery patterns influence not only adjacent fascial and muscular tissues but also condition the blood supply to the breast through branches such as the internal thoracic artery and intercostal arteries. The detail of embryonic and morphologic knowledge of the arteries contributes to a complete understanding of thoracic and breast anatomy and assists practitioners in avoiding potential pitfalls when performing procedure or diagnostic imaging in the chest and breast region (Figure 5.8).

5.4.1. Structure of Breast Tissue

The breast's complex architecture is a consequence of both its embryological development and integration into the thoracic wall. Mammary glandular tissue, instead of the conventional anatomical descriptions of a haphazard distribution, is actually localized to a single membrane-bound central structure known as the corpus mammae. This organization is contrary to past models of anatomy in emphasizing a compact glandular core surrounded by specialized fascial layers. The superficial Camper's fascia and deep Scarpa's fascia, which are the large components of the anterior thoracic body wall, play crucial functions in shaping the breast's structure. In embryogenesis, the mammary gland invaginates into the integument and is covered by these connective tissues to create a supportive fat pad and membranous lamellae that develop the breast's typical pocket-like configuration. These structural findings highlight the breast as an integrated, discrete unit and not as a tissue mass in a non-specific form, foregrounding the importance of fascial boundaries to provide breast integrity (Hall et al., 2024). Posterior fixation of the breast also brings into focus its complex relationship with the thoracic wall. Scarpa's fascia, extending from the anterior body wall, forms a circummammary ligament that is a stabilizing framework for the breast, supporting it securely but elastically against the chest wall. This ligamentous framework not only provides physical support for the breast but also permits its movement relative to the underlying ribs and musculature to facilitate necessary physiological and positional changes. Also, suspensory ligaments, traditionally classically thought to be attached to the skin directly, are actually retinaculae cutis to the fascial lamellae, and these ligaments permit uniform distribution of tension without violating the integrity of the skin. This anatomical specificity highlights the capacity of the breast to maintain both shape and function as it adapts to dynamic mechanical stresses within thoracic life (Hall et al., 2024). Knowledge of the structural dynamics of the breast is essential, especially in clinical situations such as chest wall reconstruction or oncology. If extensive tissue resection requires reconstruction, anatomical differentiation between the breast structures and adjacent thoracic fascial layers determines the selection of surgical methods. While musculocutaneous flaps were once popular for their robust coverage, advancements in fasciocutaneous flaps, particularly thoracoabdominal regions—offer promising alternatives that are amenable to the layered nature of the breast without compromising functional elements of the thorax. Procedures involving these flaps capitalize on the anatomical awareness of the fascial planes of the breast and suspensory attachments to restore thoracic wall integrity effectively in addition to breast contour maintenance or reconstruction. These operations underscore the clinical relevance of the understanding of breast tissue anatomy in its thoracic context.

5.4.2. Location and Significance of Mammary Glands

In the superficial fascia of the thorax's anterior wall, the mammary glands are anatomically located over the pectoralis major muscles, vertically between the second and sixth ribs, and from the sternum to the midaxillary line. As positioned, the mammary glands can not only be exocrine glands that secrete milk but also natural components in the female breast's shape and physiology. The glandular tissue is embedded in a dense connective tissue matrix interspersed with adipose tissue, which is influenced by hormonal status and age. Anterior to the thoracic cage, these glands are supported by suspensory Cooper's ligaments, which suspend the breast and impart structural integrity. The close relation of mammary glands to the thoracic wall underscores their susceptibility in pathological processes so that their accurate anatomical knowledge becomes paramount in clinical diagnoses and surgeries concerning the breast. In addition to their location, the mammary glands are physiologically and pathologically very important. Their only biological role is lactation, which is an extremely endocrine-sensitive process, as evidenced by associations found between endocrinological abnormalities and benign breast diseases (Rathlawath et al., 2017). Hyperprolactinemia and hypothyroidism were shown to be associated with proliferative breast pathology, suggesting the sensitivity of the glands to endocrinological abnormalities at a systemic level. It shows how mammary glands represent a dynamic interface between systemic physiological activity and the thoracic wall. This clinical significance extrapolates to breast pathology, where pathological glandular function or form may be causative of a spectrum of benign and malignant processes, and for successful treatment, close knowledge of their hormonal and anatomical environment is necessary. The anatomic location of mammary glands also intersects to a significant extent with oncologic problems, particularly breast cancer, which remains a leading health burden among women globally. Triple-negative breast cancer (TNBC), a tumor type with no receptors for estrogen, progesterone, and HER2, illustrates the virulent malignancies originating from mammary gland tissue (Sankar et al., 2017). The anatomical location of the breast makes it suitable for palpation of tumors and imaging evaluation, key to early detection. Moreover, the heterogeneously cellular glandular environment of the glands, consisting of ductal and lobular tissue within thoracic wall architecture, is a multifaceted environment open to disparate neoplastic alterations. Understanding the anatomical and physiological nuances of these glands is not only critical for surgical extirpation and reconstructive planning but also for planning directed therapy to maximize prognosis in virulent subtypes of breast carcinoma (Figure 5.9).

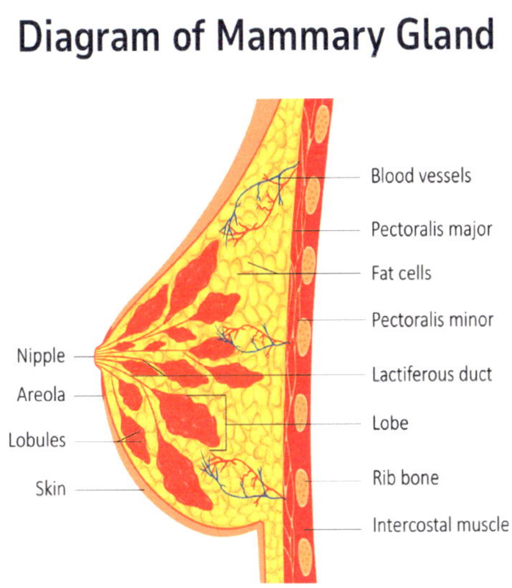

Figure 5.9. Location and significance of mammary glands.

Source: GeeksforGeeks. (2024). *Diagram of Mammary Gland.*

5.4.3. Role of Connective Tissue in Breast Support

The structural integrity of the breast largely depends on the specialized connective tissue that weaves together the glandular and adipose components. Such connective tissue is primarily composed of collagen and elastin fibers, forming a supportive framework that maintains and upholds breast shape and resists gravity. The fibrous support, also known as Cooper's ligaments, not only functions as a passive support system but also plays an active role in anchoring the breast to the underlying thoracic wall. The ligaments extend from the dermis to the pectoralis fascia and create a tension network that distributes mechanical loads and stabilizes the breast during movement. Alteration or weakening of this connective tissue can lead to ptosis or sagging, and its importance therefore in cosmetic and functional breast management. Understanding the biomechanical characteristics of the tissue explains its critical role in surgical and non-surgical management of breast disorders in the thoracic space. Not only does the breast connective tissue provide static support, but also it takes a dynamic role in healing after surgery and in structural restoration. This is particularly so in postoperative situations such as mastectomy, where thoracic wall stability needs to be ensured to prevent complications. Suction drainage methods on continuous suction have been observed to minimize postoperative seroma, hence allowing the reattachment of skin flaps and deep muscles through connective tissue remodeling (Hall et al., 2024). Elimination of dead space offered by the negative pressure favors the process of adhesion, which is highly reliant on the regenerative capacity of connective tissue. Thus, the optimal healing and maintenance of breast contour after surgery greatly rely on the structural and functional integrity of this connective tissue matrix, further emphasizing its pivotal role in the results of thoracic wall and breast surgery. The engagement of the connective tissue with the surrounding musculoskeletal (MSK) structures further stabilizes the support of the breast through biomechanical alignment. Pectoralis minor muscle, intimately associated with the anterior wall of the thorax, influences the position of the scapula and therefore indirectly regulates breast posture and movement (Morais & Cruz, 2016). Tension or contraction in this muscle can modify thoracic wall dynamics that may further modify mechanical stresses put on the breasts' connective framework. Therefore, the network of connective tissue must not only address intrinsic forces within the breast but also react to extrinsic forces developed by skeletal and muscular mechanics. MSK balancing rehabilitation techniques, like pectoralis minor stretching, enhance the preservation of connective tissue integrity, enhancing overall breast function and support. This combined perspective validates the connective tissue as a central player in the delicate anatomical and functional ensemble made up of the thoracic wall and the breast.

Test Your Knowledge

1. Where are the mammary glands located within the breast, and what is their function?
2. Why is the anatomical knowledge of the breast important in clinical examinations and procedures?

5.5. Blood Supply and Innervation of the Breast

Learning Outcome

1. Focus on Arterial Supply to the Breast
2. Explain Venous Drainage of the Breast
3. Discuss Nerve Supply and Its Implications for Breast Health

The vascularization of the breast is its complex nature and is central to an understanding both of its functional physiology and its surgical complications relating to the thoracic wall and the breast. Its principal supply is from the internal thoracic artery, and also from branches that perforate the pectoral fascia to supply the medial aspect of the breast. Collateral supply to the lateral and superior segment comes from lateral thoracic and thoracoacromial arteries. This wide anastomotic channel is responsible for sufficient perfusion, which is essential for processes like lactation and tissue repair. The venous return is similar to the arterial course and ultimately drains into the axillary and internal thoracic veins, which is a means of effective return of blood. Maintenance of this vascular integrity becomes particularly critical in procedures like mastectomy, where disruption can lead to complications such as flap necrosis and seroma, a problem managed by continuous suction modalities (Hall et al., 2024). Beyond vascular complications, the innervation pattern of the breast is accountable for its sensory and functional role in the thoracic region. Sensory innervation is largely from the second to sixth intercostal nerves' anterior and lateral cutaneous branches. The nerves enter the intercostal spaces, the fascia, and the chest wall musculature to access the skin and parenchymal breast tissue and the nipple-areolar complex. Autonomic nerve control is also present in the regulation of the breast, influencing vasomotor tone, and facilitate glandular secretions . The correct anatomy of these nerves is significant in surgical procedures to preserve sensation and minimize neuropathic pain in the postoperative process. This is relevant to approaches aimed at enhancing the outcomes of patients after breast-conserving therapies or mastectomies (Karacaoglu et al., 2019). An understanding of the dynamic interaction between blood supply and the nerve innervation of the breast is crucial in thoracic wall clinical procedures. The delicacy of achieving adequate perfusion while maintaining neural channels is the cornerstone of surgical success and post-surgical recovery. For instance, post-mastectomy continuous suction drain tube methods reduce complications like seroma by avoiding fluid buildup without affecting vascular supply or nerve function (Vinoth et al., 2017). Furthermore, reconstructive techniques after extensive resections also rely greatly on the integrity of the local vasculature for the blood supply of the flap in attempting to preserve sensory nerve supplies to enhance aesthetic and functional rehabilitation (Karacaoglu et al., 2019). Therefore, anatomical and physiological differences in the blood and nerve supply of the breast have a critical impact on therapeutic as well as reconstructive planning throughout the thorax (Figure 5.10).

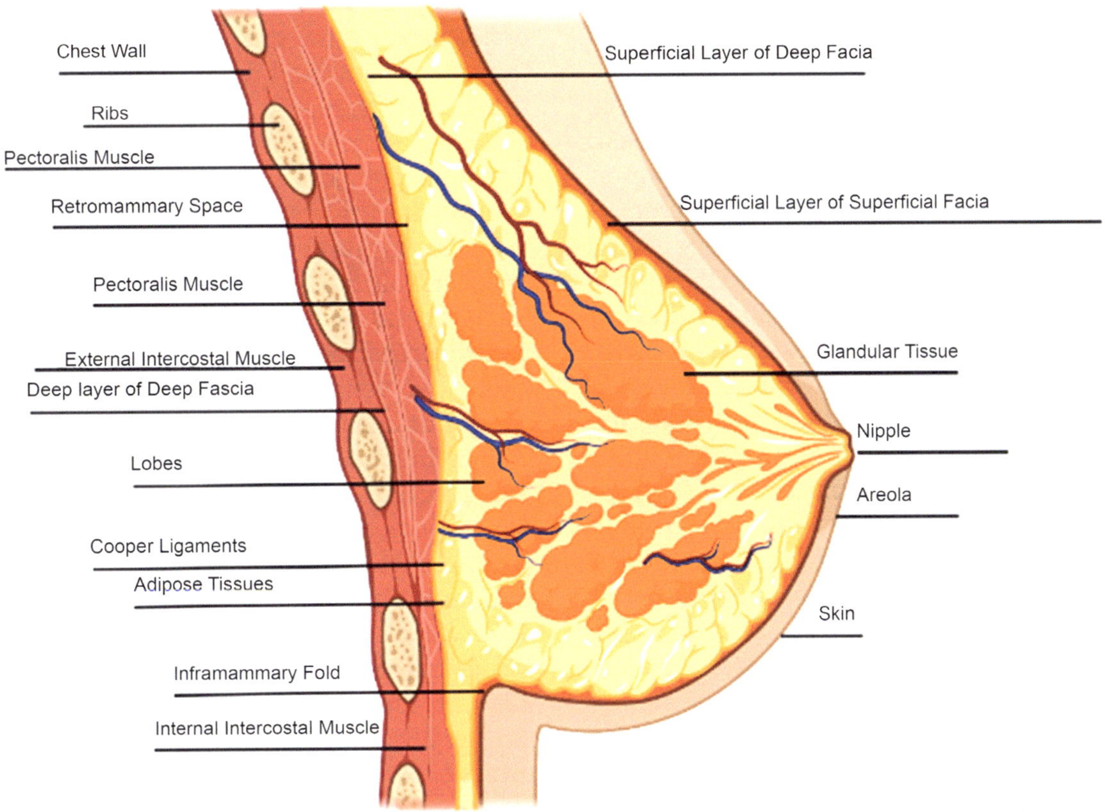

Figure 5.10. Blood supply and innervation of the breast.

Source: Galbreath S, Goswami T. Biomechanical Behavior of Female Breast—A Review. *BioMed*. 2025; 5(1):5. https://doi.org/10.3390/biomed5010005

5.5.1. Arterial Supply to the Breast

The fine vascular network in the thorax is tasked with supplying oxygenated blood to the thoracic wall and breast. Of all these vessels, the arterial supply to the breast is most significant because of its role in the viability of tissues and assisting in physiological functions like lactation. The primary arterial contributors are the internal thoracic (mammary) artery, lateral thoracic artery, and the branches of the thoracoacromial. These arteries form an anastomotic network that ensures a rich vascular supply. In addition, using perforating branches of the internal thoracic artery, blood supply to the medial and central regions of the breast is provided. This vascular pattern facilitates efficient delivery of nutrients and waste removal, which is necessary for the health and responsiveness of breast tissue to hormonal changes. Understanding this pattern in clinical practice involving breast surgery or pathology is crucial, where arterial compromise directly influences outcomes (Halvorsen et al., 2022). In addition to the primary arteries, the breast is also supplied by smaller branches that supply arteries, offering collateral circulation and redundancy. The lateral thoracic artery, which branches from the axillary artery, predominantly nourishes the lateral regions of the breast, justifying the close anatomical relationship of axilla and breast tissue. The thoracoacromial artery, yet another branch of the axillary artery, provides branches that also supply the upper regions of the breast. This redundancy of arterial supply justifies an evolutionary feature, providing the breast with adequate perfusion despite potential vascular obstruction. The role of these vessels is significant in pathological conditions such as ischemia or in surgical interventions such as mastectomy, where blood supply maintenance influences healing and recovery. Therefore, the arterial supply to the breast is not just extensive but strategized to provide tissue resistance (Hall et al., 2024). Clinically, knowledge regarding arterial supply to the breast is significant in surgeries and radiologic assessment. Surgeons must navigate these arteries carefully in an attempt to restrict intraoperative blood loss while preserving as much vascular integrity as can be safely preserved to facilitate postoperative healing. For example, internal thoracic artery perforators are typically spared in reconstructive surgery to secure perfusion. Secondly, the angiographic analysis relies on this exhaustive understanding in guiding interventions such as embolization for tumors or hemorrhages. Arterial supply variations can influence lymphedema and wound complication risks, emphasizing the necessity for personalized pre-procedure assessments. Finally, mastery of overall breast arterial anatomy supports maximizing patient results in the thoracic wall and breast therapies (Hall et al., 2024).

5.5.2. Venous Drainage of the Breast

The extensive vascular plexus of the breast is crucial to tissue viability and ensuring physiological function. An integral component of this plexus is the venous system, which serves the role of returning deoxygenated blood from the breast tissue to the central circulation. Venous return of the breast is essentially a mirror image of its arterial supply, along the internal thoracic, lateral thoracic, and intercostal veins, for efficient removal of metabolic waste products. Such an anatomical layout is critical for both the physiology of the normal breast and disease states, such as tumor metastasis along the venous tracts. Understanding the venous drainage pathways is also important in clinical practice, offering safe surgical planning and accurate imaging interpretation to avoid misdiagnosis or procedural complications (Jesinger et al., 2014). Because the venous drainage interconnects superficial and deep venous systems, it enables dynamic changes in blood flow related to hormonal cycles and physical activity. The venous channels of the breast are very variable and complex, reflecting the diversity of individual anatomy and physiological status. The superficial subcutaneous venous plexus communicates with the deep veins and establishes several anastomoses through which collateral circulation is facilitated. This network occurs within the fatty and fibroglandular tissue of the breast whose composition varies at different ages and hormonal status and adds to the venous architecture as well. The internal thoracic vein, together with the internal thoracic artery, is a good drainage channel, channeling blood medially to the brachiocephalic vein. Lateral to the former is the lateral thoracic vein together with the respective similarly named artery, channeling blood laterally to the axillary vein. Draining blood from the posterior surface are the intercostal veins, further highlighting the venous contribution of the thoracic walls to the overall drainage of the breast (Jesinger et al., 2014). The redundancy of this vascular pattern helps in maintaining functional drainage during even localized venous obstruction. Clinically, knowledge of the breast venous drainage is important in surgical and diagnostic procedures involving the thoracic wall and breast. Anatomical variations of venous anatomy can affect the management of mastectomy, breast reconstruction, or minimally invasive procedures for breast disease.

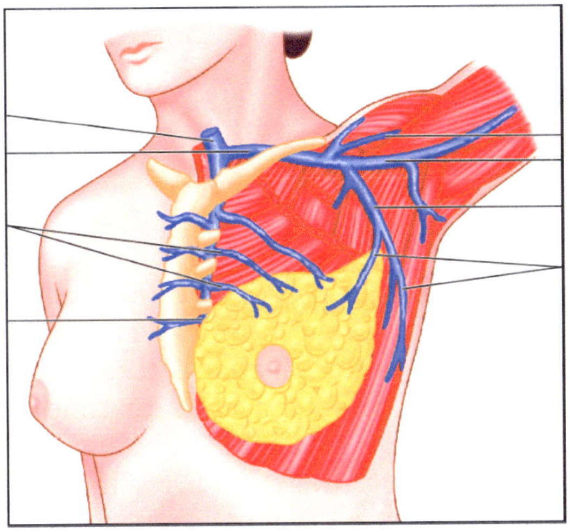

Figure 5.11. Venous drainage of the breast.

Source: Kaushik, R. (2018). *Venous Drainage of the Breast.*

For instance, incidental injury to the internal thoracic or lateral thoracic veins during a procedure may lead to hemorrhagic complications or venous return impairment, adverse tissue healing and increased morbidity. Imaging modalities that benefit from contrast enhancement are greatly reliant on accurate knowledge of venous courses to be able to differentiate normal vascular anatomy from abnormal lesions. Moreover, the venous system may also serve as a route for the hematogenous spread of cancer cells, and therefore its knowledge is necessary to integrate into staging and treatment planning. Standardization and agreement on surgical procedures, with the basis of thorough knowledge of anatomy, can optimize patient benefit and reduce procedural risk in breast surgery and intervention (Jesinger et al., 2014) (Figure 5.11).

5.5.3. Nerve Supply and Its Implications for Breast Health

The complex relationship between nerve supply and breast health is of more than theoretical significance; it is of major clinical significance. Innervation of the breast by sensory nerves is predominantly from the second to sixth intercostal nerves, which provide vital tactile and proprioceptive feedback. During surgery on the breast, e.g., mastectomy, unavoidable transection of these nerves commonly results in impaired sensation, a complication that has a detrimental effect on patient QoL. This loss of sensation is frequently unexpected and stressful, emphasizing the importance of nerve distribution and course in the thoracic region. Preservation or restoration of nerve integrity not only enhances postoperative outcomes but also impacts psychological status and body image, emphasizing the multi-faceted function of nerve supply in breast health and reconstruction surgery (Jeske et al., 2023). Advances in microsurgical techniques have sparked renewed interest in the application of nerve coaptation to autologous breast reconstruction. Through the connection of the sensory nerves of the donor flap, which are innervated by the seventh through twelfth thoracic spinal nerves, to the intercostal nerves at the recipient site, surgeons can significantly increase the sensory return in reconstructed breasts. This technique reduces the sensory loss typically accompanying transected nerves, improving the recovery of normal sensation and thereby patient satisfaction. Significantly, nerve coaptation can be applied in both immediate and delayed reconstruction with no added significant time or risk during operation, and other donor flap sites such as the back or thigh also yield suitable sensory nerves to be utilized in innervation. All these developments indicate that effective nerve handling is important for functional as well as aesthetic rehabilitation (Jeske et al., 2023). Apart from nerve regeneration, the breast's nervous-adipose tissue coordination is also responsible for overall breast health. The breast adipose tissue is very plastic, with the capacity to transdifferentiate as per physiological demands such as pregnancy and lactation. This dynamic aspect, supplemented by the input of sensory nerves, suggests a sophisticated regulatory environment that influences breast tissue homeostasis, metabolic activity, and indeed pathology. The chronic low-grade inflammation in stressed adipocytes, macrophage-mediated and by the inflammasome mechanism, may communicate with deranged nerve signaling to affect conditions ranging from insulin resistance to even tumor microenvironments in the breast. The understanding of nerve supply is not only pivotal in reconstructive success but also for general breast well-being, potentially leading to new therapeutic strategies.

Test Your Knowledge

1. Which arteries are primarily responsible for the blood supply to the breast?
2. How can damage to the nerve supply of the breast affect its function and sensation?

5.6. Clinical Considerations

Learning Outcome

1. Discuss the Common Diseases Affecting the Thoracic Wall
2. Explain Breast Cancer: Risk Factors and Prevention
3. Focus on Surgical Interventions Related to the Thoracic Wall and Breast

Careful examination of the breast and thoracic wall reveals complex clinical issues with the richly organized anatomy of this area. The thoracic wall includes vital components such as intercostal muscles, ribs, and neurovascular bundles whose structural integrity is the most important for respiratory function and structural support. Pathologies or trauma of these structures result in diagnostic and therapeutic issues in the clinical setting. For instance, rib trauma can lead to secondary complications like pneumothorax or pulmonary contusions, and appropriate clinical assessment must be done to determine appropriate interventions. Similarly, breast tissue with its lymphatic and glandular components is liable to a range of pathologies from benign cysts to cancerous tumors. The common symptomatology and anatomical associations require clinicians to employ systematic examination methods and imaging studies, carefully trading sensitivity and specificity for optimal patient benefit. This regard for detail underscores the need for multidisciplinary collaboration and integration of patient history with clinical decision-making (Halvorsen et al., 2022). The application of advanced imaging technology has changed clinical procedures in thoracic wall and breast diseases, facilitating accurate diagnosis and personalized treatment planning. Techniques such as mammography, ultrasound, MRI, and CT scans ensure accurate visualization of skeletal and soft tissue structures that are vital in detecting abnormalities early on. However, clinical application remains advanced, because tissue density, lesion type, and patient variables influence diagnostic proficiency. More advanced developments in AI, and, more particularly, deep learning algorithms, have been shown to enhance the interpretation speed and variability of images. Such algorithms have the ability to detect faint signals that may not be visible to human readers and enable earlier and more subtle interventions. However, the deployment of AI in everyday practice must be undertaken cautiously to support that ethical concerns, data quality, and interpretability are addressed appropriately to facilitate clinical trustworthiness and efficacy (Zhou et al., 2021). Effective treatment of thoracic wall and breast pathologies must be attained through a multidisciplinary clinical practice covering surgical, medical, and rehabilitative expertise. Operative issues are focused on structural stability while achieving oncological control in breast cancer cases of mastectomy or reconstruction. Radiation and chemotherapy regimens should be tailored to minimize collateral injury to tissues, given the location of the thoracic wall beside critical organs such as the lung and heart. Post-treatment surveillance is similarly important since complications from treatment later on, for example, lymphedema, chest wall abnormality, and functional loss could significantly impact QoL. Patient education and follow-up care are essential in the control of such late sequelae. Clinical considerations hence extend beyond acute treatment with an emphasis on holistic patient-centered care that supports both physiological restoration and psychological well-being during the course of disease (Zhou et al., 2021; Halvorsen et al., 2022) (Figure 5.12).

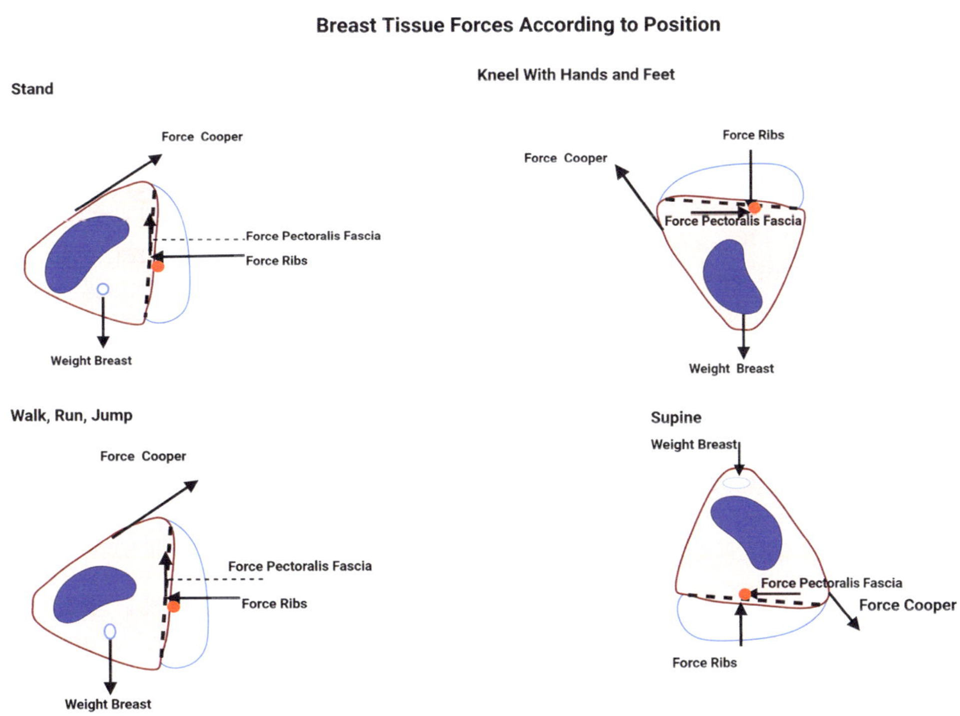

Figure 5.12. The thoracic wall and breast reveal complex clinical challenges.

*Source*Galbreath S, Goswami T. Biomechanical Behavior of Female Breast—A Review. *BioMed*. 2025; 5(1):5. https://doi.org/10.3390/biomed5010005

5.6.1. Common Diseases Affecting the Thoracic Wall

The structural integrity of the thoracic wall is vital for the protection of essential organs such as the lungs and heart, but the wall is prone to a variety of diseases that have the potential to profoundly influence respiratory and cardiovascular functions. Among the most prevalent conditions are traumatic injuries, which are most often caused by road traffic accidents and interpersonal violence. The injuries commonly involve rib fractures, flail chest, and bruising that not only compromise the thoracic skeleton but also interfere with pulmonary mechanics. Epidemiology reports highlight the fact that thoracic trauma-related injuries disproportionately affect younger men, a group trend whose causal link is associated with greater exposure to hazardous environments and activities (Ndongo et al., 2010). The prevalence of such traumatic conditions highlights the necessity of widespread trauma care and preventive strategies tailored to curtail injury rates and accelerate recovery in affected populations. Inflammatory and infectious conditions also play a major role in affecting the thoracic wall and causing high morbidity. Costochondritis and osteomyelitis of the ribs are examples of focal inflammation that is typically a result of bacterial infection or autoimmune disease, leading to pain, swelling, and limitation of motion of the chest wall. Tuberculous thoracic cage disease is another consideration, particularly in settings of high tuberculosis prevalence, where the disease can extend from pulmonary sites to the sternum and ribs to produce chronic pain and deformity. Furthermore, malignant conditions such as primary chest wall tumors and metastatic breast carcinoma have a proclivity for the involvement of the thoracic wall, complicating the clinical picture with masses, ulceration, and structural destabilization. These pathologies require multi-dimensional diagnostic approaches and treatment protocols dependent upon the etiology and course of the disease. Degenerative and congenital lesions are also an important cause of thoracic wall pathology and tend to complicate clinical management of accompanying breast disease. Deformities such as pectus excavatum, where the sternum is sunk, and scoliosis, an abnormal curvature of the rib cage, not only affect thoracic appearance but can alter the cardiopulmonary function and render surgery on the breast and thoracic structures more complex. In addition, degenerative changes in the costal cartilage and joints with time can lead to chronic chest wall pain and restricted mobility, often underdiagnosed or underappreciated in clinical practice. Knowledge of these disparate mechanisms of disease is important to a full treatment plan for disorders of the thoracic wall and breast because structural defects may influence the presentation of disease and response to therapy (Cinti, 2018).

5.6.2. Breast Cancer: Risk Factors and Prevention

The relationship between the thoracic wall anatomical structures and the breast is primary when one is thinking about the pathophysiology of breast cancer along with its risk factors. The density of the breast tissue, as determined by either genetics or endocrine influences, can influence susceptibility to malignancy through modification of cellular milieus that predispose to carcinogenesis. In addition, the proximity of thoracic lymphatic chains plays an important role in the spread and staging of breast cancer, making knowledge of thoracic anatomy an important component of risk stratification strategies. Obesity, alcohol intake, and exposure to ionizing radiation are modifiable lifestyle factors that contribute to the complexity of the risk scenario. Interestingly, integrating such environmental and anatomical determinants helps to develop precise prevention mechanisms, including lifestyle modification and surveillance recommendations that could minimize risk. This multivariate approach underscores the complexity of breast cancer causation and the need for tailored risk reduction interventions (Halvorsen et al., 2022). In planning prevention, it is important to know about modifiable and non-modifiable risk factors. Hormonal exposure, from early menarche to late menopause or hormone replacement therapy, significantly affects the risk of breast cancer through prolonged estrogen stimulation, with recurrent interaction with thoracic tissue microenvironmental factors. Genetic predispositions, including BRCA mutations, also increase susceptibility and require targeted screening and prophylaxis. Preventive measures also encompass clinical interventions such as chemoprevention and surgery in high-risk individuals, founded on a thorough understanding of the anatomy of the breast and thoracic wall lymphatic drainage channels. Early detection using mammography and emerging imaging techniques is facilitated by an understanding of the nature of the breast tissue and thoracic anatomical relationships, making results easier. Equally important is supportive care and patient education aimed at minimizing risk behaviors and maximizing surveillance (Halvorsen et al., 2022). Lymphatic channels of the thoracic wall, through which metastatic spread happens, are another equally challenging part of breast cancer risk management. Prevention entails mechanisms to preserve lymphatic integrity, particularly following surgery or radiological interventions. Lymphedema, a frequent sequelae of lymphatic disruptions, detracts from post-treatment QoL and underscores the value of preventive protocols designed to minimize lymphatic damage during oncologic procedures. International consensus statements emphasize multidisciplinary approaches that weigh cancer control and thoracic wall function preservation, with early physiotherapy and patient education promoted for incidence reduction. Thus, prevention extends beyond initial risk reduction to include preservation of the lymphatic system, an important part of thoracic anatomy, to promote long-term survivorship and decrease morbidity in breast cancer survivors (Figure 5.13).

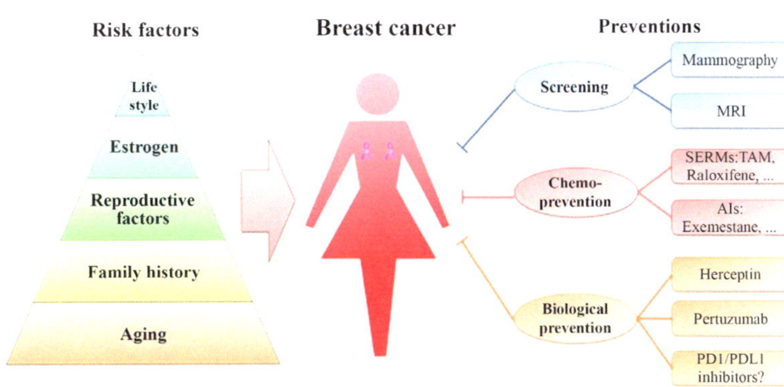

Figure 5.13. Breast cancer: risk factors and prevention.

Source: Yi-Sheng Sun et al. (2017). Risk factors and prevention strategies for breast cancer. *Int. J. Biol. Sci., 13*(11), 1387–1397.

5.6.3. Surgical Interventions Related to the Thoracic Wall and Breast

With technical improvement in breast surgery becoming increasingly focused on procedures that place equal emphasis on oncologic safety and cosmetic outcome, one such procedure of particular significance is NSM, an integral alteration of traditional mastectomy techniques with the preservation of NAC and effective management of malignant lesions. It is this delicate balance that hinges on accurate preoperative planning and anatomy awareness, specifically the preservation of anterior perforating branches supplying the vascularization of the skin. Incisions for surgery are wisely positioned at the inframammary fold or periareolar line to minimize ischemic problems and maximize cosmetic results. Retrospective analysis indicates a very minimal rate of total necrosis, emphasizing NSMs integrity when performed with utmost regard for tumor-to-skin space and incision placement (Amanti et al., 2015). Therefore, NSM is an extremely useful method of breast surgery that merges oncological attention to detail with reconstructive consideration. Congenital thoracic wall deformities such as pectus carinatum present unique challenges that often need to be corrected surgically, especially when conservative treatment fails. Although non-surgical techniques such as constant wearing of a custom orthotic brace remain the first line of treatment for teenagers, female patients complain of breast tissue compression. These discomforts result in invasive corrective surgery being considered, particularly when psychological or cardiopulmonary symptoms worsen. The design of gender-specific orthotic devices is meant to counteract such challenges with integration of customized anatomical accommodation and progressive corrective force, perhaps decreasing the indications for surgery. Nevertheless, where surgery is inevitable, reconstruction requires meticulous attention to the thoracic wall's structural support and aesthetic contouring (Mompart et al., 2024). Such procedures exemplify the complex relationship between thoracic physiology and patient QoL since it requires customized surgical planning. Surgical methods addressing the thoracic wall and breast encompass a variety of methods for restoring function and form within a spectrum of pathologies. Integrating reconstructive and corrective principles is pivotal, such as correcting thoracic deformity or post-mastectomy breast reconstruction. Surgeons will navigate complex vascular and MSK spaces to optimize outcomes, with consideration of preservation of skin perfusion and chest wall stability. Imaging and surgical design technology enhances preoperative planning, facilitating minimally invasive surgery that reduces morbidity. Moreover, interdisciplinary cooperation among oncologists, thoracic surgeons, and plastic surgeons facilitates holistic treatment protocols that rebuild form as much as they kill disease (Morais & Cruz, 2016). Cumulatively, these surgical interventions advance patient-centered care in thoracic and breast pathology.

Test Your Knowledge

1. What are the major risk factors for breast cancer, and how can it be prevented or detected early?
2. What are common surgical interventions involving the thoracic wall and breast, and when are they indicated?

SUMMARY

Thoracic wall and breast anatomical structure interaction is not just fundamental to physiological function but also to clinical interventions from diagnostic imaging to surgery. A detailed understanding of anatomical variability, such as the rare prevalence of the sternalis muscle, is significant in preventing misinterpretation and procedural issues. Such variations could influence imaging appearances, leading to potential misdiagnosis or unwanted consequences in therapeutic interventions. Furthermore, the identification of these variants provides surgeons with more reconstructive options, enhancing outcomes from the operation and reducing patient morbidity. Therefore, attention to detail and information are paramount and accentuate the necessity of continued anatomical research in order to aid in clinical decision-making and maximize patient care (Raikos et al., 2011). It is this thorough anatomy that ultimately makes possible more precise and safer treatment of thoracic wall and breast diseases. The pathological features of the breast, in the case of rare and aggressive tumors like lipid-rich mammary carcinoma, once more emphasize the complexities involved within the anatomy of the breast and its clinical correlations. These tumors reflect how subtle histological and morphological features can have significant impacts on diagnosis, treatment, and prognosis. The evolution of immunohistochemical techniques allows for more precise identification of tumor types, enhancing diagnostic precision and for more personalized therapeutic interventions. Such precision is critical as early and accurate diagnosis of uncommon malignancies influences not only surgery planning but also the extent of intervention that will be required. Therefore, a multidisciplinary expertise in breast pathology integrated with anatomical perception plays a critical role in the development of breast cancer therapy and patient survival (Gal et al., 2017). In summary, the marriage of accurate anatomical data of the thoracic wall and breast, and pathological data is the cornerstone to successful clinical practice in this area. Identification of anatomical variations and their respective clinical significance reduces diagnostic limitations and enhances surgery planning, while ongoing research into atypical breast carcinoma subtypes gives valuable insights into oncological management. Finally, the integration of pathology and anatomy enables clinicians to have a more holistic approach to the diagnosis and treatment of patients, making precision medicine possible. Education, documentation, and research are essential to advancing dynamic science, ensuring that new clinical challenges are met with knowledge-based and innovative solutions. Through such interdisciplinary efforts, patient outcomes for thoracic wall and breast diseases can be significantly improved.

Understanding the complex anatomy and physiology of the thoracic wall and breast is essential to their clinical significance and implications in disease. The thoracic wall, composed of skin, muscles, bones, and connective tissue, is of vital importance in protecting vital organs as well as facilitating respiratory mechanics. On the other hand, the breast, a homologous sweat gland, is composed of adipose and glandular tissues whose arrangement is crucial in both physiologic and pathologic conditions. Critical structural components such as the ribs, intercostal muscles, and circulation provide the background against which breast tissue is supported and dictate its vulnerability to damage and disease. The lymphatic drainage network, particularly the axillary lymph nodes, is a significant pathway for metastasis of breast cancer. Recognition of the way these physiological and anatomical features interact underlies good diagnostic and surgical techniques, enabling clinicians to anticipate probable complications and maximize patient outcomes in thoracic and breast disease (Ji et al., 2023). Metastasis via lymphatic pathways is a common denominator in breast pathology, especially in the development and staging of breast cancer. Thoracic and axillary lymph nodes are both sentinel filters and routes of tumor cell spread. Arrest of tumor cells within lymph nodes has a profound influence on immune responses and facilitates secondary spread, making lymph node metastasis an important prognostic indicator in the majority of cancers, including breast cancers. Advances in the clarification of molecular mechanisms of lymph node metastasis have enhanced clinical practice through the refinement of staging procedures and the personalized therapeutic regimen. This knowledge enables individualized medicine approaches through improved disease progression evaluation and more effective therapeutic protocols to optimize survival. Continued research in lymphatic anatomy and metastasis mechanisms is nevertheless necessary to further optimize clinical management in thoracic wall and breast cancer (Ji et al., 2023). Clinical management of thoracic and breast disease also calls for sensitivity to systemic factors and comorbidities, particularly respiratory function and tissue integrity that impact one. For instance, diseases like obstructive sleep apnea syndrome (OSAS) indirectly affect the thoracic wall by regulating upper airway mechanics and muscle function, highlighting the interconnectedness of thoracic anatomy and general well-being. Intermittent hypoxia and inflammation related to OSAS can enhance cardiovascular and metabolic disease, highlighting the importance of interdisciplinary therapeutic strategies. Understandings of these systemic interactions direct not only the management of primary breast or thoracic disease but also that of associated complications, such that individual patient assessment is promoted. By merging an understanding of regional anatomy with systemic pathophysiology, clinicians are able to create comprehensive and effective paradigms of care patient-specific profiles (Sieck & Gransee, 2012).

KEY TERMS FROM THIS CHAPTER

- Intercostal Muscles
- Sternum
- Mammary Glands
- Axillary Tail (Tail of Spence)
- Intercostal Nerves
- Ribs
- Thoracic Inlet
- Lactiferous Ducts
- Pectoralis Major Muscle
- Suspensory Ligaments

CRITICAL THINKING QUESTIONS

1. **Which muscle is the primary muscle of inspiration?**
   a. External oblique
   b. Rectus abdominis
   c. Diaphragm
   d. Internal intercostal
2. **The intercostal nerves are derived from which spinal nerves?**
   a. Cervical
   b. Thoracic
   c. Lumbar
   d. Sacral
3. **Which artery supplies the medial part of the breast?**
   a. Lateral thoracic artery
   b. Internal thoracic artery
   c. Axillary artery
   d. Intercostal artery
4. **The retromammary space lies between:**
   a. Skin and breast tissue
   b. Pectoralis major and ribs
   c. Breast and pectoralis major muscle
   d. Fascia and subcutaneous fat
5. **Which structure provides the suspensory support of the breast?**
   a. Intercostal muscles
   b. Areolar glands
   c. Cooper's ligaments
   d. Pectoral fascia

Short Answer Questions

1. Describe the anatomical layers of the thoracic wall.
2. What are the functions of the intercostal muscles?
3. Explain the significance of the retromammary space in breast anatomy.
4. What is the lymphatic drainage pathway of the breast?
5. Define the boundaries and contents of the thoracic inlet.

Answers to Critical Thinking Questions

1. (c) 2. (b) 3. (b) 4. (c) 5. (c)

REFERENCES

1. Audenaert, E., D'Herde, K., Gomes, G., Kerckaert, I., et al. (2008). 3D computerized model for measuring strain and displacement of the brachial plexus following placement of reverse shoulder prosthesis. The Anatomical Record, 291, 1173–1185 (https://core.ac.uk/download/55835228.pdf (accessed on 8th May 2025).
2. Baj, A., Moro, E., Bistoletti, M., Orlandi, V. T., Crema, F., & Giaroni, C. (2019). Glutamatergic signaling along the microbiota-gut-brain axis. International Journal of Molecular Sciences, 20, 1482. https://doi.org/10.3390/ijms20061482.
3. Bilounga, N. C., Etoundi, M. G. A., Hyder, A. A., Juillard, C. J., et al. (2010). Patterns of injury and violence in Yaoundé, Cameroon: An analysis of hospital data. World Journal of Surgery, 35(1), 1-8. https://core.ac.uk/download/323075033.pdf (accessed on 8th May 2025).
4. Boute, B., De Gersem, W., De Neve, W., Detand, J., et al. (2017). Potential benefits of crawl position for prone radiation therapy in breast cancer. Journal of Applied Clinical Medical Physics, xx, 1–6. https://core.ac.uk/download/84596109.pdf (accessed on 8th May 2025).
5. Bubberman, J. M., van Rooij, J. A. F., van der Hulst, R. R. W. 5., & Tuinder, S. (2023). Sensory recovery and the role of innervated flaps in autologous breast reconstruction—a narrative review. Gland Surgery, 12, 1094–1109. https://doi.org/10.21037/gs-23-40.
6. Chayampurath, R., Kumar, G. N. M., & Parambil, S. M. (2017). Preserving of Intercostobrachial Nerve Relieves Breast Carcinoma Patients from Postmastectomy Pain Syndrome. https://core.ac.uk/download/543135064.pdf (accessed on 8th May 2025).
7. Cinti, S. (2018). Adipose organ development and remodeling. *Comprehensive Physiology*. https://doi.org/10.1002/cphy.c170042 (accessed on 8th May 2025).
8. Clos, M. M. (2024). 3D-Printed Bracing System for Female Pectus Carinatum Treatment. https://core.ac.uk/download/613973071.pdf (accessed on 8th May 2025).
9. Demi, L., Wolfram, F., Klersy, C., De Silvestri, A., Ferretti, V. V., Müller, M., Miller, D. L., et al. (2022). New international guidelines and consensus on the use of lung ultrasound. Journal of Ultrasound in Medicine, 42, 309–344. https://doi.org/10.1002/jum.16088 (accessed on 8th May 2025).
10. Esumi, S., Kumagai, Y., Koba, Y., & Fukuda, T. (2023). Analysis of the regional anatomy of the retroesophageal right subclavian artery and surrounding structures. Folia Morphologica. Folia Morphol 2024;83(1):44-52. (accessed on 8th May 2025).
11. Gal, A. F., Cătoi, C., Marica, R., Miclăuș, A., et al. (2017). A Metastatic Lipid-Rich Carcinoma of the Mammary Gland in a Female Cat: Clinicopathological, Histopathological and Immunohistochemical Features. Bulletin UASVM Veterinary Medicine 74(2)/2017. https://core.ac.uk/download/267070439.pdf (accessed on 8th May 2025).
12. Georgakopoulos B, Lasrado S. Anatomy, Head and Neck: Inter-scalene Triangle. [Updated 2022 Nov 9]. In: StatPearls [Internet]. Treasure Island (FL): StatPearls Publishing; 2025 Jan-. Available from: https://www.ncbi.nlm.nih.gov/books/NBK544222/
13. Hall, M. I., Suarez-Venot, A., Lindvall, T., Plochocki, J. H., Grossman, A., Rodriguez-Sosa, J. R., Voegele, G. M., Valdez, D. R., & Georgi, J. A. (2024). A reinterpretation of human breast anatomy includes all the layers of the anterior body wall. Anatomical record (Hoboken, N.J. : 2007), 307(11), 3564–3573. https://doi.org/10.1002/ar.25456 (accessed on 8th May 2025).

14. Iqbal, M., & Harahap, W. A. (2021). Breasts *and Lymphatic Tissue: A Literature* Review. https://doi.org/10.25077/jom.5.2.5-13.2020 (accessed on 8th May 2025).
15. Ji, H., Hu, C., Yang, X., Liu, Y. F., Ji, G., Ge, S., Wang, X., et al. (2023). Lymph node metastasis in cancer progression: Molecular mechanisms, clinical signi*ficance and therape*utic interventions. Signal Transduction and Targeted Therapy, 8. https://doi.org/10.1038/s41392-023-01576-4.
16. Lemos, N. A. de F., & Paulinelli, R. (2024). Intraoperative physiotherapeutic approach in oncoplastic surgery: Case report. Mastology. https://www.semanticscholar.org/paper/484aed56eeb9f1021ea3c2365d760fa28454ac06 (accessed on 8th May 2025).
17. Loukas, M., Moxham, B. J., Sharma, D., Stephens, A., et al. (2020). A Core Syllabus for the Teaching of Gross Anatomy of the Thorax to Medical Students. https://core.ac.uk/download/286271196.pdf (access*ed on 8th May 2025).*
18. *Luyet, C., Eichenberger,* U., Greif, R., Vogt, A., Szücs Farkas, Z., & Moriggl, B. (2009). Ultrasound-guided paravertebral puncture and plac*ement of catheters in human cadavers: an imaging* study. British journal of anaesthesia, 102(4), 534–539. https://doi.org/10.1093/bja/aep015(accessed on 8th May 2025).
19. Lv, R., Liu, X., Zhang, Y., Dong, N., Wang, X., He, Y., Yue, H., et al. (2023). Pathophysiological mechanisms and therapeutic approaches in obstructive sl*eep apnea syndrome. Signal Transduction and* Targeted Therapy, 8. https://doi.org/10.1038/s41392-023-01496-3 (accessed on 8th May 2025).
20. López-de-Celis, C., Morgado-Águila, C., Ortiz-Miguel, S., Pérez-Bellmunt, A., *et al. (*2024). Breast Vascularization and Its Implication in Breast Reduction and Mastopexy Surgery: Anatomical Study. https://diposit.ub.edu/dspace/bitstream/2445/214529/1/jpm-14-00536.pdf (accessed on 8th May *2025).*
21. *Morais, N., & Cruz, J. (2016). The pectoralis minor muscle and shoulder movement-related impai*rments and pain: Rationale, assessment and management. Physical therapy in sport : official journal of the Association of Chartered Physiotherapists in Sports Medicine, *17, 1–13. https://doi.org/10.1016/j.ptsp.2015.10.003(accessed on 8th May 2025).*
22. *Rai*kos, A., Paraskevas, G.K., Tzika, M. et al. Sternalis muscle: an underestimated anterior chest wall anatomical variant. J Cardiothorac Surg 6, 73 (2011). https://doi.org/10.1186/1749-8090-6-73 (accessed on 8th May 2025).
23. Rathlawath, S. K. (2017). *Prevalence of Hyperprolactinemia and Hypo*thyroidism in Benign Breast Disease in Government Rajaji Hospital, Madurai. https://core.ac.uk/download/288215674.*pdf (*accessed on 8th May 2025).
24. Sankar, M. (2017). Incidence and Clinico-Pathologic*al Features of Trip***le** Negative Receptors Status in Carcinoma Breast in our Institution. https://core.ac.uk/download/288215910.p*df (accessed on 8th May 2025).*
25. *Sieck, Gary C, and Heather M Gransee. Respiratory Muscles : Structure, Function & Reg*ulation. San Rafael, Calif: Morgan & Claypool Life Sciences, 2012. Print. (accessed on 8th May 2025).
26. Smith, C. F., Finn, G. M., Stewart, J., Atkinson, M. A., Davies, D. C., Dyball, R., Morris, J., Ockleford, C., Parkin, I., Standring, S., Whiten, S., Wilton, J., & McHanwell, S. (2016). The Anatomical Society core regional anatomy syllabus for undergraduate medicine. Journal of anatomy, 228(1), 15–23. https://doi.org/10.1111/joa.12405 (accessed on 8th May 2025).

27. Vannucchi, A. M., Kiladjian, J. J., Grießhammer, M., Masszi, *T., Durrant, S., Passamonti, F., Harrison, C., et al. (2015). Ruxolit*in*i*b versus standard therapy for the treatment of polycythemia vera. New England Journal of Medicine, 372, *426–435. https://doi.org/10.1056/nejmoa1409002.*

*28. Xie, L., Kong, X., Lin, D., Song, J., Chen, X., Huang, P., & Gao, J. (*2025). Application of chest wall perforator flaps in oncoplastic breast-conserving surgery. BMC Cancer, 25. h*ttps://www.semanticscholar.org/paper/f07dea3136988ceb02*f146123d2b2cee3a7ec454 (accessed on 8th May 2025).

29. Yasmin Sánchez Delgado, Christian Enrique Soulé Martínez, Héctor Manuel Suárez Ortega, Juan Jesús Ortega Landeros, María del Rocío Barrera Figueroa, Víctor Mario Martínez Bravo, Giselle Castillo Garcia, Rogelio Rodríguez Cárdenas, César Enriq*ue Pedraza Falcón, Alvaro Sebastian* Gutierrez Macklis, Ariadna Martínez Becerril, Karla Patricia Montoya Moreno, & Fernanda Berenice Ramírez García. (2024). Thoracic Wall Reconstruction with Thoracoabdominal Flap. International Journal of Medical Sc*ience and Clin*ical Research Studies, 4(05), 842–844. https://doi.org/10.47191/ijmscrs/v4-i05-12(accessed on 8th May 2025).

LUNGS AND PLEURA

6

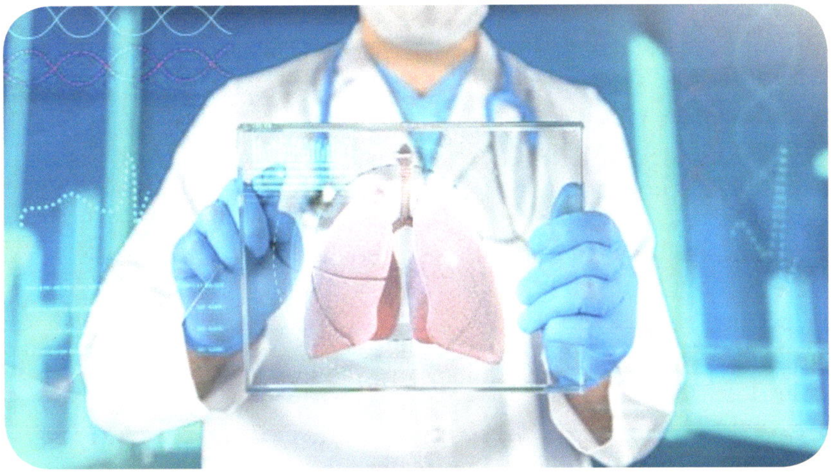

LEARNING OBJECTIVES

After studying this chapter, you will be able to:

1. Discuss the anatomy of the lungs
2. Explain the function of the lungs
3. Focus on the anatomy of the pleura
4. Learn about the function of the pleura
5. Discuss the common diseases affecting the lungs
6. Know common diseases affecting the pleura

Introduction

The human thoracic cavity harbors vital organs essential to respiration and gas exchange, with the lungs being the central organs of this complex system. The two organs are protected and supported by the pleura, which is a thin serous membrane that accommodates friction-free lung movement against the chest cage during respiration. Understanding the structural and functional interaction between the lungs and the pleura is vital to comprehending respiratory health and pathology. This data is particularly relevant in the clinical setting, such as radiotherapy, where tumor localization in the lung is hard owing to respiration-induced motion. Advanced biomechanical models incorporating thoracic physiology and anatomy, such as the pleura, ribs, and skin, have been used employing methods like finite element analysis to robustly estimate lung position in real-time and maximize treatment (Didier et al., 2009). Such multidisciplinary interventions indicate the significance of careful anatomical knowledge in advanced medical interventions. The mechanism of respiration is immediately influenced by the pleura, a double- layered structure consisting of the visceral pleura that adheres to the lungs and the parietal pleura lining the inner thoracic wall. Between them lies a pleural cavity filled with a very small amount of lubricating fluid, which is responsible for reducing friction during inflation and deflation of the lungs. The negative pressure contained within this chamber is essential in keeping the lungs inflated and enabling effective ventilation. Pleural integrity interruptions, like pneumothorax or pleuritis, illustrate the essential nature of this membrane to respiratory function. Thoracic motion is coordinated by the ribcage and muscles as well, with precise coordination ensuring perfect breathing cycles. Biomechanical simulation of the structures, using external assessments like thoracic surface displacement and airflow, has been shown with high promise in modeling lung function under respiration (Didier et al., 2009). This brings the significance of the pleura beyond merely anatomical terms into consideration for necessary physiological roles. Comparative respiratory anatomy also reveals other observations concerning specialization in the pulmonary system of species, referring to evolutionary specializations that direct the morphology of the lung and pleura. For example, avian respiration possesses typical morphological characteristics, such as a huge air sac system, to cater to the extremely high metabolic demands of flight. Such adaptations reflect not only differences in lung structure but also corresponding pleural and respiratory mechanics, which are quite dissimilar from those of mammals, including humans. Bird studies, as demonstrated through bird experiments like those on the sparrow, enrich the range of respiratory physiology by revealing differences in embryology, histology, and function. Comparative study adds depth to our knowledge of pleural and pulmonary biology and advances basic information for both clinical application and evolutionary biology (Figure 6.1).

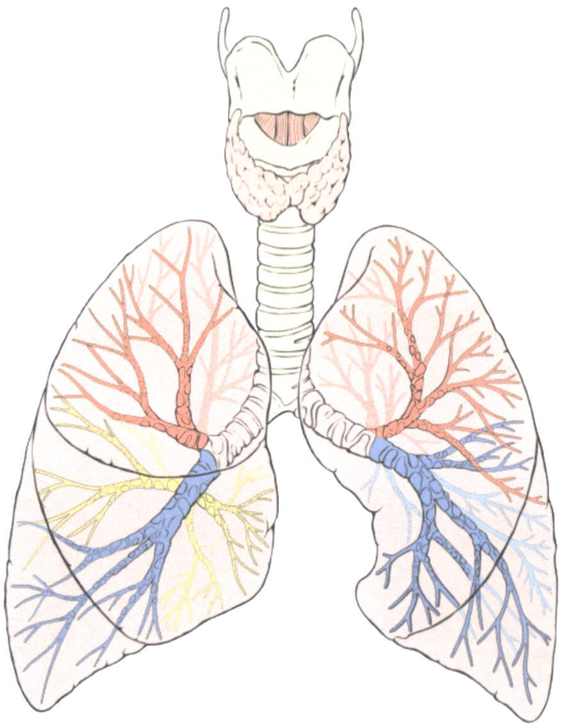

Figure 6.1. Lungs and pleura.

Source: https://en.wikipedia.org/wiki/File:Lungs_diagram_detailed.svg

Definition of Lungs and Pleura

The respiratory system plays a crucial role in sustaining life by exchanging gases essential for cellular metabolism. The system's focus is the lungs, two paired organs located within the thoracic cavity. The lungs are spongy and are made up of highly specialized tissues intended to maximize the surface area over which oxygen and carbon dioxide diffuse. The internal anatomy of the lungs contains branching airways, the bronchi and bronchioles, terminating in alveolar sacs structured for optimal gaseous exchange. The lungs provide this physiological function with a network of capillaries as well. Their functioning, however, not only demands their cellular composition but also a structural defense against encasement by protective membranes to facilitate mechanical support as well as reduce friction in respiratory motion. Understanding these fundamental characteristics of lung anatomy and physiology provides insight into their essential role in oxygenation and carbon dioxide elimination by the body. The pleura, a serous membrane surrounding the lungs, plays an essential role in respiratory mechanics through the creation of an interface that is frictionless between the thoracic wall and the lungs. This two-layered membrane is the visceral pleura, tightly in contact with the lung surface, and the parietal pleura lining the chest cavity. Between them is the pleural cavity, in which there is a thin layer of lubricating fluid that allows easy movement in lung inflation and deflation. The pleura also plays a role in the upkeep of negative intrapleural pressure necessary for each lung expansion. Sacrifice of pleural integrity in the manner of inflammation or fluid accumulation has the potential to drastically compromise respiratory effectiveness and lead to clinical states. By defining the pleura's structure and function in relation to the lungs, there is a general awareness of the anatomical and physiological harmony required for effective respiration (Logt et al., 1996). Ancient medical traditions have also recognized the complexity of respiratory organs, which were explained in terms of conceptual models such as Srotas in Ayurveda. These also encompass body channels engaged in varied metabolic and physiological activities, such as the respiratory pathway, categorized as Pranavaha Srotas. These channels integrate multiple systems, such as the cardiovascular and CNS, to enable elementary processes such as sustenance, circulation, and excretion. These integrated perspectives underscore the interconnectedness and interdependence of the lungs and respiratory tissues to general body well-being. Despite modern anatomy's maximum understanding of lung and pleura functionality, the concept of bodily channels has focused on emphasizing their role in maintaining systemic balance and ensuring the elimination of structures' importance in sustaining life beyond the mere gas exchange (Hedgde et al., 2023). This integrated view enriches existing knowledge of the lungs and pleura in respiratory medicine.

Importance of the Respiratory System

The complex interaction between the pleura and lungs is not only significant to lung function but also to health and disease prevention as a whole. The operation of the respiratory system makes gas exchange possible, oxygenation of the blood, and removal of carbon dioxide; cell metabolism and organ function are reliant upon these processes. The pleura, a double-layered membrane surrounding the lungs, reduces friction between breathing movements and provides structural reinforcement, enabling easy expansion and contraction of the lungs. Any pathological change in the lungs or pleura, such as inflammation or pleurisy, can markedly reduce respiratory efficiency, leading to compromised oxygenation delivery and complications of a systemic nature. Recognition of the complex processes of respiratory disease and health emphasizes the importance of early detection and intervention to maintain maximum pulmonary function and general health, an observation also further supported by experimentation involving the investigation of lung diseases in animal models (Logt et al., 1996).

Beyond physiological importance, the health of the respiratory system is inextricably related to broader public and animal health policy. Research into respiratory diseases such as pneumonia and pleurisy determines their huge impacts on livestock health and, as a result, food safety and economic efficiency. Studies demonstrate that farm management practices are responsible for the prevalence of respiratory diseases, indicating the efficacy of controlled environments and cleanliness in preventing infection. For instance, interventions like prudent control of yard time for lambs and hygienic housing for pigs have yielded measurable effects on disease incidence. These findings reinforce the prominence of the respiratory system not only in personal health but also in agricultural production practices toward the achievement of safe and healthy food. The systems approach to respiratory health illustrates the interconnectedness of lung function, disease prevention, and public health security (Logt et al., 1996). Furthermore, the respiratory tract serves as a defense barrier for external pathogens, particularly since the value of the respiratory system extends beyond that of gas exchange.

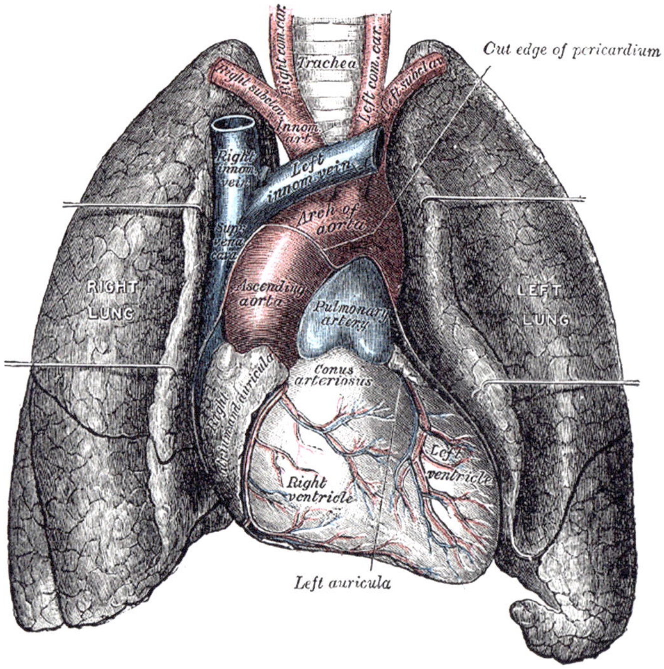

Figure 6.2. The respiratory system.

Source: By Gray's Anatomy - Gray's Anatomy at http://www.bartleby.com/107/138.html, Public Domain, https://commons.wikimedia.org/w/index.php?curid=141450

The pleura and lung together are responsible for immunological protection via air filtration upon inhalation and provision of a site for immune response vital to the prevention of infection. The pleura's sensitivity to infection-induced injury, chemical insult, or mechanical trauma means that any dysfunction will produce cascading effects along the respiratory axis. Prevention of pulmonary and pleural disease, therefore, not only preserves respiratory function but also reduces the cost of systemic infection and chronic inflammatory disease. Globally, observation of pleural conditions in animal populations has human well-being implications in promoting comparative pathology and risk management practices. The aggregation of knowledge in respiratory anatomy, physiology, and pathology emphasizes the critical role of the lungs and pleura in sustaining life and health (Logt et al., 1996) (Figure 6.2).

6.1. Anatomy of the Lungs

Learning Outcome

1. Discuss the Lobes of the Lungs
2. Explain the Bronchial Tree Structure
3. Focus on Alveoli and Gas Exchange

The elaborate structural organization of the lungs attests to their important role in gas exchange and respiration. Both lungs, suspended in the thoracic cavity, are divided into lobes by fissures; three lobes in the right lung and two in the left, to accommodate the heart. The lobes are further divided into segments, a modular design for ventilation and surgery. The bronchial tree, which begins with the division of the trachea into primary bronchi, continues to divide into smaller bronchi and bronchioles, ultimately terminating in the alveoli, the principal sites of oxygen and carbon dioxide exchange. This complexity of hierarchical branching not only maximizes surface area but also ensures efficient distribution of airflow throughout the pulmonary system. Understanding this level of detail involves full anatomical models with relations other than simple part-whole relations, including the fine-grained spatial and functional attributes necessary to characterize lung physiology and pathology (Mejino & Rosse, 2004). The lungs, other than their internal structure, are enveloped by the pleura. Notably, the anatomical closeness of the pleura to the lung tissue exposes it to a wide range of pathological processes, such as those caused by inhalation of fibrous particles. Studies emphasize how the pleura is exposed to external agents such as asbestos fibers, which can translocate and deposit here with the capability of inducing a variety of diseases ranging from benign pleural plaques to very aggressive malignancies such as mesothelioma (Agnes et al., 2011). The pleural anatomy thus represents a very significant interface between environmental exposure and lung health. Recent advances in anatomical modeling have highlighted the need for the inclusion of detailed biophysical relationships within the lung and pleural tissues to fully understand their functions and vulnerabilities. Traditional ontologies have mainly focused on hierarchical classifications and basic part-whole relationships but cannot represent complex spatial and material properties of lung tissues. The Digital Anatomist Foundational Model of Anatomy (FMA) is a symbolic framework of this nature that extends beyond mere assignments, encompassing structural relationships and physical properties required to describe human lung structure as a whole. Such a framework can result in a better understanding of how microscopic alterations, e.g., fiber retention and cellular response within the pleura, influence overall pathological outcomes (Mejino & Rosse, 2004). These findings have tremendous significance for therapeutic discovery and biomedical research in respiratory medicine (Figure 6.3).

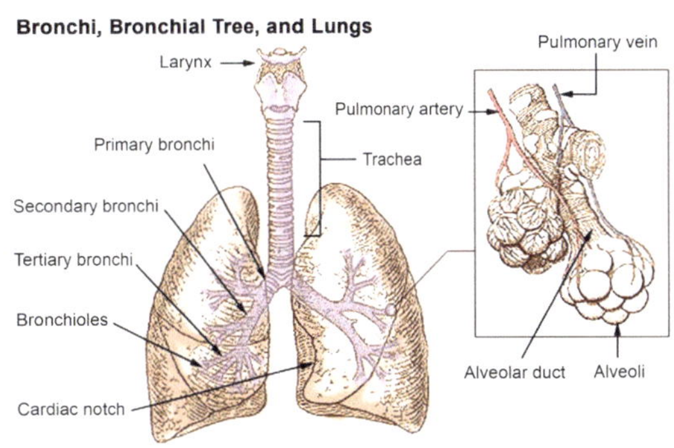

Figure 6.3. Anatomy of the lungs.

Source: Public Domain, https://commons.wikimedia.org/w/index.php?curid=789698

6.1.1. Lobes of the Lungs

The lungs' complex architecture is responsible for a significant part of their respiratory effectiveness, and the lobes play a pivotal role in segmenting lung function. Each lung is divided into lobes, with the right lung consisting of three lobes, superior, middle, and inferior, and the left lung consisting of two lobes—superior and inferior. This compartment allows for localized perfusion and ventilation, which is essential to achieve optimal gas exchange and allow the lungs to function cohesively within the pleural space. The lobar anatomy also allows for segmental isolation during surgery or disease processes, minimizing the impact on overall lung function. More recent advances in biophysical modeling have incorporated the lobar anatomy to more accurately mimic lung mechanics, revealing how the non-uniform distribution of pressures and strains takes place in different lobes during ventilation (Badrou et al., 2025). These results validate the lobes' status as more than mere anatomical compartments, as they highlight their dynamic mechanical features in respiratory physiology. The lobes of the lung are not only architectural divisions but also possess various physiological and pathological characteristics that influence respiratory health and disease processes. Separate lobes may respond variably to damage or infection, partly due to variations in blood supply, airway branching, and tissue content. Clinically, this lobe-specific vulnerability is manifested in conditions like acute respiratory distress syndrome (ARDS), where certain lobes will experience more intense inflammation or fibrosis, worsening the entire lung function. For instance, inhalation injuries to ARDS can be uneven between lobes of the lung, impacting ventilation and perfusion distribution, thus making treatment efforts more difficult. Therapeutic treatments often selectively target these damaged lobes, through ventilator settings or pharmacological interventions to most effectively oxygenate and avoid further injury (Yang et al., 2017). Understanding the distinctions between the lobes of lung injury and repair heightens the specificity of respiratory therapies and enhances prognosis in the critical care setting. Further, the interrelationship between lung lobes and overlying pleura is of paramount importance in pulmonary mechanics and pathology. The pleura, a thin layer of serous membrane covering the lungs, permits smooth gliding of lobes with breathing, reducing friction and aiding in uniform lung expansion. This relation ensures that even with segmental functional independence and movement of the lobes, they move in harmony to provide respiratory homeostasis. Computational modeling revealed that mechanical characteristics of the pleural layer influence lobar expansion and pressure distribution, and there are marked disparities in shear moduli of parenchyma, airways, and pleura itself (Badrou et al., 2025). Moreover, pleural participation in pathologic processes, e.g., pleural adhesions or inflammation, might differentially influence lobar mobility and ventilatory efficiency. In-depth information on the lobar anatomy and pleural relations is therefore required to comprehend lung physiology and guide interventions in pulmonary conditions with pleural as well as lung tissue involvement.

6.1.2. Bronchial Tree Structure

The complex respiratory system's architecture is reflective of the system's central role in facilitating efficient gas exchange. The central feature of the system is the bronchial tree, a highly branched system beginning with the trachea branching into principal bronchi to each lung. Within certain genera of mammals, such as the gray short-tailed opossum and North American opossum, the trachea consists of numerous c-shaped cartilaginous rings that ensure airway patency. These primary bronchi further branch into secondary and tertiary bronchi before gradually becoming smaller bronchioles, each level of branching having the distinctive structural and epithelial specializations. Cartilage plates present in the extraluminal bronchi provide support, whereas epithelium varies from pseudostratified ciliated columnar to simple squamous in the most distal parts and plays a variety of functions such as mucus clearance and gas diffusion. This anatomical detail ensures that air is delivered to the alveolar areas where exchange with blood is efficiently executed (Cope et al., 2001). Beyond gross structural segmentation, vascularization and innervation of the bronchial tree also conform to its functional requirements. Pulmonary lobar arteries bifurcate concurrent with bronchial architecture, controlling deoxygenated blood supply to respective lung lobes, while bronchial arteries supply oxygenated blood to the lung tissue proper. The venous return also corresponds to this lobar pattern, with veins aggregating into common trunks before returning blood to the heart. Remarkably, neural control is provided by both sympathetic and parasympathetic fibers; sympathetic nerves control airway constriction via thoracic splanchnic nerves, whereas parasympathetic innervation by the vagus nerve controls bronchial smooth muscle tone and secretions.

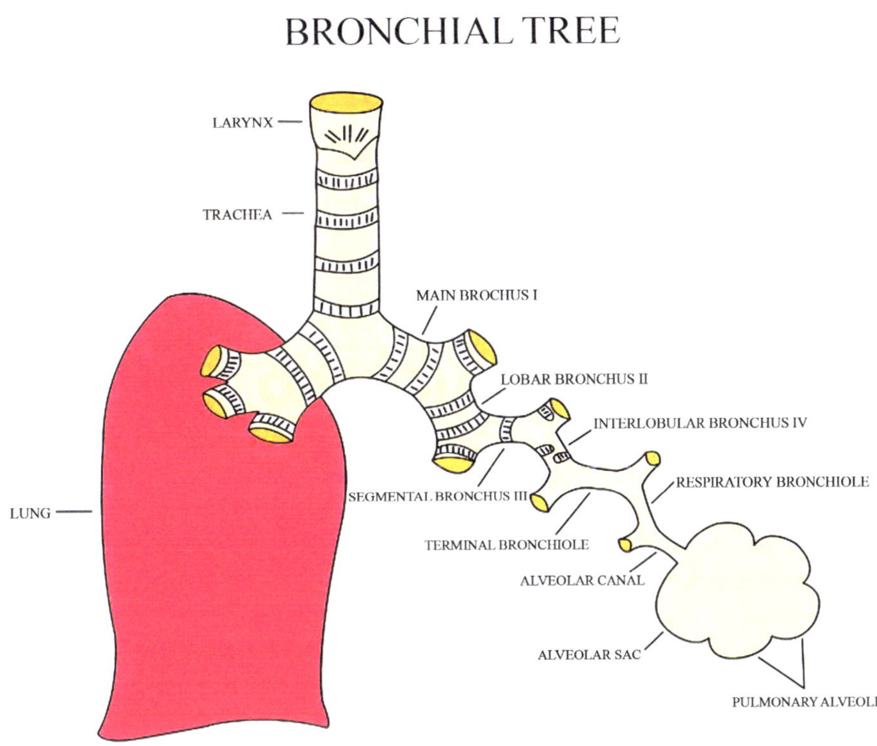

Figure 6.4. Bronchial tree structure.

Source: Dreamstime. (n.d.). *Bronchial Tree.*

Such precise neural and vascular control underscores the role of the bronchial tree not only as a mere ventilation pathway but also as an actively controlled system critical to respiratory homeostasis (Cope et al., 2001). The complex nature of the bronchial tree is also of clinical relevance with respect to pathological changes. Bronchial carcinomas, for example, often occur in the major or segmental bronchi, where epithelial and glandular tissues provide a potential field for neoplastic transformation. Macroscopic examination of these tumors reveals growth patterns that can invade mediastinal structures, underscoring the interdependence between bronchial anatomy and the pattern of disease. Mucin production and variation in tumor pathology signal the multiplicity of cellular origins within the bronchial mucosa. These neoplastic changes can obstruct airflow and jeopardize lung function, pointing to the importance of the recognition of bronchial microanatomy in the diagnosis and treatment of respiratory neoplasms. The structural intricacy of the bronchial tree therefore constitutes a foundation for normal pulmonary function and a location vulnerable to significant disease processes (Figure 6.4).

6.1.3. Alveoli and Gas Exchange

The fragile architecture of the alveoli is accountable for efficient gas exchange in the lungs. The tiny balloon-shaped alveoli are densely packed in terminal bronchioles of the bronchial tree and are surrounded by a dense network of capillaries. The alveolar walls are extremely thin, minimizing the diffusion path for oxygen and carbon dioxide between blood and air. This arrangement allows for oxygen to diffuse rapidly into the blood and carbon dioxide to escape from it, facilitating crucial respiratory functions. Advances in intravital microscopy have enhanced our understanding of alveolar dynamics by allowing researchers to observe these functions *in vivo* with unprecedented spatial and temporal resolution. The technology yields new insights into how alveolar structure and function are maintained during physiological breathing and how these can be modulated during disease states (Kuebler et al., 2020). Mechanical forces within the lung may potentially exert a significant influence on alveolar function, and thus gas exchange efficacy. The application of mechanical ventilation, while life-supporting, is associated with risks such as ventilation-associated lung injury (VALI), which has the potential to affect alveolar function and compromise gas exchange. Studies conducted via intravital microscopy have shown that certain zones of the lung, particularly where inspired gas distribution is most concentrated, are most vulnerable to injury, thus highlighting the heterogeneous character of alveolar strain and stress. These findings underscore the need for precise alveolar biomechanics at the micro-scale because inhomogeneous alveolar expansion and capillary perfusion can lead to regional damage and inflammation. With further development, even the constraints of a failure to non-invasively measure intra-acinar tissue strain hinder full appreciation of such occurrences and total understanding of the information regarding what shape respiratory support is best suited to minimize damage (Oeckler & Hubmayr, 2007). Moreover, the delicate relationship between alveolar ventilation and microvascular perfusion is essential for optimal gas exchange yet is poorly understood. The balance between air to the alveoli and blood via surrounding capillaries determines the effectiveness of oxygenation and carbon dioxide elimination. Pathologic or therapeutic manipulations that shift this balance can impair oxygenation and cause hypoxemia. Intravital microscopy studies have highlighted the complexity of this interaction, illustrating non-uniform perfusion of the alveoli and that immune responses within the alveolar-capillary unit control blood flow and ventilation. These multi-dimensional dynamics represent a difficult frontier in respiratory physiology since a better understanding of alveolar microcirculation might inform novel strategies for protecting the lungs from injury while maintaining effective gas exchange (Kuebler et al., 2020).

Test Your Knowledge

1. Describe the branching pattern of the bronchial tree from the trachea to the terminal bronchioles.
2. What is the role of alveoli in gas exchange, and how are they structurally adapted for this function?

6.2. Function of the Lungs

Learning Outcome

1. Discuss the Role in Respiration
2. Explain the Gas Exchange Process
3. Understand Regulation of Blood pH

The tortuous architecture of the lungs enables them to carry out their key task of gas exchange, which is essential for the maintenance of homeostasis. Air entering the respiratory tract travels through branching bronchi and bronchioles and eventually ends in alveoli, where oxygen is absorbed into the bloodstream and carbon dioxide is expelled. The process relies on the thin alveolar-capillary membrane that supports rapid diffusion between air and blood. The ventilatory function of the lungs also contributes to the balance of acid-base in the body by regulating carbon dioxide levels, a key buffer for physiological pH. Secondary to respiration, the lungs also perform secondary functions including the removal of microthrombi and metabolism of certain vasoactive substances. The complex interplay of lung mechanics, blood flow, and availability of surface area qualifies the lungs as more than passive organs; they are active participants in systemic balance. The interplay of the lungs with the pleura, the two-layered membrane covering each lung, becomes paramount in disease states and therapeutic interventions. The pleural space facilitates elastic lung expansion by minimizing friction through the pleural fluid, which allows effective lung compliance with each breath. In pleural illness, e.g., malignant pleural effusion, fluid accumulation can impair lung function by restricting expansion. Interestingly, pleurodesis, a therapeutic procedure aimed at eradicating the pleural space by fibrous adhesion, can stop fluid production irreversibly in such situations. Despite early concerns regarding potential restriction of lung mobility, studies indicate minimal attenuation of lung function with no significant impact on total respiratory function, even with successful pleurodesis, highlighting the physiological flexibility of lungs and pleura to alter (Bone et al., 1999). Environmental and workplace exposure reaffirms the vulnerability of lung tissue and complex defense mechanisms. Inhaled dusts and fibers can cause pathological responses in the lung, which can result in diseases such as fibrosis and carcinogenesis. Comparative toxicological studies of inhalation and intrapleural exposure are diverse in terms of the response of the lungs to different fibers and dusts.

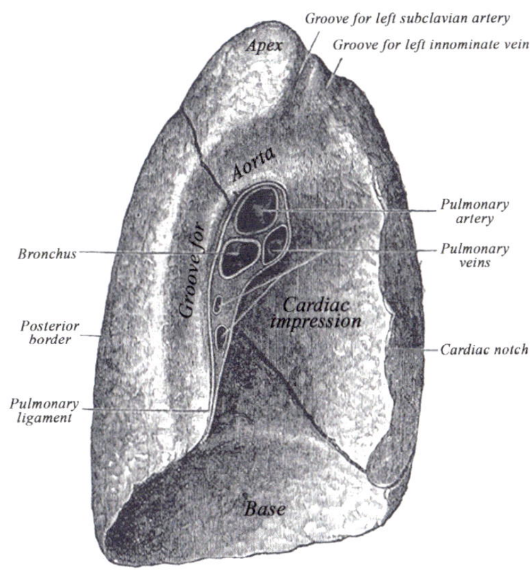

Figure 6.5. Function of the lungs.

Source: By Henry Vandyke Carter - Henry Gray (1918) Anatomy of the Human Body (See "Book" section below)Bartleby.com: Gray's Anatomy, Plate 973, Public Domain, https://commons.wikimedia.org/w/index.php?curid=566907

Notably, some intraperitoneal tests yield positive carcinogenic results that are not consistent with results from inhalation exposures, showing that direct lung exposure experiments remain the norm for health risk investigations related to pulmonary toxicity. Such clarification is significant as lung exposure to airborne toxins will have a direct impact on lung functioning and long-term integrity and therefore correct assessment methods for predicting and mitigating respiratory health hazards (Drummond et al., 2016) (Figure 6.5).

6.2.1. Role in Respiration

The complex composition of the lungs and pleura is essential for the efficient gas exchange necessary for respiration. The air's oxygen diffuses through the alveolar walls into pulmonary capillaries, while at the same time, carbon dioxide is expelled from the blood to the alveoli for exhalation. This is facilitated by the vast surface area of alveoli and their close association with capillaries, which allows for extremely rapid and efficient gas exchange. The pleura, consisting of parietal and visceral layers, also plays a significant role by creating an enclosed pleural cavity with lubricating fluid. This interaction enables proper lung inflation and deflation during the respiratory cycle while providing for the preservation of negative pressure necessary for the inflation of the lungs and preventing the collapse of the lungs. Without it, elementary gas exchange essential to the preservation of life would be radically compromised. Lungs' mechanical function in respiration is absolutely regulated by the structural relationship between the pleura and the thoracic cavity. The pleural membranes adhere closely to both lung surfaces and the chest wall, ensuring that the lungs move in synchrony with thoracic expansion during inhalation. Negative intrapleural pressure generated during this process pushes air into the lungs, aiding their role as the primary agents of respiration. The pleural fluid also reduces friction between the lungs and thoracic structures, enabling smooth respiratory movements. This biomechanical interaction is crucial, especially in pathological conditions such as lung infection or trauma, where pleural inflammation or fluid accumulation can detrimentally influence respiratory efficiency. Imaging techniques like ultrasound highlight the pleura's function, enabling diagnosis and treatment of lung disease influencing respiratory performance (Liu et al., 2020). Apart from normal respiration, the lungs and pleura are of key importance in dealing with respiratory complications developing in life-threatening diseases, like COVID-19. The lung function can be seriously compromised by inflammation, fluid buildup, and dysfunctioning gas exchange, for which therapeutic and diagnostic management is extremely reliant on lung and pleural dynamics knowledge. Ultrasound, in particular, is now an essential part of critical care, providing real-time monitoring of lung pathology and pleural status without the use of radiation. Its ease of portability and non-invasive quality allow for ready evaluation of respiratory function, guiding ventilation therapy needed to sustain compromised lungs. Therefore, the pleura and lungs not only facilitate normal respiration but also dynamically adapt to pathological loads, emphasizing their integrated role in respiratory homeostasis maintenance (Cui et al., 2020).

6.2.2. Gas Exchange Process

The efficiency of the respiratory system is subject to the fragile process in which oxygen and carbon dioxide cross through the capillary and alveolar membranes. Gas exchange plays a significant role in delivering the body's level of oxygen as well as flushing out waste products in the form of carbon dioxide. Exchange happens across a thin layer of the alveolar-capillary membrane via diffusion of oxygen into the circulatory system and diffusion out of the body via carbon dioxide. Key to this process is efficient ventilation, allowing for access of fresh air to the alveoli and perfusion, whereby efficient blood flow occurs in adjacent capillaries. Dysfunctions in either of these subjects can hinder gas exchange, leading to conditions such as hypoxemia or hypercapnia. Understanding these processes is important, especially in respiratory disease when a normal exchange is disrupted (Ernest et al., 2020). Besides, imaging during diagnosis plays a critical role in determining the structure and function of the lungs and, consequently, indirectly determining the state of the gas exchange process (Cui et al., 2020). A key determining factor of gas exchange efficiency is the accurate ventilation-perfusion ratio, also referred to as the V/Q ratio. Ideally, ventilation is coordinated with blood flow to be able to maximize oxygen intake and carbon dioxide expulsion. However, pathologies such as pneumothorax or pleural effusion create imbalances by disturbing lung expansion or reducing blood flow, which hampers the lung's ability to exchange gases. These abnormalities normally result in acute respiratory failure, where the lungs cannot meet systemic oxygen needs or effectively eliminate carbon dioxide. The pleura, as a covering membrane for the lungs, indirectly supports by providing smooth lung mobility and intrapleural pressure that is essential for optimal functioning of the lungs. Diagnosis of these dysfunctions by clinical presentation and laboratory assessment remains core to managing respiratory failure cases (Ernest et al., 2020). Advancements in medical imaging such as ultrasound have transformed lung disease assessment and management that affects the gaseous exchange mechanism. Ultrasound is a bedside, non-invasive technique used to detect abnormalities involving pleural defects in alveolar ventilation and gaseous diffusion such as effusion or thickening. The portability of this procedure coupled with the ease of decontamination renders it ideal for use within the infectious diseases community where immediate diagnosis is a prerequisite, as the COVID-19 pandemic highlighted. The ability to perform remote ultrasound consultations through modern networks also improves timely intervention, so that the disruptions in the delicate gas exchange process can be identified and addressed promptly. Such integration of diagnostic technology with an understanding of lung and pleural physiology thus offers an integrated approach to the preservation of respiratory function (Cui et al., 2020) (Figure 6.6).

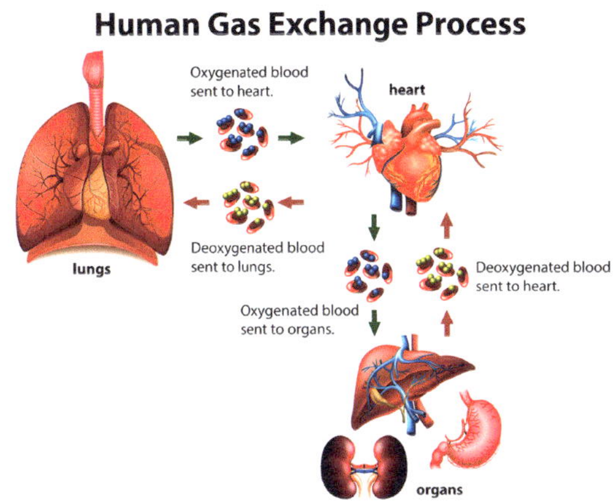

Figure 6.6. Gas exchange process.

Source: Freepik. (n.d.). *Human Gas Exchange Process Diagram.*

6.2.3. Regulation of Blood pH

The delicate balance of blood pH is crucial for the maintenance of physiological homeostasis, and its alterations can lead to severe metabolic derangements. The control of the lungs is crucial for this purpose by regulating the partial pressure of carbon dioxide (PCO_2) in the blood. CO_2, a byproduct of cellular respiration, readily dissolves in blood plasma to produce carbonic acid that dissociates into hydrogen ions and bicarbonate, thereby influencing the acidity of the blood. Through the process of ventilation, the lungs alter the exhalation of CO_2, thus affecting the acid-base status of the blood. An increase in respiratory rate, for example, actually decreases the level of CO_2 and hence avoids acidosis, while hypoventilation results in CO_2 retention and respiratory acidosis. The dynamic interaction between pulmonary function and renal compensation mechanism is an indicator of the inherent complexity of the regulatory system as part of the broad picture of respiratory physiology and pleural mechanics. Apart from the action of the respiratory system on blood pH, cellular and structural components of lung tissue are also responsible for maintaining biochemical homeostasis. Telocytes, a type of interstitial cell identified in the lung parenchyma, form a complex three-dimensional network with support for cell-to-cell communication and tissue homeostasis. These cells share intimate interactions with stem and progenitor cells, facilitating tissue regeneration and repair by means of signaling cascades that may indirectly enable proper pulmonary function and gas exchange. Proper gas exchange is essential to the removal of carbon dioxide and, thus, to systemic acid-base equilibrium. Exploring telocyte-targeting therapeutic strategies can enhance the function of lung tissue and make it more resilient, thereby improving the capacity of the lung to preserve blood pH under various physiological and pathological conditions (Bei et al., 2015). This cellular phenomenon highlights the complex regulation of acid-base homeostasis in conjunction with pulmonary and pleural integrity. While the lungs play a central role in acute pH modulation of the blood, the system itself is modulated by many external and internal stimuli, including environmental exposures and systemic disease. Both historical and contemporary research demonstrate how various agents, including inhaled pollutants and infectious agents, are capable of impairing pulmonary function and thus resultant respiratory regulation of normal pH. Chronic exposure to toxic agents or persistent infections may compromise alveolar-capillary membrane integrity, diminishing effective gas exchange and causing blood CO_2 level imbalances. Such disruptions have been linked with increased susceptibility to complex disease states, some of which are carcinogenic (Blackadar, 2016). An understanding of these risks is required to appreciate how lung and pleura health intersect with systemic acid-base homeostasis so that pulmonary function can be protected as part of an overall strategy to achieve optimal blood pH balance and overall health (Figure 6.7).

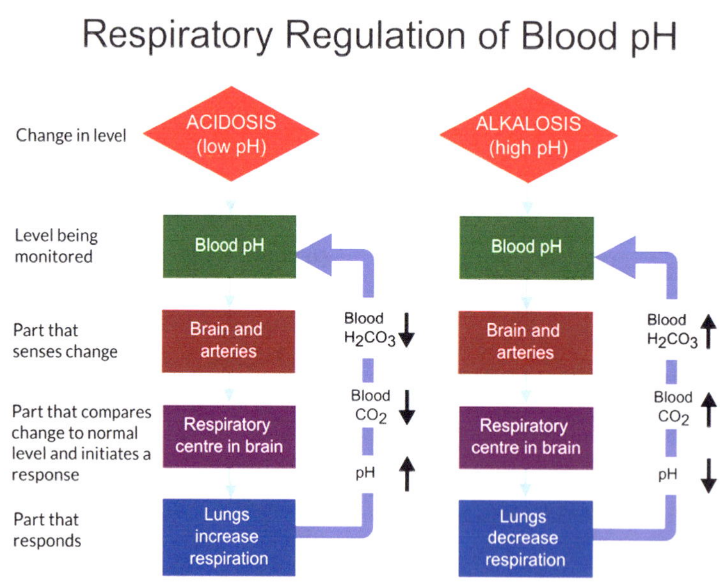

Figure 6.7. Regulation of blood pH.

Source: Let's Talk Science. (2021). *Respiratory Regulation of Blood pH.*

Test Your Knowledge

1. Explain how the lungs contribute to the process of respiration.
2. Describe the mechanism of gas exchange between alveoli and capillaries.

6.3. Anatomy of the Pleura

Learning Outcome

1. Describe the Structure of the Pleural Membranes
2. Explain the Types of Pleura: Visceral and Parietal
3. Focus on Pleural Cavity and Its Significance

The complex design of the thoracic cavity demands an effectively arranged framework to accommodate respiratory function. At the core of this framework is the pleura, a thin serous membrane that invests the lungs and lines the chest wall. The pleura consists of two layers: the visceral pleura, which closely clings to the lung surface, and the parietal pleura, which lines the thoracic cavity, diaphragm, and mediastinum. These layers create a potential space, the pleural cavity, that contains a thin layer of lubricating fluid facilitating lung motion during respiration. Anatomical relationships and three-dimensional arrangements of the pleura are of paramount importance because they dictate thoracic mechanics and respiratory function. Understanding such relationships aligns with the overall anatomical principles reflected in Terminologia Anatomica that focuses on the basic part-whole organization of anatomical structures critical to biomedical knowledge representation (Rosse et al., 2000). Beyond a mere structural boundary, the pleura also depicts complex anatomical relationships that ensure its multifunctionality in pulmonary physiology. The subdivision of the parietal pleura into several components, costal, diaphragmatic, mediastinal, and cervical, reflects an adaptation of the pleura to the varied surfaces of the thoracic wall. There are various functions for each component, such as the cervical pleura extending into the thoracic inlet and consequently forming the pleural cupula. These subdivisions and continuity illustrate the capacity of the pleura to adapt to biomechanical stresses without interfering with physiological integrity. Symbolic encoding of such relations, as advocated in advanced biomedical ontologies, aims to capture not just general partonomies but also complex anatomical relations and physical attributes necessary for a complete representation of human anatomy (Mejino & Rosse, 2004).

The pleura's anatomical complexity is also evident in its neural and vascular components, which provide for its metabolic supply and sensory innervation. The parietal pleura is innervated by somatic nerves and thus is pain-sensitive, while the visceral pleura, with autonomic innervation, is comparatively insensitive. It is supplied by adjacent systemic and pulmonary vessels, suggesting a multifaceted interaction that sustains pleural homeostasis. These physiological intricacies are reflective of the pleura as not merely a passive membrane but as a dynamic interface between the thoracic wall and the lung. Capturing these complex relationships in anatomical terminology systems is paramount to the progress of medical education and clinical practice, a goal that remains thwarted by the need for coherent and explicit anatomical representations (Rosse et al., 2000).

6.3.1. Structure of the Pleural Membranes

The complex arrangement of the pleural membranes plays a vital role in ensuring lung function within the thoracic cavity. The membranes are made up of two distinct layers: the visceral pleura, which grows directly onto the lung surface, and the parietal pleura, which lines the chest wall and diaphragm. The two layers have an intervening pleural cavity, a thin space that contains the lubricating pleural fluid, which minimizes friction during breathing movement. The intimate relationship of the visceral pleura with lung tissue facilitates the mechanism of gas exchange by maintaining surface tension that prevents alveolar collapse, while the parietal pleura provides structural support and sensory innervation. Such double-layered anatomy is fundamental in the maintenance of lung compliance and rendering ventilation dynamics effective, hence validating the functional relevance of pleural membranes in respiratory physiology.

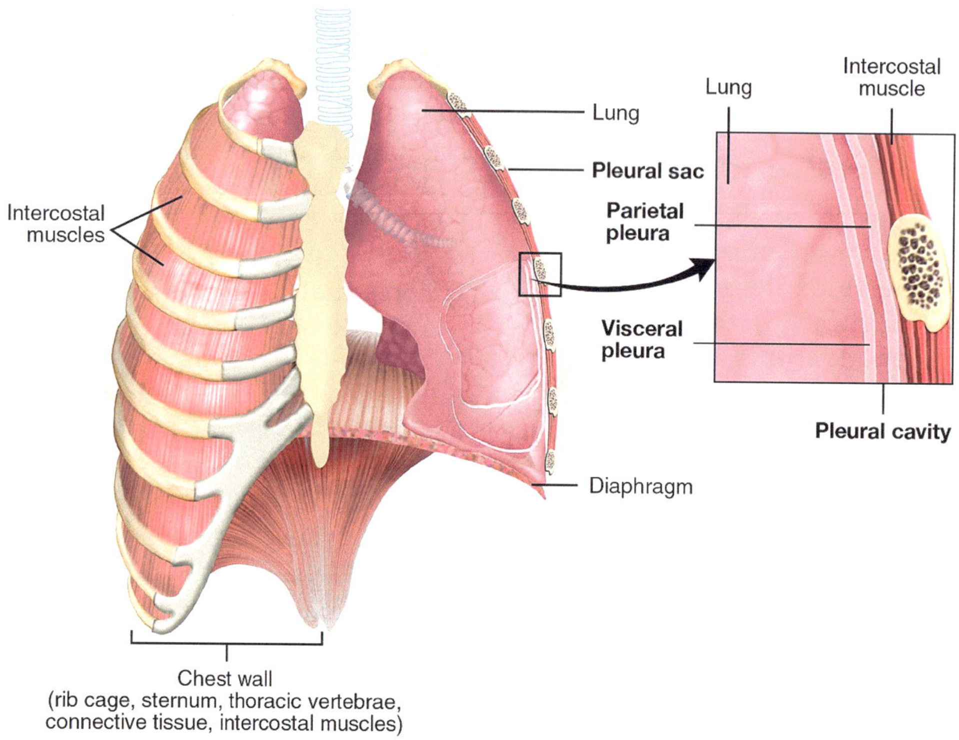

Figure 6.8. Structure of the pleural membranes.

Source: By OpenStax College - Anatomy & Physiology, Connexions Web site. http://cnx.org/content/col11496/1.6/, Jun 19, 2013., CC BY 3.0, https://commons.wikimedia.org/w/index.php?curid=30148380

Microscopically, the pleural membranes consist of a highly specialized layer of mesothelial cells that are not only smooth and frictionless but also create a dynamic barrier with the capability to exchange fluid and mount immune responses. The underlying connective tissue supporting the mesothelial cells serves as a scaffolding, which imparts elasticity and tensile strength to the membranes. The parietal pleura is richly innervated by somatic nerves, unlike the autonomic innervation of the visceral pleura that accounts for differences in pain perceptions when pathological conditions dominate. Such histological variations reflect the membranes' adaptations to both mechanical and sensory functions. Furthermore, pleural pathological alterations, such as thickening or fibrosis, may impair pulmonary mechanics, a correlation with diffuse parenchymal lung disease where pleural abnormalities correlate with compromised lung function (Ezzelregal et al., 2020). Surgical interventions on the pleural membranes, such as thoracoscopic procedures, also highlight their complex anatomy and clinical significance. Correct anatomical dissection of the pleura and surrounding mediastinal structures needs adequate knowledge of layered microanatomy to provide as little tissue damage as possible and preserve physiological function. VATS is an example in point here by utilizing magnification to recognize fine structural details of the mediastinal pleura and surrounding tissues and emphasizing the need to remain along natural anatomical planes to avoid complications such as bleeding or nerve injury (Osugi et al., 2017). These techniques emphasize the significance of the layered structure and the connective tissue architecture of the pleura not just in respiratory mechanics but also in treatment. This indicates the intrinsic role of the pleural membranes putting it between normal lung physiology and treatment procedures for thoracic diseases (Figure 6.8).

6.3.2. Types of Pleura: Visceral and Parietal

The thin membranes that surround the lungs and line the thoracic cavity are significant to both respiratory mechanics and defense. The membranes, collectively known as the pleura, are categorized into two primary forms: the visceral pleura and the parietal pleura. The visceral pleura is an essential serous covering that intimately invests the surface of the lung, circling and penetrating each fissure and curve and thereby producing a smooth, lubricated contact surface required for lung expansion in the thorax. The parietal pleura covers the inner chest wall, diaphragm, and mediastinum and anchors the lungs to keep them from collapsing into the thorax. This anatomical variation is significant because the adhesion between the two pleural layers, which is made possible by pleural fluid, allows the lungs to glide during breathing without friction or damage. The understanding of the variation in function between visceral and parietal pleura adds to the understanding of pleural pathophysiology and clinical diagnosis. The visceral pleura is richly vascularized but lacks somatic sensory innervation and thus is insensitive to pain. Conversely, the parietal pleura, innervated by somatic nerves such as the intercostal and phrenic nerves, is very sensitive to painful stimuli as a result of inflammation or trauma. It is because of this reason that pleuritic chest pain is most often caused by irritation of the parietal pleura. Furthermore, imaging studies, particularly thoracic ultrasonography, provide dynamic visualization of the pleura, detecting abnormalities such as pleural effusion or pneumothorax. However, precise pleural pathology differentiation relies upon an understanding that aeration of the lung restricts ultrasound visibility of deeper lung parenchyma, so evaluation is confined to parietal and visceral pleura surfaces (Tinti et al., 2018; Makris et al., 2019). The clinical application of visceral versus parietal pleura differentiation is a procedural intervention and diagnostic approach. For instance, pleural effusions accumulate in the space between the two layers and influence lung mechanics and gas exchange and often necessitate thoracentesis into the space adjacent to the parietal pleura. Similarly, continuity of visceral pleura with lung surface ensures that such processes as nodules or visceral pleural thickening are closely related to contiguous pulmonary disease processes. Ultrasonographic assessment uses the phenomenon of the sliding motion between the visceral and parietal pleura during respiration, which has been utilized as an indicator of lung inflation and lack of pneumothorax (Makris et al., 2019). Yet, technicalities and the expertise of the operator significantly affect the interpretation of images, affirming the need for extensive scanning of the entire thoracic region to properly assess pleural involvement (Tinti et al., 2018).

6.3.3. Pleural Cavity and Its Significance

The complex interplay of lung performance and the protective role of the pleura underscores the vital role of the pleural space. The thin, watery space between the parietal and visceral pleurae allows the easy expansion and contraction of the lung during respiration and minimizes friction. The pleural space is maintained in negative pressure, which is vital for the inflation of the lung as well as for efficient gas exchange. Disruption of this delicate environment, such as fluid build-up or inflammation, can profoundly impair respiratory mechanics. Beyond its mechanical function, the pleural space is also an active interface where immune responses can be initiated in response to foreign particles or pathogens. The clearance of airborne particulates generally involves their movement to and removal from this space and therefore emphasizes the pleural cavity's significant role not only in lung biomechanics but also in pulmonary defense. Recent studies have revealed that the pleural cavity plays a fundamental role in the pathogenesis of certain respiratory disorders related to inhaled fibrous material. The parietal pleura, in particular, was discovered to be a location of significance where long, biopersistent fibers become lodged, producing localized inflammation and, in doing so, potentially developing conditions such as mesothelioma. The investigation of high aspect ratio nanoparticles, like carbon nanotubes, demonstrates that their pathogenicity results from their inability to clear through the pleural stomata—microscopic pores that are designed to allow drainage and immune surveillance. This retention triggers a cascade of inflammatory responses, emphasizing the significance of the pleural space as an open frontline tissue vulnerable to occupational and environmental toxins. This realization alters the decades-long perception that lung parenchyma is the primary site for fiber-related pathology, and the focus is redirected to the pleural space's unique vulnerability (Donaldson et al., 2010). The reaction of the pleural cavity to the occurrence of foreign particulates has been more investigated with models developed using carbon nanotubes, whose structural resemblance to asbestos fibers is a health concern in construction work. The nanotube retention in the pleural space by length-related effects results in chronic inflammation, fibrosis, and potential tumorigenesis, replicating the disease process with asbestos inhalation. Interestingly, the inflammatory response is not only a direct effect on mesothelial cells but is also enhanced by macrophage activation and subsequent cytokine release, a phenomenon referred to as frustrated phagocytosis. These findings emphasize the dual function of the pleural cavity in disease initiation and progression and offer insights relevant to risk assessment and the design of safer nanomaterials. These studies collectively point out that the pleural space is not an inert anatomical compartment but a biologically active environment that is actively involved in both pulmonary health and disease (Murphy et al., 2012).

Test Your Knowledge

1. Describe the structural layers of the pleural membranes.
2. Differentiate between visceral pleura and parietal pleura in terms of location and function.
3. What is the pleural cavity, and why is it important for lung function?

6.4. Function of the Pleura

Learning Outcome

1. Discuss the Role in Lung Expansion and Contraction
2. Explain the Protection Against Infection
3. How to Maintenance of Negative Pressure

The pleura, a thin serous membrane enveloping the lungs, plays a critical role in respiratory mechanics beyond just being a protective cover. It provides a frictionless, smooth interface between the chest wall and the lungs so that the lungs can expand and contract freely during the breathing cycle. This is achieved through the creation of pleural fluid, which greases the pleural surfaces, preventing irritation and damage that would otherwise occur from repetitive motion. The integrity of the pleura is essential in maintaining the negative pressure within the pleural space, a force that is essential in inflating the lungs. Any disturbance, such as fluid accumulation or infection, can undermine respiratory effectiveness and gas exchange and is used here to highlight the function of the pleura in normal pulmonary function. In addition to its biomechanical functions, the pleura is an essential barrier against pathogenic invasion and a promoter of immune responses. Pathological pleural processes, such as infection with microorganisms, highlight its protective function. For instance, granulomatous inflammation of the pleuritic tissue in response to fungal infections such as cryptococcosis shows the role of pleura in host defense mechanism. The granulomas not only function towards encapsulation of the infection but are also a sign of active participation of the pleura in modulating inflammatory responses to avoid damage to lung parenchyma (Inohara et al., 1959). This immunological feature of the pleura reveals its multifaceted function beyond mechanical facilitation to essential involvement in pulmonary health. Additionally, the function of the pleura in pulmonary movement and spatial orientation is paramount for the precise administration of respiratory treatments and accurate modeling of lung dynamics. New-generation biomechanical models of the thoracic cavity incorporate the pleura as an important structural element that impinges on lung motion against ribs and chest wall. The new models, in which finite element methods investigate pleural and thoracic motions, have significant implications in clinical practice, notably in radiotherapy of lung cancer. By considering pleural elasticity and its influence on the displacement of lungs with breathing, these models improve the accuracy of treatment delivery, minimizing exposure of healthy tissues while ensuring proper targeting of the involved areas (Didier et al., 2009). Consequently, the function of pleura extends beyond physiology to influence therapy outcomes in respiratory medicine (Figure 6.9).

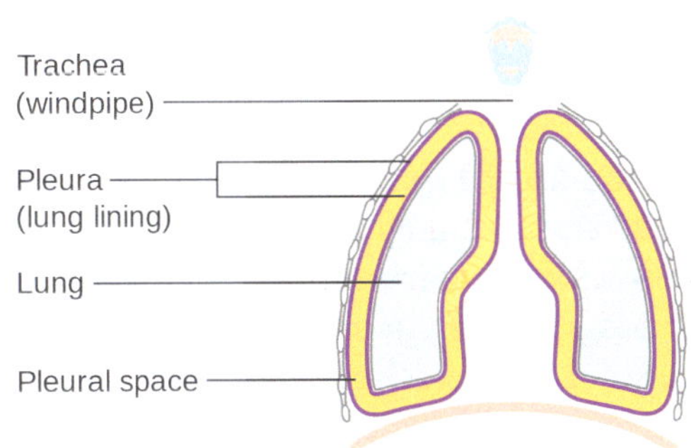

Figure 6.9. Function of the pleura.

Source: By Cancer Research UK - Original email from CRUK, CC BY-SA 4.0, https://commons.wikimedia.org/w/index.php?curid=34334105

6.4.1. Role in Lung Expansion and Contraction

The mechanism of lung inflation and deflation is inseparably dependent on the structural and functional relationship between the lungs and the pleura. The pleura, a thin but resilient serous membrane enveloping the lungs, forms a frictionless cavity that facilitates smooth respiratory movement. During inspiration, the negative pressure generated within the pleural cavity acts as a suction force, drawing the lungs outward in synchrony with thoracic expansion. This pressure gradient between the alveolar airways and pleural space aids the inflation of the alveoli and thus lung volume expansion. On exhalation, elastic recoil of the lung tissue and reduction in thoracic volume lead to deflation of the lungs. Preserving the integrity of the pleural membrane and the pleural pressure homeostasis is thus crucial to the provision of efficient lung inflation and deflation cycles and directly regulates pulmonary function and the efficiency with which breathing occurs (Ikushima et al., 2025). The efficiency with which lungs inflate and deflate is also largely dependent on underlying cellular and molecular forces acting within lung tissues, a process underscored by developments in genomics within cancer research. For instance, mutations such as MTAP deletion in lung tissue were found to be correlated with specific patterns of disease progression and drug susceptibility, suggesting molecular changes might have impacts on lung cell and microenvironment biomechanical properties (Ikushima et al., 2025). These molecular attributes can influence elastic properties of the tissue, cellular growth, and extracellular matrix composition, which could impact lung compliance and responsiveness to the respiratory cycle. These findings emphasize the intersection point of molecular pathology and lung physiology, implying that treatments aimed at particular molecular processes may also change lung mechanics, particularly in disease states when parenchyma and pleura are involved. Beyond molecular determinants, treatments that restore or enhance lung expansion and contraction illustrate the critical role of pleural health in ventilation. Therapeutic interventions, such as the use of lung-amplifying devices in conjunction with physiotherapy in patients with pleural effusion, hold the potential to improve chest wall expansion and increase pulmonary function by mitigating the restrictive impact of pleural fluid accumulation (Zunzunwala et al., 2023). The interventions not only treat symptom reduction but also attempt to restore dynamic biomechanical interaction between the pleura and lung, enabling greater ventilation. This clinical evidence highlights the critical necessity to preserve pleural integrity and to provide optimal lung-pleura interaction to ensure effective respiratory mechanics under a broad spectrum of pathological conditions.

6.4.2. Protection Against Infection

The complex defense mechanisms of the respiratory system are necessary to guard the lungs and pleura against pathogens. The lungs are continuously exposed to pathogens in the air, and thus a complex immune response is necessary to prevent infection. Among these, alveolar macrophages constitute the first line of defense by phagocytosing and killing inhaled microorganisms. Mucociliary clearance also serves to mechanically remove pathogens trapped in mucus, and tight epithelial junctions create a physical barrier. But when the mechanisms are breached by pathogens, innate and adaptive immunity act in unison to respond to the breach. Pleura, the serous covering of the lungs, also helps in immunological defense since it harbors immune cells ready to quickly act when infections penetrate pulmonary integrity. This interaction of barriers and cellular defense shows the complex protection system of the lungs and pleura to ensure respiratory health and dampen disease advancement. New evidence highlights the significant contribution of humoral immunity in the lungs and pleura under infectious challenges. In particular, B cells contribute to host defense by producing pathogen-specific antibodies that assist in neutralizing and clearing. For instance, in tuberculosis, there has been a high antibody-mediated immunity, especially among co-infected individuals with HIV, which suggests an adaptive component of the immunity to Mycobacterium tuberculosis. Studies indicate that with reduced Th1 cytokine production, humoral responses mediated by increased IgG and plasmablast activity are significant in active pulmonary tuberculosis, and this reflects an immunoregulatory shift against infection. This means that antibodies and B cell subsets are not passive bystanders but active modulators that contribute to protection and can also serve as biomarkers of disease progression and activity in lung infection (Ashenafi et al., 2013).

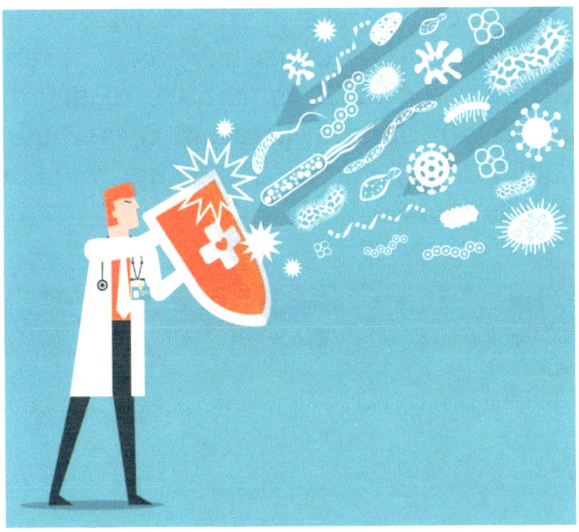

Source: Pfizer. (n.d.). *Doctor Protecting Against Pathogens with a Shield.*

Humoral mechanisms are thus crucial in complementing cellular immunity to allow for pathogen control in pulmonary tissues. The pleural space represents a strategic reservoir for effector immune cells that rapidly mobilize against pulmonary infection, underscoring its functional role in protection against infection. Recent studies have established that B1a B cells present within the pleura migrate into the lung parenchyma in the event of bacterial infection to secrete polyreactive IgM antibodies. These cells are referred to as innate response activator (IRA) B cells and regulate IgM secretion through autocrine signaling with granulocyte/macrophage colony-stimulating factor (GM-CSF). This GM-CSF-IgM axis is an early defense line, which imparts broad-spectrum antimicrobial activity before the complete activation of adaptive immunity. The capacity of these cells to produce protective IgM in a timely fashion underscores their role in immediate lung immunity and underlines the dynamic role of the pleura apart from the physical barrier. Understanding of this axis offers promise of enhancing defensive immune responses to pneumonia and other respiratory infections (Weber et al., 2015).

6.4.3. Maintenance of Negative Pressure

The delicate balance of pressures in the thoracic cavity is necessary for effective pulmonary function. The pleural cavity, between the visceral and parietal pleurae, is at a negative pressure relative to atmospheric pressure, preventing the lung from collapsing and enabling it to expand upon inspiration. This subatmospheric pressure arises due to the elastic recoil tendency of the lungs to pull inward, countered by the outward pull of the chest wall. It is physiologically crucial to uphold this negative pressure since any infringement, e.g., in pneumothorax, disrupts lung inflation and gas exchange. Technological advances, such as ex situ lung perfusion (ESLP) systems with negative pressure ventilation (NPV), better replicate physiological conditions than positive pressure counterparts. These systems highlight the importance of homogeneously distributed intrathoracic pressures in preserving lung integrity and function during transplant procedures, reducing ventilator-induced injury and edema, and thus underscoring the physiological role of negative pressure in lung maintenance (Forgie et al., 2022). These physiological processes of negative pressure in the pleural space extend beyond mechanical forces, encompassing complex biochemical and molecular mechanisms. There is now evidence that endogenously produced molecules such as sulfur dioxide (SO_2) play a regulatory role in the maintenance of vascular tone and pulmonary tissue integrity with indirect influences on pleural pressures. These gasotransmitters relax the smooth muscles and inflammatory reactions of the pulmonary vasculature, which contributes to the stability of lung tissues and their dynamic responsiveness to thoracic pressure fluctuations. By establishing structural and functional relationships among pleurae and the underlying lung parenchyma, such molecular mediators indirectly enable the maintenance of the delicate negative pressure balance essential for respiration. Additional research into endogenous molecules such as SO_2 will likely reveal novel therapeutic targets with which to enhance respiratory mechanics and oppose pathologic disruptions to pleural pressure homeostasis (Huang et al., 2021). Clinical implications of the preservation of negative pleural pressure are especially evident in mechanical ventilation or transplantation procedures. NPV, which more closely replicates normal respiration by generating subatmospheric pressure around the thorax, demonstrates advantages over PPV, in which air is pushed directly into the lungs. Pressure homogeneity in NPV minimizes ventilator-induced lung injury, inflammatory cytokine production, and pulmonary edema during ex situ lung preservation. Preservative strategies with careful modulation of ventilatory settings and perfusion pressures optimize lung viability, with special benefit in donor organs with prolonged ischemic times. The findings encourage clinical use of NPV devices in lung transplantation and critical care practice, reaffirming the basic imperative to maintain negative intrathoracic pressure to perpetuate physiological lung function and improve patient outcomes (Forgie et al., 2022).

Test Your Knowledge

1. How does the mucociliary escalator in the respiratory tract help prevent infections?
2. What structures maintain the integrity of the pleural cavity to sustain negative pressure?

6.5. Common Diseases Affecting the Lungs

Learning Outcome

1. Discuss the Chronic Obstructive Pulmonary Disease (COPD)
2. Focus on Asthma and Its Impact
3. Understand Lung Cancer and Risk Factors

The respiratory system is under continuous attack from environmental pathogens and is thus prone to a range of diseases that compromise lung function. Infectious pathogens like bacteria, viruses, and fungi may cause inflammation that results in diseases like pneumonia and bronchitis. Viral infections, notably the recent SARS-CoV-2 outbreaks, have underscored the relevance of lung pathology in global health crises. COVID-19, which was caused by this virus, showed rapid spread, acute respiratory distress, and extensive mortality, particularly in critically ill patients. Radiological methods, such as chest X-rays and computed tomography (CT), have been crucial for diagnosing and following lung involvement. Ultrasound, due to its portability and ability to be cleaned easily, has proven indispensable in checking lung pathology directly at the bedside, particularly in single or high-risk settings. These technological advances have improved clinical results by promoting early infection detection and follow-up of lung infections (Cui et al., 2020). Apart from infectious diseases, non-infectious disease conditions such as pleurisy significantly affect the pleura and lungs, typically caused by environmental and management factors. Animal model research in swine has demonstrated that poor ventilation, mixed ages, and increased movement or mixing of animals within shared airspace increase the risk for pleural inflammation. Conversely, rigorous biosecurity measures, such as all-in all-out pig flow, cleanliness, and long down time between groups, significantly reduce the incidence of pleurisy. These findings highlight the need for regulation of the environment and biosecurity in order to prevent pleural disease and illustrate the immediate impact of management protocols on the lung. Although this research might be geared toward animal pathology, the principles of disease prevention used in regulating the environment are relevant to human lung health and pleural disease management (Jäger et al., 2013).

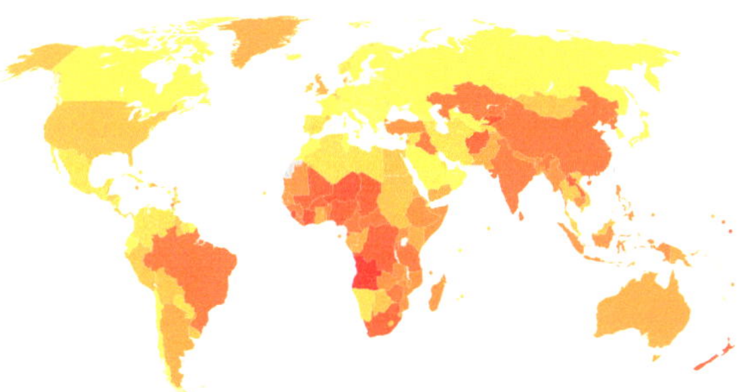

Figure 6.10. Common diseases affecting the lungs.

Source: By Lokal_Profil, CC BY-SA 2.5, https://commons.wikimedia.org/w/index.php?curid=8443662

Chronic lung illnesses such as chronic obstructive pulmonary disease (COPD) and asthma are a significant category of lung pathology with sustained health consequences. They are characterized by airflow limitation and airway inflammation leading to disturbance of gas exchange and resulting symptoms like cough and shortness of breath. Although often attributed to smoking or allergens, the pathogenesis also involves complex immune mechanisms and structural changes in the lung and pleural tissues. The chronic nature of these illnesses requires early diagnosis and multidisciplinary care to prevent advancement and improve quality of life (QoL). Pulmonary rehabilitation, drug therapy, and lifestyle modification play a crucial role in managing these chronic illnesses, indicating the necessity of continued research and clinical observation in the treatment of common diseases of the lungs and pleura (Figure 6.10).

6.5.1. Chronic Obstructive Pulmonary Disease (COPD)

The complex lung structure contains a dense vasculature and tissue network responsible for respiratory performance and immune surveillance. In COPD, structural changes extend beyond the airways to the lymphatic vessels closely associated with the lung parenchyma and pleura. Current morphometric studies illustrate a dramatic augmentation in the density of lymphatic vessels within the alveolar walls of severe COPD patients, particularly over fibrotic tissue where lymphatic density can rise exponentially. These alterations point toward an adaptive process potentially linked to elevated immune cell trafficking and modulation within the peripheral lung spaces. Moreover, bronchiolar lymphatics and their associated arteries exhibit enhanced immune molecule expression, suggesting a phenotypic change that may have implications for the progression of disease and local inflammation. Understanding these histopathologic alterations is significant as they suggest the complex nature of immune reactions in severe COPD and potentially offer new avenues for targeted treatment (Mori et al., 2013). A significant public health issue, COPD is a leading cause of morbidity and mortality in the United States, worsened by underdiagnosis and ignorance. COPD commonly manifests as emphysema, which is characterized by the pathologic and irreversible expansion of airspaces beyond the terminal bronchioles, with loss of alveolar walls and little fibrosis. This pathophysiologic characteristic reduces gas exchange and causes chronic respiratory insufficiency. Preventive interventions, under the leadership of health professionals such as Advanced Practice Nurses, focus on early disease detection through comprehensive knowledge of disease processes and risk factors. Education of patients on smoking cessation, environmental exposures, and symptoms is an important factor in preventing disease burden and progression. General management thus depends not only on pharmacological management but also on preventive patient and community measures aimed at curbing the rising prevalence of COPD (Nuxol et al., 2017). The pleura and lungs are an active interface where pathological processes of COPD may disrupt normal respiratory mechanics and immunological balance. Following the progression of the disease, the lung tissue and pleural space experience augmented inflammatory responses and structural remodeling, compromising airflow and gas diffusion. Of specific interest is the role played by altered lymphatic vessel networks to mediate immune cell trafficking to these sites which may lead to increased inflammation and fibrotic remodeling. The elevated immunoreactivity of lymph vessels to chemokines like CCL21 and scavenger receptors like D6 in the lungs of COPD patients indicates a drastic change in the immune environment of the lung, which could be responsible for both persistence of disease as well as secondary infection. Integration of such findings with the overall picture of lung pathology strengthens the conceptual framework needed to address COPD's multifaceted impact on respiratory function and provides a basis for future research initiatives aimed at modulating lymphatic involvement in chronic lung disease (Mori et al., 2013) (Figure 6.11).

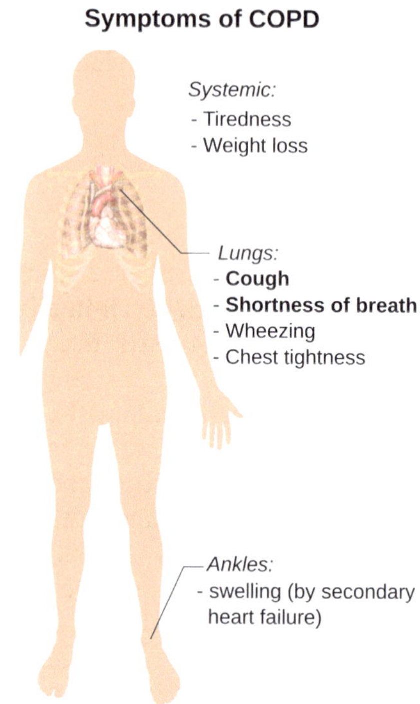

Figure 6.11. Chronic obstructive pulmonary disease (COPD).

Source: By Mikael Häggström - All used images are in public domain., Public Domain, https://commons.wikimedia.org/w/index.php?curid=27469766

6.5.2. Asthma and Its Impact

The lungs have a vital role to play in oxygenating blood and removing carbon dioxide, but useful functioning can be severely damaged by chronic diseases such as asthma. Asthma is characterized by inflammation and narrowing of the airways, which creates intermittent breathing difficulty, including wheezing, coughing, and breathlessness. This inflammation not only reduces airflow but also increases airway hyper-responsiveness, making stimuli of the environment more sensitive. Chronic inflammation of asthma can facilitate structural changes in the bronchi walls, or remodeling, that further exacerbates respiratory impairment. The changes involve both the lungs and the overlying pleura by altering normal lung mechanics, while the pleura itself is not inflamed in asthma. Understanding such pathological alterations is crucial to realize how asthma diminishes overall lung function and QoL. The impact of asthma extends past mere respiratory distress, with a substantial impact on pulmonary reserve and gas exchange efficacy. Repeated asthmatic episodes limit airflow, increasing the work of breathing and typically causing hypoxemia during extreme attacks. Pulmonary function testing most commonly demonstrates reduced forced expiratory volume and peak expiratory flow rates, highlighting airway obstruction. Obstruction may indirectly affect pleural dynamics, possibly reducing lung compliance and predisposing to ventilation-perfusion mismatch. In contrast to malignant pleural conditions for which therapies such as pleurodesis may have a minimal effect on lung function, asthmas chronic airway inflammation induces more widespread functional impairment, with a reversible and an irreversible component (Bone et al., 1999). Such abnormalities of lung function highlight the chronic and often progressive nature of asthma, classifying it as a major cause of respiratory morbidity. Moreover, the management of asthma involves its prolonged effect on respiratory function and the challenge of distinguishing its effect from other lung diseases such as lung cancer. While both lung cancer and asthma involve pathological alterations in lung tissue and supportive elements, asthma is mainly characterized by airway inflammation and remodeling but not neoplastic change (Gray et al., 2019). Nevertheless, both are capable of leading to impaired respiratory efficiency and require special treatments. Asthma's episodic, often unpredictable, course mandates careful control to prevent exacerbations and preserve lung function. Among the total respiratory system, the lungs and pleura need to be viewed as an entity to appreciate completely the complete impact of asthma's influence, making clinical management relate to ongoing research for optimal patient outcomes.

6.5.3. Lung Cancer and Risk Factors

Environmental and occupational exposures have long been a primary component of lung cancer induction, and a variety of inhaled agents have been important determinants of disease risk. At the top of this list are asbestos fibers, which are identified as particularly egregious carcinogens due to both their fibrous nature and their tendency to remain in lung tissue. Studies comparing different test methods on fibrous materials, including asbestos, demonstrate that inhalation exposure is an important determinant of pulmonary toxicity and carcinogenicity. Even though certain intraperitoneal or intrapleural administration tests are positive, these do not always forecast lung-specific cancer risks. Indeed, it has been argued that these types of tests might have the potential to clear certain fibers but are not sufficient on their own to determine inhalational carcinogenicity. This identifies the difficulty in assessing lung cancer risk from occupational exposure to fibrous dusts and demands more nuanced approaches to assessing human health risk from environmental carcinogens (Drummond et al., 2016). Tobacco smoking is the most significant risk factor for lung cancer and is responsible for the great majority of lung cancers worldwide. The carcinogens present in tobacco smoke induce genetic mutations in the lung epithelium, initiating malignant transformation. However, the pathogenesis of lung cancer is multifactorial; risks are augmented by interactions of smoking with other etiologic factors such as genetic predispositions, air pollution, and inhaled fibers. Those patients with pulmonary comorbid conditions or previous exposures, such as those necessitating special medical procedures or with cancer of pleural surfaces, also have altered disease trajectories. The role of the pleura in some metastatic processes of lung cancer highlights the requirement for integrated knowledge between pleural and lung parenchymal pathology to additionally characterize disease progression and patient prognosis (Esquivel et al., 1988). Apart from smoking and occupational exposure, accumulating evidence implicates environmental pollutants and genetic factors are associated with lung cancer. Particulate matter in the air, such as ultrafine dust and industrial fibers, can cause chronic inflammation and oxidative DNA damage, leading to tumorigenesis. Genetic polymorphisms in carcinogen metabolism or DNA repair can influence host susceptibility to these exogenous insults, leading to heterogeneous cancer incidence in populations exposed to these factors.

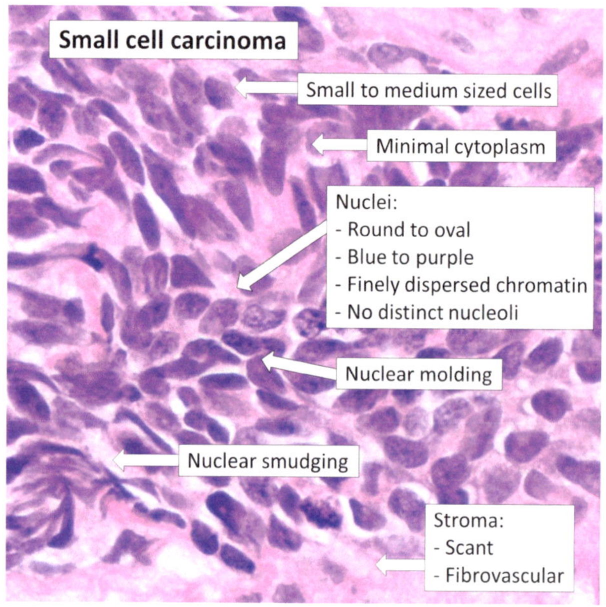

Figure 6.12. Lung cancer and risk factors.

Source: By Mikael Häggström, M.D. Author info- Reusing images- Conflicts of interest:NoneMikael Häggström, M.D.Consent note: Consent from the patient or patient's relatives is regarded as redundant, because of absence of identifiable features (List of HIPAA identifiers) in the media and case information (See also HIPAA case reports guidance). - Own work, CC0, https://commons.wikimedia.org/w/index.php?curid=141872000

Thus, risk assessment of lung cancer needs to be a multifaceted strategy incorporating environmental, occupational, and host genetic information. This multifaceted interaction complicates clinical prediction and underscores the necessity for continued research into systematic pathways of pulmonary injury and pleural involvement in order to plan prevention and targeted therapies based on diverse risk profiles (Esquivel et al., 1988; Drummond et al., 2016) (Figure 6.12).

Test Your Knowledge

1. What are the main physiological changes in the airways during an asthma attack?
2. How can early symptoms of lung cancer be misinterpreted in clinical practice?

6.6. Common Diseases Affecting the Pleura

Learning Outcome

1. Pleurisy and Its Symptoms
2. Pleural Effusion and Causes
3. Mesothelioma and Its Association with Asbestos

It is critical to understand the various conditions involving the pleura given that its precious contribution to lung function and respiratory status. Pleuritis, which is an inflammation of the pleura, is one of the most common pleural disorders and characteristically presents with sharp chest pain and limited respiratory excursion. Pathology can be caused by infections, autoimmune conditions, or physical injury, sometimes in association with bacterial pneumonia or viral illnesses. In particular, chronic suppurative pneumonia is a critical disease whereby inflammation extends to the pleura with high morbidity. Diagnosis is challenging due to overlapping syndromes with parenchymal lung illnesses, but technological advancements in imaging, such as ultrasound, have enhanced visualization of pleural disease with greater specificity, thereby enhancing early diagnosis and treatment planning (Scott, 2013). These developments stress the importance of combining clinical assessment with modern diagnostic techniques in the management of pleural conditions. In addition to inflammation, pleural effusion is a frequent pleural disorder where there is an accumulation of excess fluid in the pleural space. It may be due to congestive heart failure (CHF), tumors, infections, or injury, all of which have distinct clinical and therapeutic features. The pleural fluid disrupts the normal pressure balance, undermining lung expansion and respiratory distress. In today's clinical practice, imaging technologies like ultrasound has been found to be invaluable with their portability and ability to offer real-time assessment at bedside levels, particularly in complex cases like those encountered during the COVID-19 pandemic (Cui et al., 2020). This allows for instant intervention by starting thoracentesis and monitoring the fluid changes. Recognition of pleural effusions of multifactorial origin and application of focused diagnostic approaches are essential steps in reducing complications and improving patient outcomes. Pneumothorax, or the presence of air in the pleural space, is a serious condition that affects the pleura by causing lung collapse and impaired gas exchange. It can be spontaneous or following trauma, invasive procedures, or underlying lung disease. Clinical presentation may involve acute chest pain and dyspnea, which require immediate recognition and treatment to avoid respiratory failure. Advanced imaging aids in correct diagnosis, while therapy ranges from conservative management to chest tube placement based on the severity. The prevalence of highly contagious respiratory illnesses, such as COVID-19, highlights the complexity of managing pleural complications because infection-related pleural disease can exacerbate pneumothorax risk and complicate treatment avenues (Cui et al., 2020). It is therefore important to grasp the mechanisms and clinical significance of common pleural diseases in optimizing respiratory care in the general picture of pulmonary health.

6.6.1. Pleurisy and Its Symptoms

The pleura, a thin serous membrane enveloping the lungs and lining the chest cavity, plays a crucial role in permitting smooth respiratory motion. Inflammation of the pleura results in the condition of pleurisy or pleuritis, which, in general, leads to severe pain. This inflammation disrupts the otherwise frictionless apposition of the parietal and visceral layers, clinically being manifested as point tenderness over the chest that is typically worsened with deep breathing or coughing. Apart from this primary symptom, patients may also show secondary findings such as fever and dyspnea, which are an expression of the underlying inflammatory or infectious processes. The magnitude and character of these findings typically guide clinicians early during the diagnostic workup, emphasizing symptom detection in the treatment of pleural diseases. The pathogenesis of pleurisy is diverse with infectious, neoplastic, and autoimmune processes, each carrying unique implications in the clinic. Of the infective causes, purulent or empyemic pleurisy, that is, bacterial pleurisy, needs to be treated immediately since it can severely impair lung function and threaten patient outcome. Clinical practice stresses that patients present with chest pain and fever, and imaging tests such as chest X-rays and CT reveal fluid between pleural layers. Bacterial infections such as tuberculosis comprise the most frequent etiologic factors in the majority of cases, and they need prompt, focused intervention to reduce complications and improve outcomes (Benjelloun et al., 2025). Awareness of these etiologic factors serves a crucial function in tailoring treatment protocols and facilitating optimal recovery of patients in pleural inflammatory conditions. Complications of pleurisy can significantly influence patient care and prognosis if pleural fluid collection or malignancy occurs with inflammation. In malignant pleurisy, therapeutic interventions such as pleurodesis are employed to prevent recurrent pleural effusion and related respiratory dysfunction before the application of systemic therapies. This is particularly relevant in thyroid carcinoma patients, where malignant pleurisy can be a risk for pneumothorax during targeted therapy, a rare but fatal complication that entails the presence of air in the pleural space. The susceptibility of the pleural tissue in such cases renders surgery and these complications highlight the need for precautions against negative outcomes (Sakamoto et al., 2024). Hence, understanding the overlapping zone of signs of pleurisy and its complications is paramount for comprehensive lung and pleural treatment (Figure 6.13).

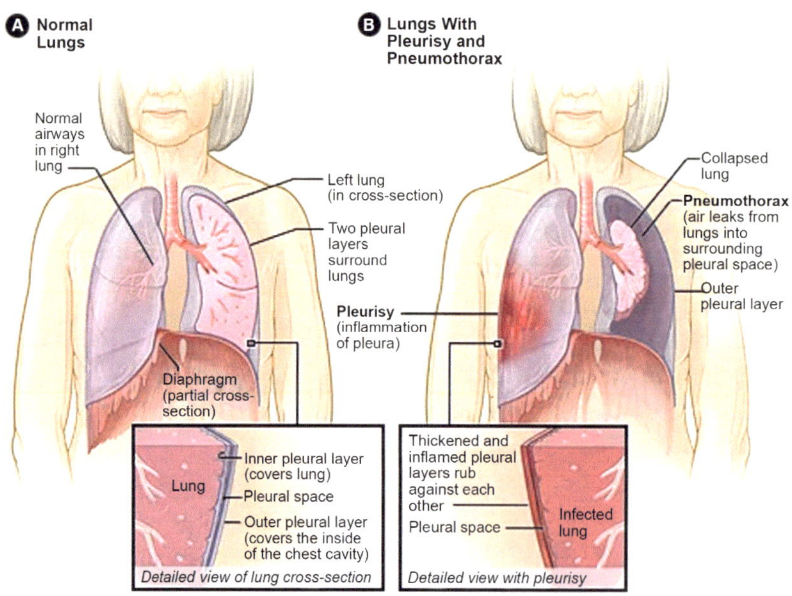

Figure 6.13. Pleurisy and its symptoms.

Source: By National Heart Lung and Blood Institute - National Heart Lung and Blood Institute, Public Domain, https://commons.wikimedia.org/w/index.php?curid=29583160

6.6.2. Pleural Effusion and Causes

Excess accumulation of fluid in the pleural space is a significant pathological condition that tends to complicate a wide range of pulmonary and systemic diseases. The accumulation of fluid referred to as pleural effusion results from an imbalance in the production and resorption of pleural fluid. Normally, there is a thin layer of lubricating fluid coating the pleural space, allowing for free expansion of the lungs during inhalation. However, alterations of vascular permeability, lymphatic drainage, or integrity of pleural membranes lead to fluid accumulation. Pleural effusions are clinically manifested by dyspnea, pain, or cough but can remain silent with minor effusions. Diagnostic imaging, particularly ultrasound, offers a convenient and helpful means of detecting and categorizing pleural effusions. Portability and real-time visualization capability of ultrasound are imperative in the acute or critical care setting, allowing better patient evaluation and management without exposing the patient to radiation (Cui et al., 2020). Etiologies of pleural effusion are multifactorial, ranging from infectious and neoplastic diseases to systemic diseases and cardiac disease. Infectious causes, especially bacterial pneumonia, may cause exudative effusions through increased vascular permeability and inflammation of the pleura. Similarly, tuberculosis remains a significant etiologic component in endemic regions. Malignancy involvement, typically by primary lung cancer or metastatic disease, may lead to malignant pleural effusion with proteinaceous fluid and tumor cells in the pleural space. Furthermore, CHF is a common cause of transudative effusions due to increased hydrostatic pressure with consequent fluid leakage but little inflammation. Awareness of such diverse etiologies assists clinicians in ordering appropriate diagnostic studies and treatment (Liu et al., 2020). In intensive care, the identification and management of pleural effusions necessitate prompt and precise clinical assessment because they may have potential impacts on respiratory mechanics and oxygenation. Ultrasound-guided thoracentesis is now a routine procedure, balancing diagnostic efficiency with safety by preventing complications, especially in critically ill patients. Additionally, critical care ultrasonography allows bedside pleural fluid detection to monitor disease progression and response to therapy dynamically. With experience acquired in treating patients with serious respiratory infections and complications such as COVID-19, bedside imaging approaches allow real-time monitoring and prompt interventions. This targeted use of ultrasound emphasizes its central position not only in the diagnosis of pleural effusions but also in making interventional procedures easier, thereby improving patient outcomes in the intensive care unit (Ernest, 2020; Liu et al., 2020) (Figure 6.14).

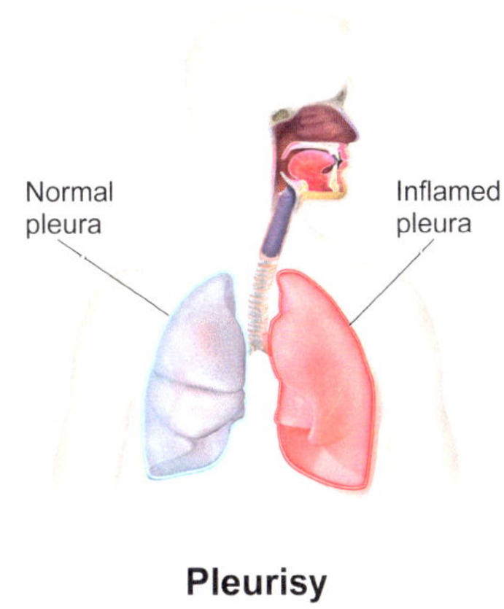

Figure 6.14. Pleural effusion and causes.

Source: By BruceBlaus - Own work, CC BY-SA 4.0, https://commons.wikimedia.org/w/index.php?curid=44806587

6.6.3. Mesothelioma and Its Association with Asbestos

The interaction of inhaled fibrous particles with the lung cellular environment represents a foundation in the context of occupational respiratory disorders. Asbestos fibers are one of these, and they have been highly implicated in the occurrence of extreme pathological changes by virtue of their resistant and biopersistent nature. Various experimental investigations of comparison between inhalation models and intraperitoneal and intrapleural injections illustrate the complexities of carcinogenicity triggered by fibers. While some fiber tests produce equal results across test modes, asbestos is the sole substance that shows positive carcinogenic responses in both inhalation and intrapleural tests, indicating its highest pathogenicity. Comparing these testing routes has enhanced knowledge of how asbestos fibers cause pulmonary toxicity, especially by causing malignant transformation. Despite a few methodological deficiencies, these findings highlight the need for placing more emphasis on inhalation exposure measurements in determining lung and pleural disease resulting from industrial fibers like asbestos (Drummond et al., 2016). The pleura, particularly the parietal pleura lining the thoracic cavity, plays an important role in the pathogenesis of asbestos-induced mesothelioma. Recent research advances involve data from studies of high aspect ratio nanoparticles, such as carbon nanotubes, to maximize the understanding of asbestos fiber behavior in the pleural microenvironment. The parietal pleura contains specialized stomata that are designed to remove particles; nevertheless, asbestos fibers block passage through these pores mechanically. Mechanical retention causes chronic inflammation and remodeling of tissue, which provides a niche for the transformation of mesothelial cells. In addition, clinical observations by thoracoscopy have identified the origin location of pleural mesothelioma primarily in the parietal pleura, redefining traditional concepts that identified tumor incidence primarily with lung parenchymal fiber burden. The comprehensive mechanistic model bears a strong implication of identifying correctly asbestos-related mesothelioma pathogenesis and spatial pathology between the layers of the pleura (Donaldson et al., 2010). In order to understand the pathogenic mechanisms of asbestos-induced mesothelioma, one has to adopt a three-dimensional perspective taking into consideration fiber biopersistence, anatomical retention, and cellular response dynamics. The pathogenesis of mesothelioma due to asbestos exposure is based on the ability of the fibers to evade clearance, remain retained in pleural tissues, and induce oxidative stress and genetic damage. This pathway culminates in malignant mesothelial cell proliferation as pleural mesothelioma, a disease with very limited therapies and unfavorable prognosis. Mechanistic studies, combined with epidemiological evidence, maintain that the pathogenesis of the disease lies not just in fiber inhalation but also in the resulting fibrotic and inflammatory consequences compartmentalized within the pleural space. Knowledge of such processes is critical to deploying more effective preventive strategies and treatments aimed at reducing the global morbidity of asbestos-related mesothelioma in affected groups (Donaldson et al., 2010; Drummond et al., 2016).

Test Your Knowledge

1. What do you understand pleural effusion and causes?
2. Explain the mesothelioma and its association with asbestos.

SUMMARY

The complex physiology and anatomy of the pleura and the lungs are of paramount importance for effective respiration and general homeostasis. Through comprehension of their structural components and pathways, it is evident how alterations within these systems lead to significant clinical impacts. Pathologies affecting either the pulmonary parenchyma or the pleural cavity place physiological dysfunctions, which usually lead to obstructed gas exchange, inflammation, or fluid collection. The application of diagnostic criteria, as described in contemporary studies, assists clinicians in efficiently diagnosing and treating such conditions in order to optimize patient outcomes. In addition, advances in radiological and histopathological techniques have improved our ability to study pathology at macroscopic and microscopic levels to obtain comprehensive information on lung and pleural diseases (Ernest, 2020). These multidisciplinary approaches emphasize the sophistication and the necessity of continuous study in respiratory medicine. Improvements in biomedical technologies over the last few years have further clarified lung and pleural physiology by enabling precise modeling of physiological and pathological processes. Amongst these, organ-on-a-chip platforms represent a paradigm shift, mimicking the microenvironment of pulmonary tissue with high fidelity. Through integrating cell biology, engineering, and biomaterial science, such systems mimic the biomechanical and biochemical stimulation of the lungs and allow researchers to study interactions between the alveolar and pleural spaces within controlled conditions (Wu et al., 2020). This biomimetic technology not only accelerates drug development and toxicity screening but also offers insight into disease development and possible treatments, thereby bridging gaps between *in vitro* research and clinical applications. The capacity to replicate a living lung microenvironment is a promising frontier in respiratory research and individualized medicine. In reconciling the complex information available on the lungs and pleura, it is clear that advancing our fundamental knowledge and technological capabilities is essential. Combining traditional clinical approaches with cutting-edge bioengineering technologies stimulates a more holistic vision for understanding lung wellness and disease. Thus, future research must address advancing more accurate diagnostic methods and developing new therapeutic modalities to treat enduring problems in pulmonary therapy. The incessant interplay among profound anatomical studies, pathophysiological knowledge, and cutting-edge technology can potentially revolutionize therapeutic strategies and patient QoL. In this regard, the ongoing development of respiratory science goes hand in hand with managing the complex issues surrounding lung and pleural diseases (Ernest, 2020; Wu et al., 2020).

An understanding of the complex anatomy and physiology of the lungs and pleura provides a foundation for appreciating their vital role in respiratory health and disease. The lungs facilitate gas exchange, which is necessary for oxygenating the blood and removing carbon dioxide. Enveloping the lungs, the pleurae—two thin sheets—conform to a closed, lubricated space that decreases friction during breathing. Disruptions of this balance, such as air into the pleural space leading to a pneumothorax, can severely compromise lung function. Successful clinical management relies on identifying these disruptions promptly and being aware of the pathophysiology that underlies them. Current guidelines stress individualized approaches to spontaneous pneumothorax treatment, with special attention to maneuvers that best promote recovery and reduce recurrence. These clinical strategies emphasize the pleura's central interaction with lung mechanics and the imperative of evidence-based treatment paradigms grounded in contemporary research (Roberts et al., 2023). Advances in critical care ultrasonography have largely made bedside diagnosis and monitoring of pulmonary and pleural diseases possible. Lung ultrasound, in reality, has become a valuable tool for intensivists with the ability to provide quick, non-invasive assessment of pleural fluid, consolidation of lung, and pneumothorax. The consensus view has established the essential skills of complete lung and pleural ultrasonography such that it is applied consistently and correctly in the most important environments. These guidelines not only advance diagnostic precision but also aid in improved patient outcomes with timely interventions. Integrating imaging and clinical evaluation is a multidisciplinary approach that reflects the complexity of pleural and lung disease and the importance of lifelong professional development (Robba et al., 2021). As the summation point for pulmonary and pleural anatomy, physiology, pathology, and management, it is apparent that a multifaceted understanding is necessary to maintain competent clinical practice. The pleura and lungs collaborate to provide respiratory homeostasis, and disruptions result in acute and chronic morbidities that require early diagnosis and treatment. Optimal practice for conditions like spontaneous pneumothorax involves patient-centered, sensitive care that balances conservative and operative management (Roberts et al., 2023). Additionally, the development of bedside ultrasonography as a daily diagnostic tool enhances clinical precision and guides therapeutic decisions (Robba et al., 2021). Briefly, integrating anatomical knowledge, clinical practice, and technological advancement forms the basis for effective management programs in pulmonary and pleural medicine (Broaddus et al., 2011).

KEY TERMS FROM THIS CHAPTER

Visceral Pleura	Parietal Pleura	Pleural Cavity
Pleural Fluid	Costodiaphragmatic Recess	Hilum of Lung
Pulmonary Artery	Pulmonary Vein	Primary Bronchus
Bronchopulmonary Segments	Oblique Fissure	Horizontal Fissure
Lobes of the Lung	Apex of Lung	Base of Lung
Lingula	Diaphragmatic Surface	Mediastinal Surface

CRITICAL THINKING QUESTIONS

1. **Which pleura covers the surface of the lungs?**
   a. Parietal pleura
   b. Mediastinal pleura
   c. Diaphragmatic pleura
   d. Visceral pleura
2. **How many lobes does the right lung have?**
   a. One
   b. Two
   c. Three
   d. Four
3. **The costodiaphragmatic recess is located between:**
   a. The diaphragm and mediastinum
   b. The ribs and diaphragm
   c. The lungs and heart
   d. The pleura and pericardium
4. **Which structure is not found at the hilum of the lung?**
   a. Pulmonary artery
   b. Pulmonary vein
   c. Bronchus
   d. Esophagus
5. **The left lung has a distinctive feature called:**
   a. Oblique fissure only
   b. Horizontal fissure
   c. Lingula
   d. Apex notch

Short Answer Questions

1. What is the significance of the pleural cavity?
2. Describe the root (hilum) of thc lung and its contents.
3. Define the costodiaphragmatic recess and state its clinical relevance.
4. Explain the bronchopulmonary segments and their surgical importance.
5. Describe the nerve supply of the pleura.

Answers to Critical Thinking Questions

1. (d) 2. (c) 3. (b) 4. (d) 5. (c)

REFERENCES

1. Arnowitz, Ben Peter, *"A Study of the* Respiratory System of the Sparrow (Passer domesticus)" (1943). Bachelors' Theses. 162. https://epublications.marquette.edu/bachelor_essays/162 (accessed on 8th May 2025).
2. Bei, Y., Wang, F., Yang, C., & Xiao, J. (2015). Telocytes in regenerative medicine. Journal of Cellular and Molecular Medicine, 19, 1441–1454. https://doi.org/10.1111/jcmm.12594 (accessed on 8th May 2025).
3. Benjelloun, H., *Amir, A., Chhen, I., Harraz, H.,* Chaanoun, K., Zaghba, N., & Yassine, N. (2025). Epidemiological, etiological and evolutionary profile of purulent pleurisy: About 91 cases. Scholars Journal of Medical Case Reports. https://doi.org/10.36347/sjmcr.2025.v13i03.022. https://www.semanticscholar.org/paper/ed515fa7013ea7c6cbc*dd61a0f264e4ad80c38e*c *(a*ccessed on 8th May 2025).
4. Blackadar, C. B. (2016). Historical review of the causes of cancer. World Journal of Clinical Oncology, 7(1), 54–54. https://doi.org/10.5306/wjco.v7.i1.54 (accessed on 8th May 2025).
5. Broaddus, V. C., Everitt, J. I., Black, B., & Kane, A. B. (2011). Non-neoplastic and neoplastic pleural endpoints following fiber exposure. Journal of toxicolo*gy and environmental health. Part B, Critical* reviews, 14(1-4), 153–178. https://doi.org/10.1080/10937404.2011.556049 (accessed on 8th May 2025).
6. Donaldson, K., Murphy, F. A., Duffin, R., & Poland, C. A. (2010). Asbestos, carbon nanotubes and the pleural mesothelium: a review of the hypothesis regarding the ro*le of long fibre retention in the pariet*al pleura, inflammation and mesothelioma. Particle and fibre toxicology, 7, 5. https://doi.org/10.1186/1743-8977-7-5 (accessed on 8th May 2025).
7. Drummond, G., Bevan, R., & Harrison, P. (2016). A comparison of the results from intra-pleural and intra-peritoneal studies with those from inhalation and intratracheal tests for the assessment of pulmonary responses to inhalable dusts and fibres. Regulatory toxicology and pharmacology : RTP, 81, 89–105. https://doi.org/10.1016/j.yrtph.2016.07.019(accessed on 8th May 2025).
8. Gray, M. E., Meehan, J., Sullivan, P., Marland, J. R. K., Greenhalgh, S. N., Gregson, R., Clutton, R. E., Ward, C., Cousens, *C., Griffiths, D. J., Murray, A., & Argyle,* D. (2019). Ovine Pulmonary Adenocarcinoma: A Unique Model to Improve Lung Cancer Research. Frontiers in oncol*ogy, 9, 335. https://doi.org/10.3389/fonc.2019.00335 (accessed on 8th May 2025).*
9. Hegde RR, Geetha B Markande, Prashanth Jain. Pragmatic Analysis of Pranavaha Srotas. J Ayurveda Integr Med Sci [Internet]. 2023Nov.9 [cited 2025Jun.19];8(9):93 -97. Available from: https://jaims.in/jaims/article/view/2657 (accessed on 8th May 2025).
10. Hieba, E. G., Shaimaa, E. E., Dina, S. S., & Noha, A. O. (2020). Diffusion lung capacity for carbon monoxide correlates with HRCT findings in patients with diffuse parenchymal lung disease. The Egyptian Journal of Bronchology, 14. https://www.semanticscholar.org/paper/0e20331a7059aa69eeaeb1fcb7f8cbebe56*dbeeb (accessed on 8th May 2025*).
11. https://www.semanticscholar.org/paper/a8b0f49cbf0105c8535eca61b4719c0053dc3ffb (accessed on 8th May 2025).
12. Huang, Y., Zhang, H., Lv, B., Tang, C., Du, J., & Jin, H. (2022). Sulfur Dioxide: Endogenous Generation, Biological Effects, Detection, and Therapeutic *Potential. Antioxidants & redox*

*signali*ng, 36(4-6), 256–274. https://doi.org/10.1089/ars.2021.0213 (accessed on 8th May 2025).

13. Ikushima, H., Watanabe, K., Shinozaki-Ushiku, A., Oda, K., & Kage, H. (2025). Abstract 1122: Pan-cancer clinical and molecular landscape of MTAP deletion in nationwide and internation*al comprehensive genomic data.* Cancer Research. ESMO Open, Volume 10, Issue 4, 104535

14. Inohara, T., Kanamoto, A., Kuroda, K., Murase, K., et al. (1959). Cryptococcus: Pathological Observations of Five Autopsy Cas*es and One Biopsy Case. https:*//core.ac.uk/download/12548640.pdf (accessed on 8th May 2025).

15. José L.V. Mejino and Cornelius Rosse. 2004. Symbolic modeling of structural relationships in the Foundational Model of Anatomy. In Proceedings of the First International Conference on Formal Biomedical Knowledge Representatio*n - Volume 102* (KRMED'14). American Medical Informatics Association, Bethesda, MD, 48–62. (accessed on 8th May 2025).

16. Kuebler, W. M., Matuszak, J., & Tabuchi, A. (2020). Ventilation and Perfusion at the Alveolar Level: Insights *from Lung Intravital Microscopy. https://core.ac.uk/download/333952469.pdf (acces*sed on 8th May 2025).

17. Mori, M., Andersson, C. K., Graham, G. J., Löfdahl, C. G., & Erjefält, J. S. (2013). Increased number and altered phenotype of lymphatic vessels in peripheral lung compartments of patients *with COPD. Respiratory research, 14(1), 65. https://doi.org/10.1186/1465*-9921-14-65 (accessed on 8th May 2025).

18. Oeckler, R. A., & Hubmayr, R. D. (2007). Alveolar microstrain and the dark side of the lung. Critical ca*re (London, England), 11(6), 177. https://doi.org/10.1186/cc6160 (accessed on 8th May 202*5).

19. Raghu, G., Rémy-Jardin, M., Ryerson, C. J., Myers, J. L., Kreuter, M., Vašáková, M., Bargagli, E., et al. (2020). Diagnosis of hypersensitivity pneumonitis in adults: An official ATS/JRS/ALAT clinical practice guideline. American Journal of Respiratory and Critical Care Medicine, 202, e36–e69. https://doi.org/10.1164/rccm.202005-2032st (accessed on 8th May 2025).

20. Roberts, M., Rahman, N. M., Maskell, N., Bibby, A., Blyth, K. G., Corcoran, J., Edey, A., et al. (2023). British thoracic society guideline for pleural disease. Thorax, 78, s1–s42. https://doi.org/10.1136/thorax-2022-219784 (accessed on 8th May 2025).

21. Rosse, C. (2000). Terminologia Anatomica; Considered from the Perspective of Next-Generation Knowledge Sources. https://core.ac.uk/download/pdf/9412243.pdf (accessed on 8th May 2025).

22. Scott P. R. (2013). Clinical presentation, *auscultation recordings,* ultrasonographic findings and treatment response of 12 adult cattle with chronic suppurative pneumonia: case study. Irish veterinary journal, 66(1), 5. https://doi.org/10.1186/2046-0481-66-5 (accessed on 8th May 2025).

23. Vergel, E. (2020). Respiratory Failure: Classification, Epidemiology and Etiolog*y Review. https://core.ac.uk/download/326559563.pdf Ernest, V.* (2020). Respiratory failure: Classification, Epidemiology and Etiology Review. Journal La Medihealtico, 1(2), 15-20. https://doi.org/10.37899/journallamedihealtico.v1i2.96 (accessed on 8th May 2025).

24. Weber, G. F., Chousterman, B. G., Hilgendo*rf, I., Ro*bbins, C. S., Theurl, I., Gerhardt, L. M., Iwamoto, Y., Quach, T. D., Ali, M., Chen, J. W., Rothste*in, T. L., Nahrendorf, M., Weissleder, R.,*

& Swirski, F. K. (2014). Pleural innate response activator B cells protect against pneumonia via a GM-CSF-IgM axis. The Journal of experimenta*l medicine, 211(6), 1243–1256. https://doi.org/10.1084/jem.20131471 (*accessed on 8th May 2025).

25. Wu, Q., Liu, J., Wang, X., Feng, L., Wu, J., Zhu, X., Wen, W., et al. (2020). Organ-on-a-chip: Recent break*throughs and future pro*spects. BioMedical Engineering OnLine, 19. https://doi.org/10.1186/s12938-020-0752-0 (accessed on 8th May 2025).

26. Xi Liu, MD, Yang Hai, MD, Bin Ma, MD, Weelic Chong, BA, Ji-Bin Liu, MD. Critical Care Ultrasonography and Its Application f*or COVID-19. Advanced Ultrasound* in Diagnosis and Therapy, 2020, 4(2): 43-49.(accessed on 8th May 2025).

27. Zunzunwala, S., & Vardhan, D. (2023). Efficacy of lung boost device on pulmonary function and chest expansion in pleural effusion patient: A randomized control trial protocol. *F1000Research*. https://www.semanticscholar.org/paper/fe86c61dea1d4423d11cf17bf383accb82f6b961 (accessed on 8th May 2025).

HEART AND PERICARDIUM

7

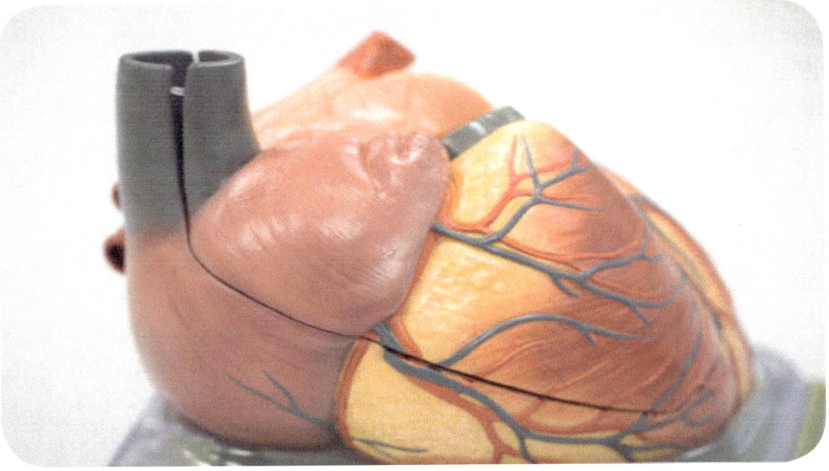

Introduction

The cardiovascular system is vital for maintaining life, and the heart acts as its center, which is tasked with pumping blood through the body. The efficiency of the heart is not only because of its muscle but also because of surrounding structures, which include the pericardium, usually underrated but a crucial component. The pericardium acts as a protective sac, giving mechanical support and lessening friction during cardiac cycles. Understanding of the heart in isolation provides only partial insight; consideration of pericardial tissues, with which it exists together, completes the picture and provides full insight into functional dynamics. Progress in anatomical terminology as well as in classification also tends to highlight the need for systematic classification as part of improving anatomical and clinical knowledge (Kayed et al., 2016). Consequently, a preliminary observation of both the heart and pericardial covering is critical in appreciating their interacting functions in cardiac physiology. Microscopically, the heart and pericardium are constituted by complex tissue structures

LEARNING OBJECTIVES

After studying this chapter, you will be able to:

1. Focus on anatomy of the heart
2. Discuss the function of the heart
3. Explain the anatomy of the pericardium
4. Focus on the function of the pericardium
5. Know common diseases of the heart
6. Understand common diseases of the pericardium

underlying their mechanical and physiological attributes. The pericardium consists mainly of collagen, a fibrillar protein whose hierarchical structure influences tissue strength and elasticity. Research has shown that pericardial type I collagen fibers are cross-linked naturally by glycosaminoglycans and synthetically by substances like glutaraldehyde, affecting their nanostructure and mechanical behaviors. The cross-links would have critical effects on the mechanical behavior of the pericardium, sustaining the heart function by regulating the orientation and strain of fibrils under load. Defining differences between biochemical and mechanical attributes of the pericardium not only casts its protective nature but also identifies the basis of clinical uses including tissue grafting and bioprosthetics made to simulate intrinsic cardiac support (Kayed et al., 2016). It speaks again to the nuances beyond mere muscular contraction that describe the environment within which the heart lives. A realistic portrayal of the heart and pericardium anatomy necessitates the use of terminological frameworks that are consistent, enabling both educational clarity and clinical communication. Anatomical literature has in the past provided extensive lists of terms; however, term-to-term relations, part-whole relations and hierarchical relations, are usually not stated and presented only implicitly. This deficiency poses challenges to both students and computational tools in anatomy, which are increasingly demanding machine-readable, precise models. Recent research shows that promoting anatomical terminologies to cover well-defined semantic relationships would result in better understanding and interoperability among biomedical systems. Consequently, integrating systematic anatomical knowledge and establishing progress standards is critical in research and clinical practice on the heart and its protective membranes (Rosse et al., 2000). Such bottom-line clarity finally enables better diagnosis, treatment, and innovation in cardiac therapy (Figure 7.1).

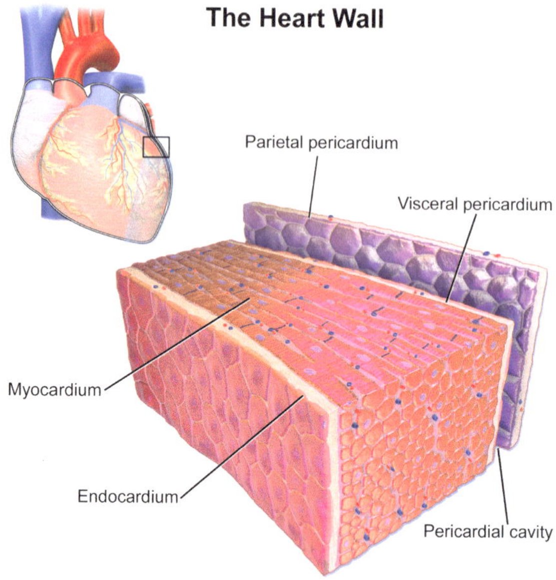

Figure 7.1. Pericardium.

Source: By BruceBlaus. When using this image in external sources it can be cited as:Blausen.com staff (2014). "Medical gallery of Blausen Medical 2014". WikiJournal of Medicine 1 (2). DOI:10.15347/wjm/2014.010. ISSN 2002-4436. - Own work, CC BY 3.0, https://commons.wikimedia.org/w/index.php?curid=28761820

Definition of the Heart and Pericardium

An understanding of the general anatomy of the heart involves realizing that it is a muscular organ whose job is to pump blood to and from the body. The position of the organ in the thoracic cavity and its complex structure are of great significance to its process. The heart is a largely cardiac muscle tissue, thus causing it to contract rhythmically and persistently. It has four chambers: two atria and two ventricles, which work in combination to facilitate circulation. Anatomically, it is contained within the pericardium, a membranous sac providing protection and mechanical support. The precise interrelationships among these structures can be better appreciated through the means of a well-organized anatomical nomenclature. Anatomical terminologies used currently tend to imply more than they say, limiting access and computational use of anatomical data (Rosse et al., 2000). Thus, a complete understanding of the heart requires anatomical and semantic precision to illuminate its structure and position in the body. The pericardium itself, a fibroserous double-layered sac, is worthy of close attention because of its functional role. It consists of an outer layer of fibrous tissue and an inner serous layer, which is further split into visceral and parietal layers. The main roles of the pericardium are to fix the heart in the mediastinum and reduce friction with cardiac motion by coating it with lubricating serous fluid. This spatial and part-whole relationship between the pericardium and heart is necessary for maintaining cardiac physiology and protecting the heart from exterior forces. However, anatomical ontologies will have vagueness between these kinds of parthood and location relations, which prevents uniform reasoning about anatomical structures and their interactions (Donnelly et al., 2006). Clarification of such formal spatial relations allows better understanding and enables better integration of anatomical data in biomedical research and in clinical applications. In addition to its anatomical borders, the existence of the heart in biomedical ontologies and terminologies relies on whether its spatial and part-whole structure is formally expressed. The heart and the covering structures like the pericardium need to be hierarchically classified and defined precisely for computational modeling and knowledge representation. These difficulties today are the outcome of the sporadic explicit portrayal of these associations in core anatomy resources, and they affect interoperability between biomedical terminologies. For example, differences between discrete classes of spatial associations, such as inclusion and adjacency, may not necessarily be explicitly portrayed, leading to the possibility of misinterpretation (Rosse et al., 2000; Donnelly et al., 2006). Hence, we need to advance and standardize the official definitions of the pericardium and heart within anatomical vocabularies to advance education as well as technology use, like diagnostic algorithms and clinical decision support systems.

Importance of Studying the Heart and Pericardium

It is of utmost importance to realize the dynamic interaction between the heart's electrical activity, mechanical function, and fluid dynamics to advance cardiovascular science. The heart is not just a muscular pump but a dynamic system where cardiac mechanical contractions are brought about by electrical signals to transport blood. The tissue that encloses the heart, the pericardium, and the blood within the chambers of the heart are also significant in the modification of cardiac deformation and function. The pericardium confines the epicardial surface whereas the blood imposes forces over the endocardium, creating a dynamic interaction essential for the proper functioning of the heart. This complex interaction underscores the necessity of coupled models that consider electrophysiology, solid mechanics, and fluid dynamics simultaneously. Recent computational advances toward the simulation of such complexity mirror the fineness of the physiology of the heart and pericardium, making mechanistic diagnosis and management of cardiac disease more accurate (Santiago et al., 2018). The penetration into the anatomical and histological fineness of cardiac structures such as the heart outflow tract reveals their essential role in regulating blood flow and hemodynamic stability. In vertebrates, cartilaginous fishes, and bony fishes, this tract connects the ventricle with the aorta and possesses specialized valves that do not allow the backflow of blood in the cardiac cycle. Throughout history, morphologic variation and functional specializations of this region have been areas of extensive study, demonstrating the evolutionary progression of cardiac anatomy in species. Understanding such differences not only illuminates developmental and evolutionary biology but is also applied in comparative studies, which can be used for research on the heart in humans. The anatomical complexity and function of cardiac support structures such as the pericardium are investigated in research that becomes the foundation necessary for the diagnosis of pathological change and optimizing operative and therapeutic measures (Garcia et al., 2019).

The clinical significance of research on the heart and pericardium extends beyond the theoretical, having an impact on clinical practice and biomedical device technology. By integrating the electrical, mechanical, and fluid components of cardiac performance into computational models, researchers can more accurately simulate normal and diseased states, such as conduction blocks and ventricular dysfunctions. These models enable therapeutic interventions like cardiac resynchronization therapy (CRT) and pacemaker implantation to be evaluated, which require precise knowledge of the heart's biomechanical environment and pericardial constraints (Figure 7.2).

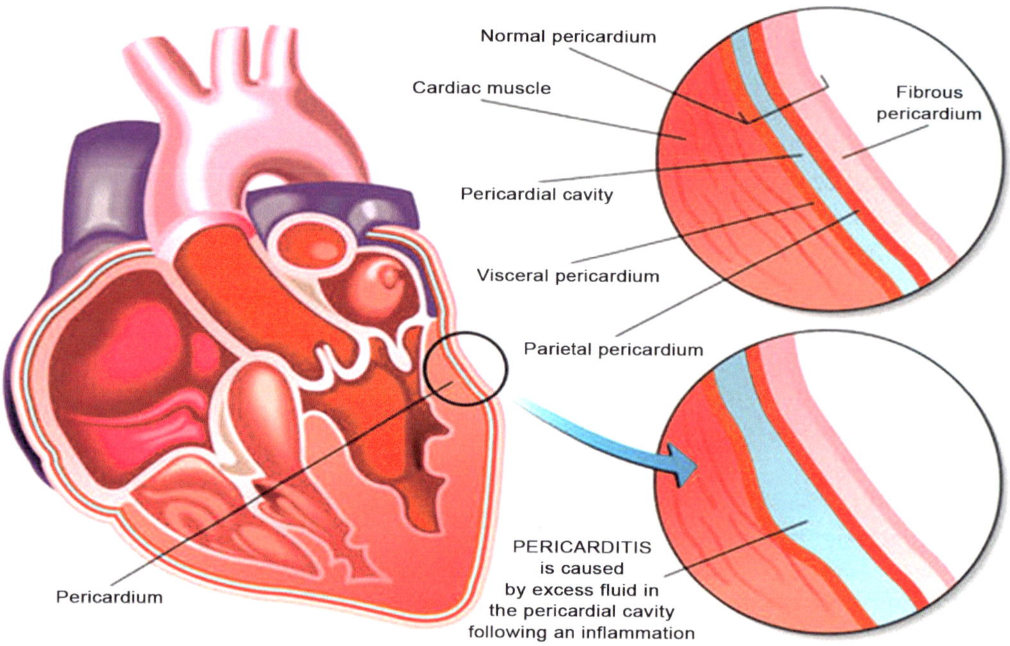

Figure 7.2. The heart and pericardium.

Source: PW Live. (n.d.). *Heart and Pericardium.*

7.1. Anatomy of the Heart

Learning Outcome

1. Describe the Structure of the Heart Chambers
2. Explain the Major Blood Vessels Associated with the Heart
3. Focus on Heart Valves and their Functions

The detailed anatomical organization of the heart is an excellent example of a complicated interaction between anatomical structures that maintains its performance as a muscular pump. Located in the mediastinum, the heart consists of four cavities: two atria and two ventricles, each of which supports unidirectional blood movement that is vital for systemic and pulmonary circulation. The heart walls consist of three layers: the epicardium, myocardium, and endocardium, of which the myocardium is the contractile, thick muscle that pumps blood. Valves between chambers, including the mitral and tricuspid valves, permit unidirectional flow and prevent backflow during contraction. Valuing such relationships highlights the part-whole relations inherent to cardiac anatomy underwriting the idea that anatomical terminologies must explicitly model such hierarchical and functional relations to enhance the clarity and efficiency of communication in medical discourse (Rosse et al., 2000). Such a systematic view facilitates both clinical and biomedical informatics. Supporting this muscular framework lies the pericardium, a double-walled sac providing protection as well as lubrication for cardiac motion. The fibrous pericardium stabilizes the heart against surrounding structures, and the innermost serous layer is further separated into parietal and visceral layers, generating a potential pericardial space filled with lubrication fluid. This organizational pattern confers frictionless contractions and prevents pathological cardiac displacement during physiological activities. Moreover, the close relation of the pericardium with critical nerves and vascular entities underscores the cardiac system's interdependency in the thoracic cavity. Although traditional medical literature has provided detailed structural descriptions, it remains to be put into larger physiological contexts so that enhanced diagnostic and therapeutic approaches can be realized. The synergistic functions of the heart and pericardium demonstrate the subtle integration necessary for cardiovascular disease and health control (Rosse et al., 2000). While macroscopic anatomy of the heart and coverings is well-studied, recent advances in neuroanatomy and imaging have established intriguing links beyond conventional descriptions. For example, the nervous system's control over the performance of the heart, demonstrated through autonomic modulation, challenges erstwhile compartmentalized views of the heart as merely a mechanical pump. These neuroanatomic principles resonate with contemporary interpretations of ancient principles of medicine, like acupuncture, where channels analogous to the nervous system interact with abdominal organs like the heart. Using today's visualization technologies to embryological anatomy, researchers suggest that ancient assumptions regarding meridians might also be depicting neuroanatomic pathways influencing cardiac physiology. This integrative perspective not only enhances our conceptualization of cardiac anatomy but also connects traditional and biomedical models with a focus on interdisciplinary approaches to disease and health.

7.1.1. Structure of the Heart Chambers

The complexity of the heart's function is directly in the specialized structure of its chambers, which allow for efficient circulation of blood throughout the body. Both atria and ventricles possess specialized structural features that adapt them to specific functions in the cardiac cycle. The atria possess thinner walls suited for receiving returning blood to the heart, while the ventricles possess thicker muscular walls to generate the force required to propel blood into the pulmonary and systemic circuits. Segmentation of these chambers by valves allows unidirectional blood flow and hence averts regurgitation and sustains hemodynamic stability. Furthermore, the myocardium tissue of each chamber is organized to facilitate synchronized contraction, which is energized by electrical impulses that are essential for rhythm and pumping effectiveness. It is this complex structure-function relationship that sustains the heart's ability to meet physiological demands in varying conditions (Battista et al., 2017). The ventricular chambers, in particular, exhibit notable structural adaptations that enable them to cope with high-pressure blood propulsion. The left ventricle of systemic circulation has the thickest wall because it must overcome greater resistance than the right ventricle, which pumps blood into the pulmonary circuit, a lower pressure system. The asymmetry in wall thickness reflects the disparity in workload and mechanical tension to which each chamber is exposed. The ventricles are lined internally by trabeculae carneae, irregular muscular ridges that increase contractile force without significantly thickening the wall. In addition, the septum interventriculare structurally and electrically separates the ventricles and plays a role in synchronous contraction that is necessary for effective pumping. An appreciation of such details highlights the design accuracy of the heart chambers in accommodating cardiovascular function under normal and pathologic states (Battista et al., 2017). Beyond mechanical function, the structural integrity of the heart chambers is closely integrated with tissue engineering attempts to model their complex features for therapeutic purposes. The pericardium and heart valves must maintain complex interfaces with these chambers to maintain function, and tissue engineering strategies hinge on the creation of scaffolds capable of mimicking the biomechanical and cellular environment of native heart tissues. Scientists emphasize the need for endothelial cell attachment maximization on the valve scaffolds for preventing immune response and thrombosis thus enhancing durability and biocompatibility. These advancements are being developed to replace or repair the diseased heart chambers and respective valves with precision and with no interruption of physiological flow patterns and chamber contraction. Current studies illustrate the relevance of combining material science with cellular biology in replicating the heart chamber structure for clinical application (Figure 7.3).

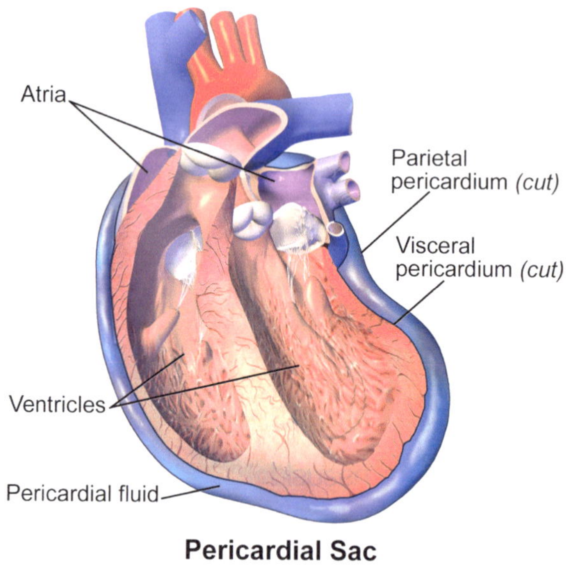

Figure 7.3. Structure of the heart chambers.

Source: By Blausen Medical Communications, Inc. - see ticket for details, CC BY 3.0, https://commons.wikimedia.org/w/index.php?curid=26986788

7.1.2. Major Blood Vessels Associated with the Heart

The heart is the focal organ of the circulatory system, prompted by a system of main blood vessels that facilitate uninterrupted blood circulation within the body. The vessels can be broadly categorized into arteries and veins, each having differing but complementary functions essential to cardiovascular welfare. The aorta, the biggest artery, originates from the left ventricle, distributing oxygenated blood to the systemic circulation through its various branches. Conversely, superior and inferior vena cavae transport oxygen-deficient blood from the upper and lower body, respectively, to the right atrium. This complex arrangement ensures constant oxygen and nutrient supply to tissues, facilitating homeostasis. Identification of these vessels' precise anatomical sites and physiological roles provides critical information regarding cardiovascular health and predisposing pathologic conditions of cardiac function (Korenkov et al., 2018). Apart from the vena cavae and aorta, the pulmonary veins and arteries also play significant roles in the heart, specifically with respect to gas exchange. Unlike in systemic arteries, the pulmonary arteries transport deoxygenated blood from the right ventricle to the lungs for oxygenation. The pulmonary veins return oxygenated blood to the left atrium to complete the pulmonary circuit. This two-way exchange highlights the heart's reliance on these vessels to facilitate adequate oxygenation systemically. Notably, the coronary arteries, which are branches of the aortic base, supply the myocardium itself with oxygenated blood, highlighting the heart's autonomy and vulnerability. Defects in coronary circulation are prone to result in catastrophic cardiac consequences, hence the clinical significance of the vessels (Korenkov et al., 2018). Emerging advancements in cardiac pacing and electrophysiology technology identify the importance of studying great vessels beyond circulation. For example, CRT utilizes the coronary sinus—a venous channel in parallel to the left atrium—as the pacing lead site aimed at reinstating synchronized ventricular contractions of critical significance in the therapy of congestive heart failure (CHF). The coronary sinus is a great venous structure intimately related to cardiac function and therapeutic interventions. Further, vascular access by way of these heart-related arteries provides new therapies like epicardial pacing for left ventricular stimulation, which requires detailed anatomical knowledge for safe use. These developments demonstrate anatomy and clinical innovation crossing over to enhance patient benefit by targeting the cardiac vascular system with therapies.

7.1.3. Heart Valves and their Functions

The heart's efficiency as a pump relies heavily on the structure and function of its valves, which provide coordinated unidirectional blood flow and prevent regurgitation. The valves—the aortic, pulmonary, mitral, and tricuspid valves—act as dynamic gates that open and shut in sync with cardiac cycles. The pulmonary valve, for instance, permits blood flow from the right ventricle to the pulmonary artery while posing unique challenges due to its exposure to congenital defects. Both repair and replacement of this valve are undermined by the limitations of current prosthetic material, especially in pediatric patients, such that advances in valve durability and biocompatibility are required. The development of living tissue valves by fibroblast seeding from the patient into decellularized scaffolds is a promising avenue for the creation of valves with the potential for continued matrix maintenance and the reduction of immunological complications (Hoskins , 2022). This approach highlights the delicate balance between mechanical demands and biological integration necessary for valve longevity. The valvular function is not simply structural but also closely tied to cellular processes that maintain the valve's extracellular matrix and surface integrity. The aortic valve, a highly significant site for cardiovascular morbidity, demonstrates the need for replacements that mimic native tissue function to minimize complications such as thrombosis and immune response. Tissue-engineered valves aim to restore the cellular components of the native valve, including endothelial and interstitial cells, that guide continued remodeling and repair. Among the greatest challenges in this endeavor is the achievement and maintenance of a confluent endothelial cell monolayer on decellularized valve scaffolds to prevent thrombogenicity and inflammation. New approaches involving protein substrates like laminin and fibronectin combined with hydrogels and dynamic seeding have exhibited enhanced endothelial cell adhesion and viability under physiologic shear stress, with the prospect of more functional and durable valve constructs (Fontaine et al., 2015). The challenges in recreating the complex functions of the valve in the cardiovascular system are underscored by these advances. The heart valves perform the essential function of maintaining pressure gradients that drive efficient blood flow to the body. Any valvular dysfunction—stenosis, regurgitation, or atresia—can cause severe hemodynamic derangements leading to heart failure or systemic hypoperfusion. The mitral and tricuspid valves regulate blood flow between the atria and ventricles to achieve competent ventricular filling and ejection. Because of their life-critical functions, valve repair and replacement strategies must consider not just mechanical function but biological compatibility and the potential for regeneration. Seeding of patient cells into valve scaffolds holds the promise to circumvent shortcomings of current mechanical and bioprosthetic valves, such as limited durability and the need for lifelong anticoagulation. Ongoing innovation in valve tissue engineering, supported by the likes of bioreactors to test hemodynamics and cell function, is key to creating valves that can meet the physiological demands throughout a patient's lifespan (Hoskins, 2022). This highlights the critical functional interplay between valve structure, cell viability, and systemic circulation (Figure 7.4).

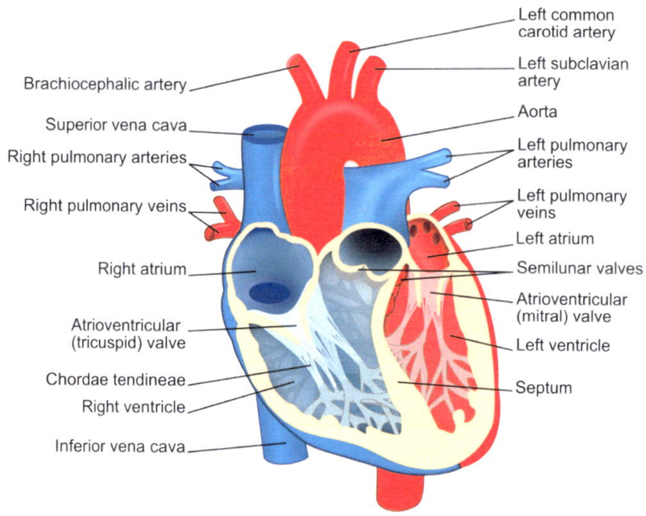

Figure 7.4. Heart valves and their functions.

Source: By ZooFari - Own workSupporting references↑ [1] (cache)↑ [2] (cache), CC BY-SA 3.0, https://commons.wikimedia.org/w/index.php?curid=9841860

Test Your Knowledge

1. Which veins return deoxygenated blood to the right atrium of the heart?
2. What is the primary function of the atrioventricular valves during the cardiac cycle?

7.2. Function of the Heart

Learning Outcome

1. Discuss the Mechanism of Blood Circulation
2. Explain the Role of the Heart in Maintaining Homeostasis
3. Focus on Electrical Conduction System of the Heart

The efficiency of the cardiovascular system is based on the heart's unique property to function as a dynamic pump, controlling ceaseless blood circulation within the body. Pumping action delivers oxygen and vital nutrients to tissues and permits the removal of metabolic waste, facilitating cellular life. The heart's chambers and valves are structurally equipped to control the one-way flow of blood, maintaining pressure gradients for circulation. Its rhythmic contractions are regulated by electrical impulses from specialized cardiac cells, enabling accurate synchronization. Anatomical familiarity with the position of the heart within the thoracic cavity and its relationship to surrounding structures such as the pericardium is significant. The pericardium does not only provide support to the heart but also makes the environment around it friction-free, thus showing how anatomical context influences function. While Terminologia Anatomica categorizes these anatomical relationships with strict classification, it refers to the interrelatedness that is the foundation for cardiac function and offers a paradigm for comprehension of these complex dynamics (Rosse et al., 2000). The effective cardiac function also depends on the coordination of neurophysiologic mechanisms to modulate heart rate and contractility according to body needs. The autonomic nervous system accomplishes this by delivering sympathetic and parasympathetic inputs that govern cardiac output to create homeostasis under varying conditions. Modern science suggests that so-called principal meridians as classically conceived in Chinese medicine could be the same as neuroanatomic structures that control such physiologic responses. This convergence of classical and modern views suggests that the regulation of function by the heart encompasses complex neuroanatomic networks, closing the millennial gap between clinical experience and present-day science (Dorsher, 2009). These insights reaffirm the appreciation of the heart as more than a mechanical pump, placing it within a larger systemic interaction necessary for wellness. In addition, the function of the heart is not only mechanical and neurophysiologic but also adaptation potential and resistance in physiological and disease states. Cardiac tissues adjust to alterations in load and metabolic demands through mechanisms that control stroke volume and heart rate with evidence of intrinsic regulatory processes. The pericardium provides structural support and limits hypercardiac dilation, therefore contributing to maximal mechanical efficiency and protection of the heart from external trauma. Impairment of pericardial function or integrity could have adverse effects on cardiac function, highlighting the functional interdependence of these anatomical structures to maintain cardiovascular stability. Such a coordinated overview of the heart and pericardium explains how their concurrent action sustains life by creating appropriate circulation and protecting vital structures (Rosse et al., 2000).

7.2.1. Mechanism of Blood Circulation

The complex anatomy of the heart and its ability to maintain rhythmic contractions are fundamental to incessant circulatory flow in the body. Circulation of blood is ensured by the heart's double-pump mechanism in the form of right and left ventricles functioning in concert to circulate blood in pulmonary and systemic circuits, respectively. Electrical impulses and muscular contractions must be coordinated for effective cardiac output.

This extremely synchronized system is under various influences, such as the electric conduction paths controlled by the sinoatrial (SA) node and atrioventricular (AV) node. Emerging developments in CRT emphasize the importance of ventricular synchrony, especially in diseased states like CHF, where impairment to this synchrony disrupts physiological blood circulation and tissue perfusion (Hawkins et al., 2010). It is thus crucial to understand the electrical and mechanical interaction of the heart to know the process of blood circulation in the cardiovascular system. Circulation of blood in the vascular and heart systems is not merely a mechanical process but is inherently associated with electrophysiological activity resulting in contraction of the myocardium. Propagation of action potential in cardiac tissue generates contractions in the muscle fibers that create the movement of blood resulting in pressure gradients. Advanced modeling studies have demonstrated the correlation of electrical stimulation with muscle force generation and fluid dynamics to produce effective pumping activity in the embryonic heart, illuminating healthy cardiac function and developmental abnormalities (Battista et al., 2017). The models reveal the complex feedback between electrophysiological signals and mechanical pumping and how alterations in electrical conductivity can produce varying flow regimes, from peristaltic-like motions to dynamic suction pumping. This biophysical understanding contributes to our knowledge of how the heart successfully controls circulation from cellular to systemic levels. The structural complexity of the heart, including the covering pericardium, plays an important role in optimizing circulatory mechanics. The pericardium provides a protective enclosure and a friction-free space in which the heart can contract and relax efficiently within the thoracic cavity. In this confined space, the hemodynamic forces generated by the synchronized contractions permit one-way blood flow maintained by valvular structures. Developments such as the epicardial satellite pacemaker system, where remotely controlled pacing leads are coupled directly onto the surface of the heart, serve to emphasize new therapeutic strategies toward restoring synchronized ventricular contractions to improve cardiac output and overall circulation in disease states (Hawkins et al., 2010). Thus, the interaction between cardiac electrical control, its mechanical function, and the supporting anatomy given by the pericardium enables effective blood propulsion required to sustain life (Figure 7.5).

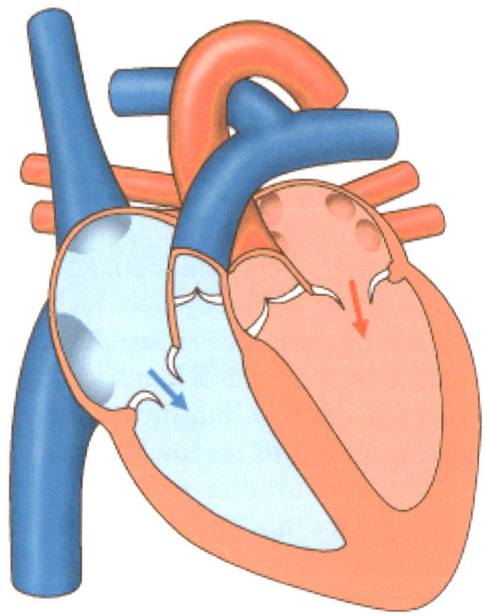

Figure 7.5. Mechanism of blood circulation.

Source: By josiño - Own work, Public Domain, https://commons.wikimedia.org/w/index.php?curid=9396374

7.2.2. Role of the Heart in Maintaining Homeostasis

The complex interaction between cardiac function and systemic homeostasis highlights the intrinsic function of the heart in ensuring homeostasis. Besides its direct function of circulating blood, the heart also regulates blood pressure, oxygenation, and delivery of nutrients to provision cells with essential factors for metabolism. Rhythmic contractions of the myocardium regulate changing physiological demands by modifying stroke volume and cardiac output accordingly. This dynamic regulation allows the cardiovascular system to make a correct response to acute stimuli such as exercise or stress, with maintenance of internal equilibrium. Further, the heart works in collaboration with neural and hormonal systems, which offer precise control of heart rate and vascular resistance to achieve homeostatic equilibrium. Derangement of these processes, either due to pathological processes or due to toxic effects from therapy like chemotherapy, can lower cardiac function and impair systemic homeostasis, emphasizing the position of the heart at the center of the regulatory system of the body (Vasiliadis et al., 2014). In addition to its mechanical work, the heart is also a participant in homeostasis through its protective covering, the pericardium, which ensures cardiac integrity and facilitates optimum heart function. This two-layer sac minimizes friction and prevents excessive cardiac movement such that the heart is able to contract properly within the thoracic cavity. Structural and functional stability is essential for unbroken blood flow and perfusion of tissues. Progress in cardiac repair, including biocompatible tissue scaffolds utilized during valve replacement, underscores the importance of preserving homeostatic mechanisms at the cellular and tissue levels. For example, the recent developments in living pulmonary valve implants, pioneered by seeding patient-derived fibroblasts onto decellularized scaffolds, illustrate the way maintaining cellular viability and matrix homeostasis can prolong cardiac stability and function (Hoskins, 2022). Such developments illustrate the way that the heart not only needs to be supported mechanically but also a conducive microenvironment to provide systemic equilibrium. Cardiovascular integrity goes beyond pump function, influencing vascular tone control and endocrine signaling required for homeostasis. Vasodilation, flow, and pressure, all coordinated with cardiac rhythm, are locally and hormonally regulated by hormones and local molecules such as nitric oxide, which are released from the endothelium. Vascular homeostasis disruption or interference with processes of vascular signaling, as is seen with certain anti-cancer treatments targeting vascular endothelial growth factor, can provoke cardiovascular side effects and challenge the ability of the heart to assure homeostasis (Vasiliadis et al., 2014). Therefore, the contribution of the heart towards homeostasis is its resistance to biochemical and mechanical stressors, its extracellular and cellular milieu maintenance, and its facilitation of coordinated communication with other systems. This double function highlights the central importance of the heart to ensuring physiological stability throughout life.

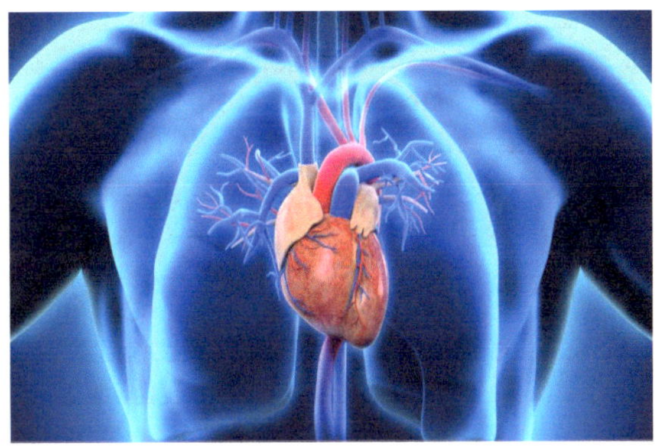

Source: Aster DM Healthcare. (2023). *Anatomy of the Heart.*

7.2.3. Electrical Conduction System of the Heart

The rhythmic muscle contractions of the heart, required for effective blood pumping, are managed by a very complex electrical conducting apparatus. This elaborate network initiates electrical stimuli that coordinate myocardial contraction, causing the heart to function as a solitary pump. Central to this is the SA node, often called the natural pacemaker of the heart, which initiates spontaneous electrical impulses. These impulses move from the atria, which have been made to contract, and then to the AV node. It goes on through the bundle of His, bundle branches, and Purkinje fibers to ultimately lead to ventricular contraction. The propagation of electrical activity in the atria and ventricles has been accurately represented using computational models with detailed atrial and ventricular anatomies and ionic activity, illustrating the richness of electrical conduction in health and disease (Bayés et al., 2015). Such models are important in explaining normal cardiac function and the mechanisms of arrhythmias. Cardiac electrical synchrony is crucial for the efficient circulation of blood and is typically lost in cardiac diseases such as CHF (CHF). Desynchronized ventricular contraction hampers efficient pumping in CHF, thereby reducing cardiac output. Treatment strategies in such a situation typically focus on the restoration of electrical conduction harmony. CRT stands out as a classic example of this by employing pacing methodology to restore synchronous ventricular activation. This therapy frequently utilizes a master pacing device that is implanted transvenously on the right heart, synchronizing ventricle and atrial activities. With some of the developments in CRT, there is the use of an epicardial satellite pacemaker placed over the epicardium of the left ventricle, which offers concentrated pacing to enhance synchronization and cardiac output (Hawkins et al., 2010). These advances place in context the central role that the electrical conduction system plays in the physiology and clinical management of heart disease. Understanding the conduction pathways and their physiological link to cardiac anatomy, particularly within pericardium, remains a foundation of cardiovascular science. The electrical activity is not only the result of intrinsic nodal function but also influenced by the mechanical and structural properties of the heart within the pericardium. The pericardium provides a protective environment, which can affect the conduction of electrical impulses because it places mechanical constraints and influences myocardial geometry. Complex simulations of the heart's electrical activity have brought together ventricular and atrial surfaces with the body, simulating body surface potentials and electrocardiograms (ECGs) in agreement with clinical recordings. Such equipment plays a very significant role during the investigation of conduction defects noted in Wolff-Parkinson-White syndrome or bundle branch blocks and, therefore, continue to enlighten the complex connection between cardiac electrical conduction, pericardium that wraps around the myocardium, and the myocardium itself (Bayés et al., 2015).

Test Your Knowledge

1. How does the heart contribute to the regulation of blood pressure and tissue perfusion?
2. How does the atrioventricular (AV) node contribute to coordinated heart contractions?

7.3. Anatomy of the Pericardium

Learning Outcome

1. Describe the Structure and Layers of the Pericardium
2. Understand Location and Attachment of the Pericardium
3. Focus on Pericardial Fluid and Its Significance

The protective sheath around the heart is crucial to its peak performance and mechanical efficacy. Amidst this sheath is the pericardium, a sac made of fibroserous covering the heart and the rootings of important vessels. The pericardium is structurally made up of two general layers, namely the outer fibrous pericardium that confers stiffness and anchors the heart within the thoracic cavity, and the inner serous pericardium, whose structure consists of a parietal and visceral layer. The visceral layer, or epicardium, makes direct contact with the surface of the heart and creates a smooth interface under which cardiac motion occurs with minimal friction. This anatomic arrangement offers mechanical support and infection or trauma protection, most importantly in supporting the heart in its position and in keeping from over-expansion during diastole. Behind the fibrous and serous pericardial layers lies the pericardial cavity, a slit-like, fluid-filled space through which the heart may make ongoing movement within the thoracic cavity. The serous fluid within the cavity acts as a lubricant, reducing friction immensely as the heart pumps and runs through its allied tissues. Notably, pericardium is intimately associated with epicardial adipose tissue, an active metabolically fat depot that encircles the coronary arteries and the heart. It offers anatomical and physiological support to the heart and is increasingly appreciated in cardiovascular disease diagnosis and cardiovascular health profiling. Novel imaging modalities, such as those applied in low-dose CT, utilize the anatomical localization of the pericardium to measure epicardial fat and provide useful biomarkers that enhance cardiovascular risk profiling (Liu, 2024). In clinical applications, the anatomy of the pericardium also parallels device manufacturing and clinical device durability, particularly bioprosthetic heart valves. Bovine pericardial tissue, with its preferred mechanical strength and biocompatibility, is used to construct such valves. However, anatomical and biochemical characteristics of the pericardium present obstacles, such as calcification of the tissue that could lead to failure of the valve after some time. Gaining insight into pericardium's complex tissue structure, particularly its collagen matrix and cellular component—has pointed the way for research into methods to prevent calcification, with treatments like the use of dimethyl sulfoxide to dissuade calcium deposits. In addition to making valves more resilient, such a development also speaks to the centrality of understanding the fine detail of pericardial tissue anatomy in medicine and therapeutic interventions (Parekh et al., 2015) (Figure 7.6).

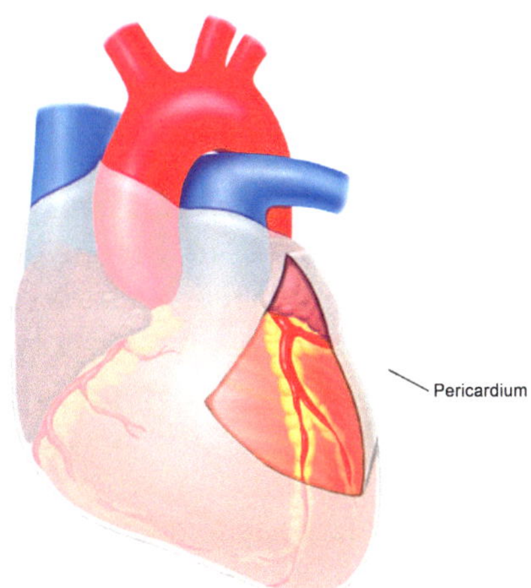

Figure 7.6. Anatomy of the pericardium.

Source: UpToDate. (n.d.). *Pericardium Anatomy.*

7.3.1. Structure and Layers of the Pericardium

The encasing protective sac around the heart is a fragile entity vital to its maximal functioning and stability within the thoracic cavity. The pericardium, the encasing entity, serves both as a mechanical guard and an initiator of the cardiac movement, providing positional integrity while allowing for required movement within the cardiac cycle. The pericardium structure is constructed of discrete compartments, each serving specialized purposes toward overall cardiovascular health. Understanding hierarchical and spatial relations among these layers reveals how the pericardium maintains the mechanical demands of the heart and interacts with surrounding tissues. Such structural intricacies are typically mapped and encoded with anatomical terms that favor part-whole relationships, enhancing clinical knowledge and applications in medical informatics (Rosse et al., 2000). Beneath its fibrous outer covering, the fibrous pericardium is a tough, inelastic sac providing tensile strength to the outside rim of the heart. This layer anchors the heart to adjacent structures like the diaphragm and sternum so that they do not over-distend during hemodynamic stress. Internally, the serous pericardium again splits into parietal and visceral layers. The parietal layer closely clings on the interior to the fibrous pericardium, but the visceral, or epicardial, layer intimately invests in the myocardium itself. There is room between these two serous layers, which is the pericardial cavity and in which is stored lubricating serous fluid that reduces friction when cardiac contraction takes place. This advanced system of layering allows for a harmonious integration between protection, adaptability, and structural support essential to dynamic cardiac function (Rosse et al., 2000). The interaction of the pericardium with surrounding anatomical structures also acts to increase its functional complexity. For example, the ascending aorta, closely enveloped by the pericardium, demonstrates how pericardial stiffness influences cardiac mechanics and vascular stress distributions. Numerical simulations simulating the aorta within its pericardial environment show that the pericardium exerts a degree of mechanical constraint, which in turn modulates vessel diameter and stress patterns it is subjected to. However, oversimplification in the guise of pericardial support only might overstate this limitation, implying that pericardial compliance must be put into the context of surrounding tissues to render biomechanical measurements valid. Such mechanistic insight underlies the pericardium's role beyond containment, directing stress responses both in normal and disease cardiovascular conditions.

7.3.2. Location and Attachment of the Pericardium

The anatomical position of the pericardium is closely associated with mediastinal structures within the thoracic cavity, serving as a protective membranous sheath that envelops the heart. This placement is important in that the pericardium is centrally placed within the mediastinum, located behind the sternum and in front of the vertebral column, defining the heart's spatial arrangement with surrounding thoracic organs. Such positioning not only assists in the mechanical stability of the heart but also offers efficient interaction with other structures like the lungs and great vessels. Pericardial attachments to these adjacent structures assist in the containment of the heart to prevent over-movement during cardiac cycles. Of note, the model rat does not have adhesions to other pleural organs and suggests species-specific variation that may dictate how the pericardial location impacts both physiological function and surgical accessibility in experimental models. Both clinical and research techniques need this information. In addition to its proper position within the thoracic cavity, the pericardium possesses specialized attachments that fix it in position and allow for necessary flexibility during cardiac motion. The fibrous pericardium, the outermost layer, is attached superiorly to the adventitia of the great vessels, including the aorta and pulmonary trunk, securing the heart in relation to vascular support. Here, it is attached to the central tendon of the diaphragm, with a tense yet dynamic attachment that transmits diaphragmatic activity to influence cardiac movement. Furthermore, ligaments such as the sterno-pericardial ligament provide additional stabilization by attaching the pericardium at the posterior of the sternum.

This ligament, particularly emphasized in rat anatomical studies, prevents excessive movement and assists in locating the heart in its proper mediastinal position (Ameri et al., 2024). These diverse attachments reveal the balance of structural support and functional mobility. The clinical significance of the location and attachments of the pericardium is significant, especially in pathological processes and surgical intervention. Because the pericardium is linked with vital thoracic structures, pathological cystic lesions such as hydatid cysts can develop within or outside the pericardium, complicating diagnosis and treatment. For instance, radiologic accidental findings of cysts in the pericardium necessitate careful differential diagnosis since they can involve lethal complications, for instance, hydatid cysts affecting several organs such as the heart and pericardium (Ameri et al., 2024). In these circumstances, both awareness of pericardial attachments as well as the position of the pericardium is important to prepare for surgical resection, especially where cardiac involvement necessitates careful consideration to prevent great vessel and myocardial damage. Such anatomical knowledge of pericardial tethers thus serves to facilitate successful management of the condition and improve prognosis in severe cardiac conditions.

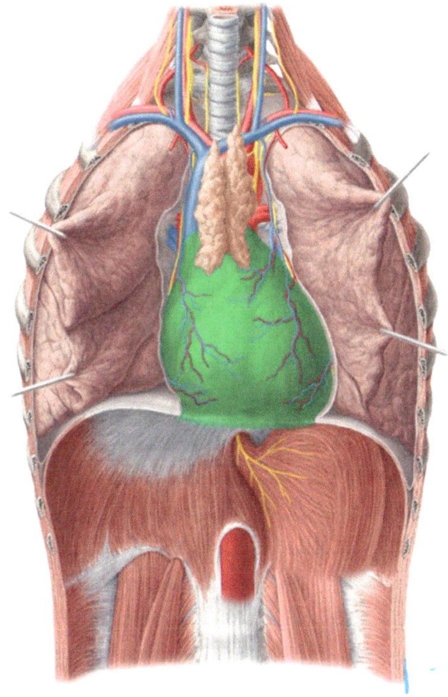

Source: Kenhub. (n.d.). *The Pericardium*.

7.3.3. Pericardial Fluid and Its Significance

The complex environment of the heart is essential to its optimal function, and pericardial fluid is vital to cardiac health. Pericardial fluid is a serous lubricating fluid found inside the pericardial cavity that cushions the heart and reduces friction generated by the cardiac movement against surrounding tissues. Beyond its mechanical function, pericardial fluid acts as a medium for immune surveillance and biochemical exchange, which is vital in preserving the microenvironment of the heart. Its chemical composition can be dramatically changed in disease states to reflect primary illnesses such as infection or inflammation. For instance, in tubercular pericardial effusion, pathological pericardial fluid accumulation not only jeopardizes cardiac function but also reflects systemic infection and inflammation. Thus, pericardial fluid is not just a physical protector but also a marker of diagnosis and pathophysiology, highlighting its multi-faceted significance in cardiovascular medicine (Motalib et al., 2024). The pericardial fluid's immunological environment is an interactive interface between systemic and cardiac local immunity, highlighting its significance over lubrication. Recent research has highlighted the presence of small extracellular vesicles (sEVs) in the pericardial fluid that are involved in intercellular communication, significantly influencing immune cell phenotypes. The vesicles carry microRNAs and other molecular cargo that actively modulate macrophage function, constituent cells in inflammatory and reparative processes. MicroRNA profile alterations carried by pericardial fluid-sEVs in coronary artery disease (CAD) have been shown to diminish macrophage anti-inflammatory functions and provoke a pro-inflammatory microenvironment in the cardiac microenvironment. These findings attest that pericardial fluid is involved in the modulation of immune homeostasis in the heart and might impact the progression of disease and recovery from injury, thereby presenting novel mechanisms for therapeutic target development (Ben-Aicha et al., 2024). With these multifunctional processes, analysis and management of pericardial fluid are most critical in clinical cardiology. Abnormalities in the volume or composition of pericardial fluid are most likely the reflection of serious pathologies such as pericardial effusion, which is secondary to infections such as tuberculosis, autoimmune diseases, or malignancies. Biochemical and immunological characteristics of pericardial fluid can thus help in differential diagnosis and guide therapy protocols. For example, management of tubercular pericardial effusion in large volumes in patients with concomitant states of heart failure and diabetes must be handled multidisciplinary, including both infectious disease management and cardiovascular management. Pericardial fluid diagnostic and therapeutic significance determines the significance of careful clinical evaluation to obtain the optimal outcome for the patient and prevent harmful complications from abnormal pericardial status (Motalib et al., 2024) (Figure 7.7).

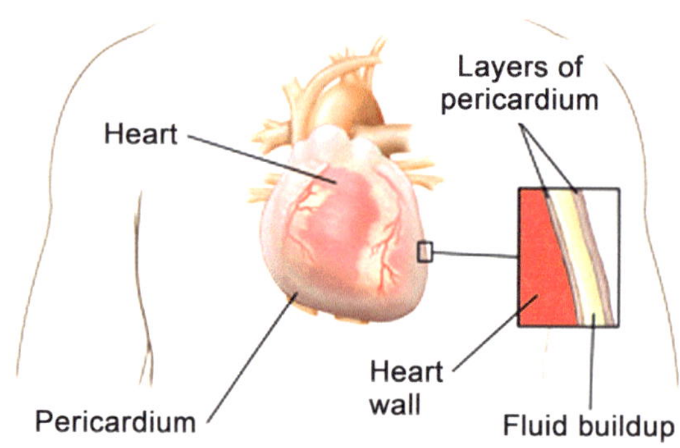

Figure 7.7. Pericardial fluid and its significance.

Source: Krames Patient Education. (n.d.). *Layers of Pericardium and Fluid Buildup.*

Test Your Knowledge

1. Where is the pericardium located in relation to the thoracic cavity and diaphragm?
2. What are the potential consequences of excess fluid accumulation in the pericardial cavity (pericardial effusion)?

7.4. Function of the Pericardium

Learning Outcome

1. Discuss the Protective Role of the Pericardium
2. Focus on Role in Reducing Friction during Heartbeats
3. Explain the Contribution to Heart Stability and Positioning

The pericardium also plays an essential role in providing mechanical stability for the heart within the thorax, providing a supporting framework that ensures the heart is in its optimal position. Its fibrous outer layer adheres to the surrounding structures firmly, preventing the excessive movement of the heart upon body movements or posture adjustments. This support structure is necessary, as it allows the heart to contract and relax properly without being exposed to abnormal torsion forces or overstretch. Further, the ability of the pericardium to limit acute cardiac dilation during acute volume or pressure overload safeguards myocardial integrity so that the heart can resume efficient hemodynamic function. This containment and support function underscore the importance of the pericardium as not merely a passive covering but as an active participant in cardiac mechanics and overall cardiovascular homeostasis (Rosse et al., 2000). Apart from its mechanical regulation, the pericardium also plays a central physiological function by secreting pericardial fluid into its serous layers. This lubricating fluid minimizes friction between the visceral and parietal pericardial layers as the heart pumps relentlessly, thereby facilitating smooth myocardial movement. The fluid acts as a cushion, absorbing minute shocks and safeguarding against the risk of inflammation or mechanical injury during cardiac cycles. The regulated fluid environment also assists in thermal insulation as well as the metabolic exchange that maintains the myocardium's sensitive tissue metabolism. The presence of this fluid layer underscores the pericardium's functional role not only as a structural barrier but also as a preservative for function, essential to the survival and ongoing function of the heart during varying physiologic states (Rosse et al., 2000). The immunological and sensory properties of the pericardium also contribute to its functional category, placing it in relation to systemic processes outside of anatomical containment. Pericardial nerve sensory fibers carry pain and mechanoreception to the CNS, involved in cardiovascular reflexes and conscious sensations of cardiac suffering. This neuroanatomical coherence is in harmony with ancient concepts of body interconnectedness in practices like acupuncture, which recognize the pericardium's function in autonomic regulation and systemic homeostasis. In addition, the pericardium is involved in immune surveillance through macrophages and lymphatic vessels, possibly regulating inflammatory reactions during infection or pericardial disease. Therefore, the pericardium represents not only a physical barrier and lubricant but also an active organ involved in defending cardiac function via neural and immunological mechanisms, further substantiating its critical role in the cardiothoracic system.

7.4.1. Protective Role of the Pericardium

The biomechanical context of the heart is critically dependent on surrounding tissues immediately around it, which control its function and protection. Among these, the pericardium is a significant protective form since it serves as a mechanical buffer that minimizes cardiac displacement within the thoracic space. It's a fibrous sac surrounding the heart and roots of large vessels, thereby limiting overexpansion during the extremes of increased intracardiac volume. In addition, the pericardial fluid that fills the space between the parietal and visceral layers reduces friction during cardiac cycles, making smooth myocardial relaxations and contractions possible. Such protective functions highlight the importance of the pericardium in ensuring efficiency and stability in the heart. Its structural and fluid dynamics create a functioning barrier that protects the heart both from external trauma and mechanical stress, which is essential in optimizing cardiac performance under physiological and pathological states (Alexander et al., 2022). Beyond the mechanical, the pericardium is essential in regulating metabolic interactions between the heart and neighboring tissues. The epicardial adipose tissue, which is situated between the visceral pericardium and myocardium, is a stereotypical illustration of this double role of metabolic as well as protective. Under physiological conditions, in this fat depot, in addition to acting locally as an energy reservoir by supplying free fatty acids to the myocardium, also releases protective adipokines like adiponectin with anti-inflammatory and cardioprotective effects. These attributes are aimed at safeguarding the myocardium from mechanical stress and hypothermia as well as complying with energetic demands (Michał et al., 2022). These interactions depict the role of the pericardium not just as a passive defensive barrier but as an active participant in cardiac homeostasis, citing its multifunctional role in cardiovascular health. In safeguarding the heart, adaptive changes in pericardial tissues, including epicardial adipose tissue, have the potential to cause cardiovascular diseases. Under disease states such as obesity, metabolic syndrome, or diabetes mellitus, there is inflammatory transformation of the epicardial fat which detracts from its protective function, leading to atherosclerosis and aggravation of cardiac conditions. This shift makes the pericardium-related tissue convert from a guardian into a potential culprit for cardiac failure. Detection of such a shift is important in understanding the balance maintained by the protective function of the pericardium and the pathological consequence when this balance is disrupted. Thus, ongoing research on the role of the pericardium within the cardiovascular system can inform therapeutic strategies of adipose tissue regulation to preserve the protective role of the pericardium (Alexander et al., 2022; Michał et al., 2022).

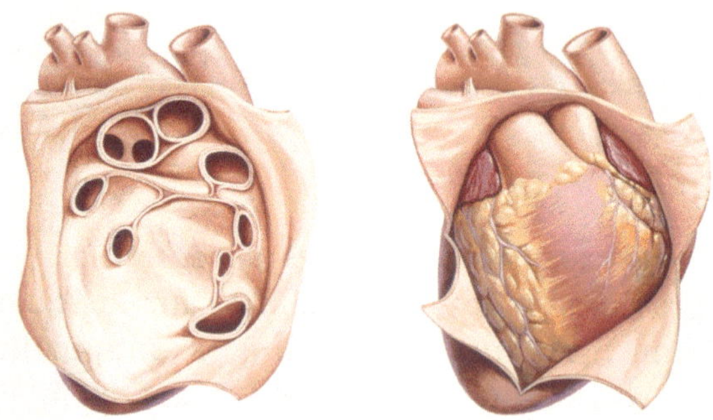

Source: Bailey, R. (2021). *Anatomy of the Heart: Pericardium.*

7.4.2. Role in Reducing Friction During Heartbeats

The cyclical rhythmic contraction and relaxation of the heart require an extremely efficient mechanism to prevent mechanical resistance within the thoracic cavity. The pericardium, a double-layered fibroserous sac enveloping the heart, is a key factor in accomplishing this by providing a lubricated environment that assists in reducing friction between heartbeats. The parietal and visceral layers of the pericardium enclose a thin film of pericardial fluid, a biological lubricant that enables the heart to slide smoothly through the mediastinum. The frictionless motion ensures the stability of the structure of the heart while accommodating the dynamic fluctuations in pressure and volume in each cardiac cycle. Over-disturbance of this delicate equilibrium may lead to inflammation and impaired cardiac performance, highlighting the central role of the pericardium in cardiac biomechanics. The anatomy and physiology of the pericardial fluid are extremely specialized to achieve maximum lubrication and protect the muscular motions of the heart. Its serous nature allows it to absorb shear stresses due to the continuous myocardial motion, thus preventing mechanical damage to the surfaces of the heart. Furthermore, the pericardial fibrous layer offers structural strength and averts undue diastolic dilation, otherwise increasing the frictional forces. Recent evidence of molecular interaction at the pericardial interface also focuses on how cellular components and ion channels interact in maintaining tissue homeostasis in conditions of stress. While the precise biochemical processes reducing arrhythmogenic potential involve complex ionic exchanges, they demonstrate interdependence between mechanical and electrophysiological stability for frictionless and uninterrupted heartbeats, a factor important to ensure unbroken normal cardiac rhythm (Salzer, 2019).

The impact of compromised friction reduction extends beyond mechanical disturbance to affect cardiac physiology and development in general. Work such as environmental toxicant work has revealed mechanisms, whereby chemicals like methylmercury, have detrimental effects on heart development and function, suggesting that even minor interference with pericardial lubrication and myocardial motion can have an appreciable influence on it. Model systems demonstrate that toxins causing the reduction in heart rate and motion indirectly highlight the significance of pericardial lubrication to sustain the intrinsic biomechanical environment. This study validates the thesis that functional impairment in heart movement is partly a result of malfunctioning mechanisms of friction reduction within the pericardium, which secondarily may initiate larger physiological abnormality. An understanding of such interactions reinforces the requirement for lubricative function by the pericardium as fundamental to both cardiac well-being and embryogenesis (Aguilar et al., 2015).

7.4.3. Contribution to Heart Stability and Positioning

The dynamic nature of the thoracic cavity necessitates multiple anatomical structures working together to keep the heart stable and in its correct position. The pericardium acts as a major fibroserous sac that envelops the heart, limiting its movement while forming a critical lubricated space that minimizes friction during cardiac cycles. In encapsulating the heart in this way, it permits it to possess a fixed spatial relationship with other organs within the thorax. Besides, the pericardium also acts as an infectious and physical shield, which indirectly guarantees the stability of the heart. The operation of inserting the left ventricular assist devices (LVAD) into the heart necessitates a thorough understanding of the location of the heart since the anatomical distinction and previous history of operation make the spatial orientation and stability of the heart complex. Surgeons must plan these procedures carefully to allow for the natural mobility of the heart and its pericardial support to achieve optimal patient outcomes (Loforte et al., 2021). Heart stability is also lost in certain cardiac surgeries, particularly those involving beating heart methods such as off-pump coronary artery bypass (OPCAB). Such procedures require temporary enucleation or positioning maneuvers to access coronary arteries, which will compromise the positional integrity and hemodynamic stability of the heart. It requires cooperative teamwork between surgical and anesthetic teams with meticulous coordination to achieve optimal positioning without compromising the function of the heart. The restraining effect of the pericardium even during such maneuvers is an important factor in providing resistance to over-displacement and maintaining orientation intact. Furthermore, effective management of myocardial ischemia under surgery demonstrates the delicate balance between mobility and stability, emphasizing the function of the pericardium in sustaining cardiac function through mechanical support and anatomic continuity (Chassot et al., 2017). The dynamic aspect of cardiac surgery emphasizes ensuring the position and stability of the heart during complex interventions. Advances in device miniaturization and intrapericardial design have taken advantage of the native pericardial space to accommodate assist devices without interfering with the anatomical fixation of the heart. Such integration between the location of device placement and native heart stabilization ensures postoperative recovery and preserves physiological interactions critical for cardiac function. Moreover, the multidisciplinary approach to cardiac surgery, imaging, surgical technique, and hemodynamic monitoring, aims to respect and utilize the pericardium as a stabilizer. This blended strategy not only optimizes surgical techniques but also enhances postoperative cardiac function long-term by maintaining the heart's precise location and protective setting within the thoracic space (Loforte et al., 2021) (Figure 7.8).

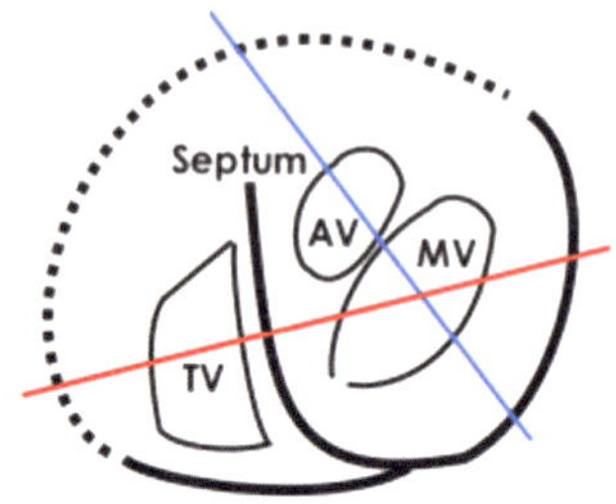

Figure 7.8. Contribution to heart stability and positioning.

Source: By Kjetil Lenes - Own work, CC BY-SA 3.0, https://commons.wikimedia.org/w/index.php?curid=3705979

Test Your Knowledge

1. How does the diaphragm assist in stabilizing the heart's location during respiration and movement?
2. What is the function of the pericardial fluid between the serous layers of the pericardium?

7.5. Common Diseases of the Heart

Learning Outcome

1. Discuss the Coronary Artery Disease
2. Understand Heart Failure
3. Focus on Arrhythmias

The complex anatomy and continuous activity of the heart make it vulnerable to many pathological processes reducing its efficacy. Of these, valvular heart diseases are notable for their impact on one-way blood flow and cardiac output. Degenerative changes, congenital lesions, and infections are all able to impair valve function with ensuing stenosis or regurgitation. New advances in tissue engineering provide new regenerative paradigms for heart valve repair, where decellularized heart valve scaffolds induce recipient cell repopulation, leading to autologous-like tissue formation. The method promises adaptive and long-lasting valve function with the ability to accommodate patient growth while reducing the rate of repeated interventions. Such environmental friendly options hold particular importance for pediatric and geriatric patients with the aim of overcoming challenges inherent in prosthetic replacements through the availability of off-the-shelf biodevices that become fully integrated into the heart's native tissue (Gerosa et al., 2015). Inflammatory pericardial diseases represent another critical category of heart disease frequently complicating diagnosis and management given the diverse etiologies. Tuberculous pericarditis continues to be common in the developing world and can result in ominous complications like constrictive pericarditis. The pericardial tuberculosis inflammatory environment is characterized by localized immune reactions that are marked by high levels of cytokines and chemokines. Treatment with adjunctive corticosteroid therapy with prednisolone has shown effectiveness in altering these immune responses by lowering pro-inflammatory mediators like IL-6, IL-1beta, and IL-8 in different bodily fluids within hours of administration. These findings highlight the significance of immunomodulation in the regulation of pericardial inflammation and prevention of fibrotic sequelae, thereby preserving cardiac function and improving clinical outcomes in pericardial diseases (Shenje et al., 2017). Along with valve and pericardial diseases, ischemic heart disease and cardiomyopathies constitute a vast majority of current heart diseases that are commonly the result of a complex interplay of genetic, environmental, and lifestyle determinants. CAD, typically due to atherosclerosis, impairs myocardial perfusion and can cause myocardial infarction, arrhythmias, or heart failure. Cardiomyopathies, dilated, hypertrophic, or restrictive, impair myocardial contractility and structure and are the causes of significant morbidity and mortality. A thorough understanding of these conditions necessitates an integrated approach from tissue-level interventions to systemic treatments. Ongoing developments in regenerative medicine and immunotherapy, in addition to conventional pharmacologic and surgical treatments, continue to unfold, offering promise for enhanced therapy for the multifaceted issues posed by common heart diseases.

7.5.1. Coronary Artery Disease

The complex relationship between cancer therapy and cardiovascular disease has attracted significant attention since the enhancement of the survival of cancer patients and the consequent evolution of late cardiac complications. Of these complications, CAD represents a significant challenge, particularly because it can develop several years after radiation therapy. The pathophysiological substrate involves radiation damage to coronary arteries, accelerating atherosclerosis and inducing ischemic heart disease. It is this type of vascular injury that typically occurs insidiously, rendering early detection difficult and optimal management problematic. Hence, cancer survivors require meticulous cardiovascular follow-up to recognize and treat these complications promptly, which can significantly improve their quality of life (QoL) and prognosis. The need for routine screening programs in post-radiation patients has been emphasized to reduce morbidity and mortality resulting from CAD in this special category of patients (Nabiałek-Trojanowska et al., 2020). Chemotherapeutic medications further complicate the CAD situation with several cardiotoxicity effects, emphasizing how delicately balanced the therapeutic and cardiovascular safety needs to be for physicians. Other medications have been linked to cardiac adverse effects of various sorts, including arrhythmias, myocardial necrosis, and coronary vasospasm, all of which actually cause or exacerbate CAD. Of most importance is an endothelial injury resulting from chemotherapy agents that undermine vascular integrity and promotes thrombosis and ischemic damage. This cardiotoxicity is augmented in vulnerable populations such as the elderly or those with an underlying cardiovascular disease. Understanding these multifaceted drug-induced pathologies is necessary to create personalized treatment regimes that minimize cardiac damage without compromising oncological efficacy (Vasiliadis et al., 2014). The long-term consequences of CAD in cancer patients point towards the necessity of multidisciplinary care by oncologists and cardiologists to prevent and manage cardiac and pericardial complications. Angiogenesis inhibitors, though revolutionary, contribute to the risk factors of hypertension and left ventricular dysfunction, being causal agents of CAD progression. The interaction between advanced cancer care and cardiovascular well-being demands continuous assessment and development in therapeutic and diagnostic modalities. Ultimately, a combined strategy taking into account the long-term cardiovascular side effects of anticancer treatment can optimize survival and quality of life, highlighting a top priority for clinical investigation and medical policy decision-making (Vasiliadis et al., 2014; Nabiałek-Trojanowska et al., 2020) (Figure 7.9).

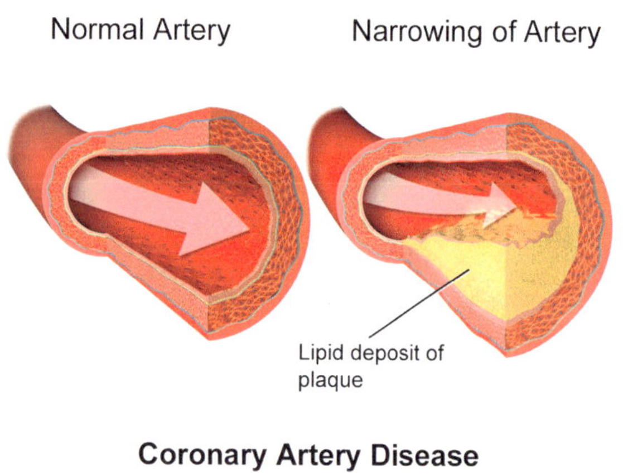

Figure 7.9. Coronary artery disease (CAD).

Source: https://en.wikipedia.org/wiki/File:Blausen_0259_CoronaryArteryDisease_02.png

7.5.2. Heart Failure

The relationship between the pericardium and the heart assumes a central role in the case of heart failure, where the physiological and mechanical interactions of the cardiac cycle are severely disturbed. Heart failure is most frequently due to abnormal myocardial function, and this may be added to by pericardial disease such as constriction or effusions. Both conditions increase external pressure on the myocardium and thereby affect ventricular filling and output. Understanding the role of the pericardium is crucial because changes in pericardial compliance or effusion directly influence cardiac preload and afterload and contribute to the worsening of the functional defect in heart failure. Management requires a close assessment of these factors to enable proper therapeutic maneuvers and to prevent further hemodynamic compromise. Successful perioperative management of patients with concomitant pericardial and myocardial disease emphasizes the significance of this interrelation within clinical practice (Oliveira et al., 2019). Recent advances in cardiovascular magnetic resonance (CMR) have provided useful information about heart failure, particularly in patients with concomitant pericardial involvement. CMR allows precise characterization of pericardial effusion to differentiate simple fluid accumulation from more complex inflammatory or fibrotic diseases, which could worsen symptoms of heart failure. Through the application of molecular imaging techniques such as T1 mapping, the volume and composition of the pericardial fluid may be analyzed non-invasively by physicians, resulting in better diagnosis and personalized therapy. Furthermore, CMR allows detailed examination of ventricular interdependence – a critical feature of constrictive pericarditis, where impaired septal motion inhibits diastolic filling and worsens heart failure. Diagnostic features of such kind increase understanding of heart failure mechanisms in the context of pericardial disease, with improved prognostic and therapeutic options (Thalén et al., 2024). The clinical importance of heart failure with pericardial abnormality extends beyond diagnosis to profoundly influence therapeutic planning and results. Pericardial diseases such as tamponade and constriction may induce or exacerbate heart failure by disrupting cardiac filling pressures and reducing effective stroke volume. Therapeutic intervention, for example, pericardiocentesis or surgical pericardiectomy, must be carefully timed and sequenced to relieve pericardial constraint without causing circulatory collapse. In addition, the concomitant organ dysfunctions frequently complicate management, demanding multicontinental treatment to restore the optimal perioperative and long-term results. Anesthetic care in these patients is a complex understanding of pathophysiology for maintaining stable hemodynamics during surgery, which creates the imperative of detail-oriented assessment and coordinated treatment in heart failure with pericardial disease (Oliveira et al., 2019).

7.5.3. Arrhythmias

The complex relationship between the heart and its enveloping tissues is at the core of the pathophysiology of cardiac disorders such as arrhythmias. Not only the inherent properties of myocardial cells but also the microenvironment created by the pericardium, governs the electrophysiological stability of the heart. Disruption of this environment, whether through structural defects or functional interventions, will result in abnormal electrical conduction pathways and hence arrhythmogenic behavior. Targeted delivery of drugs via the pericardial space, for example, has been investigated due to its proximity to the myocardium, allowing for local therapeutic effects with less systemic toxicity. Intrapericardial administration of antiarrhythmic medications is one of such strategies that utilizes this anatomical proximity to optimize pharmacokinetic profiles and limit side effects throughout the cardiovascular system (Ho et al., 2022). This approach underlines the necessity to preserve both the pericardial structural integrity and the understanding of its function in the modulation of cardiac rhythm. Anatomical anomalies of the pericardium can significantly impact the arrhythmia risk factor and management, particularly in complex cases with congenital malformations. For instance, the correction of congenital diaphragmatic hernia and associated anomalies such as pericardial absence pose unique challenges to thoracic surgical interventions. The absence or alteration of the pericardium also increases the susceptibility to mechanical trauma of cardiac tissues and may be a cause of arrhythmogenic potential by interfering with the natural electrophysiological environment of the heart. Minimally invasive procedures, like the modified thoracoscopic approach that was adapted in patients with such congenital defects, emphasize careful visualization and manipulation of cardiac structures to avoid exacerbation of arrhythmias or cardiac complications (Timman et al., 2016). These clinical observations underscore the importance of considering pericardial status in evaluating arrhythmia risks and tailoring therapeutic interventions accordingly. The development of cardiac arrhythmia therapy increasingly recognizes the pericardium as an attractive therapeutic access route, with innovative solutions beyond traditional systemic therapies.

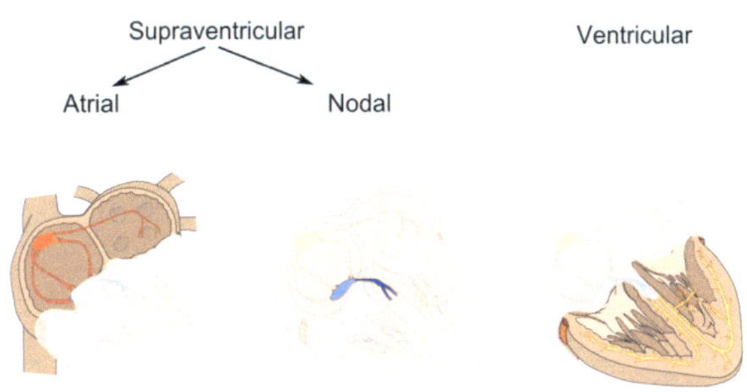

Figure 7.10. Arrhythmias.

Source: By CardioNetworks: Googletrans - CardioNetworks: De-Atrial_ventricular.png, CC BY-SA 3.0, https://commons.wikimedia.org/w/index.php?curid=24370888

By exploiting intrapericardial drug and cell delivery approaches, clinicians will be in a position to treat arrhythmias more specifically, targeting injured myocardium or arrhythmogenic foci without systemic exposure. The evolution and refinement of access devices—from needles to loop catheters—have enhanced the safety and efficacy of these procedures, with generally acceptable procedural risk and only rare significant complications reported (Ho et al., 2022). As our understanding of cardiac-pericardial interactions deepens, these intrapericardial strategies may form an integral part of personalized arrhythmia management, coupling anatomical insight with pharmacological innovation to improve clinical outcomes for patients experiencing diverse cardiac rhythm disorders (Figure 7.10).

Test Your Knowledge

1. Differentiate between left-sided and right-sided heart failure in terms of symptoms.
2. What is an arrhythmia, and how does it affect the heart's rhythm and efficiency?

7.6. Common Diseases of the Pericardium

Learning Outcome

1. Discuss the Pericarditis
2. Explain the Pericardial Effusion
3. Focus on Constrictive Pericarditis

The pericardium is valuable to cardiac performance, both because it serves as a protective sheath and for its immunologic role, the latter being of particular significance when the structure comes into play during diseases. Common pericardial diseases are acute pericarditis, chronic constrictive pericarditis, pericardial effusion, and cardiac tamponade. All four are distinct from one another in pathophysiology and clinical features but can cause compromised cardiac performance and significant morbidity. The anatomical changes of fibrosis and thickening in the pericardium can be worsened by age, which complicates clinical management, especially for older patients. As vital as it is, however, there are gaps in knowledge in the randomized trial evidence that informs management plans for pericardial diseases. Where anatomical changes overlap with immune response is where pericardial diseases become infinitely complex and necessitate tailor-made therapeutic approaches that address both the structural and inflammatory components (Athar et al., 2019). Of the range of pericardial diseases, one of the most frequent and a reason for as many as five percent of all cases of chest pain admission is pericarditis. Pericarditis can be defined as inflammation of the pericardial tissues that clinically manifests as chest pain, friction rub, and characteristic ECG changes. Etiologically, pericarditis may result from infectious etiologies such as viruses and bacteria or non-infectious causes like autoimmune conditions, malignancy, or post-cardiac injury syndromes. Diagnostic workup relies heavily on blood biomarkers and various imaging modalities, which both reflect inflammatory processes as well as structural impact on the pericardium. While pharmacotherapy forms the primary treatment, in its severe form, it may require pericardial surgery, thus underlining the importance of accurate diagnosis and early intervention (Wokurka et al., 2023). Among the rarer and more serious presentations within the spectrum of constrictive pericarditis is the so-called armored heart, wherein there is the gross thickening of the pericardium in imaging studies. This subtype is representative of the challenges of pericardial disease classification, as clear-cut diagnostic criteria are lacking, and the term armored heart comes to be used subjectively. Failure to demarcate specific diagnostic criteria is a reflection of the heterogeneity in the course and presentation of the disease. Armored heart causes restricted cardiac filling from the stiff pericardium, with resulting severe clinical impairments such as heart failure manifestations. It is critical to understand this type of constrictive pericarditis to direct prognosis as well as management strategies. Additional research is needed to delineate diagnostic standards and maximize therapeutic strategies for this severe pericardial disease (Wokurka et al., 2023).

7.6.1. Pericarditis

The complex interaction between the cardiac structures and those which envelop them is crucial in maintaining normal heart function. Among these structures, the pericardium not only comes in the form of a fibrous covering sac but also has a role in cardiac mechanical regulation. When it becomes inflamed, an inflammation called pericarditis ensues, which typically becomes challenging to clinicians due to its unpredictable presentation. The symptomatology may range from acute chest pain to presentations that resemble other cardiopulmonary diseases, and hence accurate diagnosis is imperative. Even with the advancements made in cardiovascular imaging and diagnostic tools, identification of pericarditis requires careful clinical evaluation and often multimodal imaging. CMR, for example, provides both anatomical delineation and tissue characterization that are of very high value in distinguishing pericardial inflammation and assessing functional impact on cardiac filling and motion (Bogaert & Francone, 2009). This diagnostic precision is crucial in guiding effective therapeutic interventions and preventing complications. Pericarditis may present in various forms like acute, recurrent, and constrictive types with varied pathological and clinical manifestations. The disease might be produced by infection, autoimmune mechanisms, or systemic diseases, and its onset might produce pericardial effusion or even cardiac tamponade. The immunological role of the pericardium in the modulation of inflammatory responses has become increasingly significant as an active rather than passive role. Notably, inflammation may be more severe or occur in different forms in older individuals, who also experience age-related changes in the structure of the pericardium. However, due to its clinical importance, extensive randomized trials of pericarditis therapy are unavailable, thus evidence-based therapeutic decisions are highly difficult for high-risk individuals (Athar et al., 2019).

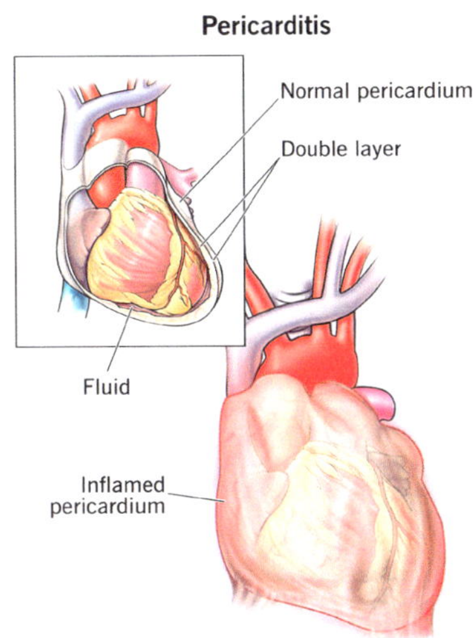

Figure 7.11. Pericarditis.

Source: Cleveland Clinic. (n.d.). *Pericarditis.*

An understanding of these nuances permits a more refined patient treatment. Prognosis and outcomes of pericarditis therapy depend largely on early diagnosis and the specific underlying etiology. Treatment in the landscape includes non-steroidal anti-inflammatory agents (NSAIDs), colchicine, and corticosteroids. In addition, where necessary, surgical intervention may include pericardiectomy. The clinical decision is very individualized secondary to the heterogeneity of presentation and balancing potential benefit against the risk of intervention. Due to limitations of discriminating between pericarditis and pericarditis mimics, exact imaging and discriminative clinical history remain management cornerstones. Furthermore, ongoing research into the pathophysiology and immunologic mechanisms of pericardial inflammation will continue to refine future diagnostic and therapeutic pathways. An interdependent strategy with advanced imaging, patient-related factors, and evolving clinical data is needed for improved outcomes in this multifactorial spectrum of pericardial diseases (Bogaert & Francone, 2009; Athar et al., 2019) (Figure 7.11).

7.6.2. Pericardial Effusion

The pericardium, a two-walled fibrous sac, specially guards and supports the heart and contains a minimal amount of serous fluid normally to avoid movement-related friction. The equilibrium may be disrupted when an excess amount of fluid gets trapped and leads to pericardial effusion. The fluid composition may range from transudative to exudative or sanguineous types based on the causative agent. This accumulation can be secondary to infection, inflammation, malignancy, or trauma to the myocardium and may manifest as a potentially serious clinical scenario if it goes undetected. The pathophysiology involves interference with regular fluid homeostasis within the pericardial sac, which in a state of normal physiology contains 15 -50 milliliters of fluid. Understanding of the etiologic factors contributing to pericardial effusion is essential for early diagnosis and treatment, thus highlighting the importance of careful evaluation in compatible presentation patients (Al-Razik et al., 2022). Pericardial changes with age also play a significant role in the susceptibility and clinical profile of pericardial effusions. As the pericardium undergoes structural and immunological alterations with advancing age, its responsiveness to inflammatory or pathological injury may be impaired. This immunological function is significant, especially in diseases such as pericarditis, which may result in effusion formation. After the established anatomy and physiology of the pericardium, evidence-based recommendations and existing studies on the management of pericardial effusions in older people are not forthcoming. This lacuna underscores the need for an individualized approach based on age-related pericardial changes, and comorbidities characteristic of the elderly. Identification of these is crucial in maximizing therapeutic interventions and clinical outcomes among multifaceted groups of patients (Athar et al., 2019).

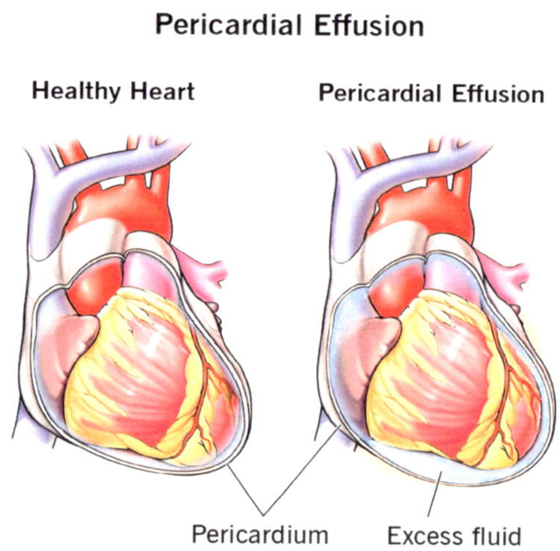

Figure 7.12. Pericardial effusion.

Source: Cleveland Clinic. (n.d.). *Pericardial Effusion: Healthy Heart vs. Excess Fluid.*

Clinical acumen is critical in the consideration of pericardial effusion as part of the differential diagnosis because of its multifarious presentation and ensuing complications, such as cardiac tamponade. Early diagnosis relies on integrating patient history, physical examination findings, and diagnostic imaging studies such as echocardiography. Analysis of pericardial fluid with laboratory studies, if present, determines its etiology and determines the appropriate treatment measures. Treatment typically ranges from conservative observation in small, asymptomatic effusions to more aggressive interventions such as pericardiocentesis in big or symptomatic effusions. An interprofessional approach by cardiologists, radiologists, and critical care teams provides coordinated care with each patient receiving individualized and maximized care. Such a collaboration helps in optimizing patient outcomes as well as reducing morbidity due to pericardial effusions (Al-Razik et al., 2022) (Figure 7.12).

7.6.3. Constrictive Pericarditis

The pericardium plays a vital role in the maintenance of cardiac function by providing a protective fibroelastic sac that surrounds the heart and regulates hemodynamics. When this structure is modified by disease, severe cardiovascular dysfunction can result. One of such disorders is constrictive pericarditis, which is characterized by the development of granulation tissue within the pericardium leading to fibrosis and loss of elasticity. This rigidity impedes ventricular filling during diastole, resulting in compromised cardiac output and the clinical manifestations of heart failure. Although usually a chronic process, exceptions such as subacute or transient constrictive pericarditis are confounding to diagnose and treat. Chronic constriction ultimately results in the heart beating within a rigid, noncompliant pericardial shell, which without treatment is accompanied by poor clinical outcomes. It is important to appreciate this altered pathophysiology to evaluate patient presentation and guide therapeutic interventions (Al-Razik et al., 2022). In oncologic practice, constrictive pericarditis is a difficult clinical condition due to its multifactorial etiology, both through direct tumor involvement as well as cancer therapy. Cancers such as lung cancer, breast cancer, and lymphoma commonly infiltrate the pericardium or cause inflammatory processes leading to constriction. Furthermore, radiotherapy and chemotherapy are significant factors that induce pericardial thickening and fibrosis, exacerbating disease progression. Diagnosis is made with a high degree of suspicion and typically requires a combination of imaging studies like echocardiography, CT, and MRI to distinguish constriction from other causes of restrictive cardiomyopathy. Early diagnosis is essential, as the condition typically carries a poor prognosis without surgery. Pericardiectomy remains the definitive therapy, with symptomatic relief and hemodynamic betterment, although postsurgical survival rates highlight the need for scrupulous multidisciplinary management (Lorenzo-Esteller et al., 2024). Management of constrictive pericarditis extends beyond surgery and involves a concerted effort between cardiologists, oncologists, and cardiothoracic surgeons to optimize patient outcomes. Medical therapy is aimed at symptomatic relief and treating potential reversible etiologies in transient types, but in most chronic cases, pericardiectomy is the cornerstone. Despite the surgical risk, treatment alleviates diastolic filling restrictions and increases functional capacity. In addition, newer approaches involve early identification using multimodal imaging and personalized immunomodulatory therapies, particularly in cancer-related cases with immune checkpoint inhibitors or inflammatory etiology. Multidisciplinary coordination streamlines clinical decision-making and promotes individualized treatment planning, with the ultimate objective of improving QoL and survival for individuals affected by this complex, progressive pathology (Al-Razik et al., 2022; Lorenzo-Esteller et al., 2024).

Test Your Knowledge

1. Differentiate between the pulmonary and systemic circulations of the heart.
2. What is the clinical significance of the transverse pericardial sinus during cardiac surgery?

SUMMARY

Advances in cardiovascular tissue engineering have opened up the possibilities for new solutions to age-old issues in valvular repair and replacement. Traditional prosthetic valves, while lifesaving, are fraught with intrinsic limitations of thrombogenicity, immune response, and lack of long-term durability, particularly in the young. These have highlighted the imperative to develop viable tissue constructs with a close approximation of native valve form and function. Recent studies demonstrate promising methods for enhancing endothelial cell attachment on acellular scaffolds through the use of protein substrates and hydrogel carriers combined with dynamic seeding techniques. In addition to increasing cellular retention, these methods also promote uniform endothelial coverage, which is essential to valve function. Integrating these strategies is a significant leap towards the creation of tissue-engineered heart valves with self-maintenance and remodeling potential, and thus resolving the degeneration and calcification issues of current prosthetics (Fontaine et al., 2015). Such developments are crucial for the advancement of cardiac therapy as well as the improvement of patient outcomes in valvular diseases. Complementing these engineering approaches, seeding of patient-derived cells into decellularized scaffolds emerges as a promising pathway to biocompatibility and long-term viability. Research in pulmonary valve reconstruction illustrates that the use of bovine pericardium and inferior vena cava as scaffolding materials imparts mechanical properties conducive to valve function. In addition, the use of novel seeding devices ensures adequate repopulation of these scaffolds with fibroblasts, promoting long-term homeostasis of the extracellular matrix. These living-valve conduits demonstrate functional competence under physiologic conditions, as evidenced by studies utilizing sterile heart valve bioreactors that mimic *in vivo* conditions. The ability to maintain cell viability and mechanical function *in vitro* is a critical step toward clinical translation, particularly for pediatric and young adult populations that receive multiple revision surgeries with existing valve replacement technologies (Hoskins, 2022). This research emphasizes the necessity for the coupling of biomechanical compatibility and biological function. In conclusion, the marriage of innovative cellular seeding techniques with suitable decellularized scaffolds is a groundbreaking step forward in the management of heart valve disease. Efforts at developing living heart valves with resistance to degeneration, calcification, and immune rejection have great promise to enhance implant durability, especially in vulnerable patient groups. While challenges remain in achieving complete endothelialization and long-term functional integrity, current research offers a compelling paradigm for continued investigation and optimization. The pursuit of bioengineered valves that reconcile structural durability and biological activity represents a fundamental advance in cardiovascular therapy, one that has the potential to transform standards of care. Continued inter-disciplinary collaboration will be required to bring these developments from laboratory completion to clinical application, with the ultimate goal of improving survival and QoL for patients worldwide (Fontaine et al., 2015; Hoskins, 2022).

The interdynamic relationship between the pericardium and heart plays a crucial role in maintaining cardiovascular health, and a number of determinants regulate their function and pathology. Recent studies on chronic rejection in transplanted hearts illustrate the complexity of immune responses on myocardial tissue and vascular structures. In model systems, arterial remodeling during the initial phases of acute rejection leads to obliterative arteriopathy later, with immune cell infiltration, endothelial activation, and lymphatic disruption. This interaction highlights how immune mechanisms underlie long-term graft dysfunction and implicates donor antigen-presenting cells in sustaining graft acceptance. Furthermore, chronic heart and pericardium inflammation is linked to structural and functional impairment that may cause rejection or disease progression, indicating the importance of immunological control for cardiac stability (Demetris et al., 1997). The results provide fundamental knowledge to advance therapeutic approaches in heart transplant survival and treatment of pericardial disease. Technological advancement to treat CAD—a phenomenon intimately connected with cardiac function, emphasizes the applicability of material science coupled with cardiovascular biology. Developments such as elastin-like recombinamer (ELR) coated stents are medical intervention advancements in arterial well-being in the vicinity of cardiac structures. These bioengineered stents exhibit physiological stress resistance under simulated implantation, mechanical stability at elevated flow, and low platelet adhesion with good endothelial cell growth. These stents' ability to maintain structural integrity while promoting endothelialization aligns with the pericardium's role of enabling the heart's optimal functioning through mechanical and immunological protection. The development of these bioactive devices, thus, can be seen to have the potential to reduce stent failure and improve patient clinical outcomes for CAD, having a direct impact on cardiac health and pericardial interaction (Oliva-Pascual-Vaca et al., 2019). In recapitulating the complex interaction of immune, mechanical, and bioengineering forces on the heart and pericardium, multidisciplinary research stands out as a prime mover in advancing cardiovascular medicine. The immune-mediated processes involved in chronic rejection of heart transplants demonstrate the need for targeted immunomodulatory therapies, while the development of stent technology speaks to the importance of biomaterials in coronary artery stabilization and preservation of the cardiac vascular environment. Both domains illustrate the delicate balance of mechanical and biological determinants necessary to maintain cardiac function and pericardial integrity. Composite knowledge of these considerations forms the basis of contemporary research and clinical practice, guiding efforts to enhance heart transplant survival and more successfully manage CAD by viewing the heart and pericardium as a pathologic and functional unit (Demetris et al., 1997; Oliva-Pascual-Vaca et al., 2019).

KEY TERMS FROM THIS CHAPTER

Myocardium	Endocardium	Epicardium
Interventricular septum	Coronary arteries	Cardiac veins
Sinoatrial (SA) node	Bundle of His	Purkinje fibers
Cardiac cycle	Systole / Diastole	Stroke volume
Cardiac output	Heart rate	Coronary circulation
Fibrous pericardium	Serous pericardium	Parietal layer

CRITICAL THINKING QUESTIONS

1. **Which layer of the heart is responsible for contraction?**
   a. Epicardium
   b. Endocardium
   c. Myocardium
   d. Pericardium
2. **The fibrous pericardium is attached inferiorly to the:**
   a. Diaphragm
   b. Sternum
   c. Lungs
   d. Esophagus
3. **Which chamber of the heart forms most of the anterior surface?**
   a. Left atrium
   b. Right atrium
   c. Left ventricle
   d. Right ventricle
4. **The pericardial cavity lies between:**
   a. Epicardium and myocardium
   b. Parietal and visceral layers of the serous pericardium
   c. Fibrous and serous pericardium
   d. Myocardium and endocardium
5. **The heart apex is typically formed by the:**
   a. Right atrium
   b. Left ventricle
   c. Left atrium
   d. Right ventricle

Short Answer Questions

1. Describe the layers of the pericardium and their functions.
2. What are the anatomical boundaries of the pericardial cavity?
3. Explain the coronary circulation and name the main arteries involved.
4. What is the significance of the fibrous pericardium's attachment to the diaphragm?
5. Describe the conduction system of the heart and its role in cardiac rhythm.
6. Discuss the nerve supply to the pericardium and associated referred pain patterns.

Answers to Critical Thinking Questions

1. (b) 2. (b) 3. (b) 4. (c) 5. (b)

References

1. *Aguilar, S. (2015). Effect of* Methylmercury Exposure on Heart and Skeletal Muscle Development in Zebrafish Embryos (Danio Rerio). Submitted to the Office of Graduate and Professional Studies of Texas A&M University in partial fulfillment of the requirements for the degree of MASTER OF SCIENCE. https://core.ac.uk/download/147242268.pdf (accessed on 8th May 2025).
2. Athar A, Dhaduk K, S. Aronow W. Pericardial Diseases in Elderly Patients [Internet]. Inflammatory Heart Diseases. IntechOpen; 2019. Available from: http://dx.doi.org/10.5772/intechopen.89473 (accessed on 8th May 2025).
3. Battista, N. A., & Miller, L. A. (2017). Bifurcations in Valveless Pumping Tec*hniques fro*m a Coupled Fluid-Structure-Electrophysiology Model in Heart Development. https://core.ac.uk/download/201720173.pdf (accessed on 8th May 2025).
4. Bogaert, J., & Francone, M. (2009). Cardiovascular magnetic resonance in pericardial diseases. Journal of cardiovascular magnetic resonance : official journal of the Society for Cardiovascular Mag*netic Resonance, 11(1), 14. https://doi.org/10.1186/1532-429X-11-14 (accessed on 8th May 2025).*
5. *Chassot, P. G., van der* Linden, P., Zaugg, M., Mueller, X. M., & Spahn, D. R. (2004). Off-pump coronary artery bypass surgery: physiology and anaesthetic management. British journal of anaesthesia, 92(3), 400–413. https://doi.org/10.1093/bja/aeh064 (accessed on 8th May 2025).
6. Demetris, A. J., Murase, N., Ye, Q., Galvao, F. H., Richert, C., Saad, R., Pham, S., Duquesnoy, R. J., Zeevi, A., Fung, J. J., & Starzl, T. E. (1997). Analysis of chronic rejection and obliterative arteriopathy. Possible contributions of donor antigen-presenting *cells and lymphatic disruption. The American journal of pathology, 150(2), 563–578.(accessed on 8th May 2025).*
7. *Dorsher,* P. The Neuroanatomic Basis of the Acupuncture Principal Meridians. Nat Prec (2009). https://doi.org/10.1038/npre.2009.3795.1(accessed on 8th May 2025).
8. Heide, Stefan & Timman, Simone. (2016). Minimally invasive repair of pectus excavatum in a 17-year-old boy *with a history of congenital diaphragma*tic hernia and lack of pericardium. Journal of Pediatric Surgery Case Reports. 9. 10.1016/j.epsc.2016.04.012. (accessed on 8th May 2025).
9. Ho, H. M. K., Craig, D. Q. M., & Day, R. M. (2022). Access routes, devices and guidance methods for intra*pericardial delivery in cardiac* conditions. Trends in cardiovascular medicine, 32(4), 206–218. https://doi.org/10.1016/j.tcm.2021.04.004(accessed on 8th May 2025).
10. Hoskins, E. (2022). Tissue-Engineered Living Pulmonary Valve for Young Adult Patients. https:/*/core.ac.uk/download/539558805.pdf* (accessed on 8th May 2025).
11. Hovde, O. H. (2024). Modeling and Simulation of Ascending Aorta, Including Influence of Tissue Change in Aneurysms. Master's thesis in Mechanical Engineering Supervisor: Bjørn Helge Skallerud Co-supervisor: Victorien Prot & Omid Ghorbani June 2024 Norwegian University of Science and Technology Faculty of Engineering Department of Structural Engineering. *https://core.ac.uk/download/646131904*.pdf (accessed on 8th May 2025).
12. https://doi.org/10.1016/j.artmed.2005.07.004.
13. Konwerski, M., Gąsecka, A., Opolski, *G., Grab*owski, M., & Mazurek, T. (2022). Role of epicardial adipose tissue in cardiovascular diseases: A review. Biology, 11, 355. https://doi.org/10.3390/

biology11030355 (accessed on 8th May 2025).

14. Liu, L. (2024). Anatomy-aided deep learning for medical image segmentation with application to epicardial adipose tissue. [PhD Thesis - Research UT, graduation UT, University of Twente]. University of Twente. https://doi.org/10.3990/1.9789036562072 (accessed on 8th May 2025).

15. Loforte, A., Gliozzi, G., Mariani, C., Cavalli, G. G., Martin-Suarez, S., & Pacini, D. (2021). *Ventricular assist devices implantation: surgical assessment and technical strategies. Cardiovascular diagnosis and therapy, 11(1), 277–291. https://doi.org/10.21037/cdt-20-325 (accessed* on 8th May 2025).

16. Lorenzale, G. M. (2019). El Tracto de Salida del Corazón de los Condrictios *y Actinopterigios. https://core.ac.uk/download/268997315.pdf (accessed on 8th May 2025).*

17. Lorenzo-Esteller, L., Ramos-Polo, R., Pons Riverola, A., Morillas, H., Berdejo, J., Pernas, S., Pomares, H., Asiain, L., Garay, A., Martínez Pérez, E., Jiménez-Marrero, S., Alcoberro, L., Nadal, E., Gubern-Prieto, P., Gual-Capllonch, F., Hidalgo, E., Enjuanes, C., Comin-Colet, J., & Moliner, P. (2024). Pericardial Disease in Patients with Cancer: Clinical Insights on Diagnosis and Treatment. Cancers, 16(*20), 3466.* https://doi.org/10.3390/cancers16203466 (accessed on 8th May 2025).

18. Maureen Donnelly, Thomas Bittner, Cornelius Rosse. A formal theory for spatial representation and reasoning in biomedical ontologies, Artificial Intelligence in Medici*ne, Volume* 36, Issue 1, Pages 1-27,

19. Motalib, M., Ali, M. Z., Islam, M. R., & Ahammed, S. (2024). Confluence of challenges: Massive tubercular pericardial effusion entangled with heart failure and diabetes mellitus – A multidisciplinary odyssey. KYAMC Journal. 10.3329/kyamcj.v15i01.75833. *https://www.semanticscholar.org/paper/f7b35a266d611405*f7793a6ddced87d2da543ced (accessed on 8th May 2025).

20. Nabiałek-Trojanowska, I., Lewicka, E., Wrona, A., Kaleta, A. M., Lewicka-Potocka, Z., Raczak, G., & Dziadziuszko, R. (2020). Cardiovascular complications after radiotherapy. Cardiology journal, 27(6), 836–847. https://doi.org/10.5603/CJ.a2018.0120 (accessed on 8th May 2025).

21. Oliva-Pascual-Vaca, Á., González-González, C., Oliva-Pascual-*Vaca, J., Piña-Pozo, F., Ferragut-Garcías, A., Fernández-Domínguez,* J. C., & Heredia-Rizo, A. M. (2019). Visceral Origin: An Underestimated Source of Neck Pain. A Systematic Scoping Review. Diagnostics (Basel, Switzerland), 9(4), 186. https://doi.org/10.3390/diagnostics9040186

22. Salzer, G. E. (2019). Pannexin 1 Channel Inhibition to Prevent Trigger*ed Arrhythmia.* https://core.ac.uk/download/640970522.pdf (accessed on 8th May 2025).

23. Santiago, A., Aguado-Sierra, J., Zavala-Aké, M., Doste-Beltran, R., Gómez, S., Arís, R., *Cajas, J. C., Casoni, E., & Vázquez, M. (2018). Fully couple*d fluid-electro-mechanical model of the human heart for supercomputers. International journal for numerical methods in biomedical engineering, 34(12), e3140. https://doi.org/10.1002/cnm.3140 (accessed on 8th May 2025).

24. Shenje, J., Lai, R. P., Ross, I. L., Mayosi, B. M., Wilkinson, R. J., Nts*ekhe, M., & Wilkinson, K. A. (2017). Effect of prednisolone on inflammat*ory markers in pericardial tuberculosis: A pilot study. International journal of cardiology. Heart & *vasculature, 18, 104–108. https://doi.org/10.1016/j.ijcha.2017.10.002 (accessed on 8th* May 2025).

25. Thalén, S. O. A. (2024). Cardiovascular Magnetic Resonance Evaluation of Effusive and Constrictive physiologies. https://core.ac.uk/download/599460664.pdf (accessed on 8th May 2025).

26. Vasiliadis, I., Kolovou, G., & Mikhailidis, D. P. (2014). Cardiotoxicity and cancer therapy. Angiology, 65(5), 369–371. https://doi.org/10.1177/0003319713498298 (accessed on 8th May 2025).

27. Wokurka, W., Węgrzyniak, A., Drobek, D., Winiarz, A., Szlendak, P., Toś, K., ... Grosman, S. (2023). Armored heart as an image of constrictive pericarditis - a review of the literature. Journal of Education, Health and Sport, *43(1), 67–81. https://doi.org/*10.12775/JEHS.2023.43.01.006 (accessed on 8th May 2025).

MEDIASTINUM

8

LEARNING OBJECTIVES

After studying this chapter, you will be able to:

1. Discuss the anatomy of the mediastinum
2. Focus on the superior mediastinum
3. Explain the anterior mediastinum
4. Know middle mediastinum
5. Understand posterior mediastinum
6. Focus on the clinical significance of the mediastinum

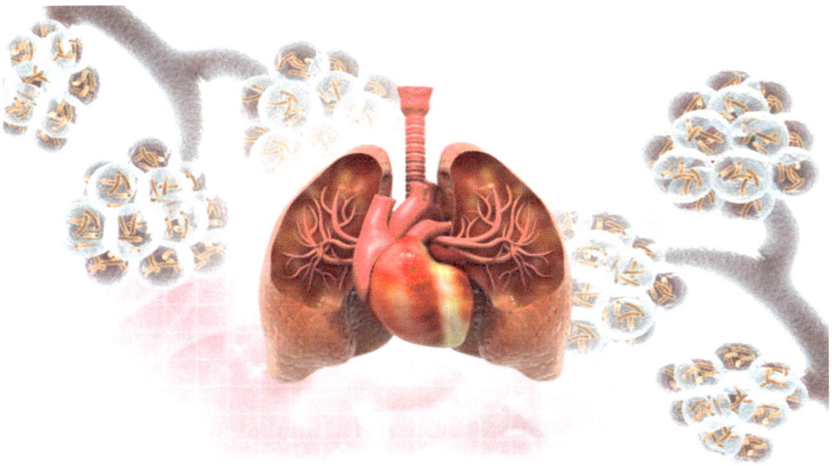

Introduction

The human organism is made up of many sophisticated structures that all work together in harmony to help preserve homeostasis and perform essential physiological processes. Of all these, the central thoracic cavity is the most notable to be an area of great clinical and anatomical interest because of its contents and the important roles it serves. The central thoracic cavity houses many vital organs and tissues, encapsulated by the rib cage but susceptible to any pathology. Understanding this central compartment's structure is relevant to both clinicians and anatomists as it addresses issues of normal physiology as well as disease states. This foundational understanding sets the stage for detailed inspection of the mediastinum, an anatomical space within the midline thorax, whose richness parallels the complex relationship among organs and structures that fill it. The mediastinum is a midline structure within the thoracic cavity that separates the two pleural sacs that contain the lungs. The mediastinum serves as a conduit and as a compartment, housing life-sustaining organs such as the heart, thymus, great vessels, trachea, and esophagus. The mediastinum is anatomically made up of an upper and lower part, the lower part being subdivided into an anterior, middle, and posterior compartment. This separation provides for a more simplified understanding of surgical and pathological processes. Due to its seemingly modest location, complex anatomical interactions of the mediastinum pose problems for diagnosis and therapy, and this necessitates full comprehension of the contents and confines of the mediastinum in health . Mediastinal exploration is not only an academic procedure but also a therapeutic necessity in radiology, surgery, and pathology. Accurate identification of the mediastinal structures is essential in diagnosing diseases as diverse as tumors and infections to vascular malformations and traumatic injury. Variations in anatomical structures, such as gender and laterality variations among ligaments within the knee (Wilson et al., 2025), can similarly influence clinical presentation and outcome of treatment in the mediastinum. Furthermore, a realization of the laws governing the flow of sensory input and signal summation, seen in other complex organ systems (Putri et al., 2023), adds to the multidisciplinary effort required for successful management of mediastinal disorders. Thus, this introduction lays the background for a thorough exploration of the mediastinum's anatomy and clinical significance.

Definition of the Mediastinum

The thoracic cavity in humans is a comprehensive anatomical compartment with the significant structures to facilitate respiratory and cardiovascular functions. In the center of the area, there is an area that separates the lungs and holds numerous significant organs like the heart, great vessels, trachea, and esophagus. The area is called the mediastinum and is a conduit for structures traveling from the neck to the abdomen. Its complex anatomical boundaries and contents make it a focal point in clinical and education environments, particularly given that it brokers the interaction and protection of these crucial organs. Understanding the arrangement of the mediastinum is vital to medical professionals in diagnostic imaging and surgery planning, where simulation and three-dimensional modeling constantly improve training and precision (Elisabetta et al., 2017). The mediastinum definition thus moves from anatomy space to an active center integral to physiology in human beings. Traditionally, mediastinum has been referred to as the middle chamber in the thoracic cavity, laterally encased by pleural sacs of the lungs. It is again separated into the superior and inferior mediastinum by a horizontal plane extending from the sternal angle to the IV disc between the fourth and fifth thoracic vertebrae. It differentiates in such a way as to assist accurate anatomical orientation and clinical diagnosis because each compartment contains structures different from the other. The higher mediastinum accommodates the thymus, great vessels, trachea, and esophagus, while the lower mediastinum is further separated into anterior, middle, and posterior areas, containing the thymus, heartand pericardium, and thoracic aorta, respectively. Such a higher-level compartmentalization indicates the complexity of the mediastinum, and it calls for a higher-level imaging examination to differentiate and assess these structures in clinical settings for effective treatment planning and interventions (Oliveira et al., 2011). Contemporary advancements in medical simulation and imaging technology have revolutionized the comprehension and application of the mediastinum in education and practice in clinical settings. Three-dimensional models with interactive visualizations and augmented reality (AR) software enable improved visualizations that ease interaction with the anatomical richness of the region. The adoption of technology not only supports cognitive learning but improves procedural proficiency through realistic simulation of clinical problems involving the mediastinum. These devices enhance diagnostic precision, especially for airway management and thoracic surgery operations. Hence, the mediastinum is not just anatomically demarcated in space but also functionally, as a result of its significance in clinical practice and teaching, wherein precise anatomical knowledge is required to achieve good outcomes (Elisabetta et al., 2017). Such an evolving concept is a testament to the mediastum's vital role in anatomical as well as clinical practice (Figure 8.1).

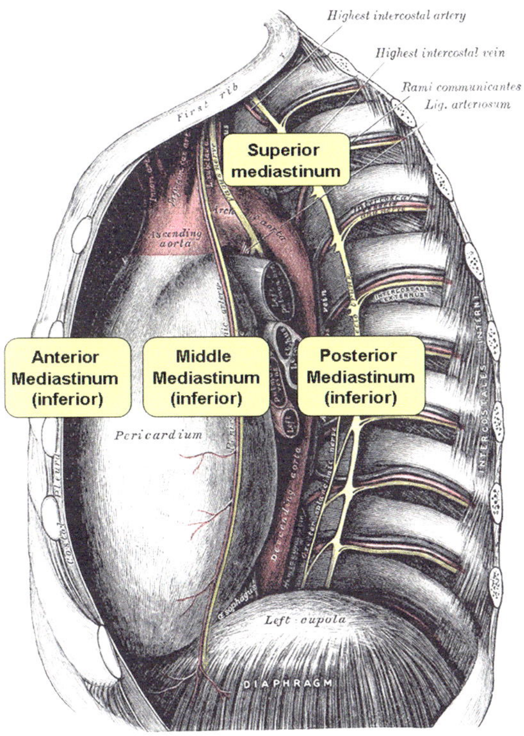

Figure 8.1. The mediastinum.

Source: Public Domain, https://commons.wikimedia.org/w/index.php?curid=1224440

Importance in Human Anatomy

The complex mediastinal architecture underscores its significance in human anatomy as a mid-compartment of the thoracic cavity housing significant structures and organs. This division between lungs houses the heart, large vessels, trachea, esophagus, and nerves, all housed by the enveloping thoracic cage. Knowledge of the spatial topology of the mediastinum is important because it influences both physiologic function and clinical diagnosis. The complexity that is present in such anatomical relationships calls for precise knowledge, particularly when it concerns the interpretation of imaging or surgical planning. With the offering of a structural and developmental model of the human thorax, anatomy offers valuable information that describes how these structures coexist and dynamically interact to offer appropriate treatment and research strategies (Rosse & Mejino, 2008). The significance of mediastinal anatomy is most noticeable when considering common anatomical variations that can arise, such as in the azygos venous system. Variations of venous pathways in the posterior mediastinum can complicate diagnostic evaluations and surgical procedures because abnormal structures can be mimicked by pathologies like thoracic aortic aneurysms, lymphadenopathy, or tumors. There is a need for a thorough anatomical understanding of such differences for radiologists and surgeons to avoid misdiagnosis and accurate identification of mediastinal structures in the case of CT or MRI scans. This awareness raises the rate of mediastinal surgeries being accurate, reducing the risk of unnecessary damage to vital vessels and thereby enhancing patients' outcomes (Geethanjali & Shivanal, 2017). Besides, the mediastinal anatomical organization serves as a general reference for clinical and research applications, coordinating across biomedical disciplines. The development of large-scale ontologies, such as the foundational model of anatomy (FMA), is one example of anatomical nomenclature and representation standardization. The ontological models enable computable and interoperable anatomical data that facilitate advanced biomedical research, clinical decisions, and education. By making the phenotypic structure of the human thorax accessible at different levels of detail, the mediastinum offers a wonderful example of how precise knowledge of anatomy underlies machine-based reasoning and artificial intelligence (AI) in medicine. This convergence of anatomy and technology demonstrates its ongoing utility in health and disease understanding (Rosse & Mejino, 2008).

8.1. Anatomy of the Mediastinum

Learning Outcome

1. Discuss the Location within the Thoracic Cavity
2. Explain the Divisions of the Mediastinum
3. Describe Key Structures Contained Within

Knowledge of the mediastinum requires a sensitivity to its complex anatomical divisions, both in the clinical evaluation and surgery. The middle thoracic compartment is generally divided into an upper and lower segment by an imaginary plane extending from the sternal angle to the intervertebral disc (IVD) between the fourth and fifth thoracic vertebrae. The inferior mediastinum is also subdivided into anterior, middle, and posterior regions, each with distinct structures that enable vital physiological functions. For instance, the middle mediastinum houses the heart in the pericardium, as well as major vessels such as the ascending aorta and pulmonary arteries. The posterior mediastinum, however, contains vital structures including the descending thoracic aorta, esophagus, thoracic duct, and sympathetic chains. This compartmentalized architecture enables clinicians to anatomically regionalize pathologies and adjust diagnostic imaging techniques more precisely, as seen in more advanced functional imaging modalities referenced in thyroid gland evaluation (Koep et al., 1980). Mediastinal outlines are defined by many anatomical borders that define its interrelationships with the encompassing thoracic and cervical structures. Anteriorly, it is bounded by the costal cartilages and sternum; posteriorly, the vertebral column; laterally, lungs and pleura; superiorly, the thoracic inlet; and inferiorly, the diaphragm. Within these boundaries, the mediastinum serves as a conduit for the principal neural, vascular, and lymphatic channels. The thoracic duct, the largest of the lymph vessels, travels unobstructed through the mediastinum to drain lymph into the venous circulation, an operation of critical immunological importance, and prolonged drainage of the thoracic duct has been investigated as an immunosuppressive complement to organ transplantation (Koep et al., 1980). Such complex interrelation of structures heralds the mediastinum's function not just as an anatomical block but also as a functional hub that integrates cardio-respiratory and immune system interactions. Understanding the complexity of the mediastinum also necessitates familiarity with its network of connective tissue and fascial planes that separate its contents and facilitate surgical resection. The mediastinal pleura invests its lateral walls and separates the contents of the mediastinum from the pleural spaces. Dense connective tissue and fat within the mediastinum provide supportive cushioning, whereas loose connective tissue allows for neurovascular bundles to travel through it. Important to mention is that mediastinal contents' arrangement determines the spread of infections, neoplasms, and fluid collections, which may spread through compartments or remain localized. While imaging modalities like scintigraphy provide functional information primarily in endocrine gland studies (Volckaert et al., 2016), cross-sectional imaging modalities like CT and MRI remain irreplaceable for careful visualization of mediastinal anatomy, pathology, and assessment of neural and vascular involvement in this essential thoracic compartment.

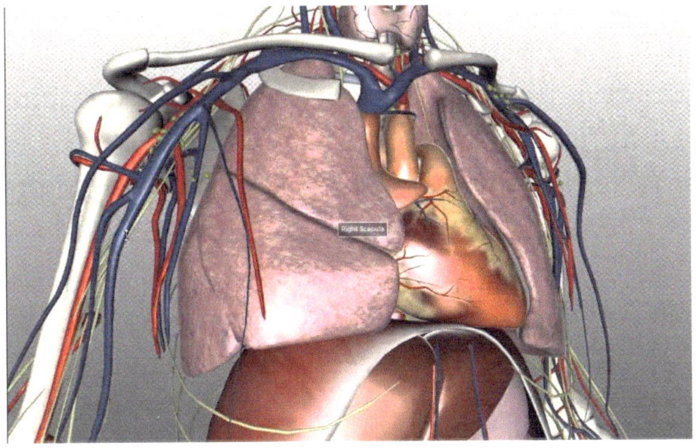

Source: YouTube. (n.d.). *Human Thoracic Anatomy Showing Lungs, Heart, and Major Vessels.*

8.1.1. Location Within the Thoracic Cavity

The thoracic cavity is a highly organized and complicated area with significant organs and structures, of which the mediastinum occupies a central position and occupies a special position. The mediastinum is situated between the two pleural cavities and extends from the sternum anteriorly to the vertebral column posteriorly and is bounded above by the thoracic inlet and below by the diaphragm. This middle compartment is also the conduit for important structures such as the heart, thymus, trachea, esophagus, and great vessels, which are all precisely located within its confines. The particular localization within the thoracic cavity enables the mediastinum to not only function as an anatomical divider but also as a protective barrier, regulating the supportive anatomy needed for cardiopulmonary and immune function. The topographical organization highlights its role in segregating the lungs bilaterally while simultaneously preserving the physiological interactions between its contained structures (Verba et al., 2023). The understanding of topography in the thoracic cavity introduces explicit divisions of the mediastinum, each with some anatomical relations and clinical relevance. The superior mediastinum is situated superior to the pericardium and includes large vascular structures such as the aortic arch and major veins draining into the heart, while the inferior mediastinum is further divided into anterior, middle, and posterior compartments based on their relative location to the pericardium. The space provides a framework for the localization and identification of the structures upon diagnostic or treatment procedures. Of particular note is the pericardium of the middle mediastinum that encapsulates the great vessels and the heart, anchoring them to their positions in the mediastinum. Experiments of the rat mediastinum attest to the pericardium being a distinct membranous structure free from adhesions and attached by ligaments, noting evolutionary conservation of structure within the mediastinum across species (Verba et al., 2023). The anatomical complexity of the thoracic mediastinum also applies to its functional coordination with nearby skeletal elements, like the thoracic sternum and vertebral column, which provide structural support as well as evolutionary specializations visible throughout species. In particular, thoracic sternum variations among various species influence the morphologies of surrounding soft tissues and their spatial relationships, defining the configuration of organs such as the heart and accompanying vascular pathways. The association of the thoracic sternums with other thoracic structures reveals profound homologies that define the position and protection of critical openings and conduits within the mediastinum. These evolutionary and developmental features augment the knowledge regarding the mediastinum's position in highlighting how the thoracic cavity's skeletal structure determines its spatial and functional dynamics, a factor highlighted in comparative anatomical research.

8.1.2. Divisions of the Mediastinum

The anatomical complexity of the thoracic cavity demands a structured approach to understanding its internal compartments. Central to this organization is the mediastinum, a compartment that extends from the sternum frontward to the vertebral column rearward, housing critical structures and organs. For purposes of clinical examination and diagnostic precision, the mediastinum has long been divided into distinct compartments. These divisions allow for more precise evaluation of pathological processes and assist in relating anatomical findings to physiology.

The older division divides the mediastinum into a superior and an inferior division, divided roughly at the sternal angle level. While this two-division grouping is useful, further subdivisions increase anatomical specificity and enable clinical communication among clinicians. There are finer subdivisions in the inferior mediastinum so that contents may be properly classified. It is subdivided into anterior, middle, and posterior mediastinum. There is predominantly connective tissue, lymph nodes, and fragments of the thymus gland, well developed in children, between the sternum and pericardium, in the anterior compartment. The middle mediastinum houses the heart in the pericardial sac, ascending aorta, pulmonary arteries and veins, and main bronchi, thus being critical in cardiovascular as well as respiratory functions. The Posteriormediastinum houses the descending thoracic aorta, esophagus, thoracic duct, and sympathetic chains, which are the structures responsible for autonomic control and digestion.

The three-way separation allows for a more accurate diagnosis of mediastinal masses and clinical interventions. The importance of identifying the mediastinal divisions extends beyond anatomy to functional and pathological conditions, affecting diagnostic imaging and surgical treatment. Radiologically, the division aids in the identification of abnormal masses or fluid collections by delineating their compartment of origin and potential etiologies. For instance, malignancies or cystic lesions are often categorized based on their mediastinal location, with prognostic and treatment implications. In addition, the incisions emphasize the anatomy of relationships crucial in procedures such as biopsies or thoracic surgery to prevent injury to the adjacent vital structures. Although not technically a component of mediastinal anatomy, cellular and structural parameter measurement in different tissues, such as the high-level histomorphometry of other biological studies, demonstrates the greater applicability of compartmental analysis to biological systems and can be utilized to report on organ function and disease (Abasi et al., 2013; Hovde, 2024) (Figure 8.2).

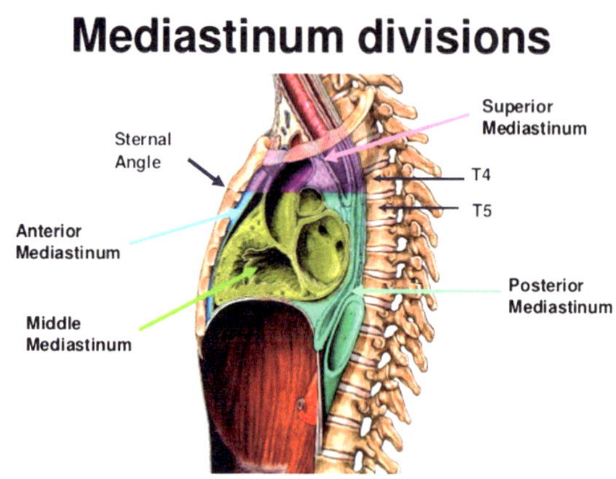

Figure 8.2. Divisions of the mediastinum.

Source: Homoeo Adda. (n.d.). *Mediastinum Divisions.*

8.1.3. Key Structures Contained Within

Contained within the middle of thoracic cavity is an area of involved anatomy known as the mediastinum, within which a number of central structures play vital roles in cardio-respiratory function. Traditionally, it has been considered superior and inferior, the latter being further subdivided into anterior, middle, and posterior regions, each possessing typical organs and tissue. Mediastinum encapsulates the heart in the pericardium, major arterial and venous tracts including the ascending aorta, pulmonary trunk, and superior vena cava, and trachea and esophagus.

The continuity of the structures has to be maintained for coordinated physiological interaction to ensure the sustenance of life. Thoracic duct courses and lymph nodes passing through this location provide space for immune surveillance as well as fluid homeostasis. Knowing these large mediastinal structures is significant, especially in the pathologic and clinical setting with trauma or pathologic conditions, where injury to one of the above structures would be capable of exerting significant effects on systemic homeostasis. Another extremely significant component of the mediastinum is also the autonomic plexus of nerves that controls thoracic and adjacent organs. Vagus nerve, recurrent laryngeal branches, and phrenic nerves course through this compartment and lead to parasympathetic control of heart rate, bronchial constriction, and movement of the diaphragm. The sympathetic chain is along the vertebral bodies and keeps fight or flight active through control of vascular tone and respiratory activity. These nerve tracts underscore the mediastinum's function of being not merely an organ container, but also a conduit for complex neurovascular communication essential to unified system function. Pathology of these nerves, via disease or injury, can lead to harmful effects such as paralysis of the vocal cords or dysfunction of the diaphragm, and this is why preservation of the nerves in the mediastinum is significant in both diagnostic or operative interventions. It contains significant endocrine and lymphatic organs that help in systemic homeostasis and protection from immune attack.

The thymus gland, which is located predominantly in the anterior mediastinum, is a significant organ during T-cell maturation in early life, reflecting the role of the mediastinum in immunologic development. In addition, the thoracic duct, the largest lymph vessel, ascends in the posterior mediastinum, taking up lymph from the majority of the body before emptying into the venous system. The presence of numerous lymph nodes along the path helps to illustrate the mediastinum's function in immune protection and screening. These mediastinal structures usually interface with the cardiovascular and respiratory mediastinal structures, and alterations such as lymphadenopathy or thymic hypertrophy are perhaps indicative of systemic disease processes. The presence of such diverse structures within the mediastinum underscores its critical role as a site of physiological regulation and defense (Landa-Garc et al., 2024; Younis et al., 2024).

Test Your Knowledge

1. Where is the mediastinum located within the thoracic cavity?
2. What are the main divisions of the mediastinum, and how are they anatomically separated?

8.2. Superior Mediastinum

Learning Outcome

1. Discuss the Major Blood Vessels Present
2. Focus on Thymus Gland and Its Function
3. Explain the Trachea and Esophagus Positioning

The region above the inlet of the thorax is significant because of its complex anatomical arrangement and the critical nature of structures that are housed in it. The superior mediastinum is a channel through which numerous neurovascular and respiratory components connect the neck and thorax. Within this compartment lie the origins of great arteries such as the aortic arch, which gives off the branches brachiocephalic trunk, left common carotid artery, and left subclavian artery. These arteries are loaded with the responsibility of providing oxygenated blood to the brain, head, neck and upper extremities, indicating the region's significance in systemic circulation. In addition, the superior mediastinum contains the thymus gland's upper portion, which is responsible for immune development during infancy. This area of anatomy is bounded in front by the manubrium and behind by the first thoracic vertebra, marking its position relative to the rest of the mediastinum and emphasizing its particular spatial arrangement (Hovde, 2024). From a functional point of view, the superior mediastinum houses several essential elements that provide respiratory and nervous system functions. The trachea traverses this location, passing from the larynx before branching into the main bronchi, thus serving as the main airway conduit. Parallel to this trachea travels the esophagus, passing posteriorly to direct ingested material to the stomach. Lying near them are the vagus and phrenic nerves, innervating thoracic and abdominal structures pivotal in autonomic control and diaphragmatic contraction, respectively. Notably, the thoracic duct, an important component of the lymphatic system, ascends through this area to drain into the venous circulation. The presence of these structures in the limited superior mediastinal space speaks well of their significance in aiding life-sustaining processes and organizing inter-system communication (Scott et al., 2013). From a clinical perspective, the superior mediastinum is noteworthy due to its susceptibility to a variety of pathological processes capable of having a profound impact on patient outcomes. Mediastinal masses such as thymomas or lymphomas can occur in this region and present symptoms by compressing overlying airways or vessels, leading to vascular congestion or respiratory compromise.

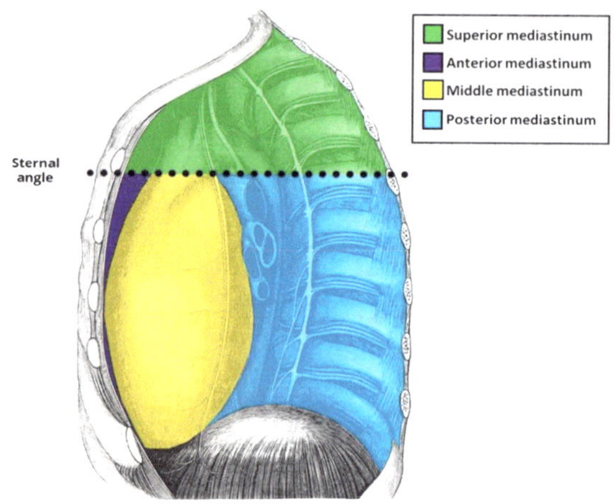

Figure 8.3. Superior mediastinum.

Source: TeachMeAnatomy. (n.d.). *The Superior Mediastinum and Sternal Angle.*

Understanding the precise anatomy of the superior mediastinum is beneficial in the surgical treatment and management of mediastinal tumors, vascular malformations, or traumatic injuries. Besides, transesophageal echocardiography as a diagnostic modality using anatomical landmarks within the mediastinum requires precise information regarding this space to evaluate cardiovascular function better during perioperative care (Scott et al., 2013;

Hovde, 2024). Thus, the anatomy and contents of the superior mediastinum are part and parcel of not only physiological normalcy but also of managing complex clinical situations (Figure 8.3).

8.2.1. Major Blood Vessels Present

The mediastinum is a central compartment of the thoracic cavity that houses key anatomical structures that are responsible for critical physiological activities. Of these, the great vessels stand out as significant conduits for systemic and pulmonary circulation. The thoracic aorta, arching across the superior mediastinum, divides into crucial arteries such as the brachiocephalic trunk, left common carotid, and left subclavian arteries, which distribute oxygenated blood to the head, neck, and upper limbs. The superior vena cava, formed by the union of the brachiocephalic veins, enables the venous drainage of the upper body into the right atrium. These vessels are situated in close relation to other mediastinal organs, necessitating a spatial relationship to provide both protection and accessibility. Their presence within the mediastinum is an evolutionary design significant to the preservation of efficient cardiovascular dynamics within the thorax (Dyl et al., 2009). By way of an examination of terminal branching and arterial course within adjacent anatomical structures, one comes to appreciate the complexity of vascular arrangements in intimate association with the mediastinum. For instance, the testicular artery's variable trajectory alongside the mediastinum testis exemplifies how major vessels adapt to their local environment to optimize functionality and supply. In humans, the artery's division into terminal branches occurs precisely at the level of the mediastinum testis, contrasting with bovine specimens where this division lies nearer to the gonad's inferior extremity. These comparisons emphasize the variability and specificity that the great blood vessels exhibit relative to their mediastinal and other surrounding structures. These observations also underscore the necessity of being cognizant of both species-specific and regional variations in vascular anatomy to understand clinical and surgical approaches at a fundamental level (Dyl et al., 2009). Besides the great arteries, the mediastinum contains significant venous conduits that are inherent to circulatory homeostasis. The azygos vein system, located on the right side of the vertebral column, drains deoxygenated blood from the thoracic wall into the superior vena cava, providing important collateral circulation in case of venous obstruction. The pulmonary arteries and veins also travel through the middle mediastinum, linking the heart and the lungs and enabling gas exchange for respiration. The intimate relationship of these vessels with the surrounding mediastinal structures, including nerves and lymph nodes, serves to highlight the mediastinum's role as something more than a mere passageway. Rather, it is a dynamic complex whereby large blood vessels not only transport blood but also come into contact with important biological systems, a complexity reflected in detailed anatomy textbooks and medical school textbooks (Korenkov et al., 2018).

8.2.2. Thymus Gland and Its Function

The complex anatomical position of the thymus gland within the mediastinum calls to attention its extremely critical role within the body's immune system. Positioned in the anterior mediastinum, the thymus is fixed to surrounding structures, especially by the sternopericardial ligament (SPL), creating a fibrous connection between the gland and pericardium. This unique attachment not only stabilizes the thymus but also isolates it from adjacent tissues since the SPL is a thickened component posterior to the thymus that tugs on the pericardium (Nakanishi & Goto, 2023). Such precise anatomical connections mean that the thymus is not a passive organ but one embedded structurally and functionally within the thoracic cavity. The location of the gland near large vessels and the heart in the anterior mediastinum highlights its significance beyond anatomy, indicating a role in systemic physiological processes that need protection and support. Beneath its anatomical complexity is the thymus gland's significant role in immune development, particularly in the maturation of T lymphocytes. Histologically, the thymus is characterized by a lobulated structure enveloped by a connective tissue capsule, with a distinct cortical and medullary region (Iman et al., 2018). The cortex is filled with immature T cells that are proliferating and undergoing positive selection, whereas the medulla contains a more mature population of T cells along with epithelial elements called Hassall's corpuscles. These microscopical features bring forth the thymus as a preeminent place for T cell education and calibration, which are pivotal in immune response as well as self-tolerance. Therefore, the thymus is more than an anatomical organ within the mediastinum but a pivotal organ responsible for producing the immune repertoire as well as immune homeostasis. The thymus position and function in the mediastinum are thus inextricably linked, highlighting its dual importance in immunology and anatomy. The gland location within the anterior mediastinum places it at the juncture of major cardiovascular and respiratory organs, and its firm anchorage, sustained by the SPL, ensures positional fixation (Nakanishi & Goto, 2023). Functionally, this allows the thymus to properly manage immune cell maturation during early life, after which its size typically declines but its immunologic imprint endures (Nakanishi & Goto, 2023). Understanding the thymus in the context of the mediastinum sheds still more light on the way structural anatomy supports dynamic physiologic functions. This coincidence of structure and function has certain implications for surgical approach, radiologic interpretation, and diagnosis of mediastinal illness including the thymus (Figure 8.4).

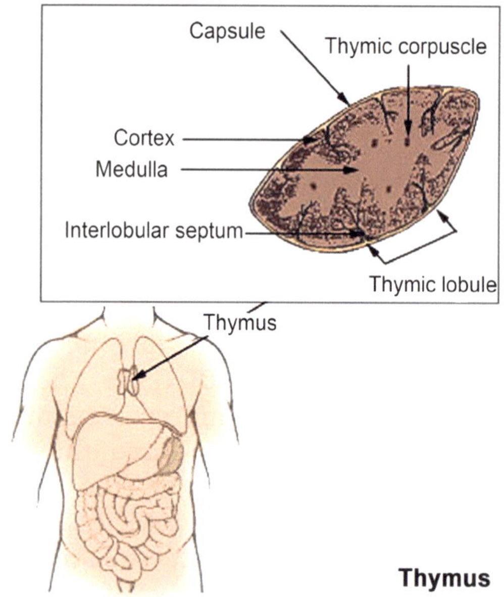

Figure 8.4. Thymus gland and its function.

Source: Public Domain, https://commons.wikimedia.org/w/index.php?curid=1394154

8.2.3. Trachea and Esophagus Positioning

The three-dimensional arrangement of thoracic elements profoundly influences their physiological interactions and their clinical significance. In the mediastinum, the trachea and the esophagus have a unique positional relationship favorable to their respective physiological activities of respiration and digestion. The cartilaginous tube called the trachea is placed anteriorly to the esophagus and extends from the larynx to the carina. This anterior positioning of the trachea allows for a clear airway, and the posteriorly positioned esophagus allows for the passage of food into the stomach without compromising respiratory function. Their side-by-side positioning in the superior and posterior mediastinum demands anatomical alignment to the very minimum to prevent compression, which can lead to such complications as dysphagia or airway compromise. Understanding of this complex anatomy serves as the foundation for mediastinal pathologies' imaging diagnostics and helps in interventions with these life-support conduits (Wietholt et al., 2008). Tracheal and esophageal mediastinal relationship takes on particular importance if one is considering pathological changes or surgery. For instance, any enlargement of mediastinal lymph nodes, tumors, or vascular malformations can interfere with the usual position of such structures, and by doing so, can compress the trachea or create fistulae. Cross-sectional imaging with computed tomography (CT) and magnetic resonance imaging (MRI) explains the spatial relationships by showing precise cross-sectional images that highlight the relative anterior course of the trachea and the posterior course of the esophagus. These imaging modalities play a crucial role in preoperative planning and surveillance of diseases that provoke angiogenic remodeling of mediastinal vessels, which indirectly may influence these structures by altering the surrounding vascular anatomy (Wietholt et al., 2008; Hovde, 2024). Beyond anatomical considerations, functional interaction between the trachea and esophagus is governed by their position within the mediastinum. The pliability of the esophagus allows it to widen during swallowing without compromising airway patency by the rigid trachea. But their normal variations in position can derange these functions. For example, mediastinal masses or inflammatory conditions can result in pressure from the front or back and compromise normal air or food passage. Enhanced imaging modalities have allowed precise evaluation of such anomalies, and early diagnosis with focused therapy is a reality. As the mediastinum contains significant structures such as the trachea and esophagus, thorough familiarity with their positions is critical for best treatment of thoracic diseases and interventions (Wietholt et al., 2008; Hovde, 2024).

Test Your Knowledge

1. What do you understand Thymus Gland and Its Function?
2. Focus on Trachea and Esophagus Positioning

8.3. Anterior Mediastinum

Learning Outcome

1. Discuss the Contents and Significance
2. Explain the Pathologies Associated with this Region
3. Focus on Surgical Considerations

The mediastinum, a mid-thoracic space, is segmented into various portions, with each of them housing important anatomical structures. One such compartment is the anterior mediastinum, located between sternum and pericardium. There are loose connective tissue, fat, lymphatic vessels, and importantly thymus gland in young individuals. Because the thymus atrophies with increasing age, it is usually replaced by fat, and therefore the anterior mediastinum remains a part of variable content throughout life. Anterior mediastinum also has internal mammary vessels and segments of the drainage system of lymphatics, which contribute to its clinical complexity. Pathologically, the anterior mediastinum is a location for typical masses such as thymomas, teratomas, lymphomas, and germ cell tumors, whose exact demarcation from neighboring structures must be done during diagnosis. Understanding its anatomy is crucial considering the range of surgical and diagnostic procedures performed in this area (Hovde, 2024). The clinical significance of the anterior mediastinum extends to perioperative and diagnostic realms, where imaging and minimally invasive techniques play pivotal roles. Contemporary intraoperative monitoring, e.g., utilitarian transesophageal echocardiography, though focused on cardiac anatomy, indirectly serves assessment of mediastinal masses and their effects on cardiovascular dynamics (Scott et al., 2013). Since the anterior mediastinum has a direct relation with the heart and great vessels, any disease in this region may produce compressive effects resulting in hemodynamic instability. Hence, proper knowledge regarding the mediastinal anatomy and contents, particularly of the anterior compartment, can enhance the efficacy of echocardiographic evaluation and surgeries. The clinician must be able to correlate imaging techniques with anatomical data to identify and treat potential complications of anterior mediastinal disease.

The anterior mediastinum is also a significant location of immunologic maturation and lymphatic drainage, especially early in life. Even as the thymus gland involutes gradually, it continues to play a crucial role in T-cell maturation, illustrating the anterior mediastinum's function beyond that of structural support. Abnormalities in this region, including congenital cysts or neoplastic masses, can impair both mechanical and immunological function. The anatomical complexity in this region necessitates an interdisciplinary appreciation involving anatomy, radiology, and pathology to optimize patient outcome. Surgical access to the anterior mediastinum, which is often complicated by the limited space and the position of vital structures, demands accuracy and experience and therefore highlights the need for in-depth knowledge of its anatomy as well as common clinical presentations (Scott et al., 2013; Hovde, 2024) (Figure 8.5).

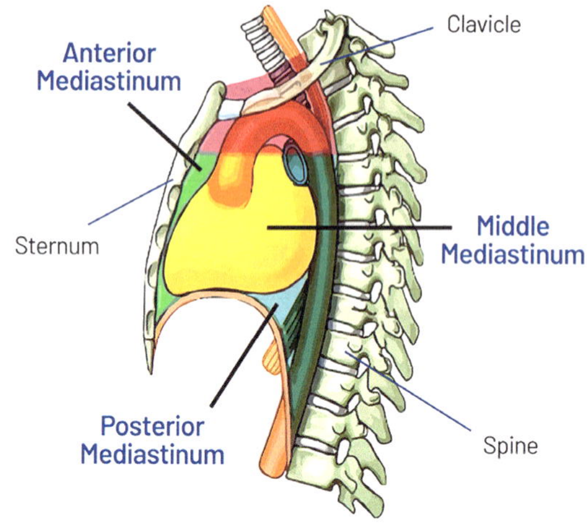

Figure 8.5. Anterior mediastinum.

Source: Saint John's Cancer Institute. (2023). *Mediastinum: Anterior, Middle, and Posterior.*

8.3.1. Contents and Significance

To understand the mediastinum, one needs to have a careful examination of the diversity of contents it holds, which consist of vital anatomical structures necessary for different physiological functions. The mediastinum, between the two pleural sacs, holds the heart, major vascular structures such as the aorta and superior vena cava, the trachea, esophagus, thymus gland, lymph nodes, and other nerves such as the phrenic and vagus nerves. These are all essential structures, the trachea facilitating airway and the heart systemic and pulmonary circulation, and they are situated such that the proximity of these structures not only signposts their respective anatomical sites but also hints at the role of the mediastinum as a consolidating area through which various systems converge, interface, and achieve homeostatic regulation. Thus, the complex mediastinal contents represent a central location of vital physiological activities, proving its irreplaceable role within the thoracic cavity. Apart from its anatomical composition, the mediastinal contents have deeper pathophysiological implications because any disarrangement risks involving several important systems simultaneously. For instance, trauma or pathologic processes such as tumors within this compartment may affect cardiac performance, respiratory effectiveness, and neurovascular integrity due to the closely packed nature of its contents. Such interdependency is highlighted in clinical conditions when mediastinal trauma causes cascading disturbances of function, which necessitates adequate knowledge of mechanical interactions among such organs. Instruments such as TRAUMAP, simulating the anatomical and physiological impacts in three dimensions, illustrate how trauma to one of the mediastinal structures indirectly impacts adjacent systems, proving the multi-systemic functional role played by the mediastinum in illness and health (Kaye, 1995). Thus, its contents do not operate in isolation but as an integrated system, necessary for sustaining life. Furthermore, the functional significance of mediastinum involves not just spatially housing organs but also supporting physiological processes. The multilayered cytological and epithelial nature found in some mediastinal regions, such as those found in the reproductive ducts depicted by similar excretory organs, suggest absorptive and secretory functions. These histological variations are an expression of specialized functions to cope with specific physiological demands, enhancing the mediastinum's dynamic role in the homeostasis of the body (Kumar et al., 1979). For example, lymphatic drainage and immune responses heavily rely on the thymus and lymph nodes of the mediastinum. Thus, the mediastinal contents are not just passive anatomical inhabitants but are themselves actively engaged in maintaining systemic health by multiple mechanisms, reinforcing its status as a multifunctional and vital anatomical compartment.

8.3.2. Pathologies Associated with this Region

The complexity of the mediastinum as a central thoracic anatomical compartment predisposes it to a variety of pathological processes that can impose significant impacts on adjacent vital structures. Among these pathologies, the mediastinal masses stand out for their diagnostic challenge and a broad spectrum of etiologies, ranging from benign cysts to malignant tumors. These masses can develop from lymphatic, thymic, neural, or germ cell tissues and typically present with nonspecific symptoms such as chest pain, cough, or dyspnea due to compression of adjacent organs. Radiologic imaging plays a significant role in identifying the nature and precise location of these masses. Advances in imaging datasets, particularly chest X-rays with careful labeling and systematized terminologies, have allowed for improved identification and differential diagnosis of mediastinal abnormalities, promoting more effective clinical management of these difficult presentations (Bustos et al., 2019). In autoimmune disorders, myasthenia gravis demonstrates the intimate relationship of the mediastinum with systemic disease through the involvement of the thymus gland. The procedure of extended thymectomy aims not only at the removal of the thymus but also at the removal of any ectopic thymic tissue dispersed in the mediastinal fat. This ectopic tissue, present in more than half of MG patients undergoing surgery, can have a role in disease recurrence or persistence. These areas include the anterior mediastinal fat, pericardiophrenic angles, and aortopulmonary window, among others. The presence of this ectopic tissue is linked to poorer clinical prognosis after thymectomy, highlighting the need for wider surgical approaches beyond central thymic resection to improve prognosis (Li et al., 2019). Neoplastic and inflammatory processes also make the spectrum of mediastinal pathologies complex. Lymphomas and thymomas are the two prominent malignant neoplasms arising in the mediastinum, not uncommonly in the anterior compartment. They can cause local bulk effects and systemic symptoms such as night sweats, weight loss, and fever, which are due to their aggressive nature. Inflammatory processes such as mediastinitis and sarcoidosis cause diagnostic difficulty because of overlapping radiographic manifestations with neoplastic processes. Mediastinal lymph nodes frequently reflect metastatic diseases, emphasizing the mediastinum as a pathway for malignancies that occur in the lung and other thoracic structures. As such, the complex anatomy and diverse pathology of the mediastinum necessitate meticulous diagnostic assessment and multidisciplinary treatment strategies to optimize patient outcomes.

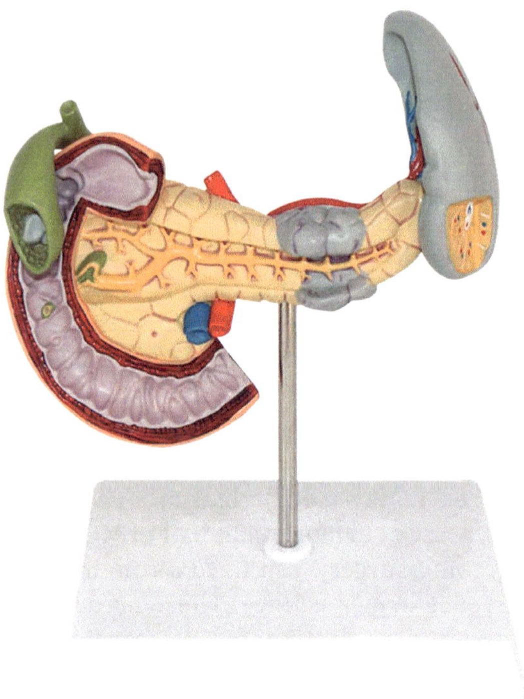

Source: IndiaMART. (2024, February). *Caput Succedaneum Nursing Chart Model.*

8.3.3. Surgical Considerations

Surgical intervention within the mediastinum requires meticulous preoperative planning due to the complex anatomy and vital structures contained within this area. The proximity of the heart, great vessels, trachea, esophagus, and lymph channels requires careful consideration to prevent intraoperative risk as well as postoperative morbidity. Perioperative management has undergone significant strides that have served to encourage more optimal results in cardiac and mediastinal operations. These developments cross anesthetic techniques, hemodynamic monitoring, and postoperative care to allow patients to have better recovery trajectories. Moreover, advanced surgery technologies, including high-level imaging machines and improved surgical instruments, offer greater precision and less invasiveness, an aspect that is incredibly significant in handling mediastinal tumors or vascular malformations (Hovde, 2024). Together, these considerations highlight the importance of a multidisciplinary paradigm that unites surgical expertise with perioperative technologies in the pursuit of optimizing patient safety and procedural efficiency in mediastinal surgery. Minimal invasive techniques have been a commanding development in mediastinal surgery, matched by experience from gastro-esophageal and other thoracic operations. Employment of laparoscopic and thoracoscopic surgery results in lesser operative trauma, negligible blood loss, and more rapid postoperative recovery, factors paramount to consideration because the mediastinum's short and vulnerable anatomic compartment constrains freedom. As much evidence for these methods remains a continuum, initial experience suggests minimally invasive techniques to deliver oncologic and functional security at the cost of not affecting patient quality of life (QoL) over the traditionally applied open methodologies. However, skill acquisition and the learning curve for surgery are significant challenges that have been proven to need the attainment of proficiency often with the undertaking of numerous procedures to attain operative uniformity and decrease complications. These factors highlight the importance of good surgical training programs and ongoing monitoring of outcomes in institutions performing mediastinal minimally invasive surgery (Gemmill, 2025). Apart from surgical technique and method, patient-specific factors play an immense role in mediastinal surgical planning. The presence of comorbidities, history of thoracic surgery, mediastinal pathology location, and type determine the selection of technique. The optimization of complete resection, particularly in malignancy, and preservation of critical structures is a paramount consideration. For example, superior vena cava or pulmonary artery involvement may necessitate major reconstruction or special preoperative techniques. Furthermore, intraoperative choice-making is facilitated by imaging and intraoperative monitoring improvements that enable real-time assessment of vascular integrity and tissue involvement. These considerations along with developments in perioperative care algorithms minimize mortality and morbidity post-surgery, highlighting that successful mediastinal surgery is an interactive union of technological support, surgical dexterity, and personalized patient assessment (Hovde, 2024; Gemmill, 2025).

Test Your Knowledge

1. What symptoms might suggest a mediastinal pathology compressing nearby structures?
2. Why is knowledge of mediastinal anatomy critical during thoracic surgeries?

8.4. Middle Mediastinum

Learning Outcome

1. Discuss the Heart and Pericardium Overview
2. Explain the Major Bronchi and Pulmonary Vessels
3. Focus on Lymphatic Structures and Nodes

It is a sophisticated understanding of the thoracic compartment that necessitates a thorough investigation of the middle mediastinum, a middle division within the mediastinal cavity filled with vital cardiovascular structures. It is bounded anteriorly by the anterior mediastinum and posteriorly by the posterior mediastinum and represents a crucial region via which the heart and major vessels traverse. The midline spatial organization permits protective but not static accommodation of the heart, pericardium, ascending aorta, pulmonary trunk, and superior vena cava. Recent anatomical studies employing high-technology imaging modalities and digital reconstructions have significantly enhanced knowledge of the complex three-dimensional organization of this area. These models have explained the precise relations and geometric forms of these vital organs, enabling improved surgical planning and diagnostic accuracy in thoracic medicine (Dyl et al., 2009). Therefore, the middle mediastinum not only serves as a conduit for cardiovascular structures but is also an important region that influences worldwide thoracic physiology. The middle mediastinum contains the vascular structures that exhibit significant anatomical variations demanding careful attention in clinical interventions. The superior vena cava, ascending aorta, and pulmonary arteries are the major vascular structures housed here, all of which are covered by the fibrous pericardium. Notably, the pericardium offers a morphologic border that assists in positioning the heart and provides a low-friction environment for its continuous rhythmic movement. Detailed anatomical investigations demonstrate that the contact between the vascular structures of the mediastinum and adjacent connective tissue plays a critical role in maintaining hemodynamic stability. Furthermore, the anatomical variability of the adjacent structures, including variations in the course and ramification of arteries supplying the mediastinum, emphasizes the importance of individualized assessment in surgical and diagnostic procedures (Dyl et al., 2009). These findings highlight the clinical and anatomical intricacy of middle mediastinum vascular anatomy in cardiothoracic surgery. Beyond its cardiovascular content, the middle mediastinum has significant neural and lymphatic components whose complex functional importance contributes to the region's overall significance.

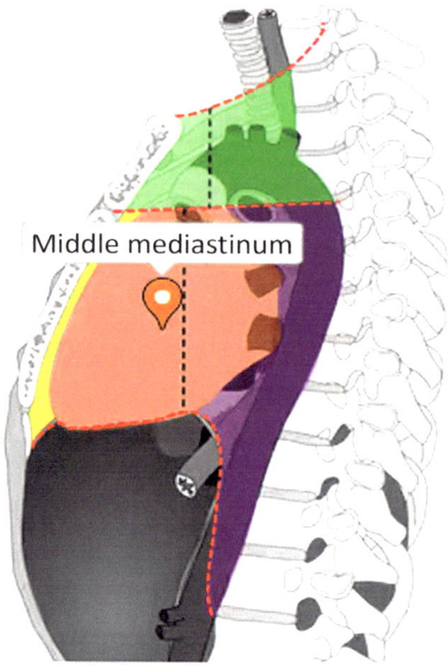

Figure 8.6. Middle mediastinum.

Source: IMAIOS. (n.d.). *Middle Mediastinum.*

The phrenic nerves, which provide motor innervation of the diaphragm, are laterally positioned within this compartment, and vagus nerves contribute to parasympathetic innervation of the heart and lungs. In addition, the middle mediastinum holds lymphatic structures such as the tracheobronchial lymph nodes, which are responsible for immune protection and are of particular interest in oncological investigations. The accurate segmentation and three-dimensional visualization of these neural and lymphatic structures within the middle mediastinum, as made possible by cutting-edge imaging software, have made a considerable impact on anatomical education and clinical practice (Xie et al., 2013). Recognition of the presence and course of these vital non-vascular structures is crucial to avoiding iatrogenic trauma with mediastinal interventions, emphasizing the vast anatomical complexity typical of the middle mediastinum (Figure 8.6).

8.4.1. Heart and Pericardium Overview

The complex relationship of the heart with adjacent structures is central to the preservation of cardiovascular function in the mediastinum. The heart's position is stabilized by the pericardium, a fibrous sac that encloses the organ and offers a protective and supportive sleeve. The enclosure not only restricts excessive cardiac distension but also facilitates unencumbered cardiac motion by reducing friction between the heart and the adjacent mediastinal tissues. The pericardium consists of two layers: the outer fibrous pericardium and the inner serous pericardium, which is further divided into parietal and visceral layers. The double layers mechanically support while encompassing lubricating fluid for promoting optimal cardiac function. Such information is initial when considering pathophysiological conditions such as aneurysms or pericardial diseases that can undermine the delicate balance within the mediastinal space and the mechanical function of the heart. Significant insights into the mechanical environment of the heart and aorta have been obtained through biomechanical modeling, such as the contribution of the pericardium to vascular support and stress distribution. For example, geometrical modeling of the ascending aorta with and without the support of simulated surrounding tissue has demonstrated that the pericardium confers essential stiffness to the vessel, but exclusive dependence on this structure as support may lead to overestimation of its real biomechanical contribution. Finite element analysis demonstrated that the pericardium restrains aortic enlargement, moderating diametric changes, an aspect having relevance in understanding pathologic conditions like aneurysm development. Those aneurysms that are characterized by dilatation and deterioration of the wall alter tissue qualities like the dispersion of collagen fibers that significantly determine the local stress distribution and predispose the vessel to rupture. Hence, cardiac and pericardial structures intertwine within the mediastinum underpins vital biomechanical function as well as disease processes (Hovde, 2024). Clinical outcomes further place emphasis on the integral part played by the integrity of both the pericardium and heart in the regulation of life-threatening complications. For example, left ventricular pseudoaneurysm is a serious complication typically secondary to myocardial infarction in which the heart wall rupture is confined only by the adherent visceral or parietal pericardium. This containment is a two-edged sword: it will prevent abrupt cardiac tamponade but has a high tendency to rupture with a fatal result. Diagnosis remains challenging due to the stealthy presentation of the pseudoaneurysm, but the advancement of non-invasive imaging modalities has improved detection. Early surgical intervention remains the treatment of choice to prevent death, emphasizing the pericardium's two roles as protector and also a potential cause of pathology within the mediastinal compartment. Understanding the structural and functional dynamics of the heart and pericardium, therefore, is at the center of the management of mediastinal cardiovascular disease (Aminorroaya et al., 2021).

8.4.2. Major Bronchi and Pulmonary Vessels

The thoracic cavity is complex and is defined by the positioning of life-giving structures, the most significant of which are the primary bronchi and pulmonary circulation which are found centrally in the mediastinum. Emerging from the trachea at the level of sternal angle, the right main bronchus and left main bronchus are the two primary air passages that transport inhaled air to each lung. These dichotomously branching bronchi are closely invested by pulmonary veins and arteries that facilitate bidirectional blood transportation towards and away from the lungs. Their positioning along with vessels is critical since this facilitates maximum respiratory gas exchange in the confined mediastinal space. Clinical interventions and thoracic pathology diagnosis need an understanding of the precise anatomical positioning of these structures (Bumeister et al., 2016). This fact makes them important in maintaining respiratory and circulatory system relationships within the mediastinum. The pulmonary arteries coexist with the bronchi, running through the lung roots with deoxygenated blood from the right ventricle to the lungs. Such vessels are specifically adapted to accommodate changes in blood pressure and flow at the interface of systemic and pulmonary circulations. Tracing with the pulmonary arteries are the pulmonary veins, which return oxygenated blood to the left atrium. Their arrangement in relation to the bronchi is asymmetrical; therefore, the right pulmonary artery lies in front of the right main bronchus, whereas the left pulmonary artery crosses over the left main bronchus. This organization of anatomy in the mediastinum is a well-designed architecture facilitating proper function and is a milestone in thoracic surgery and imaging (Korenkov et al., 2018). The pulmonary vessels and great bronchi encircle crucial vascular and airway pathways and form an intrinsic network that decides the mediastinal root. Their close proximity to each other poses both anatomical challenges and clinical significances, especially in diseases like bronchogenic carcinomas or vascular malformations that can encroach upon these structures. Surgical exposure to the mediastinum requires detailed knowledge of the passage of the bronchi along the pulmonary arteries and veins to prevent injury. Moreover, the lymphatic drainage around these bronchi and vessels within the mediastinum involves them in immune defense and pathological dissemination. Comprehensive anatomical studies, complemented by didactic materials, underlie the way in which such structures find common purpose as a functional unit within the mediastinum (Bumeister et al., 2016; Korenkov et al., 2018). This interconnected interrelationship provides the basis for both normal physiology and disease processes that act upon the thoracic cavity (Figure 8.7).

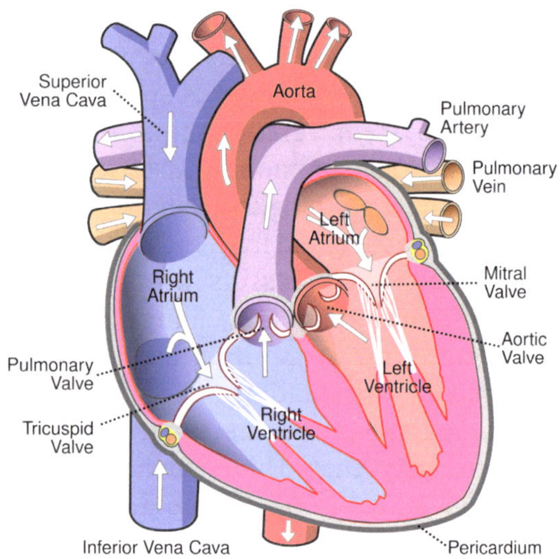

Figure 8.7. Major bronchi and pulmonary vessels.

Source: By Wapcaplet - Own work, CC BY-SA 3.0, https://commons.wikimedia.org/w/index.php?curid=830253

8.4.3. Lymphatic Structures and Nodes

The complex mediastinal lymphatic network is absolutely vital for immune monitoring and fluid balance. Lymph nodes, placed strategically along the course of lymphatic vessels, serve as dynamic sieves where antigens and immune cells converge to initiate immune responses. Their specialized microanatomy segregates immune cells such as B lymphocytes in the follicles and T lymphocytes in the paracortex to foster discrete interactions that are imperative for pathogen recognition and clearance. Moreover, mast cells, although less in number, invade several nodal compartments, governing immune cell migration and supporting mechanisms such as lymphangiogenesis through the secretion of molecules such as VEGF-C and VEGF-D. These interactions between mediastinal lymph nodes emphasize a dense immunological environment that not only screens lymphatic fluid but co-ordinates systemic immune response tailored to the thoracic region's unique exposure to respiratory and cardiovascular antigens (Elieh-Ali-Komi et al., 2025). Operatively, lymph vessels and nodes of the mediastinum form an integrated system responsible for interstitial fluid drainage, removal of cellular debris, and trafficking of immune cells. Placing such nodes in key pathways will enable effective capture of antigens from the lung, heart, and esophagus and ready immune activation. The specialized structure of lymph nodes creates a scaffold where antigen-presenting cells, such as dendritic cells, can present processed antigens to naive lymphocytes to bridge between innate and adaptive immunity. This efficiency of this system is also boosted by the active role of lymphatic endothelium to regulate the entry and exit of immune cells, hence ensuring homeostasis under normal conditions. Disruptions or pathological alterations of mediastinal lymphatic structures may trigger major immune dysfunctions, affecting responses against infections, malignancies, and inflammatory diseases that involve thoracic organs (Elieh-Ali-Komi et al., 2025). Knowledge of the anatomical and functional subtleties of mediastinal lymphatic structures takes on added importance in the light of clinical uses including cancer staging, surgical procedures, and immunotherapy. The mediastinal lymph nodes, routinely assessed in malignancies such as lung or esophageal carcinoma, are pivotal in understanding disease spread and metastasis. Anatomical differences in lymphatics, depending upon physiological measures and body habitus, can change lymph node drainage and distribution, making surgical precision and radiologic assessment more difficult. Additionally, the adaptive immune response housed within these nodes can be modulated by external agents, such as therapeutic drugs directed against mast cells and other immune mediators. Appropriate interpretation of these lymphatic tissues is therefore essential to optimize diagnostic accuracy and therapeutic modalities for mediastinal disease.

Test Your Knowledge

1. What is the difference in structure and orientation between the right and left main bronchi?
2. Which major lymph nodes are associated with the lungs and hilum?

8.5. Posterior Mediastinum

Learning Outcome

1. Discuss the Aorta and Its Branches
2. Explain the Thoracic Duct and its Role
3. Focus on Nerves and their Functions

Deep within the thoracic cavity lies the posterior mediastinum, an area situated behind the pericardium and in front of the vertebral column. The compartment is an anatomically complex region with essential structures such as the descending thoracic aorta, esophagus, thoracic duct, and other significant autonomic nerve fibers including the vagus and sympathetic trunks. The complex structure of these organs necessitates a thorough understanding, particularly in clinical cases where pathological processes such as tumors, infections, or vascular anomalies may arise. Because of the restricted spatial environment of the posterior mediastinum, any mass effect or enlargement can readily influence respiratory and cardiovascular function, requiring precise diagnostic imaging and thorough anatomical knowledge in the treatment of posterior mediastinal conditions (Hovde, 2024). The descending thoracic aorta, the continuation of arch of aorta, in the posterior mediastinum is the major pathway for oxygenated blood circulation from the heart to the lower regions of the body, coursing in association with significant autonomic nerve plexuses that regulate thoracic and abdominal viscera. The esophagus, also located within this compartment, is an essential component of the digestive system by transporting ingested material from the pharynx into the stomach. This close relationship of anatomy highlights the clinical significance of the posterior mediastinum when investigating symptoms of dysphagia or unexplained chest pain. Furthermore, lymphatic structures such as the thoracic duct traverse this area to ensure transport of lymph and immune function, thus making the posterior mediastinum a zone of interest for both vascular and immunologic disease (Scott et al., 2013). Surgical interventions in the posterior mediastinum require meticulous perioperative assessment, in most instances using advanced imaging methods and intraoperative surveillance through transesophageal echocardiography to evaluate adjacent cardiovascular structures. The intimate arrangement of structures within the constricted space renders it difficult to manage conditions such as aneurysms of the descending aorta, esophageal malignancies, and neural tumors. Clinicians are invited to adopt a multidisciplinary approach, covering thoracic surgery, radiology, and anesthesiology expertise to achieve optimal patient results. The dynamic function of imaging and monitoring technologies allows for detection of disease processes and guidance of treatment plans within posterior mediastinum, highlighting the synergy of anatomical complexity with clinical precision (Scott et al., 2013; Hovde, 2024) (Figure 8.8).

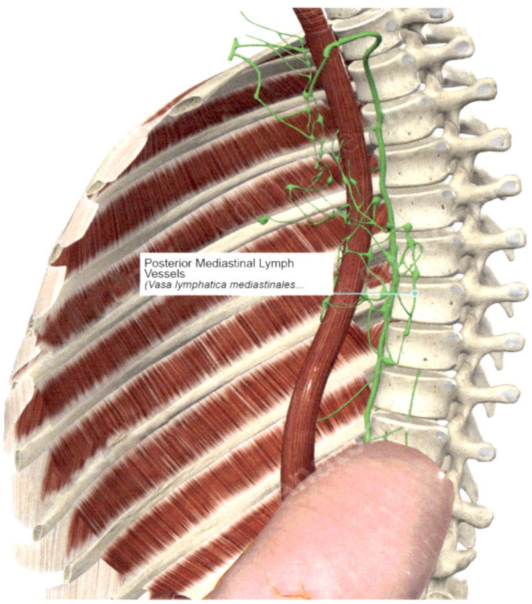

Figure 8.8. Posterior mediastinum.

Source: 3D4Medical. (n.d.). *Posterior Mediastinal Lymph Vessels (Vasa Lymphatica Mediastinales).*

8.5.1. Aorta and Its Branches

Within the complex thoracic cavity, the aorta represents a principal vessel for oxygenated blood, coursing through the mediastinum in a tortuous course and branching to provide vital supplies to the different thoracic and systemic structures. Originating from the left ventricle of the heart, the ascending aorta ascends momentarily to form the aortic arch, which curves posteriorly and to the left. It gives rise to three major branches, the brachiocephalic trunk, the left common carotid artery, and the left subclavian artery. These vessels are significant in their role to supply the head, neck, and upper limbs with blood, and also to further facilitate the mediastinum's role as a central location for vital circulatory tracts. Three-dimensional reconstructions and high-resolution imaging of these thoracic structures, including the aorta and its branches, have facilitated enhanced anatomical understanding and surgery (Xie et al., 2013). As the aorta extends from the aortic arch, it forms the descending thoracic aorta in the posterior mediastinum, where it provides blood supply to the thoracic wall and viscera such as the esophagus and lungs. Along its path, various smaller yet important branches originate, such as the intercostal arteries, bronchial arteries, and esophageal arteries. These branches infiltrate the surrounding tissues to ensure their vascularization and functional integrity, highlighting the aorta's function beyond the simple transport of blood. Current imaging modalities, such as multidetector computed tomography (CT), provide exquisite visualization of these vessels and their spatial relationship, an aspect that is vital in the diagnosis of vascular disease and preoperative planning of complex thoracic interventions (Bertolini & Angeloni, 2017). The aortic branches thus emphasize the mediastinum as a key crossroads for cardiovascular and systemic health. Understanding the anatomical intricacies of the aorta and its mediastinal branches is necessary for clinical practice, particularly in cardiovascular surgery and diagnostic radiology. The intimate relationship of the thoracic aorta with many critical structures, including the esophagus, trachea, and thoracic duct, necessitates thorough study to avoid complications in medical procedures. Contemporary three-dimensional imaging and modeling techniques have transformed this knowledge by allowing for accurate definition of the aortic wall, origins of branches, and surrounding tissues (Xie et al., 2013). In addition, the constant evolution of CT technology keeps improving the visualization of vascular abnormalities and pathologies of the aorta and its branches to facilitate quick and correct diagnoses (Bertolini & Angeloni, 2017). This evolving data solidifies the mediastinum's role not only as an anatomical compartment but also as a centerpiece in cardiovascular medicine (Figure 8.9).

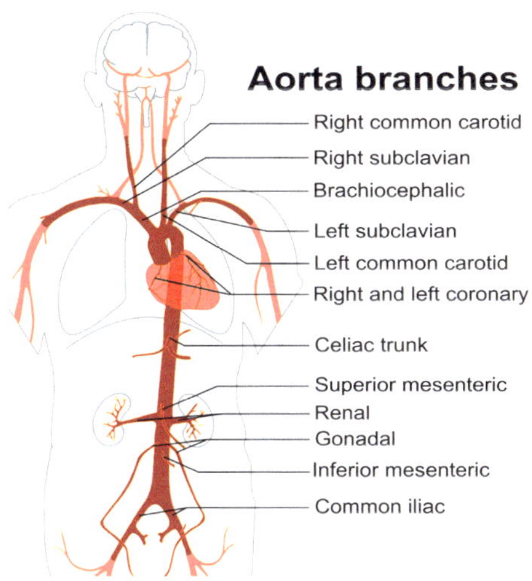

Figure 8.9. Aorta and its branches.

Source: Wikimedia Commons. (n.d.). *Aorta Branches*.

8.5.2. Thoracic Duct and its Role

In the mediastinum, the thoracic duct is a significant vessel in the lymphatic return pathway that brings back lymph and chyle from the abdomen, lower limb, and thoracic space to the venous blood. Its anatomical position alongside the aorta and esophagus makes it clinically significant, particularly with its long course from the cisterna chyli in the posterior mediastinum to the intersection of the left subclavian and internal jugular veins. The duct's role in establishing fluid balance and immune surveillance in the thoracic space goes far in accounting for why disruption of its structure, either from trauma or surgery, might result in severe complications such as chylothorax or lymphedema. Its complex anatomical relationships thus demand full understanding on the part of practitioners, especially in thoracic surgery and critical care medicine. This information is crucial for mediastinal and lymphatic drainage apparatus interventions (Koep et al., 1980). Beyond its anatomical position, the thoracic duct plays a priceless physiological function by draining fat-laden, protein-laden, and immune cell-filled lymph that is collected from most of the body. This lymphatic return facilitates interstitial fluid clearance, dietary lipid uptake, and transport of antigen-presenting cells, thus linking immune system function to circulatory function. Clinically, prolonged thoracic duct drainage has been studied as an immunosuppressive adjunct to organ transplantation, highlighting its role in systemic immunity and fluid homeostasis. The success of this procedure in 96 % of the reported cases helps to elucidate the function of the thoracic duct not just as a passive conduit but as an active mediator in immune regulation with important implications for management and care postoperatively and for treating immune-related disease in the mediastinum (Koep et al., 1980). Pathologically, the role of the thoracic duct in mediastinal disease processes goes further to illustrate its critical importance. Trauma or neoplasms on the duct may compromise lymph flow, leading to conditions such as chylothorax, where there is an accumulation of lymph within the pleural space leading to respiratory failure. Its closeness to large vascular and neural tissues within the mediastinum also exposes it to risk during tumor resections within the mediastinum or thoracic procedures, for which careful surgical planning is necessary to prevent accidental damage. Understanding the delicate topography and functional importance of the thoracic duct contributes to diagnostic accuracy as well as to therapeutic approaches in mediastinal illness. Such information, coupled with educational programs targeted for clinicians, ensures optimal incorporation of the complexity of the thoracic duct into clinical practice (Korenkov et al., 2018) (Figure 8.10).

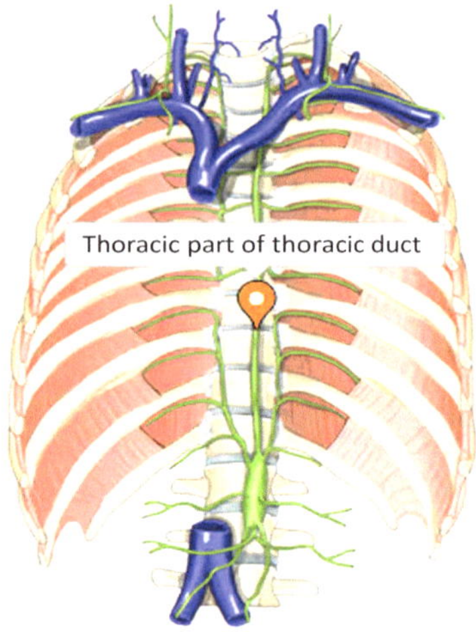

Figure 8.10. The thoracic duct and its role.

Source: IMAIOS. (n.d.). *Thoracic Part of Thoracic Duct.*

8.5.3. Nerves and their Functions

The complex network that supports communication between the central nervous system (CNS) and mediastinal structures is responsible for significant physiological mechanisms. Mediastinal nerves are conduits for the conduction of sensory data and motor messages vital for maintaining homeostasis and organ functioning. These nerves are both autonomic and somatic in nature and reflect the mediastums' multi-faceted role for heart, respiration, and digestion control. In particular, the vagus nerve, a significant component of the parasympathetic nervous system, traverses the mediastinum, controlling heart rate and bronchial constrictions. These neural tracts are meant for instantaneous reflexive compensation to circulating demands, which proves the integration of the nervous system with mediastinal organs. Understanding these interactions is key to comprehension of pathological states in which neural insufficiency leads to deregulated organ function, and the general applicability of mediastinal nerve anatomy to the clinical sphere (Rosse & Mejino, 2008; Korenkov et al., 2018). Anatomical examination reveals that the mediastinum is richly innervated by several key nerves, which illustrate differentiated functions in autonomic and somatic control. Sympathetic trunks, located along vertebral bodies, influence vasomotor tone and cardiac contractility through postganglionic fibers to the heart and great vessels. Phrenic nerves, originating from cervical spinal roots, descend through the mediastinum to supply the diaphragm, highlighting their pivotal function in respiratory mechanics. Their injury may cause inefficient respiration or abnormal cardiovascular reactions, proving their functional versatility. Such complex neuroanatomical organization is an excellent example of the integrational function of the nervous system in the mediastinum, its importance for physiological homeostasis, and for potential surgical intervention involving the mediastinal structures (Rosse & Mejino, 2008; Korenkov et al., 2018). Functional neuroanatomy in the mediastinum also encompasses reflex arcs that consolidate autonomic responses to survival. Afferent fibers from the lungs and heart relay information to the brainstem via nerves within the mediastinal space, where integration results in modulations of heart rate, blood pressure, and respiratory rhythm. These feedbacks allow the nervous system to react dynamically to external and internal stimuli to ensure cardiovascular and pulmonary homeostasis. In addition, pathological activation of mediastinal nerves, such as compression or inflammation, can disrupt these regulatory feedback loops and produce clinical manifestations such as arrhythmias or shortness of breath. The foundational understanding of such neural mechanisms coupled with detailed anatomical models and teaching resources provides essential insights to medical students and clinicians for diagnosing and managing mediastinal neuropathies (Rosse & Mejino, 2008; Korenkov et al., 2018).

Test Your Knowledge

1. Which areas of the body are drained by the thoracic duct?
2. Which part of the autonomic nervous system is involved in sympathetic innervation of the heart and lungs?

8.6. Clinical Significance of the Mediastinum

Learning Outcome

1. Mediastinal Disorders Discuss the Common Diseases Affecting the Mediastinum
2. Explain the Diagnostic Imaging Techniques
3. Focus on Treatment Options for

The clinical importance of the mediastinum is underlined by its being an axial anatomical compartment housing essential structures such as the heart, great vessels, trachea, and esophagus. Pathologic processes originating or extending into this compartment may generate complex clinical conditions, often necessitating advanced diagnostic techniques. For example, nuclear imaging modalities that evaluate autonomic nervous system dysfunctions have been found to be variably reliable in differentiating neurodegenerative disorders affecting mediastinal ganglia, and this has been seen to necessitate careful interpretation in clinical practice (Skowronek et al., 2019). Despite the promise of such diagnostics, noncorresponding clinical presentations and imaging findings reveal the complex mediastinal role in systemic illness and the challenge in its evaluation, thus the need for correlating multimodal diagnosis with full clinical evaluation to make proper decisions. Infections involving or extruding into the mediastinum are health-replete dangers because they can rapidly progress to life-threatening processes. Deep neck and mediastinal infection usually originate from odontogenic or oropharyngeal sources, demonstrating mediastinum's connection with fascial planes in the cervical region as a route for infection spreading. Recent studies have identified that early and accurate imaging, commonly carried out with MRI, has an important role in determining the size of infection and organizing surgical treatment (Velhonoja, 2024). Failure to early detect and treat mediastinal infections results in severe complications, underlining the clinical significance of the mediastinum as an anatomic entity but, above all, as a central region in the pathogenesis of infectious processes and the determination of therapeutic approaches. The mediastinum's implication in systemic diseases further accentuates its clinical relevance, particularly when structural and functional impairments are implicated in deranging fundamental physiological processes. Autonomic innervation disorders in the mediastinal spaces can be variable in their presentation, which complicates diagnosis and management. The nature of mediastinal disease necessitates a multidisciplinary team approach that involves clinical evaluation, state-of-the-art imaging modalities, and judicious interpretation of results to achieve optimal patient outcomes (Skowronek et al., 2019). In addition, addressing predisposing factors such as poor oral hygiene, leading to infection with mediastinal extension, illustrates the importance of combined preventive strategies in the reduction of morbidity and mortality from mediastinal diseases (Velhonoja, 2024). The mediastinum, thus, remains a field of clinical vigilance and intervention in multiple medical specialties (Figure 8.11).

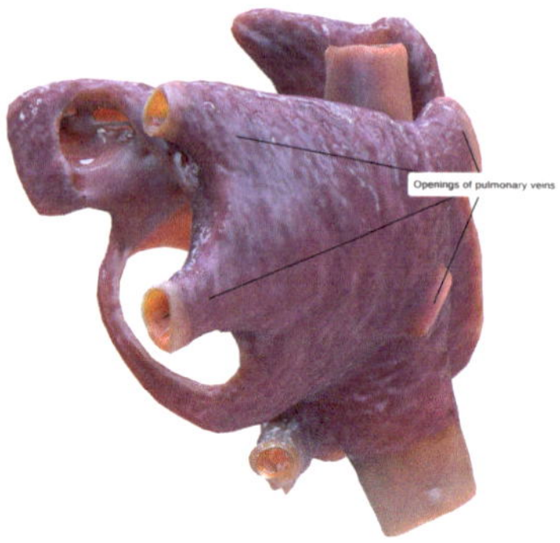

Figure 8.11. Clinical significance of the mediastinum.

Source: By xranatomy.com - Own work, CC BY-SA 4.0, https://commons.wikimedia.org/w/index.php?curid=147210728

8.6.1. Common Diseases Affecting the Mediastinum

The mediastinum, a median compartment of the thoracic cavity, is the repository of vital structures such as the heart, great vessels, trachea, and esophagus, and is thus susceptible to a wide range of diseases that can significantly impact patient morbidity and mortality. Among them, non-neoplastic benign diseases are commonly diagnostically perplexing due to their overlapping clinical and imaging presentations. Large vessel vasculitis, including Takayasu arteritis and giant cell arteritis, affects the vessel walls within the mediastinum, leading to inflammation and vascular compromise. These conditions present with systemic symptoms along with the localized symptoms, and hence, diagnosis becomes even more difficult early in the disease. The pathophysiology and epidemiology need to be understood because early management can avoid catastrophic complications. Current reviews emphasize the necessity of combining clinical suspicion with modern imaging and laboratory data to maximize diagnostic yield and patient outcomes in these difficult disorders (Farooq et al., 2024). Infectious processes also account for a significant source of mediastinal diseases, most commonly as a result of spread of infection either hematogenously or via contiguous extension. Mediastinal infections range from acute mediastinitis, most frequently postoperative or traumatic in origin, to chronic granulomatous infections such as tuberculosis and histoplasmosis. Infections cause inflammatory reactions that can lead to fibrosis and scarring, sometimes progressing to fibrosing mediastinitis, a rare but disabling disease with thick fibrous tissue encasing mediastinal structures. The covert nature of these infections can delay the diagnosis, emphasizing the need for a high index of suspicion, especially in endemic areas or immunocompromised individuals. The correlation of microbiological studies with radiological assessment remains the cornerstone of effective management and in preventing irreversible complications (Farooq et al., 2024). Benign or malignant neoplastic lesions constitute another large category of mediastinal disease, but benign processes may cause considerable clinical concern because of their potential proximity to vital thoracic organs. The most frequent benign mediastinal tumors are thymomas, cysts, and neurogenic tumors, each with distinctive features and clinical behavior. While interest is typically directed at neoplastic processes, inflammatory and granulomatous pathology with tumor-like presentation on imaging studies must be recognized, for which careful differential diagnosis is necessary. Multimodal approaches utilizing laboratory studies, imaging modalities, and biopsy if appropriate have an important role in distinguishing these pathologies to tailor therapy. Although neoplasms are often highlighted, the focus should not be distracted from non-neoplastic benign mediastinal illnesses whose early diagnosis and treatment are crucial to the reduction of complications and mortality (Farooq et al., 2024).

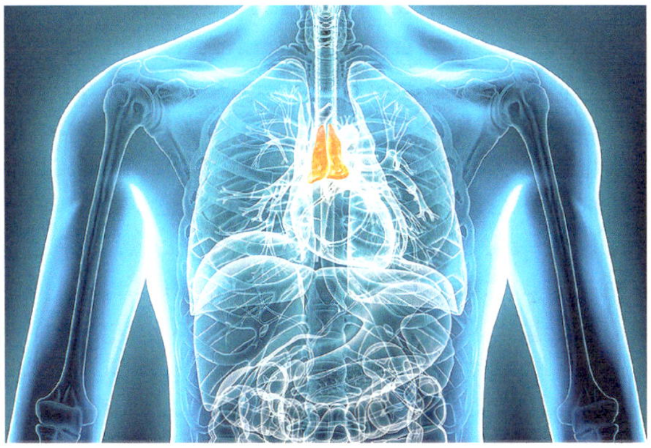

Source: Saint John's Cancer Institute. (2023). *Thymoma Tumor Anterior Mediastinum*.

8.6.2. Diagnostic Imaging Techniques

Advances in imaging technology have had a tremendous impact on the diagnostic approach to mediastinal abnormalities, with an increased ability of clinicians to detect and characterize lesions effectively. Cross-sectional imaging techniques, particularly CT and MRI, form the initial approach towards the evaluation of masses or lymphadenopathy in the mediastinum. CT, with its superior spatial resolution, facilitates the identification of the size, location, and interaction of mediastinal structures, while MRI offers improved soft tissue contrast, enabling vascular, cystic, or solid element differentiation. Along with anatomical imaging, functional imaging techniques have further enhanced diagnostic sensitivity. For instance, positron emission tomography (PET) combined with CT enables metabolic assessment, making benign versus malignant lesion differentiation feasible. This multimodal imaging strategy is the cornerstone of mediastinal assessment, providing comprehensive data to direct subsequent intervention or observation. The application of nuclear medicine techniques in mediastinal imaging has particularly improved the diagnostic trajectory for specific pathologies. For familial syndromes such as familial paraganglioma with SDHD mutations, whole-body imaging with PET-CT using radiotracers like 18F-DOPA is now the gold standard for lesion detection and staging. These functional imaging examinations not only identify lesion localization but also assist in tumor characterization and prognostication because uptake patterns correlate with biological aggressiveness. Other agents, such as 123I-MIBG, provide therapeutic predictive information, especially when determining radiometabolic treatment plans. Furthermore, new PET radiopharmaceuticals, including 68Ga-peptides, show excellent diagnostic accuracy in initial studies, although validation by larger cohorts remains necessary.

The combination of biochemical study and routine imaging monitoring creates a robust model for early diagnosis and treatment of mediastinal tumors in genetically predisposed populations (Puliani et al., 2020). Minimally invasive techniques have also transformed mediastinal evaluation, particularly in malignancy staging where accurate lymph node assessment is crucial. Endobronchial ultrasound (EBUS) guided transbronchial needle aspiration (TBNA) is an example of this type of innovation, offering real-time mediastinal and hilar lymph node sampling without surgical biopsy morbidity.

It has expanded the ability to accurately stage lung cancer, with significant effects on prognosis and treatment planning. EBUS has high sensitivity and specificity with a great safety profile, and it is the first-line investigation in the absence of distant metastases. Furthermore, it has been found to be useful for applications other than lung cancer, including other intrathoracic cancers necessitating the assessment of mediastinal lymph nodes. The speed, precision, and minimally invasive application of EBUS TBNA highlight its central position in today's mediastinal diagnostic algorithms (Bilocca et al., 2016) (Figure 8.12).

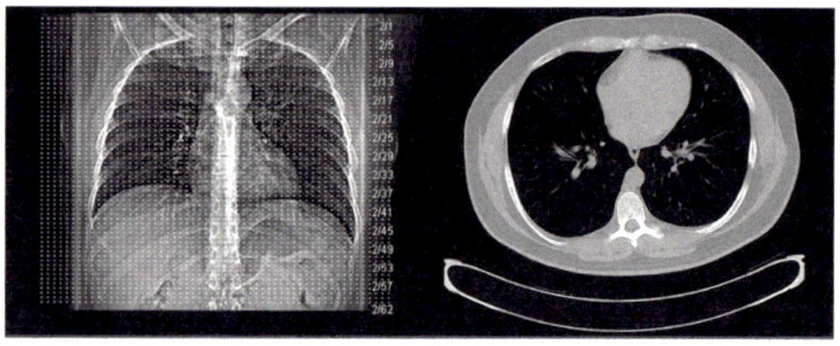

Figure 8.12. Diagnostic imaging techniques.

Source: By Ptrump16 - Own work, CC BY-SA 4.0, https://commons.wikimedia.org/w/index.php?curid=123692659

8.6.3. Treatment Options for Mediastinal Disorders

Treatment approaches for mediastinal disease are highly dependent on the specific diagnosis, location, and type of underlying disease. Surgery still is a mainstay, especially for mediastinal masses like thymomas, cysts, or tumors endangering critical structures. Video-assisted thoracoscopic surgery (VATS) and other minimally invasive methods have become popular due to lower morbidity versus classic open thoracotomy. Moreover, radiation therapy is often employed as an adjunct or substitute for surgery when surgical resection is contraindicated or not possible, especially in cancers like lymphomas or thymic carcinomas. The choice of treatment should be multidisciplinary with respect to potential complications due to the intimate relationship of the mediastinum with the heart, lungs, and great vessels, highlighting the importance of precise preoperative imaging and planning. In inflammatory or granulomatous mediastinal illnesses such as sarcoidosis, treatment is primarily medical. Corticosteroids are the preferred form of treatment, effectively reducing inflammation and preventing fibrosis that can destabilize mediastinal structures. Of special interest is neurosarcoidosis, a presentation of the nervous system, in which there is a very great requirement for treatment, with over 90% of patients requiring drug therapy due to the significant symptoms of meningitis and cranial neuropathy, which significantly affect QoL (Voortman, 2019). Refractory or when the side effects of steroids become significant can be the use of immunosuppressive drugs. These regimens require careful monitoring and prolonged treatment courses, emphasizing the need for individualized therapy for each patient. Emerging treatment strategies continue to shape the therapy of mediastinal diseases, with enhancements in targeted therapy and immunotherapy being the most promising, especially for thymic carcinoma and lymphomas. Supportive care to palliate symptom burden and overall quality of life in patients has also become increasingly necessary. Fatigue, mental impairment, and pain, especially prevalent in systemic diseases like sarcoidosis, necessitate an integrated treatment plan through multidisciplinary teams of neurologists, pulmonologists, and mental health practitioners (Voortman, 2019). Resources compiled in medical literature and faculty publications provide a foundation for ongoing research and evidence-based practice improvement. By merging technical innovations and global care patterns, therapeutic treatments of mediastinal disorders constantly change, improving prognosis and QoL in patients with the conditions.

Test Your Knowledge

1. How does the esophagus relate anatomically to the mediastinum?
2. What are the boundaries of the posterior mediastinum?

SUMMARY

Examination of the mediastinum reveals its internal importance via thoracic anatomy and clinical practice, with a focus on the complex interrelation of structures demanding careful attention at the time of diagnosis and treatment. The function of the mediastinum extends beyond simple anatomical definition; it is a conduit for major biological cardiovascular, respiratory, and lymphatic elements, and integrity becomes paramount to overall physiological homeostasis. With proper observation, clinicians can realize the manner in which lesions, infections, or cancers in this compartment may impact remote organs and systems. Such thorough knowledge translates to increased diagnostic specificity and therapeutic results, positioning the mediastinum not only as an anatomical compartment but also as a critical target for multidisciplinary medical management. In integrating available medical data, it is apparent that technological advances in imaging and diagnostic modalities have significantly enhanced the capability to evaluate mediastinal disorders accurately. They facilitate early diagnosis of abnormalities, which guides more targeted interventions. Finally, synchronizing clinical practice with developing research, including data from artificial intelligence (AI) technology, would also have the potential to further optimize healthcare providers' capacity to manage mediastinal pathologies successfully. But caution is warranted, because variation in test outcomes and compounded anatomy necessitate continuous education and training. Implementation of new equipment should augment, not replace, detailed anatomical and clinical expertise to produce optimal patient outcomes. Ultimately, research confirms the necessity of integrating anatomy with emerging clinical practices and pedagogical strategies. The continuous evolution of medical education, facilitated by interdisciplinarity research and technological advancements, holds the promise of increased competence in the management of mediastinal disorders. However, one must not overlook the human factors inherent in this process, such as the cognitive and affective abilities of healthcare professionals, which affect diagnostic accuracy and patient care. As research in nearby fields continues, such as the contribution of AI to inclusion in medical assessments (Liu, 2024) and the relationship between empathy and burnout during medical training (Cairns et al., 2024), the mediastinum remains a current example where the field of anatomical knowledge, clinical skill, and human factors all converge to improve health outcomes.

The mediastinum, a mid-space compartment of the thoracic cavity, houses vital structures such as the heart, thymus, esophagus, trachea, and great vessels. Understanding its anatomical boundaries and subdivisions is the cornerstone of clinical diagnosis and surgical management. The anterior, middle, and posterior mediastinal divisions serve as a paradigm for localizing disease and selecting treatment modalities. Understanding the complex anatomy of the mediastinum helps to interpret imaging tests and evaluate diseases such as tumors, infections, or vascular abnormalities. Highlighting anatomical accuracy decreases the incidence of iatrogenic injuries with invasive techniques, highlighting the clinical relevance of advanced mediastinal knowledge to clinical practice. Discussing the clinical relevance of the mediastinum in relation to research, there is a need to emphasize the variability of the pathologies affecting the space. Mediastinal masses, including cysts, lymphadenopathy, and neoplasms, are difficult to diagnose and treat due to their proximity to critical organs. Mediastinal involvement in cardiovascular and respiratory disease requires a multidisciplinary onslaught of radiology, surgery, and pathology. Technical innovations in imaging modalities such as CT and MRI have enhanced the characterization of mediastinal lesions with improved accuracy. These advances facilitate early detection and tailored treatments, resulting in improved patient outcomes. Thus, a clear understanding of mediastinal disease and its management remains central to thoracic medicine. Condensing key points about the mediastinum emphasizes the need to separate structural and functional characteristics into categories to guide clinical practice. Like more complex clinical specialties, establishing established guidelines for diagnosis and management guarantees consistency and quality of care. Building on the analogies from fields like treating temporomandibular disorder, where clear-cut key points direct practitioners, mediastinal treatment would also benefit from abstracted protocols to enhance decision-making (Manfredini et al., 2024). Moreover, emerging regenerative medicines and cellular technologies are poised to be the solution for treating mediastinal organ injury, mirroring regenerative solutions on the horizon in cardiovascular medicine (Kyryk, 2024). Long-term research and interdisciplinarity collaboration will be essential in formulating next-generation comprehensive mediastinal treatment models, eventually enhancing patient safety and therapeutic efficacy.

KEY TERMS FROM THIS CHAPTER

- Central thoracic cavity
- Diaphragmatic contraction
- Foundational model of anatomy (FMA)
- Histomorphometry
- Inferior mediastinum
- Mediastinal anatomy
- Clinical diagnosis
- Fluid homeostasis
- Heartand pericardium
- Immunologic development
- Intervertebral disc (IVD)
- Mediastinal architecture

CRITICAL THINKING QUESTIONS

1. **Which of the following structures is found in the superior mediastinum?**
   a. Heart
   b. Thymus
   c. Descending aorta
   d. Esophageal plexus
2. **The transverse thoracic plane, dividing the mediastinum into superior and inferior parts, passes through which vertebral level?**
   a. T2–T3
   b. T4–T5
   C. T6–T7
   d. T1–T2
3. **The middle mediastinum contains which of the following structures?**
   a. Esophagus
   b. Heart
   c. Thoracic duct
   d. Azygos vein
4. **The posterior mediastinum is located:**
   a. Behind the sternum
   b. Between the lungs
   c. Behind the pericardium
   d. Anterior to the heart
5. **Which nerve passes through both the superior and posterior mediastinum?**
   a. Phrenic nerve
   b. Vagus nerve
   c. Intercostal nerve
   d. Hypoglossal nerve

Short Answer Questions

1. Define the mediastinum and explain how it is divided anatomically.
2. Differentiate between the anterior, middle, and posterior parts of the inferior mediastinum.
3. What is the clinical importance of the transverse thoracic plane (T4–T5 level)?
4. Describe the course and function of the thoracic duct in the mediastinum.
5. Which major nerves pass through the mediastinum, and what is their significance?
6. What are common pathologies that can occur in the mediastinum?

Answers to Critical Thinking Questions

1. (b) 2. (b) 3. (b) 4. (c) 5. (b)

REFERENCES

1. Abasi, M., Kiani, A., Mohammadzadeh, S., Tavafi, M., (2013). *Reproductive Efficiency of an Indigenous Iranian Goat (Capra hircus)*. Animal Research International; 10(2): 1723 – 1729 https://core.ac.uk/download/478406447.pdf (accessed on 8th May 2025).

2. Ashraf H, Sadatnaseri A, Aminorroaya A, Kuhi Z, Zandi N, Karbalai Saleh S, (2021). Left Ventricular Pseudoaneurysm as a Complication of Myocardial Infarction; A Case Series and Review of the Literature. Front Emerg Med; 5(3):e30 (accessed on 8th May 2025).

3. Bertolini G, Angeloni L. Vascular and Cardiac CT in Small Animals [Internet]. Computed Tomography - Advanced Applications. InTech; 2017. Available from: http://dx.doi.org/10.5772/intechopen.69848(accessed on 8th May 2025).

4. Li, F., Tao, Y., Bauer, G., Elsner, A., Li, Z., Swierzy, M., Englisch, J., Meisel, A., Ismail, M., & Rückert, J. C. (2019). Unraveling the role of ectopic thymic tissue in patients undergoing thymectomy for myasthenia gravis. *Journal of thoracic disease*, *11*(9), 4039–4048. https://doi.org/10.21037/jtd.2019.08.109 (accessed on 8th May 2025).

5. Bilocca, D., Vella, C. & Montefort, S. (2016). Endoscopic bronchial ultrasound in mediastinal staging of lung cancer. Malta Medical Journal, 28(3), 42-49 (accessed on 8th May 2025).

6. Bustos, A., Pertusa, A., Salinas, J. M., & de la Iglesia-Vayá, M. (2020). PadChest: A large chest x-ray image dataset with multi-label annotated reports. *Medical image analysis*, *66*, 101797. https://doi.org/10.1016/j.media.2020.101797(accessed on 8th May 2025).

7. Puliani, G., Sesti, F., Feola, T., Di Leo, N., Polti, G., Verrico, M., Modica, R., Colao, A., Lenzi, A., Isidori, A. M., Cantisani, V., Giannetta, E., & Faggiano, A. (2020). Natural History and Management of Familial Paraganglioma Syndrome Type 1: Long-Term Data from a Large Family. *Journal of clinical medicine*, *9*(2), 588. https://doi.org/10.3390/jcm9020588 (accessed on 8th May 2025).

8. cholar.org/paper/f0aba3ac56c9b6ae9738e472b0ea5467b048f09a

9. Cianfanelli, E., Corbetta, L., Goretti, G., Malpelo, M. L., & Pelosini, L. (2017). *SAM – Simulation Airways Models*. https://core.ac.uk/download/599305241.pdf (accessed on 8th May 2025).

10. Wietholt, C., Roerig, D. L., Gordon, J. B., Haworth, S. T., Molthen, R. C., & Clough, A. V. (2008). Bronchial circulation angiogenesis in the rat quantified with SPECT and micro-CT. *European journal of nuclear medicine and molecular imaging*, *35*(6), 1124–1132. https://doi.org/10.1007/s00259-007-0684-y (accessed on 8th May 2025).

11. Oliveira, D.A., Feitosa, R.Q. & Correia, M.M. Segmentation of liver, its vessels and lesions from CT images for surgical planning. *BioMed Eng OnLine* **10**, 30 (2011). https://doi.org/10.1186/1475-925X-10-30 (accessed on 8th May 2025).

12. V. Volckaert, E. Vandermeulen, S. Daminet, J.H. Saunders, K. Peremans (2016). *Hyperthyroidism in Cats, Part I: Anatomy, Physiology, Pathophysiology, Diagnosis and Imaging*. Vlaams Diergeneeskundig Tijdschrift, 2016, 85. https://core.ac.uk/download/74658457.pdf (accessed on 8th May 2025).

13. Elieh-Ali-Komi, D., Maurer, M., & Siebenhaar, F. (2025). The Impact of Mast Cells on the Anatomy, Cellular Communication, and Molecular Immune Network of Lymph Nodes. *Clinical reviews in allergy & immunology*, *68*(1), 35. https://doi.org/10.1007/s12016-025-09050-5 (accessed on 8th May 2025).

14. Geethanjali, H. T., & Shivanal, U. (2017). *Anomalous Azygos Veins – Its Embryological Basis and Clinical Significance*. https://core.ac.uk/download/544391733.pdf (accessed on 8th May 2025).

15. Gemmill, E. H. (2025). *Minimally Invasive Gastro-Oesophageal Surgery for Cancer: Current Evidence and Practice*. https://core.ac.uk/download/161526134.pdf (accessed on 8th May 2025).

16. Hovde, O. H. (2024). *Modelling and Simulation of Ascending Aorta, Including Influence of Tissue Change in Aneurysms*. Master's thesis in Mechanical Engineering Supervisor: Bjørn Helge Skallerud Co-supervisor: Victorien Prot & Omid Ghorbani June 2024 Norwegian University of Science and Technology Faculty of Engineering Department of Structural Engineering(accessed on 8th May 2025).

17. Putri, Giovani & Soehartono, & Astiarani, Yunisa. (2023). Exploring The Tasting System and Clinical Significance of Taste Disorders: A Narrative Review: Clinical Significance of Taste Disorder. Journal of Urban Health Research. 1. 22-36. 10.25170/juhr.v1i3.4476. (accessed on 8th May 2025).

18. Kaye, J. (1995). *TrauMAP – Integrating Anatomical and Physiological Simulation.* Dissertation proposal. https://core.ac.uk/download/76363490.pdf (accessed on 8th May 2025).

19. Kumar, A., Prakash, A., & Prasad, M. R. N. (1979). *Light Microscopic Features of the Rete Testis, the Vas Efferens, the Epididymis and the Vas Deferens in the Adult Rhesus Monkey*. https://core.ac.uk/download/pdf/291525863.pdf (accessed on 8th May 2025).

20. Kyryk, V. (2024). Stem cell therapy for cardiac regeneration: Key points. *Cell and Organ Transplantology*. https://www.semanticscholar.org/paper/6a1b536f3691ad0d162e4187a4a2e2ffd1507b5f (accessed on 8th May 2025).

21. Skowronek, C., Zange, L., & Lipp, A. (2019). Cardiac 123I-MIBG Scintigraphy in Neurodegenerative Parkinson Syndromes: Performance and Pitfalls in Clinical Practice. *Frontiers in neurology*, *10*, 152. https://doi.org/10.3389/fneur.2019.00152 (accessed on 8th May 2025).

22. Rosse, C., Mejino, J.L.V. (2008). The Foundational Model of Anatomy Ontology. In: Burger, A., Davidson, D., Baldock, R. (eds) Anatomy Ontologies for Bioinformatics. Computational Biology, vol 6. Springer, London. https://doi.org/10.1007/978-1-84628-885-2_4 (accessed on 8th May 2025).

23. Nakanishi, K., & Goto, H. (2023). Fascial structure of the anterior mediastinum: The surgical figure of the sternopericardial ligament and the role of affixing the thymus to the pericardium. *Journal of Thoracic Disease, 16*, 1044–1053. https://www.semanticscholar.org/paper/452463d788f2752e98d0756d599ef9a0cc3d0db6 (accessed on 8th May 2025).

24. Touro College & University System. (2019). 2018 Touro College & University System faculty publications. https://core.ac.uk/download/226776536.pdf (accessed on 8th May 2025).

25. Velhonoja, J. (2024). *Severe Orofacial and Neck Infections – Predisposing Factors, Changing Characteristics, and Advanced Diagnostics*. https://core.ac.uk/download/596767156.pdf (accessed on 8th May 2025).

26. Voortman, M. (2019). *The Burden of Neurosarcoidosis and Small Fiber Neuropathy Associated Symptoms*. https://core.ac.uk/download/323359046.pdf (accessed on 8th May 2025).

27. Wilson, S., Awazi, A., Gray, T., Cooper, C., Sadacharan, C., Mendoza, M., Ayala, M., & Tippen, S. P. (2025). Morphometric Evaluation of the Anterior Meniscofemoral Ligament in Human Cadaveric Knees: Anatomical Variations and Clinical Significance. *Cureus*, *17*(2), e79013. https://doi.org/10.7759/cureus.79013(accessed on 8th May 2025).

ABDOMINAL WALL AND INGUINAL REGION

9

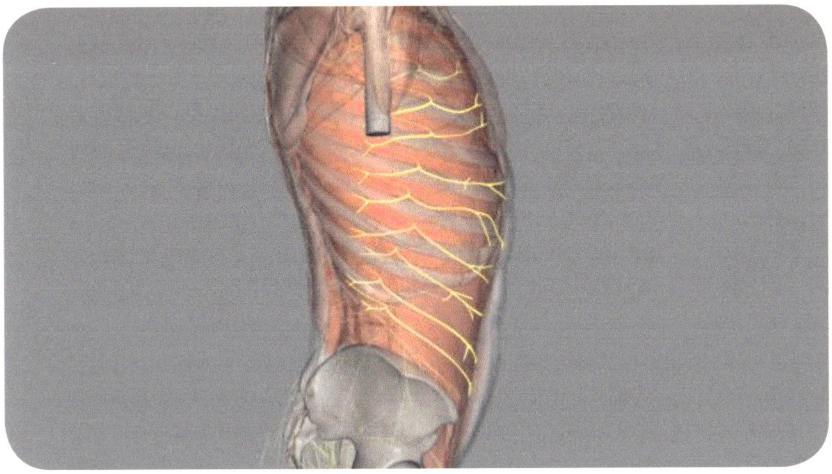

Introduction

An appreciation of the complex anatomy of the lower torso puts into perspective the crucial role played by the tissues enveloping the abdominal cavity. The wall of the abdomen, composed of several layers of muscles, fascia, and membranes, safeguards internal organs while maintaining integrity and pressure necessary for body functions such as respiration and locomotion. Adjacent to this complex structure is the inguinal region, a region in which defects in the musculofascial compartment are frequently responsible for the production of hernias. These hernias are caused by protrusion of intra-abdominal contents through weakened areas of fascia, underlining this region's clinical and functional significance. With its global prevalence and clinical management implications, the pathobiology of the abdominal wall and inguinal region not only directs operative management but also continues to enhance the understanding of common pathologies to impact patient health. Surgical repair of defects in the region has evolved substantially over time, with more recent advances being contingent upon advances

LEARNING OBJECTIVES

After studying this chapter, you will be able to:

1. Focus on the anatomy of the abdominal wall
2. Explain the functions of the abdominal wall
3. Discuss the inguinal region anatomy
4. Know inguinal hernias
5. Understand surgical interventions
6. Learn about the clinical significance

in anatomical appreciation and technology. Inguinal area hernia repair is still one of the most frequent operative procedures worldwide, with consequences extending across demographics and economic boundaries. The transition from older open repair methods to minimally invasive laparoscopic surgery is a classic case in point. Laparoscopic inguinal hernia repair (LIHR) is now viewed as an optimum option based on its association with less postoperative pain, reduced hospital stays, and lower recurrence. It is crucial to appreciate this evolution to understand current standards of care and the reasoning behind current surgical practices in the inguinal area and abdominal wall (Hasslinda, 2010). The therapeutic imperatives and diagnostic challenges of inguinal hernias are underscored by atypical clinical presentations, e.g., interstitial inguinal hernias, where the hernia sac lies between muscle layers rather than outward protruding. These rare conditions pose a diagnostic and management challenge, necessitating meticulous surgical methods. Laparoscopic and minimally invasive repairs, for example, using specialized mesh placement, have been effective in the management of these rare defects with minimal patient morbidity. Refinements in imaging and surgery technology further enhance our ability to visualize and treat such hernias. This ongoing evolution highlights the dynamic relationship between clinical practice and anatomical information in the abdominal wall and inguinal region (Glaser et al., 2011).

Definition of the Abdominal Wall

The human body structure relies primarily on protective and elastic tissue layers, particularly in the trunk. Of these, the abdominal wall is significant in covering and shielding the internal organs of the abdomen. It is composed of multiple muscular and fascial layers that work synergistically to provide intra-abdominal pressure, maintain posture, and facilitate bending and twisting movements. Abdominal wall complexity results from the component arrangement since it consists of skin, superficial fascia, muscles, and deep fascia that, together, form a strong yet flexible envelope. Its anatomical disposition is not only required for the mechanical safeguard but also for physiological roles like respiration and viscera retention under varying pressures, thus demonstrating its indispensable function in human anatomy. Deeper, the muscle components of the abdominal wall include primarily the rectus abdominis, external oblique, internal oblique, and transversus abdominis muscles. The muscles are arranged in layers, with specific mechanical properties and strength. Fascial layers like the aponeuroses of muscles weave centrally at the Linea alba, creating a fibrous seam that offers tensile strength. There are also neurovascular elements running through these layers, supporting their function and survivability. It is a crucial organization, particularly in the clinical context when disease or surgery compromises the integrity of the abdominal wall. Understanding the layered anatomy is the basis for choosing incisions, repair techniques, and prevention of postoperative complications. The abdominal wall is therefore a dynamic anatomical structure that is best suited to meet different biomechanical demands. Clinically, the definition of the abdominal wall transcends static anatomical description into its role in surgical anatomy and pathology, specifically incisional hernias (IH) and laparoscopic surgery. The risk of hernia formation varies with midline incisions or trocar sites, highlighting the clinical importance of precise knowledge of layers of the abdominal wall and their contribution to structural integrity. Surgeons must consider these anatomical realities in their efforts to optimize closure techniques, reducing such complications as surgical site infections (SSIs) that disproportionately impact abdominal wall integrity (David et al., 2023). Furthermore, advances in newer imaging technologies like ultrasound and CT scans have enhanced visualization of the morphology and pathology of the abdominal wall to drive optimal clinical management. These advancements underscore the need for a multidisciplinary understanding of the abdominal wall in both anatomical composition and practical use within clinical practice (Lee et al., 2023) (Figure 9.1).

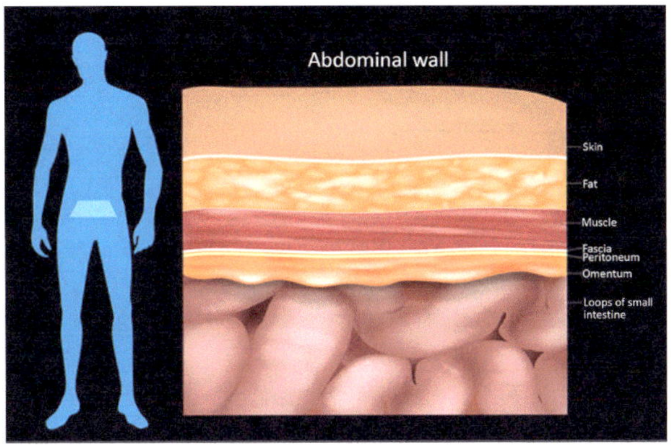

Figure 9.1. The abdominal wall.

Source: FT Creations. (n.d.). Abdominal Wall Anatomy Illustration

Importance of the Inguinal Region

The inguinal region is of utmost anatomical and clinical significance due to its complex structural composition as well as serving as a passage for numerous vital factors. An inguinal canal exists in this area, which serves as a passage for the spermatic cord in males and the round ligament in females. Its unique anatomy, bounded by fascial and muscular layers of the abdominal wall, makes it a location at risk for herniation, particularly inguinal hernias, when the contents of the abdomen protrude through defects here. Recognition of the boundary of inguinal areas and contents is essential not just for surgery but also for diagnostic examination. These facts make discrimination between indirect and direct inguinal hernias possible and direct approaches to repair, paying special attention to the interrelation of anatomy and clinical practice. This active role of this field, considering its impact on abdominal wall integrity and intra-abdominal pressure, underlines its obligatory role in physiological as well as pathological states (Lee et al., 2023). Besides, from the surgical perspective, the groin region is demanding and rewarding in terms of results for operations involving the lower abdominal wall. Due to the proximity between neurovascular structures, i.e., the femoral vessels and the ilioinguinal nerve, finesse is needed to avoid complications like vascular compromise, chronic pain, or nerve damage. The importance of the region is heightened in minimally invasive hernia repair and colorectal operations, in which developed anatomical know-how can reduce operative risk and optimize patient recovery. Anatomical variation within the region also affects clinical presentations, making tailored examination necessary. In addition, the inguinal region is at the center of oncologic consideration, particularly in the context of lymphatic drainage pathways and sentinel node evaluation for cancers in the lower abdominal and pelvic regions (Halvorsen et al., 2022; Lee et al., 2023). This reflects the region's significance extending beyond mechanical stabilization, into systemic disease control.

The clinical importance of the inguinal region continues in the application of diagnostic imaging and staging where precise anatomical delineation is vital. The advancement in imaging modalities such as MRI has enhanced the capability of clinicians to evaluate the tissues within this region with improved benign versus pathological differentiation. For instance, high-definition imaging facilitates soft tissue mass differentiation, local tumor invasion assessment, and surgical intervention planning. Such precision results in personalized therapeutic interventions, including watchful waiting or organ preservation in individual cases. As detailed in current radiologic nomenclatures, mention of anatomical landmarks in reports guarantees the best interdisciplinary communication and treatment results, especially in the case of rectal and lower abdominal cancers (Lee et al., 2023).

Thus, the structural and functional significance of the inguinal regions transcends into various medical specialties, affirming its central role in abdominal wall anatomy and patient management (Figure 9.2).

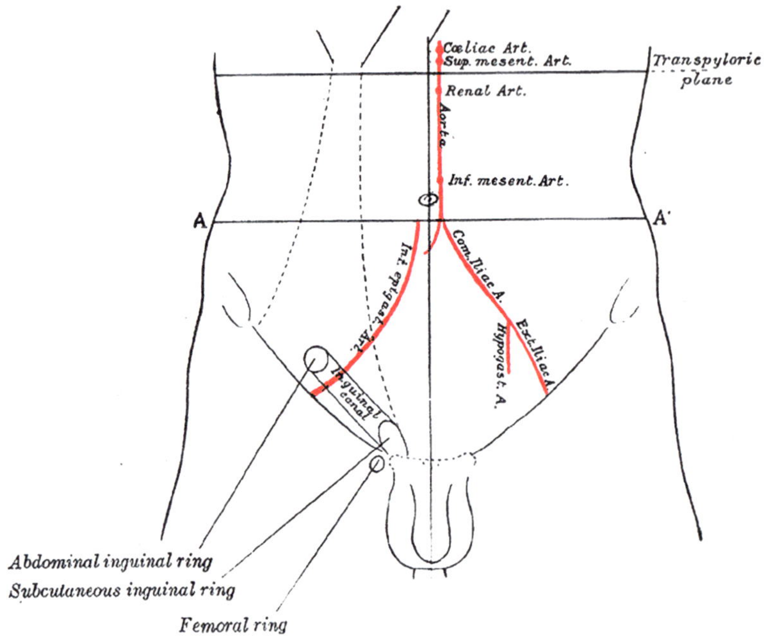

Figure 9.2. The inguinal region.

Source: By Henry Vandyke Carter - Henry Gray (1918) Anatomy of the Human Body (See "Book" section below)Bartleby.com: Gray's Anatomy, Plate 1227, Public Domain, https://commons.wikimedia.org/w/index.php?curid=564843

9.1. Anatomy of the Abdominal Wall

Learning Outcome

1. Discus the Layers of the Abdominal Wall
2. Explain the Muscles Involved in the Abdominal Wall
3. Focus on Blood Supply and Innervation

The abdominal wall is a complex and vital structure that is responsible for both intraperitoneal organ protection and intra-abdominal pressure regulation. Its layers are precisely stacked, beginning most superficially with the skin, followed by multiple fascial layers wrapping around the musculature beneath. The musculature consists primarily of the external oblique, internal oblique, and transversus abdominis muscles in combination that form a solid yet compliant barrier. These muscles are buttressed by their aponeurotic enlargements, which interlock in the midline to form the Linea alba. This composite structure enables the abdominal wall to provide support for movements such as flexion, rotation, and lateral bending and be an important aspect of respiratory mechanics and pressurized abdominal elevation during activities such as coughing or defecation. It is crucial to comprehend this layered complexity to be able to understand the clinical significance of this topic, especially when managing conditions like hernias that breach the integrity of the abdominal wall. Beneath the muscle layers, the transversalis fascia and peritoneum are additional protective interfaces between the abdominal contents and the outside world. The vascular supply and innervation of the abdominal wall are closely related to its functional needs, which are largely supplied by the lower intercostal nerves and abdominal aortic branches.

This complex vascular system allows proper perfusion and supports the healing mechanisms upon injury or surgery. From a clinical perspective, this information aids in surgical procedure planning, especially in herniotomy or laparoscopic surgery. The inguinal region, an area of anatomical weakness of the lower abdominal wall, highlights the importance of precise anatomical knowledge due to its susceptibility to herniation. Present surgical techniques, like laparoscopic inguinal hernia repair (LIHR), have been evolved to circumvent such anatomical challenges, with less invasive approaches and shorter recovery times (Hasslinda, 2010). To enhance the understanding of surface anatomy, innovative learning techniques such as body painting have been employed, with good effects in achieving a more thorough understanding of topographical relationships of the abdominal wall. Interactive learning techniques such as these facilitate students to gain a hands-on concept of muscular and fascial landmarks, which is advantageous in clinical assessment and diagnosis. This pedagogical strategy highlights the importance of anatomical knowledge not only as a theoretical foundation but as a functional one in practice. The precision with which one can map the abdominal wall on the surface is a reflection of its internal complexity, bridging the gap between surface anatomy and clinical application. Such innovation in teaching further enhances the anatomical basis demanded for effective patient care in pathology involving the abdominal and inguinal regions (Gomar et al., 2019).

9.1.1. Layers of the Abdominal Wall

An understanding of the composition of the abdominal wall is relevant to an understanding of its role in the protection of intra-abdominal organs and support of intra-abdominal pressure. The fine structure consists of several discrete layers that work synergistically to provide both strength and elasticity. Beginning on the surface, the skin provides the external covering layer, then an elastic layer of variable thickness of subcutaneous fat that cushions and insulates deeper tissues. Deep to this fat lies the superficial fascia, Camper's and Scarpa's fascia, which is of tensile strength and accommodates channels for neurovascular structures. The three flat muscles, the external oblique, internal oblique, and transversus abdominis, exist in overlapping layers as the layers go deeper, each of the fibers in different directions to give the abdominal wall resistance to mechanical stress. These layers of muscles become aponeuroses that form the rectus sheath over the rectus abdominis muscle, which is a primary muscle involved in trunk flexion and stabilization. More superficially, the rectus sheath consists of anterior and posterior layers formed by the flat muscle aponeuroses, over the rectus abdominis and a significant source of abdominal wall strength and integrity. The arcuate line marks an important anatomical border at which the posterior sheath ends, and the rectus abdominis is consequently positioned directly over the transversalis fascia below this landmark. The deepest of the muscle fibers are covered by the transversalis fascia, a thin but robust layer of connective tissue that provides support and helps to interpose muscle and peritoneum. The peritoneum itself, a lining of serous membrane over the cavity of the abdomen, is the innermost boundary of the abdominal wall. This layering enables the abdominal wall to be capable of accommodating increases in intra-abdominal pressure, to supply substrate for the contraction of the muscle, and to possess a barrier against herniation, such as when defects through layers of the muscle permit protrusion of contents of the abdomen, e.g., an interstitial inguinal hernia (Glaser et al., 2011). The interlayered anatomy of the abdominal wall directly influences surgical techniques for dealing with the inguinal region, particularly hernias. Given the multifaceted interface between fascial planes and muscle layers, understanding these layers is crucial for effective hernia repair and especially with laparoscopic techniques reliant on meticulous dissection and mesh placement.

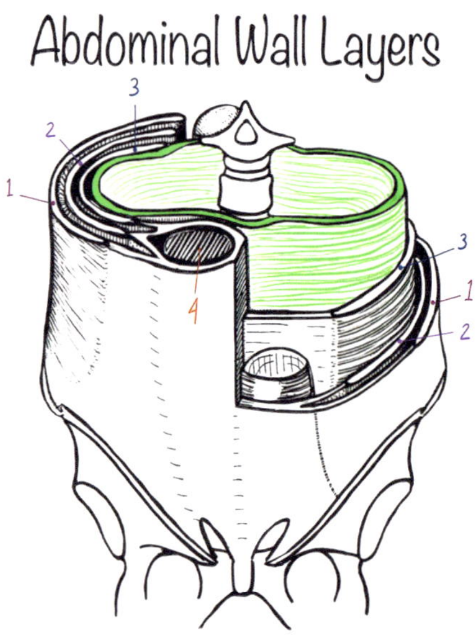

Figure 9.3. Layers of the abdominal wall.

Source: https://pbs.twimg.com/media/EI7OTGDWsAA2jpS.jpg:large.

Modern LIHR utilizes knowledge of these layers by entering the preperitoneal space, without disrupting the muscular abdominal wall, thus reducing morbidity and allowing for faster recovery. This is unlike traditional open repairs, which would disrupt these layers more severely and have longer recovery times. Minimally invasive repair methods, despite being at times accompanied by adverse outcomes, have become the preferred approach due to their superior anatomical preservation and reduced postoperative pain, underlining the vital role of a clear understanding of abdominal wall layers' anatomy in surgical innovation and patient outcomes (Hasslinda, 2010) (Figure 9.3).

9.1.2. Muscles Involved in the Abdominal Wall

The stability of the abdominal wall is, to a large extent, a function of a complex pattern of muscles which not only provide protection to the internal viscera but also facilitate various movements and contribute to the maintenance of intra-abdominal pressure. Among these muscles, external oblique, internal oblique, and transversus abdominis are of paramount significance. The external oblique muscle, located superficially, runs from the lower ribs to the iliac crest and plays a role in trunk rotation and lateral flexion. Below it is the internal oblique, which runs perpendicular to the external oblique, helping to stabilize the trunk as well as compress the abdomen. The transversus abdominis, the innermost of the three lateral muscles, runs horizontally and is significant in abdominal stabilization as well as intra-abdominal pressure increase in actions involving lifting or forced exhalation. Its major layered configuration ensures elasticity and strength to achieve body and athletic movement. The rectus abdominis and its upright positioning along the midline are central to the abdominal wall muscle structure. Tucked away as it is within the rectus sheath, which is constructed from aponeuroses of the lateral muscles, the rectus abdominis assists in flexing the lumbar spine and stabilizing the pelvis on movement. Due to the observable tendinous intersections in fit individuals, the rectus abdominis is also referred to as the six-pack muscles. The synchronization between the rectus abdominis and lateral muscles is crucial to the biomechanics of the abdominal area and is particularly significant in posture maintenance as well as resistance against abdominal protrusion during physical activity. Its role is closely interwoven with the other muscles, and the two are a dynamic complex that is essential for the integrity of the overall abdominal wall (Meyers et al., 2007). Beyond their specific functions, all of these muscles combined are utilized in the stabilization of the abdominal wall and play a tremendous role in conditions such as athletic pubalgia. The condition, typically caused by repetitive stress or imbalance of musculature, accentuates the importance of understanding such muscular interaction. A "pubic dynamic complex" is the mechanism by which the musculoskeletal (MSK) tissues encircling the pubic symphysis, including the abdominal wall muscles, act synergistically in an attempt to prevent injury. Trauma in this area can occur due to a compromise of the coordination or power of such muscles, typically in sports individuals, and may need a diagnostic and therapeutic approach suited to the complex anatomy and function of the abdominal wall and groin region (Meyers et al., 2007).

9.1.3. Blood Supply and Innervation

Understanding the abdominal wall nerve anatomy is required for both surgical intervention and clinical diagnosis. Abdominal wall innervation is primarily provided by the lower six thoracic nerves (T7-T12) and the iliohypogastric and ilioinguinal nerves that derive from the lumbar plexus, more specifically around the level of L1. These nerves run between muscle layers, giving both motor and sensory fibers enabling contraction of abdominal muscles and cutaneous perception. Surgical intervention into the abdominal wall, such as trocar insertion in laparoscopic procedures, risk injuring these nerves with resultant possible muscle paresis or sensory loss. For instance, trocar insertions near the upper lateral abdomen can injure the subcostal or the thoracic intercostal nerves, and the lower abdominal ones the iliohypogastric and ilioinguinal nerves. These injuries are typically rare, owing to the overlapping innervation and the size of the incision, but knowledge of this network is still important to avoid postoperative complications (Van Ramshorst et al., 2009). The abdominal wall is also supplied with its blood through a complex and highly anastomosed system that is pivotal to tissue viability and wound healing of any nature. The principal arteries are the superior and inferior epigastric arteries, which are branches of the internal thoracic and external iliac arteries, respectively. These vessels pass deep to the rectus abdominis muscle and supply this, together with the surrounding musculature. Other arteries such as the intercostal, subcostal, and deep circumflex iliac arteries help in collateral circulation such that blood continues to circulate even when one pathway is compromised. In the region of the inguinal area, the vascular supply not only provides nutrients to the skin and muscles but also structures passing through the inguinal canal, significant to males and females. An understanding of this blood supply assists surgeons preoperatively in planning incisions and flaps, minimizing ischemic risk and allowing for effective healing. Other than vascular and somatic innervation, visceral innervation of the region reflects the complex embryologic formation of its structures, such as the testes and associated structures. Visceral pain from regions like the testis classically localizes to the lower abdomen or groin based on affected nerve pathways, most notably through spinal segments T10 to T12. Pseudolocalization of pain in initial pathologic conditions like testicular torsion may be deceptive secondary to shared afferent pathways for cutaneous and visceral fibers. This common afferent innervation of the Genito-femoral nerve and the visceral afferents direct towards the clinical significance of the information on referred pain in the inguinal region. Pain mechanism systems in this area emphasize segmental spinal organization and embryological origins in the diagnosis and treatment of pain syndromes of the lower abdomen and the inguinal region (McNair, 1960) (Figure 9.4).

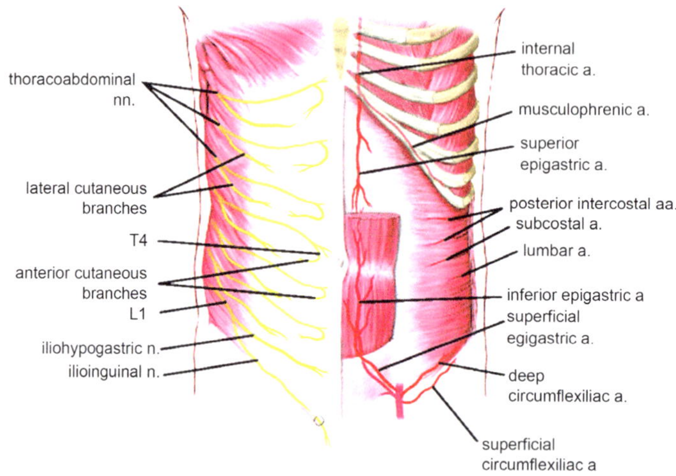

Figure 9.4. The blood supply and innervation of abdominal wall

Source: Prendergast, P.M. (2013). Anatomy of the Anterior Abdominal Wall. In: Shiffman, M., Di Giuseppe, A. (eds) Cosmetic Surgery. Springer, Berlin, Heidelberg. https://doi.org/10.1007/978-3-642-21837-8_4

Test Your Knowledge

1. How do the external and internal oblique muscles contribute to abdominal compression and rotation?
2. What is the role of the lower intercostal and subcostal nerves in abdominal wall innervation?

9.2. Functions of the Abdominal Wall

Learning Outcome

1. Discuss the Protection of Internal Organs
2. Explain the Role in Respiration
3. Describe the Contribution to Posture and Movement

The structural organization of the abdominal wall is not only a covering for intraperitoneal organs but also a significant function in controlling intra-abdominal pressure and mobility of the trunk. This structure consists of several layers including muscles, fascia, and tendinous components working synergistically to accommodate functions such as respiration, posture stabilization, and body movements such as twisting and bending. Particularly within the region of the inguinal canal, the abdominal wall possesses a complex architecture formed by the internal oblique muscle and transverse abdominal muscle and their respective aponeuroses, which form the posterior wall of the inguinal canal together. This muscle-tendon apparatus is both tensile and flexible, functionally countering pathological bulging such as hernias by supporting the structural integrity of the inguinal canal. Interestingly, the transverse fascia, though in intimate anatomical relation, contributes minimally to this resistance, emphasizing the functional support role of muscular and aponeurotic layers (Xiao et al., 2024). Apart from its protective and mechanical functions, the abdominal wall is also involved in physiological functions that are critical for core stability and modulation of intra-abdominal pressure. This modulation is essential for processes such as forced expiration, coughing, defecation, and parturition, where a build-up of pressure due to the contraction of abdominal muscles is required to enable such processes. For the inguinal region specifically, coupled action of muscles such as the internal oblique and transversus abdominis and their function in the cremaster muscle helps both functional support and spermatic cord and testicular thermoregulation. Therefore, the abdominal wall not only forms a stabilizing barrier but also includes complex muscular interactions that allow reproductive and visceral health. Such interaction of components ensures the inguinal canal is strong as well as functionally flexible to physiological demands (Xiao et al., 2024). Whenever surgery or surgical trauma results in large defects in the abdominal or inguinal wall, functional reconstruction becomes crucial to prevent complications and maintain patient quality of life (QoL). Emerging reconstructive techniques such as the keystone flap utilize local tissue for the reconstruction of large defects without requiring distant tissue transfer, thus maintaining abdominal wall integrity and function. This reconstructive method is very effective for maintaining the abdominal wall functions of protection, regulation of pressure, and mechanical support using tissue of identical biomechanical properties to the native structures. By restoring proper closure with low morbidity, keystone flaps restore abdominal wall's resistance to protrusion and core stability following surgery, allowing global patient recovery and function preservation in the inguinal and more extended abdominal areas (Figure 9.5).

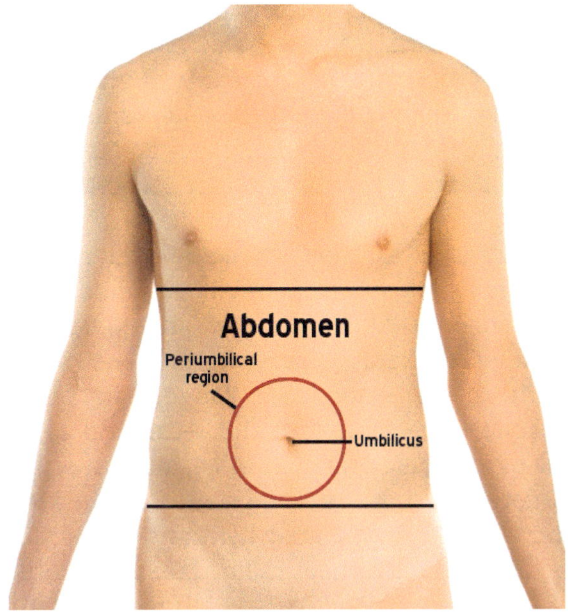

Figure 9.5. Functions of the abdominal wall.

Source: By 7mike5000 - Own work derivative of File:Upper body front smiling.png by User:Mikael Häggström, CC BY-SA 3.0, https://commons.wikimedia.org/w/index.php?curid=34551275

9.2.1. Protection of Internal Organs

The structural composition of the abdominal wall plays a crucial role in safeguarding the internal organs within the abdominal cavity. It is composed of many layers, skin, subcutaneous tissue, muscular layers, and the peritoneum, which together form a solid barrier against external trauma. All of these layers need to be intact to facilitate abdominal organ placement and prevent protrusions that can lead to pathological processes, such as herniation. Muscles like the rectus abdominis and the obliques are also not just responsible for wall strength but also for dynamic control of intra-abdominal pressure, which is crucial in maneuvers like lifting or straining. This equilibrium between the static and dynamic elements in the wall is an evolutionary measure to safeguard sensitive visceral structures without compromising essential body functions. Breakdown of this protective mechanism often leads to clinical conditions demonstrating the need for balanced abdominal wall anatomical and functional properties. A key site in the abdominal wall, the inguinal canal, demonstrates the delicate balance between structure and protection requirements. It has important structures such as the spermatic cord in males and the female round ligament, and thus serves as a weak point for possible abdominal wall weaknesses. Notably, increased intra-abdominal pressure—whether from congenital factors, lifestyle, or physical exertion—can add to the risk of inguinal hernias, in which internal organs thrust past the weakened abdominal muscle. The classic symptoms of herniation, including the feeling of intestines falling into the scrotum and the occurrence of swelling and pain, emphasize the repercussions of abdominal wall defense compromise (Bumeister et al., 2015). The clinical, as well as theoretical, importance of these pathologies lies in the manner in which they demonstrate the abdominal wall's protective function may be influenced by both intrinsic genetic and extrinsic environmental factors. Beyond human anatomy, comparative anatomical studies in other mammals continue to highlight the evolutionary significance of organ protection mechanisms. Studies of the reproductive organs of various mammalian species, including bats, illustrate structural variations that fulfill specialized physiological demands while preserving the integrity of critical organs (Bumeister et al., 2015). These morphological differences further work to emphasize how anatomical protection is adapted based on species-specific behavior and environmental stresses, ranging from reproductive behavior to hibernation patterns. This variation provides valuable insight into how the composition of protective zones within the body, like the abdominal wall and its weaknesses such as the inguinal canal, have developed to be optimized. This perspective provides depth to our knowledge regarding how structural weakness versus protective function in the abdominal region is traded off across species.

9.2.2. Role in Respiration

Apart from its well-characterized structural and protective functions, the abdominal wall plays a multifunctional role in respiratory mechanics. Synergistic contraction of abdominal wall muscles elevates intra-abdominal pressure, which supports the descent of the diaphragm during forceful expiration. This supports effective ejection of air from the lungs, particularly with activities that necessitate increased respiratory effort, such as exercise or coughing. Abdominal muscles stabilize the trunk and allow optimal lung volume through their opposition of passive thoracic expansion. This relationship of abdominal wall with the structures of the respiratory system emphasizes its function not only in ventilation but also in providing core stability, essential to successful respiratory mechanics. Furthermore, the inguinal region, a complex anatomical area of the lower abdominal wall, indirectly influences respiratory function through the impact it has on abdominal pressure relationships and musculature. Dysfunction or weakening in this region, as with inguinal hernias, is capable of altering the coordinated contraction of the abdominal muscles to be effective for breathing. Abdominal wall integrity disruption decreases the abdominal wall's ability to generate the pressure necessary for effective ventilation, particularly during forceful expiration. This points to the clinical significance of structural competence being preserved in the inguinal region to enhance respiratory effectiveness and overall functional well-being, demonstrating the interdependence between localized anatomical structure and systemic physiological process. Physiological pathways for the promotion of non-shivering thermogenesis and respiratory processes further demonstrate a preeminently critical role of the abdominal wall in respiration. While brown adipose tissue and its lipolytic activity have long been considered linked to thermogenesis, more recent information suggests that effective delivery of substrates and cardiac function are as central to the support of energy-extracting processes like respiration. This highlights that metabolic function and mobilization of nutrients in regions such as the abdominal wall helps facilitate respiratory muscles under increased demand. Understanding these stratified physiological interactions is key in integrative patient care, particularly cardiopulmonary and metabolic disease management (Jean-Ricco et al., 2017; Schreiber et al., 2017). The abdominal wall's role, therefore, is not merely mechanical, involving cardiovascular and metabolic thought critical for respiration.

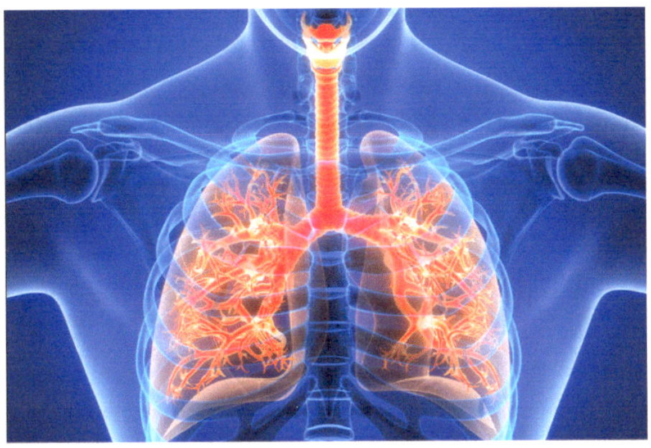

Source: RobinAge. (2024). Respiratory System Illustration.

9.2.3. Contribution to Posture and Movement

The abdominal wall is a major structure in the support of upright standing through the coordinated action of its connective tissues and its musculature. Rectus abdominis, external and internal obliques, and transversus abdominis muscles work synergistically to stabilize the trunk, especially under dynamic movement or static posture of long duration. Through the increase in intra-abdominal pressure, the abdominal wall stabilizes the lumbar spine, reducing load and hyperextension or excessive lordosis. This biomechanical function facilitates even weight distribution and spinal orientation necessary for efficient locomotion and less MSK strain. The region of the inguinal canal, being a transition zone, is preferred for this mechanical stability, as it allows for regulated hip and pelvic movement necessary for posture and gait. Thus, the structural and functional integrity of the abdominal wall is crucial in static and dynamic postural control. Initiation and regulation of movement are in great part reliant on the interaction of the abdominal wall with the rest of the core structures, playing its key function in the coordinated motion of the body. Under bending, twisting, or lifting movements, contraction of the abdominal muscles provides torsional stability and contributes to the production of force through the trunk and lower extremities. This interaction gives the pelvis and spine a stable platform, which facilitates the efficient transfer of muscular forces generating movement. The inguinal region also offers structures that react to pressure change and affect lower limb biomechanics, with effects on gait and stability. This might be compromised by weaknesses or hernias, causing inefficiencies in movement and posture. Therefore, the abdominal wall and inguinal region as a functional unit enable continuous execution of complex motor patterns necessary for everyday activities. In addition to mechanical participation, the abdominal wall and the inguinal region contribute to posture and movement through their interaction with vascular and neurological factors. Increased abdominal adiposity can put pressure on the inguinal area, and this can alter venous return as evidenced by changes in femoral vein diameter and tissue pressures during sitting positions (Wall, 2011). While this primarily affects circulatory dynamics, physiological changes such as these can affect muscle function indirectly by altering tissue oxygenation and fatigue resistance. Furthermore, proprioceptive feedback from abdominal wall muscles plays a part in postural reflexes, facilitating balance adjustment during movement. Though very little specific information is available concerning neurological control in the region (Mair, 1945), it is evident that the abdominal wall as well as the inguinal area is inclusively involved in posture maintenance and effective movement by structural, vascular, and neuromuscular means.

Test Your Knowledge

1. Discuss the Protection of Internal Organs
2. Explain the Contribution to Posture and Movement

9.3. Inguinal Region Anatomy

Learning Outcome

1. Discuss the Boundaries of the Inguinal Region
2. Describe the Structures Within the Inguinal Canal
3. Differentiate Between Male and Female Inguinal Anatomy

The inguinal region is complex because it is a transition zone between the abdominal cavity and the lower limb, which houses structures of paramount significance such as the inguinal canal to permit passage of the spermatic cord in men and the round ligament in women. This canal is created by the folds of the lower abdominal musculature and their aponeuroses, hence creating a passage of necessity for reproductive and vascular requirements but also one which is a possible site of weakness in the abdominal wall. The anatomy of this region lies at the heart of an understanding of the frequent clinical situations like inguinal hernias, which occur due to the bulging of contents of the abdomen through a weak inguinal canal. Despite advances in surgery, such anatomical vulnerability remains of relevance to patient management, as highlighted by the innovation of laparoscopic repair aiming to reinforce the canal with less morbidity and healing time (Hasslinda, 2010). The functional anatomy of the abdominal wall, especially the inguinal region, needs proper pedagogical approaches so that medical professionals can diagnose and treat related pathology correctly. The traditional anatomical education has the tendency to underestimate the surface anatomy for clinical practice, which relies on palpation and visual observation of deep structures. Innovative strategies of teaching, for instance, body painting, have demonstrated efficacy in the appreciation of space for this area by allowing students to observe musculature, vascular channels, and the intricacies of the inguinal canal on living subjects. This experiential education also appropriately aligns with the requirements of surgery training, facilitating increased recognition of anatomical landmarks throughout operations such as hernia repair and informing improved patient outcomes (Gomar et al., 2019). The correlation between anatomical complexity and clinical practice is particularly evident in the management of inguinal hernias, one of the most prevalent surgical diseases globally. Surgical techniques have progressively evolved from open to less invasive laparoscopic surgery that aims at the recovery of the patient and reduces postoperative complications. Knowledge of the layered anatomy of the region—the external oblique aponeurosis, internal oblique, transversus abdominis, and the transversalis fascia—is crucial for successful hernia repair. Modern practice affirms the value of learning anatomy to avoid nerve injury and offer long-term support of the posterior inguinal canal wall. Therefore, the anatomy of the groin remains a pillar in abdominal surgery and also in medical training (Hasslinda, 2010) (Figure 9.6).

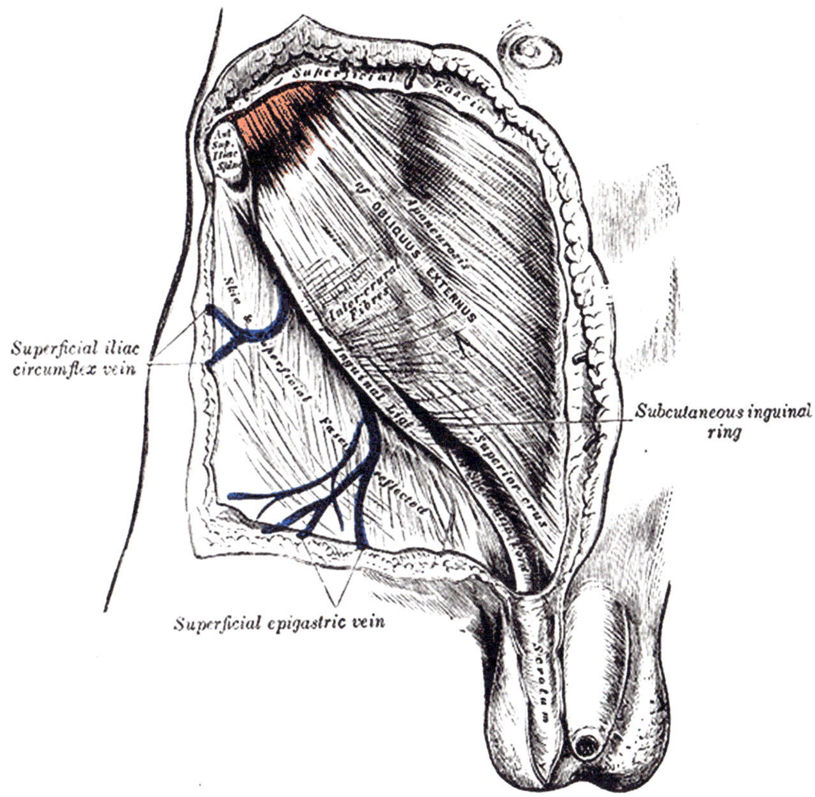

Figure 9.6. Inguinal region anatomy.

Source: By Henry Vandyke Carter - Henry Gray (1918) Anatomy of the Human Body (See "Book" section below)Bartleby.com: Gray's Anatomy, Plate 393, Public Domain, https://commons.wikimedia.org/w/index.php?curid=561483

9.3.1. Boundaries of the Inguinal Region

An understanding of the topography of the lower abdominal wall is vital for appreciating the complexity of the inguinal region, most notably in the clinical and surgical context. The inguinal region is an important site of intersection between the lower limb and abdomen, demarcated by several significant structures marking its border. Superiorly, the region is limited by the lower border of the abdominal wall, the inguinal ligament connecting the anterior superior iliac spine to the pubic tubercle. It is the base of the inguinal canal, a vital channel for the neurovascular components and the spermatic cord in males or round ligament in females. The lateral border is demarcated by the iliac crest, and it constitutes a structural framework that lies deep into the broader abdominal wall musculature, which plays an essential function in ensuring abdominal integrity (Hasslinda, 2010). Moving medially, the limits of the inguinal area are demarcated by the Linea semilunaris and the pubic tubercle, acting as indicators of the medial border of the inguinal canal. Behind it comes the transversalis fascia, a deep layer of the abdominal wall between the muscular layers and the peritoneum. It is involved in the formation of the posterior wall of the inguinal canal and thereby influences the susceptibility of this region to herniation. In addition, the conjoint tendon—a layer of the internal oblique and transversus abdominis muscles—represents a support on the medial aspect of the posterior wall that helps to reinforce this border to be more robust and resilient. The boundaries of the region in their entirety create a complex anatomical compartment essential for structural stability and passage of essential structures, making a thorough understanding of these boundaries essential to medicine (Hasslinda, 2010). Clinically, demarcating the borders of the inguinal area is very crucial, especially in the diagnosis and management of groin pathologies.

The proximity of the area to the pelvic viscera and lower limb circulation necessitates precise anatomical knowledge in the handling of conditions such as hernias, where abdominal contents protrude through the defects in the borders. The inguinal canal, demarcated by these borders, is a location of indirect and direct hernias, common clinical presentations requiring surgery. MRI and other imaging modalities have facilitated enhanced visualization of the anatomic structures of the inguinal region to better characterize these borders and disease processes. While much of the imaging interest lies in gynecologic cancer and local spread within the pelvis, anatomical boundary identification principles in the inguinal region continue to remain important to ensure appropriate treatment planning for a wide range of abdominal and pelvic pathologies.

9.3.2. Structures Within the Inguinal Canal

The inguinal canal is a significant channel in the inferior abdominal wall between the abdominal cavity and the external genitalia. The contents of males and females vary but contain some significant structures that are significant for physiological function and clinical importance. In the male, spermatic cord within the inguinal canal contains structures such as vas deferens, testicular artery, pampiniform plexus of veins, lymphatics, and autonomic nerves. These passages play a role in testicular function and temperature. In women, the round ligament of the uterus has its course through the passage, supporting the uterine support mechanism. The ilioinguinal nerve also makes its course and is involved in the sensory innervation of the groin. The intimate arrangement and proximity of these structures are the reasons why the inguinal canal is particularly susceptible to hernias, especially abdominal pressure dynamics cases (Autieri et al., 2015). Apart from supporting the reproductive and nervous elements, the inguinal canal also contains the cremasteric muscle fibers from the internal oblique muscle. These fibers encircle the spermatic cord in males and also cause the cremasteric reflex, which elevates the testes upon stimulation, helping to protect the testes from mechanical trauma and temperature changes. The canal itself is encased by several anatomical layers such as the external oblique aponeurosis, which constitutes the superficial inguinal ring, and the transversalis fascia, which constitutes the deep inguinal ring. This multi-layered structure offers a physiologically meaningful tunnel for the passage of structures and, simultaneously, a site of mutual vulnerability for weaknesses that render one vulnerable to herniation. Understanding these structures of the inguinal canal is critical in surgical management, particularly with the advent of laparoscopic techniques enhancing visualization and repair (Hasslinda, 2010). Clinically, the anatomy of the inguinal canal becomes very important while dealing with pathologies like inguinal hernias, which is one of the most common surgical disorders worldwide. The relationship between the contents of the canal and covering fascial layers will decide how and what type of hernias are presented to us. Direct hernias go through medial to the inferior epigastric vessels through the Hesselbach's triangle, and indirect hernias go through the course of the spermatic cord through the deep inguinal ring. These are important in using proper surgical repair techniques, especially in consideration of the likelihood of bladder involvement in massive hernias in older patients, where entities such as chronic bladder distention are involved in hernia formation (Autieri et al., 2015). Advances in technology in LIHR have improved results through the preservation of these complex frameworks and the reduction of complications, underlining the significance of detailed anatomical knowledge for effective treatment (Hasslinda, 2010) (Figure 9.7).

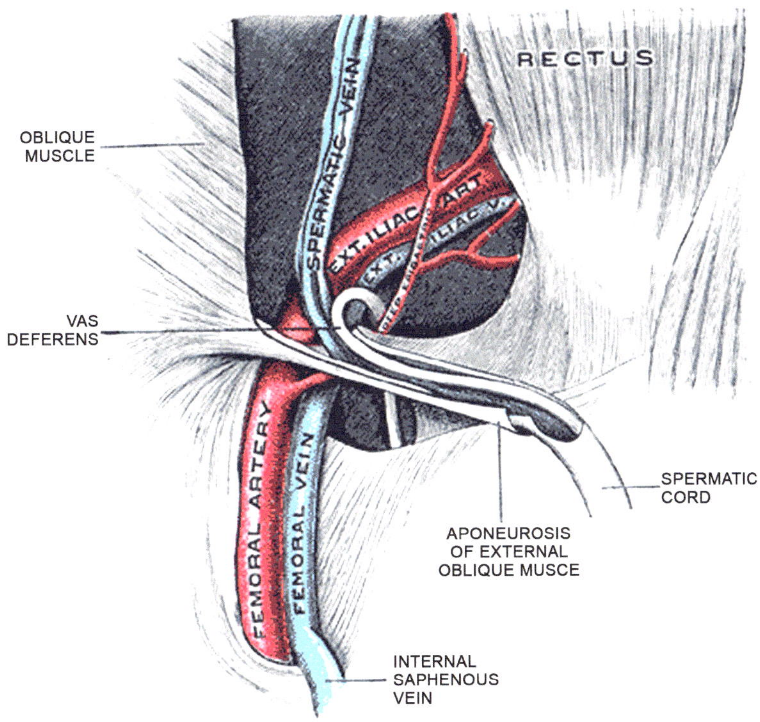

Figure 9.7. The inguinal canal.

Source: By Henry Vandyke Carter - Henry Gray (1918) Anatomy of the Human Body (See "Book" section below)Bartleby.com: Gray's Anatomy, Plate 1146, Public Domain, https://commons.wikimedia.org/w/index.php?curid=567115

9.3.3. Differences Between Male and Female Inguinal Anatomy

The deep inguinal structures differ markedly between the sexes, mainly due to their dissimilar reproductive anatomy. The spermatic cord, with the vas deferens, blood vessels, lymphatics, and nerves, is a significant conduit within the male inguinal canal. The canal itself is typically larger and more conspicuous due to the process of testicular descent during fetal development. However, in females, the inguinal canal is narrower and primarily transmits the round ligament of the uterus, which is not as large as the spermatic cord. This differential anatomy not only affects the canal's physical dimension but also its vulnerability to certain clinical conditions. The wider and more complex male inguinal canal makes men more susceptible to inguinal hernias, a pathological protrusion of intra-abdominal contents through the damaged canal,the role of gender-specific anatomy in clinical phenomena. The borders and supportive structures delimiting the inguinal canal further exhibit sexual differences crucial to its stability and integrity. In the man, the external oblique aponeurosis and internal obliques form a tight anterior wall, reinforced to hold within itthe spermatic cord structures. The deep inguinal ring, an opening in the transversalis fascia, is better developed in the man, to permit the passage of the spermatic cord. In the woman, these muscular and fascial elements are smaller by comparison, to match the minute round ligament. This anatomical difference affects the dynamic support of the inguinal region upon physical stress. The male inguinal canals complexity then demands increased muscular support against pathological weakening. A knowledge of these differential structural configurations is thus necessary in the diagnosis of such pathologies as athletic pubalgia, or sports hernia, and suitability of appropriate interventions, thereby emphasizing the importance of sex-specific anatomical knowledge in the clinic (Meyers et al., 2007). Beyond structural and functional variability, diagnostic techniques must also consider the unique ultrasonographic features of the inguinal region by sex. Imaging protocols identify hernias and other pathologies in both men and women, but anatomical variations necessitate individualized interpretation. For instance, the greater diameter and complex contents of the inguinal canals in men produce variant sonographic landmarks compared with women. The smaller diameter of the female inguinal canal and simpler content create less distinct imaging profiles, making accurate diagnosis more challenging. These reference values have been improved in research involving animal models to differentiate between normal variation and pathological change in both males and females (Gómez Martin et al., 2024). This quiet insight enables correct clinical assessment, ensuring appropriate identification of abdominal wall and inguinal region-related injuries in women and men, required for effective management and correct therapeutic choices.

Test Your Knowledge

1. What structure passes through the inguinal canal in females?
2. How does the content of the inguinal canal differ between males and females?

9.4. Inguinal Hernias

Learning Outcome

1. Definition and Types of Inguinal Hernias
2. Identify of Causes and Risk Factors
3. Focus on Symptoms and Diagnosis

Anatomy of the lower abdominal wall is a unifying principle to the pathophysiology of inguinal hernias. Inguinal space, with its complex interrelated muscle group, fasciae, and ligaments, imparts structural rigidity and areas of susceptibility through which contents of the abdomen can herniate. Especially noteworthy is that the inguinal canal contains a conduit through which the spermatic cord is in males and the round ligament in females, and, consequently, these can be the site of commonly recurring hernial development because they represent a relatively weak posterior wall due to natural weaknesses. Both susceptibility to and susceptibility from the anatomical structure as against intra-abdominal tension would determine an imbalance. Anatomical knowledge that is based on basic principles and clinical correlations increases insight into this balancing act, emphasizing the value of accurate anatomical instruction in clinical practice (Dagur et al., 2017). This basic knowledge is essential for accurate diagnosis and successful surgical repair of inguinal hernias. In clinical terms, inguinal hernias are marked by presentation and classification into direct and indirect types, each caused by varied anatomical defects. Indirect hernias go via the deep inguinal ring, along the path of the inguinal canal, often with an accompanying patent processus vaginalis, while direct hernias protrude through a weakening of the transversalis fascia in Hesselbach's triangle. Both distinctions are essential, as both the likelihood for complications of incarceration or strangulation and the mode of surgical treatment depend upon them. Diagnosing issues may be challenging because the conditions may share similar symptoms with other groin conditions, and hence proper evaluation methods are crucial. For example, some of the fluid accumulations such as hydroceles need to be differentiated from hernias so that they are not treated inappropriately, and hence proper clinical and imaging methods are crucial (Dagur et al., 2017). Therefore, the mixture of anatomy with clinical presentation is superior to patient outcomes in treating inguinal hernia. Treatment of inguinal hernias generally involves a multidisciplinary approach with surgical expertise in pathogenesis and patient-related factors.

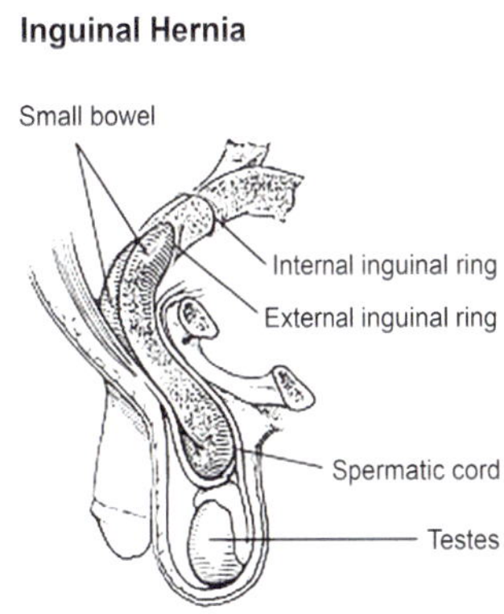

Figure 9.8. Inguinal hernias.

Source: By National Institutes of Health - http://digestive.niddk.nih.gov/ddiseases/pubs/dictionary/pages/e-k.htm, Public Domain, https://commons.wikimedia.org/w/index.php?curid=1819589

The laparoscopic and open repair will often reinforce the weakened abdominal wall, typically with mesh to reduce recurrence. Surgical technique development is driven by improvements in anatomical research and practice guidelines. Postoperative complications like chronic pain or mesh issues must also be carefully considered. In addition, patient education about risk factors, including increased intra-abdominal pressure from lifting heavy loads or being overweight, is a cornerstone of prevention strategies. Comprehensive care is improved through adherence to standardized anatomy curricula to aid trainees in having the depth of knowledge needed for competency in hernia repair, as promoted by educational consensus models (Hasslinda, 2010). Lastly, an integration of anatomical understanding with clinical skills enables increased therapeutic success and reduced morbidity of inguinal hernias (Figure 9.8).

9.4.1. Definition and Types of Inguinal Hernias

The abdominal wall plays an important role in holding the abdominal contents in place, but its anatomical weak points render certain areas of the wall more susceptible to herniation. Among these, the inguinal region is most susceptible to hernias due to the complex anatomy involving the inguinal canal, through which run structures such as the spermatic cord in males and the round ligament in females. An inguinal hernia happens when abdominal contents, usually parts of the intestine, protrude through an abdominal wall defect or weakness in the lower area near the inguinal canal. The protrusion may result in discomfort, pain, or complications if the hernia is strangulated or incarcerated. The clinical significance of the identification and classification of inguinal hernias is their prevalence and the need for their adequate management because the hernias account for a large proportion of abdominal wall hernias encountered by surgeons (Halvorsen et al., 2022). Inguinal hernias are primarily of two kinds: direct and indirect, depending on their anatomical relationship with the inferior epigastric vessels. Indirect inguinal hernias occur when abdominal contents enter the inguinal canal through the deep inguinal ring, lateral to the inferior epigastric vessels, typically along the track of the descended testes in males. Indirect inguinal hernias are usually congenital and result from a patent processus vaginalis. Direct inguinal hernias, on the other hand, protrude medial to the inferior epigastric vessels, arising from a posterior wall inguinal canal weakness in Hesselbach's triangle. These are more typically present later in life secondary to acquired factors, such as increased intra-abdominal pressure or degeneration of the abdominal musculature. Recognition of these distinctions is extremely important in surgical planning and prognostic assessment (Halvorsen et al., 2022). Both diagnosis and classification of inguinal hernias have important clinical implications given their changing symptomatology. Many patients are asymptomatic or minimally symptomatic, and a great many discover their hernia incidentally on medical exams. Acute pain secondary to bowel obstruction or strangulation, however, warrants urgent attention. It has been shown that while femoral hernias more frequently initially present with strangulation, inguinal hernias remain the most frequently surgically treated type worldwide, with advances in surgical technique significantly reducing recurrence rates. Management of asymptomatic hernias remains contentious; the evidence now stands confirming that elective repair can improve QoL and prevent significant complications without risk of chronic postoperative pain, emphasizing the importance of individualized treatment based on hernia type and patient status.

9.4.2. Causes and Risk Factors

The anatomy of the abdominal wall and inguinal area predisposes the area to some pathological conditions, arising from an interplay of intrinsic as well as extrinsic factors. Abnormalities in pelvic vasculature, for example, such as anomalous vessels taking off via the canal of the inguinal canal, create atypical presentation of pain and hematoma mimicking gynecological emergencies. Vascular anomalies may disturb normal circulation and result in compromised perfusion leading to acute presentation. One documented case was that of a patient with torsion accompanying an ovarian cyst whose presentation was complicated by an unusual blood vessel causing an inguinal hematoma.

Such anatomical variations depict the degree to which variation in pelvic and abdominal vascular anatomy is accountable for significant risk factors affecting the function and integrity of this region (Stallworth et al., 2025). Such vascular anomalies must be well understood to make an appropriate diagnosis and provide appropriate surgical care. The other significant cause of inguinal and lower abdominal wall morbidity is the development of hernias, which is mostly brought about by chronically increased intra-abdominal pressure. When the intra-abdominal pressure exceeds the tensile strength of the abdominal wall or contaminates standard anatomical openings such as the inguinal canal, protrusions of visceral content arise, hence leading to hernias. Indirect inguinal hernias, more common in men but occasionally seen in older women, typically result from such pressure gradients with congenital or acquired weakness of the inguinal region. Clinical practice demonstrates how hernias with bowel loops can produce life-threatening complications like bowel obstruction by compression of the vessels and ischemia of the hernia sac. These findings emphasize elevated intra-abdominal pressure as a significant risk factor in hernia development, under the influence of chronic coughing, heavy lifting, or straining (Hany et al., 2021).

Also, surgery performed on the abdominal or groin region can also present risks through tissue injury or iatrogenic trauma. Surgical procedures such as hernia repair or ablations can result in hematomas or inadvertent vascular injury as complications, particularly with unrecognized anomalous vessels during surgery. Postoperative hematomas of the inguinal region, although rare, have serious clinical implications, particularly if they mimic other acute pathologies such as adnexal torsion. This clinical overlap requires heightened sensitization and extensive imaging to distinguish postoperative complications from benign pelvic or abdominal emergencies. Anatomical variation and iatrogenic cause, therefore, must be considered significant etiologies of abdominal wall and inguinal area illnesses (Stallworth et al., 2025).

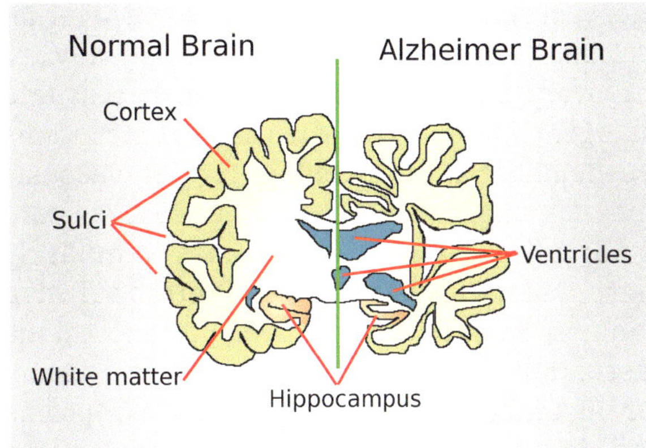

Source: By Garrondo - Own work, Public Domain, https://commons.wikimedia.org/w/index.php?curid=4387759

9.4.3. Symptoms and Diagnosis

The disorders of the abdominal wall and inguinal region can present with difficult clinical presentation and overlapping symptomatology of various conditions. The patients can also present with pain, swelling, or discoloration in the affected part, which can mimic other intra-abdominal pathology. For example, abnormal bruising or hematomas of the inguinal region can at times be a confusing symptom, which needs to be properly differentiated. On a few occasions, as indicated by a bizarre presentation with anomalous pelvic vasculature, symptoms such as acute pelvic pain with ipsilateral subcutaneous inguinal hematoma after physical exertion or intercourse. This indicates the importance of suspecting vascular anomalies on clinical examination because such presentations can also lead one to suspect gynecological emergencies such as ovarian torsion initially. Therefore, a careful history and physical examination with a focus on the onset, nature, and duration of symptoms can guide the diagnostic process in this anatomically challenging area (Stallworth et al., 2025). Diagnostic imaging is important to elucidate the cause of abdominal wall and inguinal-related symptoms. Ultrasonography, in particular transvaginal ultrasound, plays a significant role in evaluating adnexal structures and vascular perfusion. In suspected ovarian torsion, the absence of arterial blood flow to the ovary can both diagnose and necessitate emergent intervention. When atypical symptoms are hematomas or swelling, further vascular imaging might be required to demonstrate abnormal vessels or hematomas simulating more common pathologies. Intraoperative findings, such as the discovery of anomalous vascular branches within the inguinal canal, for instance, explain unexpected symptoms and improve outcomes when acted upon appropriately. Diagnostic studies, thus, need to be applied sparingly to discern typical from atypical causes of inguinal and abdominal wall pathology (Stallworth et al., 2025). In postoperative assessment and in the management of surgical defects in the abdominal and inguinal region, observation of symptoms may reveal complications or the success of attempts at reconstruction. In procedures like tumor excision, patients may present with distress because of large tissue defects that need to be reconstructed with reliable and low-morbidity techniques. Techniques such as the keystone flap have proven effective in the closure of large abdominal wall and inguinal wall defects, with enhanced symptom resolution and return of function. Careful follow-up of wound healing, pain, and development of infection or hematoma formation is crucial to ensuring flap viability and patient recovery overall. Thus, the addition of postoperative symptomatology to diagnosis and treatment planning ensures comprehensive care in the management of complex pathologies in this anatomical area.

Test Your Knowledge

1. How does increased intra-abdominal pressure contribute to hernia formation?
2. How does the location of the hernia sac relative to the inferior epigastric vessels help distinguish the two types?

9.5. Surgical Interventions

Learning Outcome

1. Discuss the Indications for Surgery
2. Focus on Common Surgical Techniques
3. Explain the Post-Operative Care and Recovery

Surgical intervention in the abdominal and inguinal walls must be based on a sophisticated understanding of the underlying pathology to most optimally deal with patient outcomes. Where conservatively managed treatments prove unhelpful or complications arise, the technique becomes critical. Inguinal disruption, for instance, and often referred to as a "sportsman's hernia," lacks a true hernial sac but exists as abnormal tension and micro-tears around the inguinal ligament and the external oblique aponeurosis. Surgical treatment applies relief of this tension, often supplemented with mesh or suture closure, aiming to re-establish mechanical stability without increasing tissue stress. This treatment emphasizes the need to treat anatomical defects and restore function. Individualized surgical methods such as these represent a trend toward multidisciplinary evaluation, allowing for precise diagnosis and targeted intervention for optimal recovery and return to function (Sheen et al., 2014). Controversy in abdominal wall surgery typically revolves around the application of mesh in hernia repair, particularly in the inguinal and femoral regions. Prosthetic mesh incorporation is now a norm in preventing the recurrence of hernias but is balanced against potential complications such as chronic pain, infection, or foreign body reaction. Comparative studies contrasting mesh with non-mesh closure techniques demonstrate mesh to have a significant relative benefit in terms of durability of long-term repair. Patient-related factors, including comorbidities and type of hernia, influence operative decisions significantly. Thus, the use of materials and techniques for repair must be individualized based on empirical data as well as clinical practice to minimize recurrence and maximize postoperative QoL (Lockhart et al., 2015). The dynamic topography of abdominal wall surgery also emphasizes the necessity of an integrated, holistic approach, particularly in complex inguinal disruption.

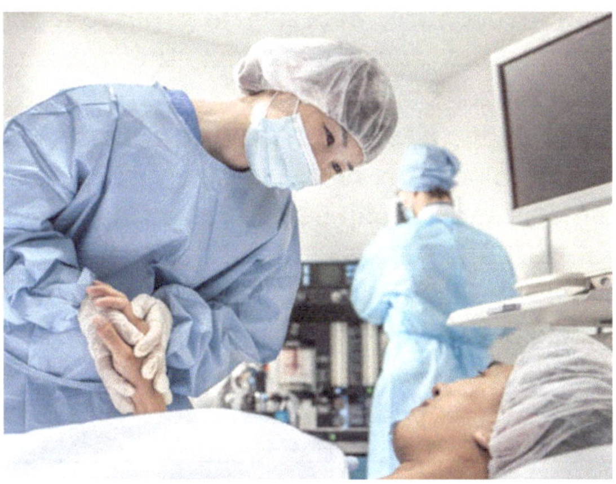

Source: Stridewell. (2021). Surgical Interventions.

The interface with physiotherapy and MSK radiology facilitates the preoperative assessment and postoperative rehabilitation, leading to better functional outcomes. Surgical repair is now viewed not as a single textural repair but as one part of an integrative continuum of treatment. The development of consensus protocols and national registries of surgical outcomes further underscores this trend, with standardized data at hand to refine techniques and optimize patient-centered care. This interdisciplinary intersection of surgical excellence with rehabilitative care is striking the new paradigm for treating disorders of the abdominal wall and inguinal region (Sheen et al., 2014).

9.5.1. Indications for Surgery

Surgical exploration of the abdominal wall and groin space is most commonly prompted by the clinical presentation of palpable lumps or swellings that may be simulating more common pathologies such as hernias. In a patient presenting with enlarging or persistent lumps, especially if accompanied by pain or signs of incarceration, the complete evaluation must not only consider common hernias, but less common ones such as soft tissue tumors. Misdiagnosis can lead to inappropriate management plans, as in the case of tumors like mammary-type myofibroblastoma being initially misdiagnosed as hernias. With obstructive or irreducible presentation, surgery then becomes necessary not only for symptom resolution but also for definitive diagnosis and treatment to avoid complications resulting from tumor growth or mismanagement (Kawakami et al., 2024). Clinical suspicion and imaging then help refine surgical indications in the region. In non-emergent situations, the presence of the abdominal wall and inguinal mesenchymal tumors is another principal reason for surgical intervention. While such tumors often encompass liposarcomas, leiomyosarcomas, and soft tissue sarcomas of other types, they are most often treated with radical surgical resection to achieve oncological control. Due to the presence of potential vascular and osteoarticular complications, surgical intervention should be highly preoperative-planned and carried out by a multidisciplinary group of surgeons with the participation of plastic and vascular surgeons. The technical challenge of such resections commonly necessitates sophisticated reconstructive approaches to attain abdominal wall integrity while preserving function. Tumor recurrence as a result of inadequate timely or effective intervention can develop into progression, rendering the course complicated and survival compromised (Jari et al., 2024). Suspected or established diagnosis of malignancy in this anatomic location therefore remains a strict surgical indication. Moreover, recurrence and chronicity of abdominal and inguinal wall diseases play a central role in making a patient suitable for surgery. Persistent lesions, recurrent hernia, or tumors with local aggressiveness are indications for an operation to prevent loss of function or complications such as obstruction or necrosis. Multidisciplinary therapy provides maximized outcomes by means of oncological security, preservation of function, and aesthetic reconstruction. Expert centers that can carry out these delicate resections emphasize referral to sarcoma centers or multi-surgical teams to achieve optimal patient outcomes. The necessity for surgery thus transcends imminent peril to encompass long-term functionality and QoL in individuals with disorders of the abdominal wall and groin (Jari et al., 2024; Kawakami et al., 2024).

9.5.2. Common Surgical Techniques

Inguinal surgery typically demands a multifaceted understanding of anatomical layers and the physiology of hernia formation. One of the key techniques employed in inguinal hernia treatment is open herniorrhaphy, which often entails reconstruction of the posterior wall of the inguinal canal. Among the various methods, the Modified Bassini's repair stands out due to its widespread application, particularly in regions with limited resources or where mesh availability is constrained. This technique involves suturing the transversalis fascia and conjoint tendon to the inguinal ligament, effectively reinforcing the posterior wall. The enduring relevance of the procedure is evidenced by a study noting its predominant use in over 79% of procedures in certain clinical settings, delivering a uniform combination of efficacy and cost-effectiveness. Surgical strategy under these circumstances is guided by the presentation of the patient and the infrastructure of health, influencing the choice of anesthesia, typically spinal, to optimize outcomes (Mabula & Chalya, 2012). Besides routine primary hernia repairs, surgeons need to be cognizant of atypical cases such as bladder hernias, which account for a minority but clinically significant proportion of inguinal hernias. These hernias also have a specific tendency to affect older patients and are attended by risks inherent in urinary obstruction and chronic bladder distention. Operative technique must therefore be modified not only to the hernial sac but also to the involved anatomy and pathology with bladder inclusion. In such a scenario, careful dissection to preserve bladder integrity is necessary to avert postoperative complications. The presence of pericystitis and protrusion of perivesical fat may complicate the repair procedure, necessitating personalized interventions. For this reason, the operation may extend beyond merely approximating tissues to include reduction and repair of the bladder, in support of the value of preoperative diagnosis and intraoperative versatility (Autieri et al., 2015). Mesh techniques, specifically the tension-free Lichtenstein repair, revolutionized inguinal hernia surgery by significantly reducing recurrence and postoperative pain. Despite its advantages, application is variable across the globe depending on the resource availability, and in a few centers, there has been minimal application of mesh repairs. Where used, the Lichtenstein procedure involves closure of the posterior wall defect using a synthetic mesh in a tension-free manner to permit tissue ingrowth and mechanical strengthening. While mesh repairs allow for quicker recovery and elective procedural success, emergent cases may require other actions, such as potential bowel resection in the context of strangulation or obstruction. Results after surgery are directly linked to timing, patient condition, and procedure type; elective mesh procedures under spinal anesthetic thus dominate where feasible, underlining the benefit of early intervention in minimizing complication rates and hospitalization durations (Mabula & Chalya, 2012).

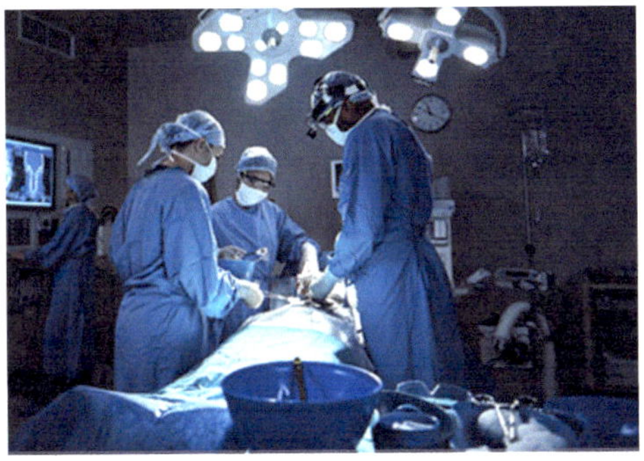

Source: Johns Hopkins Medicine. (n.d.). Common Surgical Procedures.

9.5.3. Post-Operative Care and Recovery

Successful outcomes from the abdominal wall and inguinal region operations rely on meticulous post-operative management to minimize complications and enhance patient outcomes. The evolution of specialized surgical programs, such as the robotic abdominal wall service (AWS), has demonstrated the benefit of dedicated teams focusing exclusively on hernia repairs to achieve optimal outcomes. These programs focus on regular follow-ups, personalized pain management strategies, and mobilization at an early point to restrict the dangers of wound infection and deep vein thrombosis. As complex and variable as these procedures are, lengthy post-operative protocols must address physical in addition to psychological arenas to advance rehabilitation. This coordinated care has been shown to reduce hospital stay and post-operative pain, allowing earlier return to daily activities and improving patient satisfaction overall (Gilmore et al., 2025). Post-operative monitoring is necessary to identify early complications in the form of seroma formation, infection, or hernia recurrence, particularly in the inguinal region where anatomical complexity can pose special challenges. Imaging modalities like ultrasound are especially crucial during this phase because high-resolution sonography is a non-invasive, accurate method of assessing wound healing and detecting residual or emergent pathology without exposing patients to ionizing radiation. Researchers have noted the legitimacy of ultrasound for verifying intraoperative findings and guiding clinical decision-making during the recovery. This diagnostic tool augments clinical examination, enabling precise evaluation of the surgical site and allowing for early intervention when indicated, eventually contributing to improved patient outcomes (Saran et al., 2024). Postoperative care in addition to clinical surveillance should comprise patient education regarding restriction of activities, wound care, and symptom recognition to empower patients during recovery. Those undergoing minimally invasive procedures, such as robot-assisted hernia repairs, have less pain and earlier mobilization compared to traditional open techniques but still require adequate counseling to prevent complications. The commitment of multidisciplinary teams of surgeons, nurses, and rehabilitation specialists provides a culture of cooperation and support necessary for recovery. By coupling novel surgical approaches with expert post-operative care pathways, centers of excellence can be developed by healthcare organizations that enhance long-term recovery and QoL in individuals with abdominal wall and inguinal hernias (Gilmore et al., 2025).

Test Your Knowledge

1. What factors influence the decision between elective and emergency hernia repair?
2. What are the main surgical techniques used to repair inguinal hernias?

9.6. Clinical Significance

Learning Outcome

1. Discuss the Common Disorders of the Abdominal Wall
2. How to Impact of Inguinal Hernias on Quality of Life (QoL)
3. Focus on Preventive Measures and Education

An understanding of the complex anatomy of the abdominal wall is necessary for successful operations, particularly hernia repair. The layered anatomy with transversalis fascia and preperitoneal fascia offers isolated planes that are critical during operations such as totally extraperitoneal herniorrhaphy (TEP). Accuracy of movement within the planes reduces risks such as damage to vessels or incomplete repair of the hernia. The separation between the parietal and visceral planes, given by interfascial planes theory, enables safer dissection and explains anatomical variations that occur during surgery. An example is the knowledge of the "holy plane" in the median region providing an avascular path beneficial in minimizing intraoperative bleeding. Besides, the recognition of the transition between these planes assists surgeons in managing complex hernia loops and spaces characteristic of the inguinal region, enhancing procedure precision (Li J-Wen, 2019). The clinical significance of the abdominal wall extends to include uncommon pathologies that impact this region and adjacent structures. Abdominal cocoon (AC), a disease with fibrotic entrapment of the small bowel, emphasizes the importance of full preoperative investigation, especially in patients with unusual hernias or chronic bowel obstruction symptoms. While uncommon, AC demonstrates how pathological abnormalities in or around the abdominal wall can present with common clinical presentations such as umbilical hernias, thus posing diagnostic difficulty. Imaging modalities such as computed tomography (CT) have proved to be highly valuable in the differentiation of the condition by showing typical bowel encapsulation and thickened membranes. Emergency surgical treatment through a combination of laparoscopic and open procedures enables both diagnosis and effective treatment, highlighting the increasing role of minimally invasive surgery in treating conditions of the abdominal wall (Zhang et al., 2015). Postoperative management and adhesion protection are equally significant factors that influence long-term outcomes in abdominal wall repair. The thin edge between accurate membranous dissection and avoiding irritation of the peritoneum determines the risk of adhesion-related complications such as bowel obstruction or recurrent hernia recurrence. The use of adjuvant therapies, such as anti-adhesion medications like sodium hyaluronate gel, has been encouraging to reduce postoperative fibrosis, but further work is needed to substantiate their efficacy, most notably in atypical diseases like the AC. Furthermore, appendectomy as a chance discovery during operation on the abdominal wall can reduce the likelihood of subsequent complications, showing the end-to-end process that goes into planning surgery. These strategies emphasize the balance between knowledge of anatomy, surgical expertise, and postoperative care in optimizing the patient's recovery and reducing recurrence (Li, 2019; Zhang et al., 2015) (Figure 9.9).

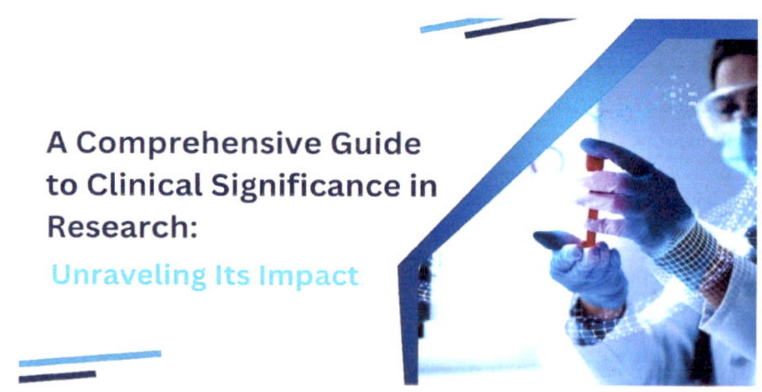

Figure 9.9. Clinical significance.

Source: LLRI. (2023). A Comprehensive Guide to Clinical Significance in Research: Unraveling its Impact.

9.6.1. Common Disorders of the Abdominal Wall

In the athletic setting, groin pain assessment often illustrates multifactorial overlapping pathologies that hinder accurate diagnosis and treatment. Athletes are particularly apt to present with chronic pain where abdominal musculature converges on the pubis, an area prone to a variety of disorders. Of these, core muscle injury, or sports hernia or athletic pubalgia, is more recognized due to its insidious onset and resistive diagnosis. The condition is most commonly linked to posterior inguinal canal wall and distal rectus abdominis tendon damage, occasionally combined with adductor longus tendinopathy. The diagnosis depends significantly on sound clinical examination due to the fact that imaging studies such as MRI are known to underestimate the severity of injury. Dynamic ultrasonography is being established as a more sensitive tool for evaluation. Conservative rehabilitation can restore function but persistent symptoms more than 12 weeks of follow-up typically necessitate surgical intervention, typically mesh repair and conjoined tendon myotomy. Early identification is of vital importance for treatment success and return to activity (Julianne et al., 2022). Hernias, also known as inguinal hernias, are another prevalent abdominal wall disorder with a high percentage of abdominal wall defects worldwide. These hernias are caused by defects in the abdominal fascial layers and musculature, which permit protrusion of intra-abdominal contents through the inguinal canal or femoral ring. Although they might first be noted as asymptomatic bulges, complications of incarceration and strangulation cause acute abdominals necessitating emergent surgical intervention. Although inguinal hernias are common after repetitive strain or degeneration of the abdominal wall with age, they can also be one of the causes of the attacks of small bowel obstruction (SBO). One must recall that in young and healthy individuals with no conventional risk factors, hernias can cause obstruction, usually complicating the clinical picture. Imaging studies like CT can identify the herniated bowel loops, contributing to diagnosis as well as treatment planning (Emily et al., 2021). Other than hernias and athletic trauma, less frequent but clinically important abdominal wall pathology includes traumatic abdominal wall defects like hematomas of blunt trauma. They, too, can masquerade as more frequent intra-abdominal illnesses, so differential diagnosis is even more difficult. Congenital weakness or defect, too, can predispose the patient to rupture of the muscle across, rupture of the fascia across, or neurovascular entrapment syndromes in the inguinal area. These pathologies highlight the importance of thorough patient history and physical examination supplemented by focused imaging. Multidisciplinary care involving surgical, rehabilitative, and sometimes interventional radiologic expertise optimizes results in each instance. Familiarity with the obscure presentations and pathophysiology of abdominal wall conditions ensures proper diagnosis and tailored therapy to restore functional integrity in impaired patients.

9.6.2. Impact of Inguinal Hernias on Quality of Life (QoL)

Early medical intervention and advancement of inguinal hernias are apt to exacerbate complications, directly influencing the general well-being of patients. Long-term presence of hernias is likely to lead to obstructions, strangulation, and irreducibility, events that not only increase morbidity but also prolong hospital stay, hence disrupting normal working and living routines. Research has indicated that the majority of patients, particularly in more resource-poor settings, present only after several years of symptoms, resulting in a high rate of emergency operations and their consequences. This plight increases the physiological and psychological burden on the individual, highlighting the crucial relationship between early intervention and QoL. Moreover, chronic pain and functional impairment related to hernias disrupt day-to-day life, exacerbate stress, and lower satisfaction with life. Early diagnosis and elective repair are underscored in studies showing reduced complications and improved postoperative recovery when procedures are done before emergency stages are reached (Mabula & Chalya, 2012). Other than mechanical symptoms, the consequences of surgical repair also present other challenges that impact patients' long-term QoL. Recurrent pain, or inguinodynia, frequently complicates open and laparoscopic herniorrhaphy based on tissue inflammation and prosthetic mesh presence. Although the majority of patients experience mild to moderate pain, a considerable percentage experience severe pain that limits normal physical activities and considerably impairs work and social life. Chronic pain negatively affects psychological well-being by causing anxiety and depression, further impairing postoperative recovery and QoL. The recurrence of inguinodynia emphasizes the need for greater diagnosis and pain control techniques, with particular attention to scrupulous anatomical care at surgery and individualized postoperative management. Pain complications must be addressed to optimize the overall impact of hernia correction on patient-reported outcomes (Ceballos-Villalva et al., 2020). Inguinal hernia-related impairment in QoL is both physical disability and psychosocial distress and reflects the complex interrelationship between clinical and personal factors. The health burden extends beyond symptomatology to impact emotional well-being, as frustration and decreased self-esteem are prevalent among patients due to activity restriction or appearance concerns. Furthermore, socioeconomic consequences can arise from prolonged absenteeism and impaired functional capacity, endangering livelihood and contributing to the cost burden of society. Evidence confirms that success with surgery is no guarantee for restored QoL; sustained support, tailored rehabilitation, and chronic pain management are crucial for complete recovery. Multidisciplinary approaches involving medical, surgical, and psychological management are therefore recommended to address the multifaceted impact of inguinal hernias and improve patient well-being in short- and long-term views (Mabula & Chalya, 2012; Ceballos-Villalva et al., 2020) (Figure 9.10).

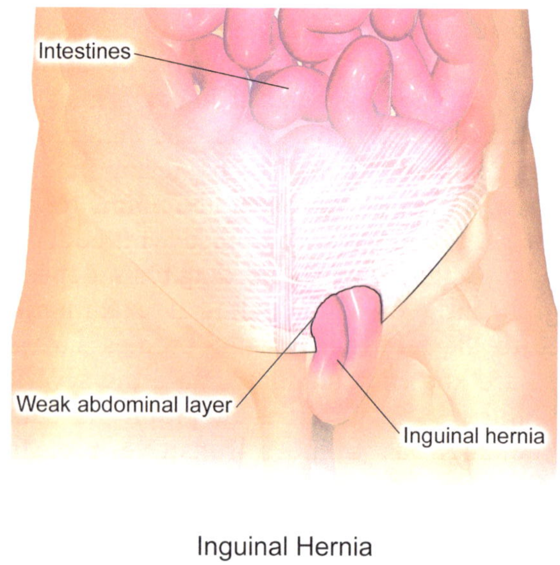

Figure 9.10. Impact of inguinal hernias on quality of life (QoL).

Source: By BruceBlaus. When using this image in external sources it can be cited as:Blausen.com staff (2014). "Medical gallery of Blausen Medical 2014". WikiJournal of Medicine 1 (2). DOI:10.15347/wjm/2014.010. ISSN 2002-4436. - Own work, CC BY 3.0, https://commons.wikimedia.org/w/index.php?curid=31118600

9.6.3. Preventive Measures and Education

Successful health provision has as much to do with greater than cure; it involves attention to prevention and patient education, particularly where rates of prevalent conditions such as the abdominal wall and the inguinal area are high. Prevention from such is at least partly founded on minimizing the risk for hernias and other abdominal wall problems through the promotion of strengthening exercises in the core and proper lifting habits. Patient education on modifiable risk factors such as obesity, smoking, and chronic cough is essential to reducing intra-abdominal pressure that causes predisposition to herniation. Along with this, awareness campaigns for early recognition of symptoms can facilitate on-time medical consultation and intervention. An overall educational model educates patients not just about anatomical susceptibility but also about lifestyle changes that guarantee the integrity of the abdominal wall. Educational programs that are structured thus occupy a central place in minimizing morbidity in abdominal and inguinal conditions, affirming that prevention is a cornerstone of care management in the anatomical region (Tong, 2018). The nature of the inguinal region, with its convoluted anatomical landmarks and novel physiological behaviors, demands tailored educational methods for both patients and clinical workers. Curriculums that emphasize anatomical data, pathophysiology, and clinical competencies improve patient outcomes and accurate diagnostics. Additionally, technology advancements in regional anesthesia approaches enabled minimally invasive procedures, reducing postoperative complications and shortening recovery but requiring clinicians to achieve superior anatomical familiarity and technical expertise beyond their usual education (Halvorsen et al., 2022). Tailored educational interventions can enhance practitioner competence in procedures such as ultrasound-guided inguinal nerve blocks, thereby optimizing prevention anesthesia protocols. By integrating anatomical education alongside the evolution of clinical practices, institutions can build safer and more efficient prevention measures. Ongoing professional development for regional anatomy is thus a primary factor in reducing iatrogenic injuries and improving patient safety for abdominal and inguinal treatment (N/A, 2022). Preventive care policies incorporate patient-centered educational outreach to address the demographic and socioeconomic disparities impacting disease prevalence in abdominal wall and inguinal regions. Research indicates that socioeconomic, provider, and patient risk profiles continually shape the utilization of preventive services (Tong, 2018). Interventions should therefore be context-dependent to promote equitable access to proper health information and screening where needed. For example, community-based prevention programs can demystify the risk of hernias and encourage earlier health encounters before complications. Of equal importance is making prevention communication culturally specific to engage diverse populations, and coupling culturally competent communication to close gaps in health literacy. Prevention is thus no longer confined to health settings but extends to public health infrastructure, aligning individual risk reduction with system-level strategies towards the alleviation of abdominal and inguinal disease burden. This integrated approach points to the necessity of integrating education as a fundamental principle of preventive health interventions (Tong, 2018).

Test Your Knowledge

1. Differentiate between direct and indirect inguinal hernias based on anatomical location.
2. What are the boundaries of the inguinal (Hesselbach's) triangle?

SUMMARY

The complex abdominal wall and inguinal anatomy underscores the importance of proper diagnosis and individualized treatment protocols. Such conditions as inguinal disruption demonstrate beyond typical hernia classifications complexities that involve defective tension and tissue integrity rather than actual herniation, which requires a delicate distinction to avoid misdiagnosis and proper application of therapy. By emphasizing a multidisciplinary team that includes surgeons, radiologists, and physiotherapists, it is ensured that individually tailored plans of care address the biomechanical and structural differences of the region. It encourages consistency in standards of care while maximizing results through combining experience from various disciplines to thoroughly understand and deal with these complex presentations (Sheen et al., 2014). Additionally, the variable clinical presentation of abdominal wall and inguinal diseases requires the clinician to be vigilant and exclude rare presentations. Inguinal hernias, for instance, may sometimes present with other abdominal wall swellings such as Spigelian hernias and thus diagnosis and management would be a challenge. Such diagnostic challenges combined with predisposing factors such as compromise of the abdominal wall in certain populations necessitates the application of high-level imaging technology combined with appropriate clinical examination to avoid misinterpretation. Understanding differential mechanisms behind such presentations is thus in favor of developing exact surgical procedures, crucial in recurrence and complication prevention. Thus, ensuring that the importance of individualized, evidence-based clinical pathways in treating abdominal wall and inguinal diseases is upheld (Diop et al., 2011). Therefore, the complex interaction between pathological processes and anatomical differences along the abdominal wall and inguinal region emphasizes the need for a strategic, evidence-based treatment approach. Consensus over nomenclature and multidisciplinary management not only properly demystifies ambiguity associated with conditions such as inguinal disruption but also promotes standardized approaches that simplify patient care. The adoption of targeted physiotherapy as a first-line measure with selective surgery as indicated is a model of forward-thinking management. Furthermore, the adoption of national registries and the promotion of continuous collaborative research are essential to the optimization of therapeutic approaches and outcomes. These high-level initiatives keep the delivery of care responsive, precise, and aligned with evolving clinical acumen (Sheen et al., 2014).

The thorough analysis of the inguinal and abdominal wall anatomy is shown to exist in complex association between the necessary anatomical structures for both clinical management and function. Improved outcomes from surgery, especially that involving inguinal hernia repair, have been made possible due to refinements in the methods of surgical approach and the use of mesh. The Swedish Hernia Register offers a vast database showing the shift in surgical methods, noting that day-case procedures have risen and recurrence rates have decreased during the past three decades. These findings illustrate the necessity of choosing appropriate surgical methods based on patient population traits, like laparo-endoscopic procedures being more advantageous to females and open mesh repair being more effective in males. Furthermore, registry data quality and quantity reinforce the robustness of these findings, with implications for decision-making in evidence-based practice (Axman et al., 2024). Apart from surgical procedures, the complex dynamic between abdominal wall integrity and patient QoL presents as a key area of interest. Incomplete abdominal wall hernias impact patients in both physical and psychosocial realms, influencing mental health, body image, and interpersonal relationships. Recent qualitative research that has employed interpretative phenomenological analysis has provided insights into how patients cope with disruptions in identity, mobility restrictions, and accommodation in social and sexual relationships. These sophisticated effects highlight the necessity of overall evaluations beyond biological restoration, such as emotional and social well-being in patient care. As such, there has been an increasing acknowledgment that current health-related quality of life (HRQOL) tools poorly reflect such complex patient experiences and a key area for future study and tool development is therefore identified (Smith, 2021). In collating the most important information concerning the abdominal wall and the inguinal area, it can be seen that patient-reported outcomes need to inform both clinical practice and research. The interplay of large-scale registries and patient-reported outcomes provides a solid foundation for assessing interventions that reduce recurrence, postoperative pain, and complications. However, this clinical focus must be followed by comprehension of what is most important to patients, particularly in complex cases where the social and emotional effect of the hernia is severe. The double emphasis on technical competence and holistic wellbeing demonstrates the evolving pattern of hernia management, toward future orientation in individualized approaches aimed at addressing not only anatomical fixation but also the general QoL needs of patients (Axman et al., 2024 Smith, 2021).

KEY TERMS FROM THIS CHAPTER

- Abdominal cavity
- Anatomical disposition
- Elastic tissue layers
- Fetal development
- Ilioinguinal nerve
- Inferior epigastric vessels
- Abdominal organ placement
- Bladder distention
- Excessive lordosis
- Gynecological emergencies
- Incisional hernias (IH)

CRITICAL THINKING QUESTIONS

1. **Which of the following is the most superficial layer of the anterior abdominal wall?**
   a. Transversalis fascia
   b. External oblique muscle
   c. Camper's fascia
   d. Rectus abdominis
2. **Which muscle contributes to the formation of the inguinal ligament?**
   a. Internal oblique
   b. Transversus abdominis
   c. External oblique
   d. Rectus abdominis
3. **The deep inguinal ring is located in which layer?**
   a. External oblique aponeurosis
   b. Internal oblique muscle
   c. Transversalis fascia
   d. Peritoneum
4. **Which of the following passes through the inguinal canal in females?**
   a. Vas deferens
   b. Round ligament of the uterus
   c. Ureter
   d. Femoral artery
5. **The conjoint tendon is formed by the fusion of:**
   a. Internal oblique and external oblique
   b. Internal oblique and transversus abdominis
   c. External oblique and transversus abdominis
   D. Rectus abdominis and transversus abdominis

Short Answer Questions

1. What is the inguinal ligament and how is it formed anatomically?
2. Define the deep and superficial inguinal rings and describe their locations.
3. What is the significance of the transversalis fascia in the inguinal region?
4. What is the conjoint tendon and what is its clinical significance?
5. Describe the contents of the spermatic cord.
6. Explain the function and innervation of the muscles of the abdominal wall.

Answers to Critical Thinking Questions

1. (c) 2. (c) 3. (c) 4. (b) 5. (b)

REFERENCES

1. Abu Hassan, Hasslinda (2010) Study of feasibility of laparoscopic inguinal hernia surgery in taiping hospital. Masters thesis, Universiti Sains Malaysia. (accessed on 8th May 2025).
2. Axman, E. (2024). Outcomes of Inguinal Hernia Surgery: Combining and Exploring Data from National Registers in Sweden. https://core.ac.uk/download/620671317.pdf (accessed on 8th May 2025).
3. Bumeister, V. I., Prykhodko, O. O., Sulym, L. H., Tkach, T., et al. (2015). Supporting and Locomotor Apparatus. Sumy : Sumy State University, 2022. – 207 p. https://core.ac.uk/download/141445231.pdf (accessed on 8th May 2025).
4. Ceballos-Villalva, J. C., Contreras-Flores, E. H., Corona-Torres, M. J., García-Olivo, A., et al. (2020). Incidence and Management of Inguinodynia After Inguinal Plasty. https://core.ac.uk/download/539913526.pdf (accessed on 8th May 2025).
5. Dagur, G., Gandhi, J., Suh, Y., Weissbart, S., Sheynkin, Y., Smith, N. L., Joshi, G., et al. (2017). Classifying hydroceles of the pelvis and groin: An overview of etiology, secondary complications, evaluation, and management. Current Urology, 10, 1–14. https://doi.org/10.1159/000447145 (accessed on 8th May 2025).
6. Diop, B., Konate, I., Ka, S., Fall, D., Sy, A., Wone, Y., & Sarre, S. M. (2011). Indirect inguinal hernia masquerading as a Spigelian hernia. Hernia : the journal of hernias and abdominal wall surgery, 15(5), 579–581. https://doi.org/10.1007/s10029-010-0698-4 (accessed on 8th May 2025).
7. Forlizzi, J. M., Ward, M. B., Whalen, J. M., Wuerz, T. H., & Gill, T. (2022). Core muscle injury: Evaluation and treatment in the athlete. The American Journal of Sports Medicine, 51, 1087–1095. https://www.semanticscholar.org/paper/db06326a61b6d0dbe8b354504768b18fb3fb613d (accessed on 8th May 2025).
8. Glaser, J., Pearl, J., Wind, G., & Sheppard, F. (2011). Laparoscopic repair of a large interstitially incarcerated inguinal hernia. Journal of surgical case reports, 2011(3), 2. https://doi.org/10.1093/jscr/2011.3.2(accessed on 8th May 2025).
9. Gómez Martin, N., Domínguez Miño, E., García de Carellán, A., & Vilalta Solé, L. (2024). Abdominal ultrasound features and reference values in healthy guinea pigs (Cavia porcellus). The Veterinary record, 194(2), e3668. https://doi.org/10.1002/vetr.3668 (accessed on 8th May 2025).
10. Halvorsen, S., Mehilli, J., Cassese, S., Hall, T. S., Abdelhamid, M., Barbato, E., De Hert, S., et al. (2022). 2022 ESC guidelines on cardiovascular assessment and management of patients undergoing non-cardiac surgery. European Heart Journal, 43, 3826–3924. https://doi.org/10.1093/eurheartj/ehac270 (accessed on 8th May 2025).
11. Lee, S., Kassam, Z., Baheti, A., Hope, T. A., Chang, K. J., Korngold, E., Taggart, M. W., et al. (2023). Rectal cancer lexicon 2023 revised and updated consensus statement from the Society of Abdominal Radiology Colorectal and Anal Cancer Disease-Focused Panel. Abdominal Radiology, 48, 2792–2806. https://doi.org/10.1007/s00261-023-03893-2 (accessed on 8th May 2025).
12. Lockhart, K., Dunn, D., Teo, S., Ng, J. Y., Dhillon, M., Teo, E., & van Driel, M. L. (2018). Mesh versus non-mesh for inguinal and femoral hernia repair. The Cochrane database of systematic reviews, 9(9), CD011517. https://doi.org/10.1002/14651858.CD011517.pub2 (accessed on 8th May 2025).

13. Mabula, J. B., & Chalya, P. L. (2012). Surgical management of inguinal hernias at Bugando Medical Centre in northwestern Tanzania: our experiences in a resource-limited setting. BMC research notes, 5, 585. https://doi.org/10.1186/1756-0500-5-585 (accessed on 8th May 2025).

14. Mair, G. B. (1945). An Investigation Into the Surgical Problems of Inguinal, Femoral, Umbilical, Ventral and Certain Other Types of Abdominal Hernia with a Description of a New Principle of Repair Using whole Skin Grafts in Place of Fascia. https://core.ac.uk/download/287590045.pdf (accessed on 8th May 2025).

15. McNair, T. J. (1960). Observations on Visceral Pain with Special Reference to Pain Originating in the Testis. https://core.ac.uk/download/429728301.pdf (accessed on 8th May 2025).

16. Meyers, William & Yoo, Edward & Devon, Octavia & Jain, Nikhil & Horner, Marcia & Lauencin, Cato & Zoga, Adam. (2007). Understanding "Sports Hernia" (Athletic Pubalgia): The Anatomic and Pathophysiologic Basis for Abdominal and Groin Pain in Athletes. Department of Radiology Faculty Papers. 20. 10.1053/j.otsm.2007.09.001. (accessed on 8th May 2025).

17. Sala, E., Rockall, A., Freeman, S., Mitchell, D. G., & Reinhold, C. (2013). The added role of MR imaging in treatment stratification of patients with gynecologic malignancies: What the radiologist needs to know. Radiology, 266, 717–740. https://doi.org/10.1148/radiol.12120315 (accessed on 8th May 2025).

18. Sanders, D. L., Pawlak, M., Simons, M. P., Aufenacker, T., Balla, A., Berger, C., Berrevoet, F., et al. (2023). Midline incisional hernia guidelines: The European Hernia Society. British Journal of Surgery, 110, 1732–1768. https://doi.org/10.1093/bjs/znad284 (accessed on 8th May 2025).

19. Sheen, A. J., Stephenson, B. M., Lloyd, D. M., Robinson, P., Fevre, D., Paajanen, H., de Beaux, A., Kingsnorth, A., Gilmore, O. J., Bennett, D., Maclennan, I., O'Dwyer, P., Sanders, D., & Kurzer, M. (2014). 'Treatment of the sportsman's groin': British Hernia Society's 2014 position statement based on the Manchester Consensus Conference. British journal of sports medicine, 48(14), 1079–1087. https://doi.org/10.1136/bjsports-2013-092872 (accessed on 8th May 2025).

20. Smith, C. F., Finn, G. M., Stewart, J. A., Atkinson, M., Davies, D. C., Dyball, R. E. J., Morris, J. F., et al. (2015). The Anatomical Society core regional anatomy syllabus for undergraduate medicine. Journal of Anatomy, 228, 15–23. https://doi.org/10.1111/joa.12405 (accessed on 8th May 2025).

21. Smith, O. (. A. M. A phenomenological study of the lived experiences of patients with complex abdominal wall hernia (CAWH). (Thesis). Hull York Medical School, the University of Hull and the University of York. https://hull-repository.worktribe.com/output/4223783 (accessed on 8th May 2025).

22. Tong, J. (2018). Influence of Patient and Provider Characteristics on the Overuse of Health Care Services. https://core.ac.uk/download/211354948.pdf (accessed on 8th May 2025).

23. van Ramshorst, G. H., Kleinrensink, G. J., Hermans, J. J., Terkivatan, T., & Lange, J. F. (2009). Abdominal wall paresis as a complication of laparoscopic surgery. Hernia : the journal of hernias and abdominal wall surgery, 13(5), 539–543. https://doi.org/10.1007/s10029-009-0473-6 (accessed on 8th May 2025).

24. Wall, Michael Lewis (2011). The effect of obesity on venous impedance and outflow measured by ultrasound. University of Birmingham. M.D. (accessed on 8th May 2025).

ABDOMEN REGION

10

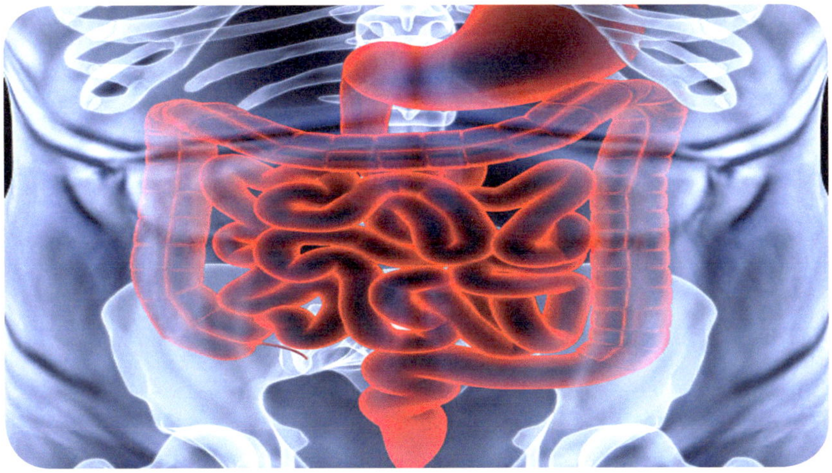

LEARNING OBJECTIVES

After studying this chapter, you will be able to:

1. Focus on the anatomy of the abdomen
2. Understand the functions of the abdomen
3. Discuss the common disorders of the abdomen
4. Know the health and wellness of the abdomen

Introduction

The human abdomen, located between the thorax and pelvis, is a significant region for different physiological processes and houses essential organs. The area not only serves digestion but also serves multiple vital functions in metabolism, immunity, and even emotional health. This muscle, fat, and connective tissue system stabilizes these organs structurally and makes them functionally effective. In addition, being aware of the different parts of the abdomen can help one realize larger health issues, as conditions of the abdomen and pain from the abdomen often act as an indicator of overall conditions. To investigate the abdomen, one needs to look into the gastronomical systems, the abdominal muscles' contribution to physical health, and how sicknesses in the area can influence overall health. Thus, proper observation of the abdomen not only enhances our understanding of human body anatomy but also tells us how important it is to maintain health and well-being.

Definition of the Abdomen Region

The abdomen, an essential region of the human body, is anatomically described as the area between the diaphragm and pelvis. This area holds essential organs of digestion, such as the stomach, intestines, liver, and spleen, together with important structures of the circulatory and endocrine systems.

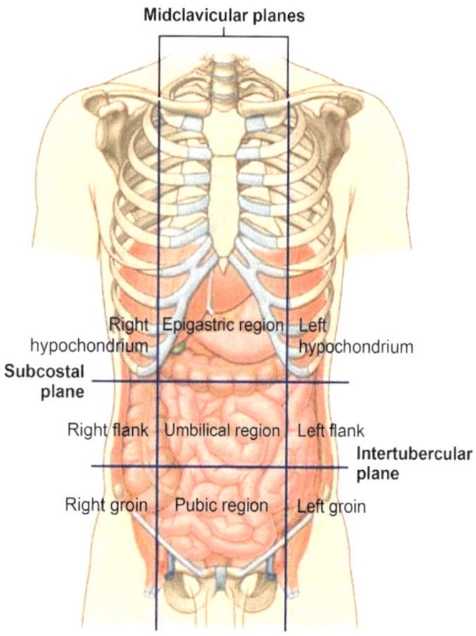

Figure 10.1. Topographic regions of the abdomen.

Source: Mehmetoglu, F. (2024). *Topographic Regions of the Abdomen.*

It is crucial not only for students of medicine but also for healthcare practitioners to know the anatomy of the abdomen to provide for the intricacy of this region in disease and in health. Effective learning strategies, including cadaveric prosection techniques, play a central role in imparting such anatomical information. Studies have shown that students learn much better with a conceptual understanding of anatomy while going through prosection material as opposed to interacting with immersive virtual reality (iVR) platforms, more so in areas like thoracic anatomy that identify the challenges faced in teaching the complex structures of the abdomen effectively (Freer et al., 2024). As the landscape of anatomy teaching changes, the efficacy of various teaching aids continues to be a matter of critical appraisal (Kalle et al., 2023) (Figure 10.1).

Importance of Studying the Abdomen

Understanding the abdomen is not only significant for physicians but also for anyone concerned with human body anatomy and health. The abdomen holds some highly crucial organs like the liver, kidneys, and intestines, each of which is crucial to the overall functionality of the body.

Knowledge of this region allows for pre-detection and management of a number of disorders, such as hepatobiliary cancers, that have shown the role of inter-disciplinary approach to therapy, according to NCCN guidelines (Benson et al., 2021). Besides, advances in diagnostic imaging technology, such as ultrasound, have significantly advanced fetal growth assessment and diagnosis of abnormalities, demonstrating the growing significance of abdominal examinations during pregnancy care (Paladini et al., 2021). By analyzing the complexities of the abdominal region, researchers and practitioners can advance their understanding of diseases, plan effective interventions, and enhance overall health status.

Overview of Abdominal Anatomy

The abdominal region entails a complex scheme of organs and structures that are necessary in digestion, absorption, circulation, and the general operation of the body. The anterior abdominal wall, peritoneum, and other body systems constitute the abdomen and are vital for storing and processing nutrients. The digestive system possesses vital components such as the stomach, small intestine, and large intestine that streamline the breakdown and absorption of food. Further, the vascular anatomy is also critical, particularly concerning the Deep Inferior Epigastric Artery (DIEA) and perforators, as emphasized by studies depicting their role in perfusion during surgery such as breast reconstruction with tissue from the abdomen (Sumadewi, 2023).

This comprehension of fundamental anatomical formations makes possible improvements in surgical procedures, as cutting-edge techniques like Natural Orifice Transluminal Endoscopic Surgery (NOTES) take advantage of these anatomical understandings for minimally invasive procedures (Barrow et al., 2016). As surgical practice develops, it is still necessary to maintain a complete understanding of abdominal anatomy to successfully practice clinically.

Common Functions of the Abdomen

Serving as a central site for many of the body's essential functions, the abdomen plays a very significant role in several physiological processes. Its primary role is digestion as it houses key organs such as the stomach, intestines, liver, and pancreas that work in concert to digest food, absorb nutrients, and eliminate waste. The liver, in particular, also functions as both an endocrine and exocrine glandular organ, secreting bile for digestion and metabolizing drugs and nutrients from the bloodstream (Sumadewi, 2023). The abdomen also takes part in respiration by supporting the diaphragm and abdominal muscles during inhalation and exhalation. This support is essential to enable adequate breathing patterns, particularly during exercise. Furthermore, the protective cage of the abdomen, as enclosed by fascia and muscle, guards these organs against trauma while allowing for the movements that must accompany their functions, demonstrating its role in overall health (Figure 10.2).

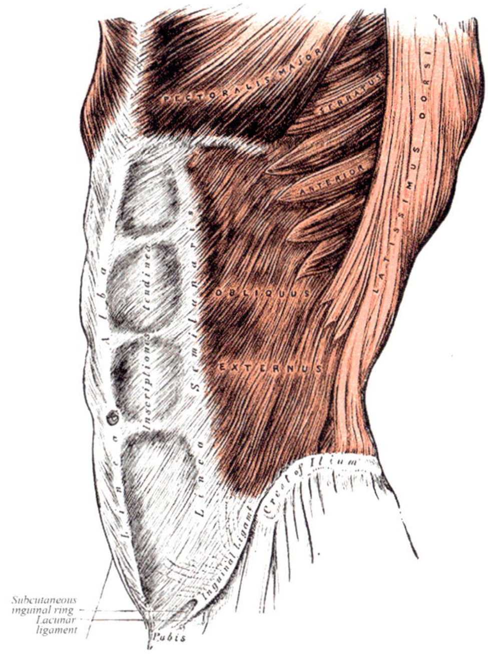

Figure 10.2. Abdominal muscles.

Source: By Henry Vandyke Carter - Henry Gray (1918) Anatomy of the Human Body (See "Book" section below)Bartleby.com: Gray's Anatomy, Plate 392, Public Domain, https://commons.wikimedia.org/w/index.php?curid=287550

Relevance to Overall Health

Maintaining abdominal organs in their optimal condition is crucial because they affect several body systems and play a role in an individual's overall well-being. Proper functioning of abdominal organs, such as the liver, kidneys, and digestive system, is necessary for efficient absorption of nutrients, elimination of waste, and metabolic processes. Increased blood levels of Epstein-Barr Virus (EBV) have been linked to specific abdominal diseases, most significantly in children with Non-Hodgkins Lymphoma, demonstrating the involvement of viral infections in complicating abdominal health outcomes (Filipovich et al., 2013). Moreover, advancement in surgical techniques, such as NOTES, demonstrates the importance of minimally invasive treatment for abdominal conditions without associated complications of traditional surgery. These developments highlight the dynamic relationship between abdominal health and overall medical progress, insisting that healthy abdomens have a crucial role in healthier individuals and effective practice of health care (Barrow et al., 2016).

Brief History of Abdominal Studies

The abdominal history over the centuries has evolved a long way from early observations to current-day advanced medicine. Early attempts at stomach ailments were typically plagued by misconceptions, with abdominal illnesses simulating hernias attributed largely to occult reasons or simple strains with unsuccessful treatments as a consequence. As medical science progressed, there started to evolve a more discerning approach to the identification of athletic pubalgia, better known as sports hernia. This condition illustrates the evolution of abdominal studies, in which scientists began highlighting the role of dynamic anatomical components such as the pubic joint. The need for accurate diagnosis focused attention on the specific mechanisms of injury and underscored the complexity of abdominal and groin injuries in athletes. Thus, the realization that the majority of injuries could be efficiently treated through individualized techniques or surgery is an important abdominal research advancement, enhancing treatment and recovery rates of the victims (Meyers et al., 2007).

Scope of the Discussion

A critical examination of abdominal illness leads to a huge collection of complex disorders that can challenge diagnosis and management. An example of such a condition is *situs inversus totalis*, which significantly renders surgical interventions such as laparoscopic cholecystectomy very challenging. As discussed in cases where surgeons had to adapt to reversed anatomical patterns, meticulous preoperative planning is essential in a bid to obtain a successful outcome (Freer et al., 2024). Equally intriguing is the relationship between temporomandibular joint (TMJ) disorders and their symptoms, which commonly involve referred pain to the ears and neck, and are associated with more widespread musculoskeletal (MSK) conditions that could have abdominal etiologies (Makeev et al., 2020). Practitioners need to be sensitized about these relationships so that they can allow for a multi-disciplinary process that acknowledges the interrelatedness of body systems. Together, the study of these varied conditions highlights the importance of taking a holistic approach to the treatment of diseases within the abdominal cavity.

10.1. Anatomy of the Abdomen

Learning Outcome

1. Explain the Major Organs Located in the Abdomen
2. Describe the Layers of Abdominal Wall
3. Focus on Quadrants of the Abdomen
4. Understand Blood Supply to the Abdomen
5. Focus on Nerve Supply and Innervation
6. Learn about Lymphatic Drainage in the Abdomen
7. What do you mean Anatomical Variations in the Abdomen?
8. Focus on Imaging Techniques for Abdominal Assessment
9. Explain the Surgical Considerations in Abdominal Anatomy

It is vital to understand the anatomy of the abdomen to comprehend its various functions and associated illnesses. The abdomen houses vital organs like the stomach, intestines, liver, and pancreas, all of which play an integral role in digestion and metabolic processes. The complex coordination of these organs, ensured by a network of muscles and tissues, facilitates body functions to function smoothly. Notably, athletic pubalgia and other conditions and injuries highlight the significance of the abdominal structures in sports, where disruption of this dynamic complex is an etiologic factor for disability and pain (Meyers et al., 2007). Besides, the core anatomy gives room for additional complex studies, e.g., on dissecting approaches in biological research, which typically require a thorough grasp of inner and outer structures (Casagrande-Jaloretto et al., 2013). Ultimately, a thorough grasp of abdominal anatomy not only accounts for medical procedures but also continues to explain physical well-being and action (Figure 10.3).

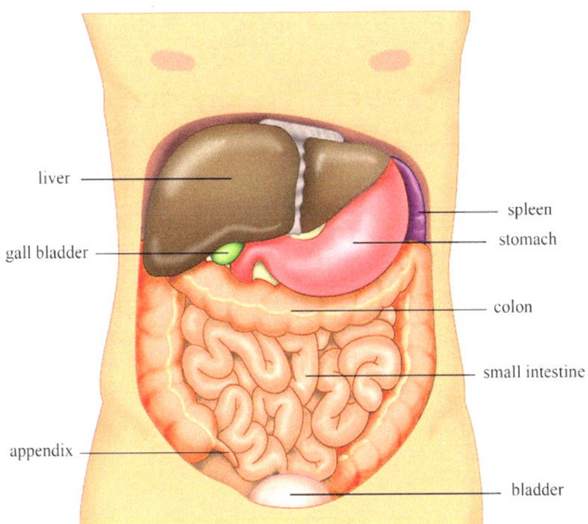

Figure 10.3. The anatomy of the abdomen.

Source: By Tvanbr - Own work, Public Domain, https://commons.wikimedia.org/w/index.php?curid=11625998

10.1.1. Major Organs Located in the Abdomen

The abdomen is a critical region with a multitude of primary organs that are crucial in numerous functions of the body. They include the digestive organs, such as the intestines and the stomach, which are critical in digestion and nutrient absorption. The liver, which has functions in metabolism and detoxification, and the pancreas, which is crucial in digestive enzyme production and hormone production like insulin, are also found in this region. Additionally, the spleen in the abdomen is important in immune response and blood purification. In the absence of vertebrates, abdominal complexity in structure is observed in other organisms, for instance, in *Oestrus ovis*, where the larval digestive and excretory systems possess specialized structures for nutrient assimilation (Martín-Vega et al., 2020). Further, several muscle systems in the abdomen facilitate movement and support, underscoring the abdomen's multi-functionality (Ziv et al., 2022). Familiarity with these organs and their functions that are interdependent is necessary to grasp basic anatomy and physiology.

10.1.2. Layers of Abdominal Wall

The abdominal wall is made up of several discrete layers, each contributing its role to its functional and protective role. The most external layer of the abdominal wall is the skin, which provides protection from the external environment and permits sensory perception. Deep to the skin is the superficial fascia, which provides the skin with support in addition to the storage of fat and the provision of thermoregulation. The deeper layers consist of the muscular layers that consist of the external oblique, internal oblique, and transversus abdominis, which collectively play a role in movement and provide structural support to the abdomen. The rectus abdominis is also crucial for flexion and trunk stabilization. It is important to know these layers, especially in clinical cases such as surgeries or trauma examinations, where the anatomy can be utilized to determine best practices. This layered structure ultimately enables the abdomen's contribution to the rest of the body functions, including respiration and digestion, to overall health (Casagrande-Jaloretto et al., 2013) (Figure 10.4).

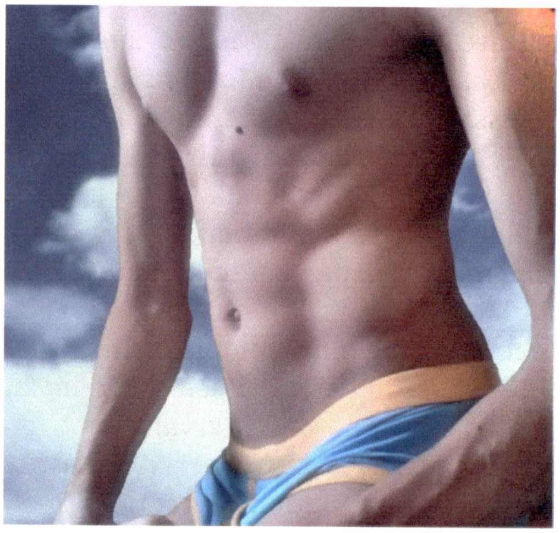

Figure 10.4. Anterior abdominal wall anatomy.

Source: By Locketudor - Own work, CC BY-SA 3.0, https://commons.wikimedia.org/w/index.php?curid=4358070

10.1.3. Quadrants of the Abdomen

Understanding the quadrants of the abdomen is essential in clinical examination and medical diagnosis. The abdomen is traditionally subdivided into four quadrants: the right upper quadrant, left upper quadrant, right lower quadrant, and left lower quadrant. The quadrants contain vital organs and structures that specialists need to consider when performing their exams. For example, the liver, which is the largest gland in the human body and performs numerous functions for metabolism, predominantly lies in the right upper quadrant, which could potentially also be the location of diseases like gallbladder disease and hepatitis (Sumadewi, 2023). Alternatively, diverticulitis problems might be the resident of the left lower quadrant as it contains segments of the descending colon. The clinicians apply this quadrantal system not only to localize the symptoms but also to differentiate among various abdominal pathologies so that the patients can be provided with correct and timely treatments (Hooria et al., 2024).

10.1.4. Blood Supply to the Abdomen

The arterial supply of the abdominal region is complex and crucial in sustaining the various organs of this region. Abdominal blood supply is predominantly supplied by branches of the abdominal aorta, such as vital arteries like the celiac artery, superior mesenteric artery (SMA) and inferior mesenteric artery (IMA). These arteries branch to provide vital circulation to the intestines, pancreas, and segments of the liver for proper functioning. Characteristic is the existence of collateral pathways among these arteries that act as a crucial backup during surgical conditions in which blood supply might be compromised. For instance, in a study, it has been shown that knowledge of the arterial supply of both mesenteric arteries is significant because they possess redundant anastomoses that preserve blood supply during conditions of ischemia (Slavu et al., 2024). Furthermore, associated structures like the omentum serve purposes other than fat storage and assist with fluid drainage and immune function, illustrating the vulnerability of vascular and anatomical structures to each other in the abdomen (Barone et al., 2016). Not only does this complex network sustain the physiological demands of the organs but it also holds important weight in abdominal surgical procedures.

10.1.5. Nerve Supply and Innervation

The nerve supply and innervation of the abdominal region are crucial in regulating various physiological functions and sensations. It is richly innervated, comprising a complex network of both autonomic and somatic nerves that provide for not only motor and visceral activities but also sensations. The convergence of the nerve fibers allows complicated communication among abdominal organs and the brain, hence making it vital in processes such as digestion and pain sensation. For instance, inflammation in the related pathways of signaling causes diseases such as low back pain (LBP), which is controlled by the condition of intervertebral disc (IVD) degeneration and its related inflammatory mediators (Feng-Juan et al., 2021). Also, while we are wont to put a premium on the face and hands when it comes to nerve content, abdominal innervation complexity remains relevant because it determines overall body functioning and contributes to perceived pain and discomfort in the abdomen (Giulia et al., 2020).

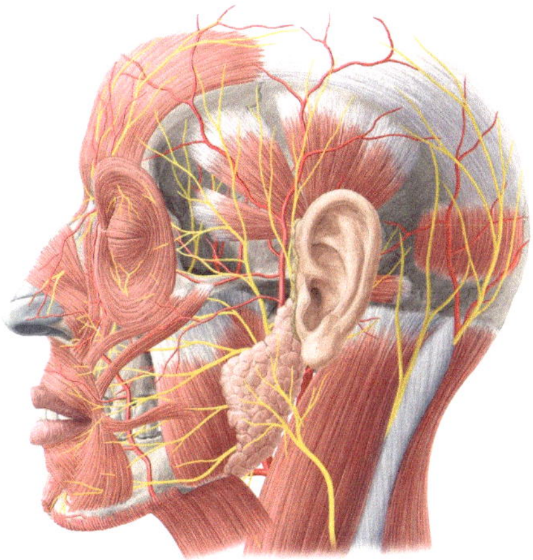

Source: Kenhub. (n.d.). *Superficial Nerves of the Face and Scalp*.

10.1.6. Lymphatic Drainage in the Abdomen

The lymphatic system plays an important role in the establishment of homeostasis in the abdominal cavity. It is the system for lymph drainage, which is high in waste products, fats, proteins, and immune cells, from the organs within the abdomen. This complex network of lymph vessels begins at the capillary level where excess interstitial fluid is taken up and passed on to larger vessels and ultimately into the thoracic duct or the right lymphatic duct for return to the blood. Effective lymph drainage is crucial not only for toxin removal but also for aiding immune function by transporting antigens to lymph nodes. This system's dysfunctions may lead to severe conditions such as lymphedema, characterized by localized swelling and tissue hypertrophy (Viitanen et al., 2014). The connection of lymphatic drainage with the general welfare of the abdomen indicates its importance in physiological function and protection from disease (Dakwar et al., 2017).

10.1.7. Anatomical Variations in the Abdomen

Abdominal anatomical variations can significantly affect clinical practice, particularly for surgery and diagnosis. The presence of accessory lobes of the liver, such as the extraordinary beaver tail liver, is a case in point, and they depict the complexity and diversity of human anatomy. This uncommon anomaly, in which the left lobe of the liver is longer and passes over the spleen, can complicate imaging interpretation and may cause misdiagnosis and potentially make it confusing with splenic injury (Freer et al., 2024). Similarly, venous variations in gonadal arteries help to highlight the importance of being knowledgeable about these anatomical variations. Studies have revealed that such variations, particularly relating to the frequency of origin, are more common in men, and this makes it essential for surgeons and radiologists to understand these abnormalities (Freer et al., 2024). It is a significant information in averting complications of intervention, leading to improved patient outcomes from interventions and abdominal surgeries.

10.1.8. Imaging Techniques for Abdominal Assessment

With advances in imaging technology in the last few years, abdominal assessment has been significantly improved, providing significant information regarding several diseases of this vital body region. The most dramatic modality is likely to be computed tomography (CT), with its clear-cut images and precise measurement of abdominal structures, including the aorta. Research brought to the limelight the fact that application of contrast-enhanced CT helps doctors effectively observe alterations in abdominal aortic measurements, which could signify severe illnesses such as ectasia and aneurysms (Rakhee et al., 2023). In addition, magnetic resonance imaging (MRI) is a valid option, particularly when employing strategies such as frequency-modulated continuous wave triggering, which can enhance abdominal scan quality without differences in image quality detectable by patients versus standard respiratory belt triggers (Qingling et al., 2024). All of these imaging techniques contribute collectively toward diagnostic accuracy and treatment planning, reinforcing their importance in contemporary medical practice (Figure 10.5).

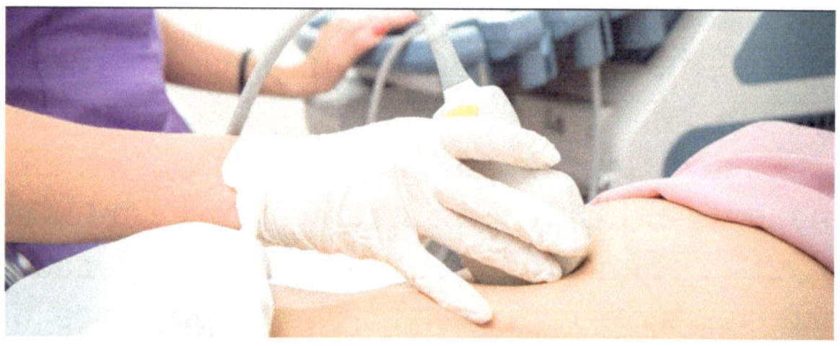

Figure 10.5. Abdominal ultrasound.

Source: UCSF Health. (n.d.). *Abdominal Ultrasound.*

10.1.9. Surgical Considerations in Abdominal Anatomy

Abdominal anatomy is also extremely relevant in surgery within the region, as the complex relationship of several structures can significantly influence results. Surgeons must deal with a complex interplay of vessels, nerves, and muscles, all of which can influence both the approach and strategy of method during surgery. For instance, incisions for hepato-pancreatic-biliary (HPB) procedures must consider muscular layers and neurovascular bundles to prevent complications such as incisional hernias (IH) or bulging, which can cause long-term adverse effect on a patient's quality of life (QoL) (Medina et al., 2023). In addition, previous lower abdominal surgery can potentially complicate future surgery as the anatomy may be distorted by adhesions and render procedures like robotic radical cystectomy with intracorporeal urinary diversion more complicated (Freer et al., 2024). Therefore, not only does a thorough knowledge of anatomy facilitate successful surgical technique, but it also minimizes the likelihood of complications (Figure 10.6).

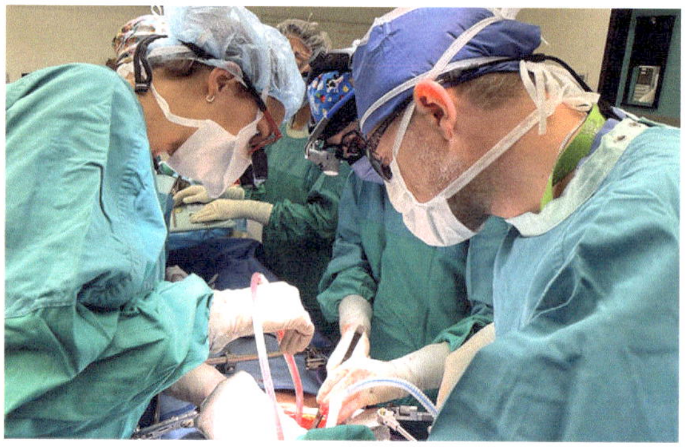

Figure 10.6. Surgeons performing hepato-pancreatic-biliary (HPB) surgery.

Source: Wixstatic. (n.d.). *Surgical Team Operating in Theater.*

Test Your Knowledge

1. Name at least five major organs found within the abdominal cavity.
2. Which abdominal organ is primarily responsible for detoxification and metabolism?
3. What is the anatomical relationship between the stomach and the pancreas?

10.2. Functions of the Abdomen

Learning Outcome

1. Discuss the Digestive Processes in the Abdomen
2. Explain the Role of the Liver in Metabolism
3. Focus on Functions of the Kidneys and Urinary System
4. Discuss the Importance of the Spleen in Immune Response
5. Know Reproductive Organs in the Abdomen
6. Discuss Role of the Diaphragm in Respiration
7. Describe how to Impact of Abdominal Muscles on Movement
8. Understand Hormonal Functions of Abdominal Organs
9. Focus on Interaction Between Abdominal Organs and Systems

The abdomen is responsible for many significant functions within the human body as a core hub for several organ systems that facilitate essential physiological processes. The abdomen houses key organs like the stomach, intestines, liver, and kidneys, which are crucial in the process of digestion and metabolism. Through the breaking down of food and absorption of nutrients, abdominal organs are involved significantly in energy balance and overall health. In addition, the region is a part of waste elimination by the urinary system and kidneys to achieve homeostasis. The region in the abdominal part is also critical for respiration because the diaphragm that lies below the ribcage assists in expansion and contraction in the process of breathing. Hence, understanding the different functions of the abdomen highlights its importance not only in digestion but also in coordinating the body, disposing of waste, and respiratory efficiency, thus making it a very essential area of study in both anatomy and physiology studies (Georgakopoulos & Lasrado, 2022; Casagrande-Jaloretto et al., 2013).

10.2.1. Digestive Processes in the Abdomen

The abdomen is a critical site for digestive processes, efficiently breaking down food and absorbing nutrients required for body function. Organs within the abdominal cavity, such as the stomach, intestines, and liver, work in concert to facilitate digestion.

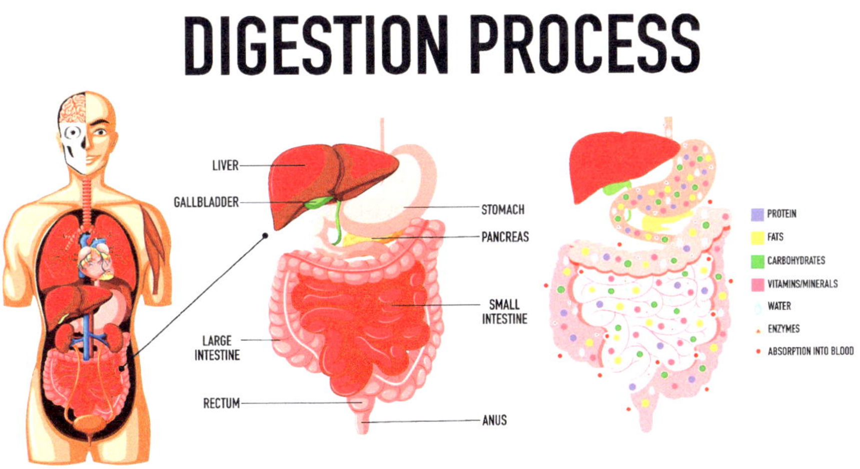

Figure 10.7. Diagram showing digestion process.

*Source*Vecteezy. (n.d.). *Diagram Showing Digestion Process.*

The stomach initiates this process by secreting gastric juices, enzymes, and acids that denature proteins and break down food particles. Once in the small intestine, the partially digested food is encountered by a number of digestive enzymes released by the pancreas and by bile of the liver. All these compounds further enhance nutrient absorption from the intestinal walls into the blood, allowing essential amino acids, fatty acids, and carbohydrates to be absorbed into the bloodstream. It is also very important to comprehend these digestive mechanisms, particularly when studying model organisms like the African clawed frog, which can be utilized to study comparative digestion (Ahn et al., 2017). Furthermore, a conservation strategy that has a very balanced approach, as highlighted by marine research, further illustrates why digestive function is at the heart of maintaining healthy biological systems that are resilient (Truitt, 1939) (Figure 10.7).

10.2.2. Role of the Liver in Metabolism

Among all the organs of the human body, the liver is a central location for metabolic functions. It controls carbohydrates, fats, and proteins to provide homeostasis and energy balance in the body. Through its function to convert excess glucose into glycogen, it serves as an essential energy reservoir. Moreover, it metabolizes fatty acids and produces other lipoproteins, facilitating lipid transport in the bloodstream. Drug metabolism evaluation also underscores the liver's function; for example, recent evidence shows that human liver fatty acid binding protein (hFABP1) can bind drugs in ternary complexes, which influence their metabolism when attached to cytochrome P450 enzymes like CYP2C9 (Yabut et al., 2024). Besides, recent findings illustrate the importance of considering factors such as alveolar echinococcosis, which can impact the liver's function and, subsequently, affect metabolic processes (Miloš et al., 2024). Therefore, the multifunctional roles of the livers highlight its supreme position in maintaining metabolic equilibrium.

10.2.3. Functions of the Kidneys and Urinary System

Urinary and kidneys are essential in the body's maintenance of homeostasis, primarily through balancing fluid and electrolyte levels. As large organs within the abdominal cavity, kidneys eliminate waste substances and excesses from the blood and produce urine to carry wastes out of the body.

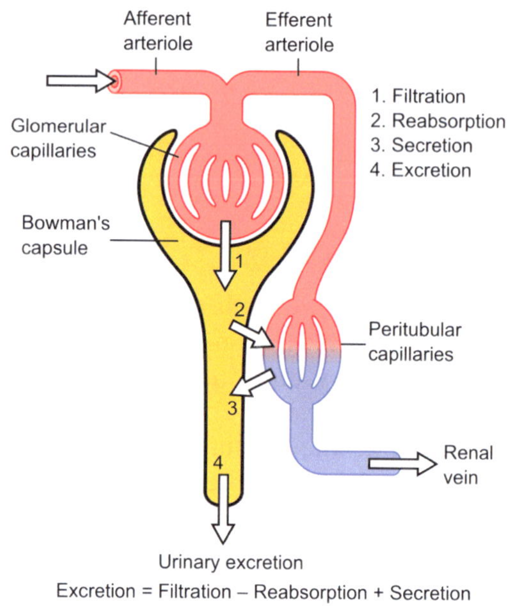

Figure 10.8. Functions of the kidneys.

Source: By Madhero88 - Own workReferenceshere, CC BY 3.0, https://commons.wikimedia.org/w/index.php?curid=9665603

Besides excretion, they are also responsible for maintaining blood pressure by regulating blood volume and secreting hormones such as renin. Additionally, the kidneys are engaged in acid-base balance by secreting hydrogen ions and reabsorbing bicarbonate, keeping the body's pH very strictly within a narrow range.

It is critical to understand these functions since kidney conditions, such as chronic infection or obstruction, may result in disease that affects the system at large, as seen in historical anatomical studies (Dogra, 1930). This underscores the importance of the kidneys not just within the urinary system but also in overall metabolic functions (Figure 10.8).

10.2.4. Importance of the Spleen in Immune Response

In the complicated universe of the immune system, the spleen is a necessary organ to assist in developing an efficient immune response. The spleen functions as a filter for the blood, identifying and removing pathogens and red blood cells that are damaged or old. The organ is divided into two general compartments: the red pulp, in which blood filtration is carried out, and the white pulp, in which lymphocytes and immune cells interact to initiate the immune response.

The compartmentalization allows the spleen to take part in both adaptive and innate immunity significantly. With its function in the proliferation and activation of lymphocytes, the spleen enhances the body's ability to develop specific reactions to antigens, enhancing overall immune defense. In addition, owing to its positioning, it can react swiftly to infection or damage, showing its relevance to the upkeep of the body's immune homeostasis (Freer et al., 2024).

10.2.5. Reproductive Organs in the Abdomen

The abdominal cavity holds vital reproductive organs that play important roles in male and female reproductive health. In females, the ovaries and uterus are central structures responsible for egg development and care for developing embryos. A deviation in these organs will lead to a range of issues, including symptomatic infertility caused by disease or infection, as is evident in studies that indicate common diseases in female rabbits such as endometritis and pyometra (Koreyba et al., 2024). Similarly, in males, the testes and associated structures facilitate sperm development and production. Besides, proper functioning of the reproductive organs is also connected with abdominal well-being, as sickness or inflammation could significantly impair fertility and general well-being. Understanding the positioning within the body and the physiological functioning of the organs is central to addressing reproductive health issues, thus abdominal well-being plays an essential role in human as well as animal biology.

10.2.6. Role of the Diaphragm in Respiration

At the core of the process of respiration, the diaphragm is the key muscle employed for exhalation and inhalation. The diaphragm is a muscular dome-shaped organ that serves as the separator between the abdominal cavity and the thoracic cavity. The diaphragm controls air pressure inside the lungs. When the diaphragm contracts, it flattens out, and this increases the volume of the thoracic cavity, and as a result, the pressure inside the lungs decreases, and this allows air to flow in. On the other hand, during exhalation, the diaphragm becomes relaxed, which helps to force air out of the lungs. The smooth interactions with adjacent structures, such as abdominal organs, are representative of its significance in ensuring respiratory efficiency as well as intra-abdominal pressure equilibrium. As discussed earlier, the asymmetry of the diaphragm with the left side lower due to the placement of the liver once again highlights the connection between abdominal structure and respiration mechanics, summarizing the complexity that goes into the action of the diaphragm during respiration (Kanwal et al., 2018).

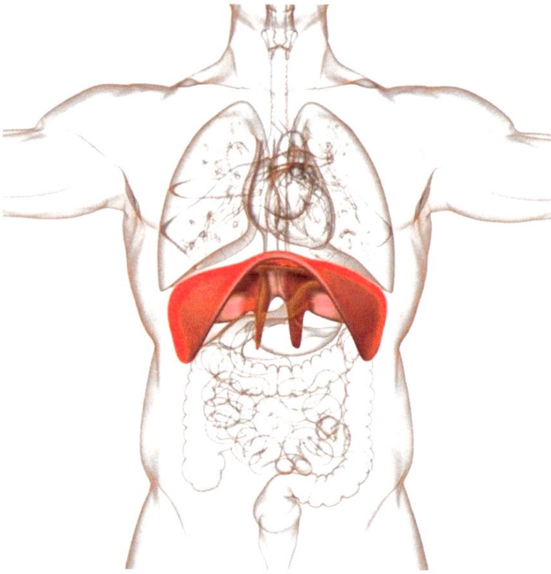

Source: LinkedIn. (n.d.). *Human Diaphragm Illustration*.

10.2.7. Impact of Abdominal Muscles on Movement

The role of the abdominal muscles to aid movement is quite significant since these muscles are a key factor in the maintenance of stability and balance in movement. A strong and good core helps support the spine, which aids in carrying out movement, from simple day-to-day movements to sophisticated sporting activities. For instance, trunk flexor fatiguing exercises have been discovered to cause local exercise-induced hypoalgesia (EIH), implying that pain perception in the region can be enhanced by having strong abdominal muscles, hence promoting overall function in movement (Bement et al., 2019). Moreover, the relationship between abdominal strength and respiratory function is evident because too much body fat can compromise respiratory efficacy, possibly limiting physical performance (Indahswari et al., 2019). Collectively, these findings underscore the key role abdominal muscles play in maintaining not just movement, but also general health and functional capacity of the individual, making them essential for both QoL and performance.

10.2.8. Hormonal Functions of Abdominal Organs

The abdomen holds several essential organs that play a role in hormone regulation and affect various physiological processes. Among the most important of these organs is the pancreas, which secretes insulin and glucagon, two critical hormones applied in glucose metabolism. The hormonal interaction regulates blood sugar levels, hence showing the abdominal organ homeostasis. The other important contributor is the adrenal gland located above the kidneys responsible for secreting hormones such as cortisol and adrenaline in response to stress and metabolic control. In addition, gut-secreted hormones such as ghrelin and leptin have a primary role in the management of appetite and energy balance. The complex system of the hormonal function supports the abdomens central role in the regulation of metabolic processes and overall health control. To understand these interactions among hormones is significant to realizing how dysfunction of any one of these organs can lead to metabolic disease and other medical disorders in the area of the abdomen.

10.2.9. Interaction Between Abdominal Organs and Systems

The complex interactions between organs and abdominal systems are essential to the maintenance of overall health and functioning. Organs that interact include the kidneys, liver, and gastrointestinal system, with the region's integral role being emphasized in functions like digestion, waste elimination, and hormonal regulation. The liver, for instance, plays a critical role in the metabolism of nutrients from gut absorption while, concurrently, detoxifying toxic substances in the body. Besides, kidneys also talk to the circulatory system to regulate blood pressure as well as fluid status, showing the inter-relationship between the systems. Such complex interaction is specifically evident during medical procedures, where knowledge of organ motion is vital for successful outcomes. Technical advancements in imaging, such as those involving MR-based navigators to track organ movement, have improved procedural safety and efficacy (Celicanin, 2014). These discoveries provide evidence of the importance of synergistic activity in the abdominal cavity and of the need for continued investigation in this active area (Tsitlakidou et al., 2022) (Figure 10.9).

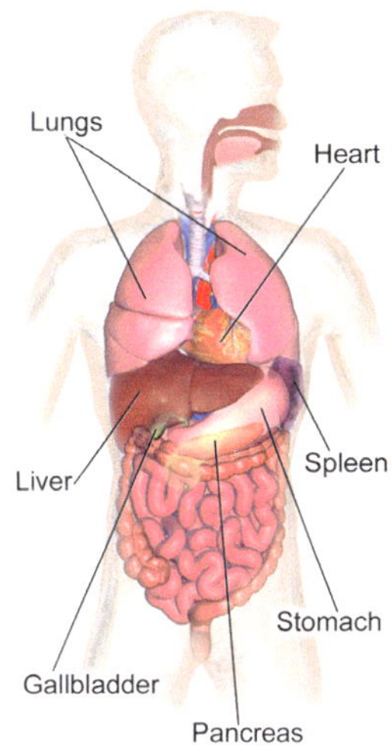

Figure 10.9. Interaction between abdominal organs and systems.

Source: By BruceBlaus - Own work, CC BY-SA 4.0, https://commons.wikimedia.org/w/index.php?curid=47113847

Test Your Knowledge

1. Which abdominal muscles assist with forced expiration and intra-abdominal pressure during actions like coughing or lifting?
2. Which abdominal organ is responsible for insulin and glucagon secretion?

10.3. Common Disorders of the Abdomen

Learning Outcome

1. Discuss the Gastrointestinal Disorders (e.g., IBS, Crohn's Disease)
2. Focus on Liver Diseases (e.g., Hepatitis, Cirrhosis)
3. Understand Kidney Disorders (e.g., Stones, Infections)
4. Know Abdominal Pain and its Causes
5. Explain the Infections Affecting the Abdomen (e.g., Appendicitis)
6. Evaluate Cancer Risks in Abdominal Organs
7. How to Impact of Obesity on Abdominal Health
8. Discuss the Hernias and their Implications
9. Describe the Diagnostic Methods for Abdominal Disorders

Abdominal disorders form a broad category of conditions that can have a critical impact on an individual's QoL. Of these, functional abdominal pain disorders tend to pose critical challenges, especially among pediatric patients. Studies indicate that the disorders are common but in most cases misunderstood, thus receiving inadequate treatment (Freer et al., 2024). Hereditary disorders form another category, such as hereditary spherocytosis, which may present in the form of infectious diseases. A case report presents the way a young man presented with jaundice and abdominal pain and was inappropriately diagnosed with dengue due to overlapping symptoms. This mistake highlights the necessity of vigorous evaluation to prevent inappropriate treatment and appropriate health care (Calcino-Cuela et al., 2024). The complexity of abdominal disorders demands interpretive understanding, the synthesis of clinical insight and patient education, to enhance better results and minimize the negative effects of the ubiquitous but variable conditions.

10.3.1. Gastrointestinal Disorders (e.g., IBS, Crohn's Disease)

The complexity of gastrointestinal disorders such as irritable bowel syndrome (IBS) and Crohn's disease complicates their diagnosis and management. IBS with its symptom complex of abdominal pain and alteration in bowel habits is prevalent in millions of individuals worldwide and often coexists with other functional gastrointestinal syndromes, leading to diagnostic uncertainty. This multidimensional nature of IBS is exacerbated by psychological features, as a notable percentage of sufferers experience co-morbid anxiety and depression that can exacerbate symptoms and impact QoL (Freer et al., 2024By way of contrast, Crohn's disease, an inflammatory bowel condition, is characterized by chronic inflammation that can involve any part of the gastrointestinal tract and often comes with catastrophic complications, including malabsorption and bowel obstructions (Hemant et al., 2016). Determining these disorders requires not just a multidisciplinary approach to symptom management but also calls attention to the need for ongoing investigation into their mechanisms and potential treatments (Figure 10.10).

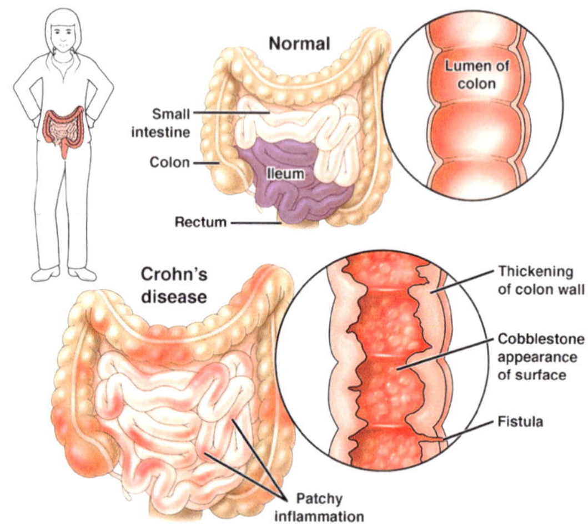

Figure 10.10. Crohn's disease.

Source: American Gastroenterological Association. (2021). *Comparison of Normal Bowel and Crohn's Disease.*

10.3.2. Liver Diseases (e.g., Hepatitis, Cirrhosis)

Among the many diseases in the abdominal region, liver illnesses such as hepatitis and cirrhosis are serious issues. Chronic hepatitis B is widespread in certain regions, particularly in Asia, indicating an enormous burden and contributing to a significant proportion of mortality due to liver cancer. In fact, chronic hepatitis B contributed 49.1% to liver cancer death in the Asia-Pacific area, a keen contrast compared to lower figures in Western countries, where alcohol consumption and non-alcoholic fatty liver disease are top causes (Jian et al., 2022). Furthermore, recent studies have identified extensive prevalence of hepatitis delta virus (HDV) infection, which complicates existing infections and leads to severe liver consequences like cirrhosis (Isaeva et al., 2022). The interplay of these factors justifies the need for comprehensive screening as well as targeted prevention programs in response to the widened prevalence of liver disease among different populations.

10.3.3. Kidney Disorders (e.g., Stones, Infections)

Kidney diseases, including stones and infections, are severe medical conditions that can significantly impact one's QoL. Kidney stones, formed through the crystallization of minerals and salts in the urine, lead to severe pain, frequently described as one of the worst feelings a person can have. They can cause complications such as urinary tract infections (UTIs) and also impede the flow of urine, resulting in further renal damage if not treated. Similarly, kidney infections, which are typically caused by untreated UTIs, have systemic effects such as fever and weakness, which complicate the patient's overall health and well-being. According to a review of abdominal complaints, patients with chronic abdominal pain and renal symptoms often present with multifactorial issues, requiring large-scale diagnostic workups (Gupta et al., 2017). It is essential to know these disorders in depth so that prompt intervention can prevent serious complications and enhance the patient's outcomes.

10.3.4. Abdominal Pain and its Causes

Abdominal pain can be a consequence of a range of underlying causes, highlighting the complexity of it as a clinical sign. In most instances, the etiology can range from relatively benign conditions like indigestion and gas to more severe conditions like organ dysfunction or systemic disease.

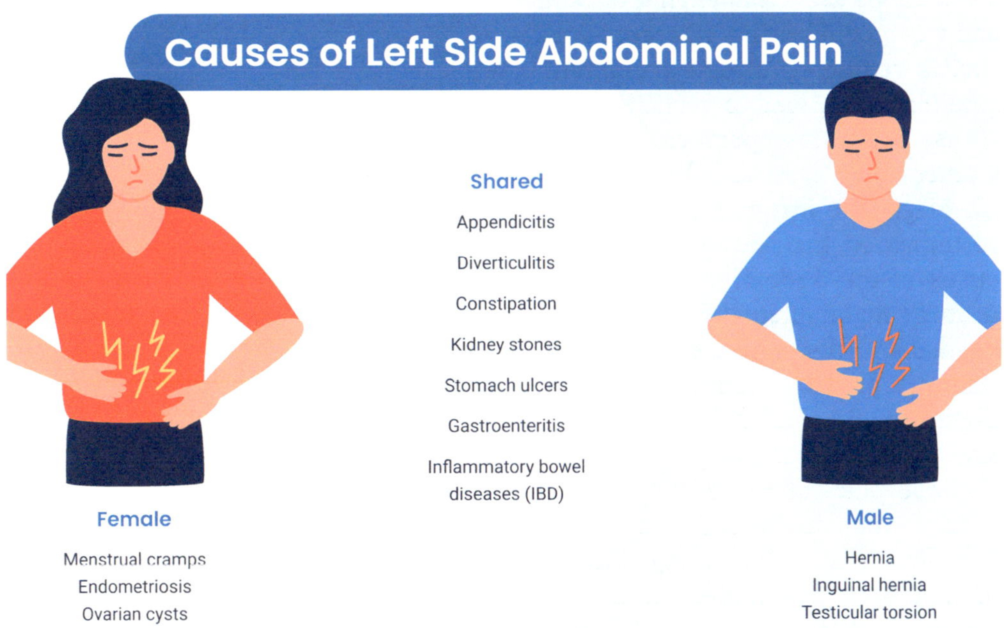

Figure 10.11. Abdominal pain and its causes.

Source: Complete Care. (2021). *Causes of Left Side Abdominal Pain.*

For instance, in adults, bowel obstructions due to conditions like tumoral growths can cause severe pain and can result in acute conditions like intussusception. As shown in a case, ileo-ileal intussusception in an elderly man aged 60 was secondary to a T3N1 neuroendocrine tumor (NET), a rare but severe underlying condition that attests to the need for proper investigation on the part of nonspecific abdominal pain (Freer et al., 2024). Secondly, interstitial pregnancies, that is, in the interstitial portion of the fallopian tube, present with similarly indeterminate features but are characterized by higher risks of complications such as internal hemorrhage (Bužinskienė et al., 2023). The identification of such varied causes is crucial for effective and timely management (Figure 10.11).

10.3.5. Infections Affecting the Abdomen (e.g., Appendicitis)

Abdominal infections are challenging to both diagnose and treat, with certain disorders such as appendicitis requiring urgent treatment. Infected appendixes can lead to certain severe complications, including perforation and peritonitis unless they are treated right away. Advances in diagnostic imaging, including CT scans, have improved the ability to diagnose various causes of the abdominal illness. For instance, a study highlighted the value of CT scans in diagnosing HIV-positive patients with acute abdomen symptoms, since the imaging can not only detect abdominal tuberculosis but also prevent unnecessary operations (Singo, 2016). It shows the importance of proper diagnosis in preventing risks from operations. With intra-abdominal infections still presenting difficult clinical cases, a sensitive understanding of presentation signs and symptoms, early imaging, and evidence-based practice for management are key to better patient outcomes. The complexity of these infections requires clinicians to be sensitive to efficient and timely interventions.

10.3.6. Cancer Risks in Abdominal Organs

The abdominal region's complexity poses a big challenge to the early detection and intervention of cancer. Various cancers such as liver, kidney, and pancreatic cancer can significantly affect the health of organs found within the belly. A frightening fact points out that pancreatic cancer, for instance, is very aggressive and diagnosed late in most instances because the initial symptoms are not revealed. Besides, advancements in imaging technology, i.e., CT scans, enhance the need for accurate organ contouring for treatment purposes. Manual segmentation is also not highly reliable and therefore indicates the need for good methodologies for better accuracy. New techniques using deep learning techniques have been found to be very effective in organ segmentation tasks and have produced mean dice scores of as high as 98.0% in organs like the liver, thus making it possible to monitor and manage cancer risk efficiently within abdominal organs (Freer et al., 2024). Thus, knowing such cancer risks is vital to improving overall outcomes for patients.

10.3.7. Impact of Obesity on Abdominal Health

Obesity directly affects abdominal health, regulating many of the body's physiological functions and disease susceptibility. Excess fat in the abdominal region, particularly visceral adipose tissue, can enhance intra-abdominal pressure and inflammation, negatively impacting organ function and imparting a greater risk for metabolic disorders. Additionally, research indicates a correlation between the percentage of body fat and lung health, as indicated by a study of a negative correlation between body fat and peak expiratory flow rates in children (Indahswari et al., 2019). This suggests that excess stomach fat may not only disrupt lung function but further aggravate other conditions. In addition, some fat stores like subcutaneous and visceral fat have different health connotations, with evidence showing that breast cancer patient's risk of death is attributed to higher subcutaneous fat (Bradshaw et al., 2019). Thus, fighting against obesity is important in guaranteeing better abdominal health and better health.

10.3.8. Hernias and their Implications

Abdominal hernias present significant clinical challenges with their various types and complications. Being most often caused by a combination of high intra-abdominal pressure and weakened tissue, hernias need strict care in order not to lead to severe complications such as incarceration or strangulation, which can result in severe medical issues. For instance, the presence of the appendix within an inguinal hernia is known as Amyands hernia, and it is a less frequent but complex condition that may require specialized surgery, demonstrating that accurate diagnosis and early treatment are warranted (Al Sulaim et al., 2024). Moreover, recent advances in surgical technique, including laparoscopic methods, have been promising to enhance outcomes in recovery as well as reduce rates of recurrence. As emphasized in the 2014 International Endohernia Society guidelines, consistent study and adjustment of evolving operating methods are needed to develop patient management and treatment for cases of hernia (Bain et al., 2019). Understanding these implications is of extreme significance to medical practitioners and patients (Figure 10.12).

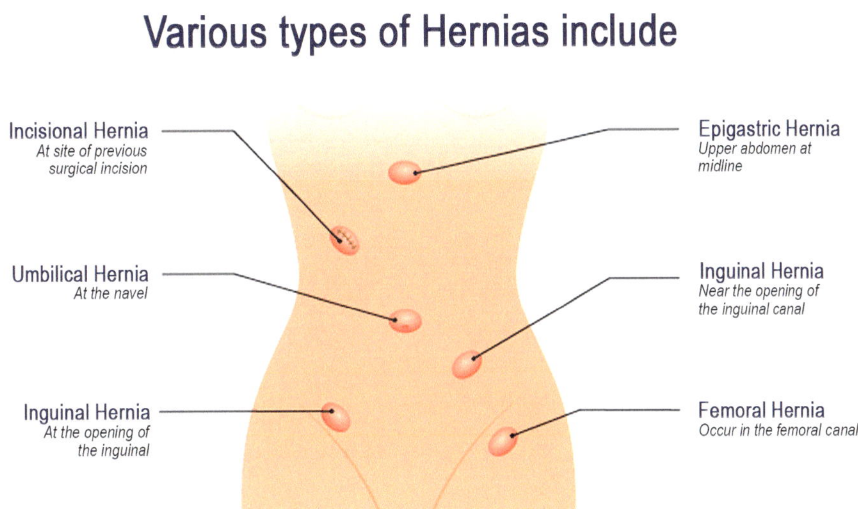

Figure 10.12. Hernias and their implications.

Source: Yashoda Hospitals. (n.d.). *Various Types of Hernias Include.*

10.3.9. Diagnostic Methods for Abdominal Disorders

Extensive diagnostic procedures are instrumental in the diagnosis of abdominal conditions because doctors must deal with a bewildering array of symptoms and probable conditions. Technologies such as ultrasound, CT, and MRI are all essential tools that give information on the function and structure of abdominal organs. Most notably, ultrasound has gained popularity based on its non-invasive nature and real-time imaging according to the European Federation of Societies for Ultrasound in

Medicine and Biology's support of gastrointestinal ultrasound (GIUS) in clinical practice (Calabrese et al., 2016). Additionally, laboratory tests and endoscopic evaluation augment these imaging tests to provide the entire panorama of both obstructive and infective diseases. For instance, abdominal tuberculosis requires surgery to be commonly carried out along with medicine, which underscores the importance of correct diagnosis for an efficient treatment (Singhal et al., 2013). A multimodal strategy thus enhances the investigative light needed for the management of abdominal illness.

Test Your Knowledge

1. What are the typical signs and symptoms of acute appendicitis?
2. What imaging techniques are commonly used to diagnose abdominal conditions?
3. How is a physical examination used to detect tenderness or guarding in abdominal infections?

10.4. Health and Wellness of the Abdomen

Learning Outcome

1. Know Importance of a Balanced Diet for Abdominal Health
2. Focus on Exercise and its Effects on Abdominal Strength
3. Explain the Role of Hydration in Digestive Health
4. Understand Stress Management and Its Impact on the Abdomen
5. Discuss the Preventive Measures for Abdominal Disorders
6. Explain the Regular Screenings and Check-Ups
7. Know Importance of Maintaining a Healthy Weight
8. Learn about Lifestyle Changes for Better Abdominal Health
9. Discuss the Role of Education in Promoting Abdominal Wellness

Prevention of optimal health and well-being of the abdomen is crucial for overall health as it influences various physiological functions and QoL. A healthy abdominal region not only facilitates digestion and metabolism but also assists in boosting the immune system. Interventions like therapeutic mineral bathing and targeted massage, which have been shown to enhance wellness tourism experiences, may also be beneficial treatments for abdominal well-being, relieving stress and promoting relaxation (Freer et al., 2024). In addition, integrating evidence-based practices within the health policy is important to improve abdomen-related health outcomes, particularly for areas with very limited access to quality healthcare (Masoud et al., 2022). Public-private partnerships may endeavor to enhance access to wellness resources for healing common abdominal ailments while promoting the overall well-being of individuals. Through putting the health and wellness of this region foremost, individuals are able to notice profound depths of improvement in their vitality and health.

10.4.1. Importance of a Balanced Diet for Abdominal Health

Good health of the abdomen is very much based on adherence to a well-balanced diet, which is crucial in the prevention of various health disorders. Dysbalance in the consumption of nutrients can result in obesity and its related diseases, for instance, insulin resistance and metabolic disorders, particularly among vulnerable individuals, for example, those with polycystic ovary syndrome (PCOS) (Ghazeeri et al., 2021). A well-balanced diet with the proper proportions of carbohydrates, proteins, and fats supports body weight control and metabolic health. Research indicates that total intake of energy and fat and carbohydrate quality are inseparably linked with body weight and waist circumference, supporting the diet-abdominal health link (Delecluse et al., 2007). Thus, placing a well-balanced diet at the forefront of the list not only helps in effective weight management but also ensures overall abdominal well-being by reducing chronic disease risk factors of unhealthy diet (Figure 10.13).

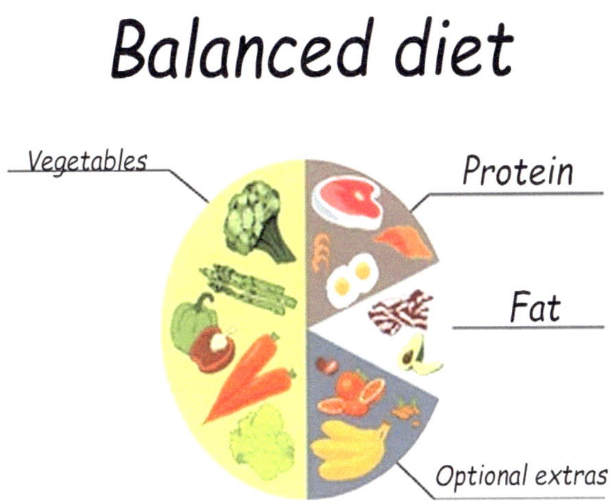

Figure 10.13. Balanced diet.

Source: Shutterstock. (n.d.). *Balanced Diet*.

10.4.2. Exercise and its Effects on Abdominal Strength

Involvement in prolonged exercise has significant implications for the stabilization of the abdominal muscles and core stability. Some exercise modalities, such as fatiguing trunk flexor exercises, have been discovered to stimulate localized EIH that can decrease pain usually associated with weakness of the abdominal muscles. Studies have indicated that postpartum women exhibit lower pressure pain thresholds, yet involvement in targeted abdominal exercise is able to induce changes in strength and pain tolerance (Bement et al., 2019). Furthermore, mat Pilates studies indicate radical body composition alterations in postmenopausal women, such as gains in muscular mass in key sites like the trunk and abdomen. This demonstrates the efficacy of exercise in not only building abdominal strength but also in attaining a healthier overall composition (Aguado-Henche et al., 2017). In total, consistent exercise is essential to the development of abdominal strength, which results in enhanced functional ability and injury prevention among various populations.

10.4.3. Role of Hydration in Digestive Health

Optimal hydration is essential for digestive health, as water is used in significant bodily functions involving the digestive system. Adequate water consumption allows for the digestion of food, allowing enzymes to function effectively within the gastrointestinal tract. It also supports saliva and mucosal secretions, which are necessary for swallowing and the protection of the digestive lining. Moreover, hydration is responsible for keeping normal bowel habits by making the stool softer, thereby preventing constipation and maximizing the overall health of the intestine.

In urban Latin American cities, as per a recent study, plain water makes only 38.4% contribution to water intake, and significant contributions come from other beverages, such as coffee and sugary drinks (Yépez et al., 2024). This blended strategy towards hydration indicates the importance of having pure water as a leading component in one's diet, as it directly contributes to digestive efficiency and overall well-being in the long run, an important consideration especially where diversity in food sources is limited (Freer et al., 2024).

10.4.4. Stress Management and Its Impact on the Abdomen

The intertwined relationship between stomach health and stress cannot be overlooked, as stress also has a tendency to manifest physically, and most commonly, in the stomach. Long-term stress makes the body release hormones such as cortisol, which can also lead to many types of gastrointestinal issues, including IBS and increased stomach pain. The need for stress management techniques is pressing, considering that psychological therapy has been proven effective in the management of such disorders, as debated in studies on anxiety and depressive disorders in children (Smith et al., 2008). Application of techniques like mindfulness, yoga, and cognitive-behavioral therapy can reduce stress and its physiological impacts. Apart from that, prevention and treatment services of the psychological health component demonstrate how emotional wellness treatment is crucial to the overall abdominal well-being (Alewijnse et al., 2016). Last but not least, prioritizing stress management is capable of enhancing both mental and physical welfare, recognizing it as an important sector in maintaining the health of the abdomen.

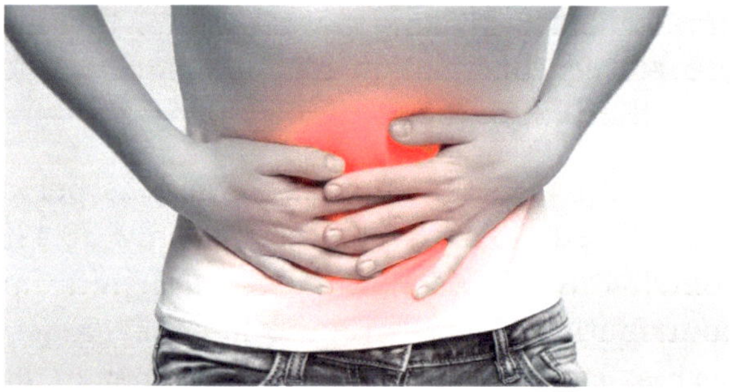

Source: PatientPop. (n.d.). *Person Holding Stomach in Pain.*

10.4.5. Preventive Measures for Abdominal Disorders

Preventive measures for abdominal ailments can significantly foster total wellness and reduce the likelihood of chronic pain onset. Key steps include the intake of a balanced diet, rich in fiber, to enhance gastrointestinal health and prevent the onset of conditions such as IBS and abdominal pain. Physical exercise, preferably consistent, is also essential; it supports digestive health and may assist in weight maintenance, thereby reducing the risk of visceral pain. In addition, the neuroplastic pain-perceiving mechanisms that lead to chronic conditions are relevant to know. According to recent studies, neuroplasticity changes were revealed to play a central role in chronic pain development from acute pain, implying the need for early intervention and pain management strategy training (Lars et al., 2017). With the active identification and management of vulnerable risk factors and these preventive strategies, it is possible to enhance one's abdominal health and QoL.

10.4.6. Regular Screenings and Check-Ups

Maintaining optimal health is often facilitated through regular screenings and check-ups, which serve as proactive measures to identify potential health issues before they become severe. Such assessments are crucial for detecting conditions that may affect the abdomen, including gastrointestinal diseases or metabolic disorders. For instance, as noted in a study of rural firefighters, consistent health screenings can reveal critical information regarding body composition, cardiovascular fitness, and overall physical health (Langford, 2019). In this context, identifying alarming changes through screenings can help initiate early intervention strategies. Similarly, the unfortunate case of a young woman experiencing respiratory failure two weeks postpartum highlights the importance of continuous medical oversight during pivotal life events like pregnancy. Regular check-ups can ensure that any underlying health concerns, such as those related to calcium metabolism and parathyroid function, are promptly addressed, thereby preventing tragic outcomes (Catani et al., 2022). Thus, regular screenings play an essential role in fostering long-term health and well-being.

10.4.7. Importance of Maintaining a Healthy Weight

Being a healthy weight is central to wellness and prevention of the development of many chronic conditions. Overweight populations are at high risk of various health conditions, including cardiovascular diseases, diabetes, and certain cancers, particularly gastric cancer, which highlights the significance of weight control as indicated in the pathogenic role of Helicobacter pylori in chronic gastritis that might progress to more severe diseases (Peter et al., 2023). The abdominal region, with visceral fat accumulation, is especially prone to health problems, further highlighting weight maintenance as critical in individuals seeking to lower their probability of acquiring related complications.

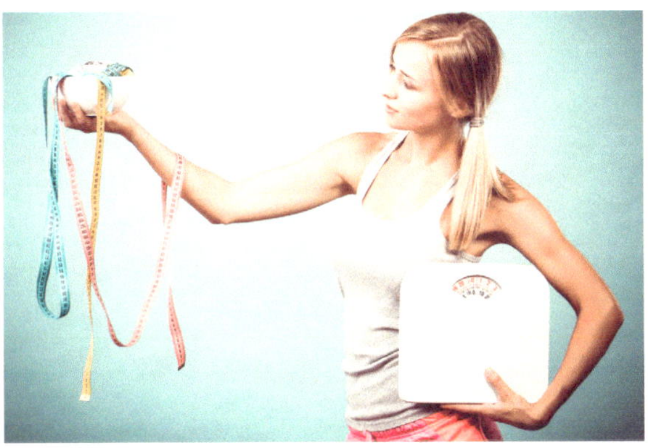

Figure 10.14. Importance of maintaining a healthy weight.

Source: Shopify. (n.d.). *Woman Holding Weighing Scale and Bowl with Measuring Tapes.*

Additionally, the association of the vagus nerve with physical and psychological well-being ensures that a healthy weight might improve mood as well as stress coping mechanisms, hence further validating the value of effective weight management techniques (Sigrid et al., 2018). Lastly, promoting a healthy lifestyle with regular exercise and mindful dietary habits is important to achieve maximum weight gain and improve QoL (Figure 10.14).

10.4.8. Lifestyle Changes for Better Abdominal Health

Adherence to lifestyle changes plays a crucial role in ensuring enhanced abdominal well-being and the prevention of related discomforts. Regular physical exercise, particularly certain exercises, greatly enhances core strength and flexibility, and this serves to assist in relieving tensions often associated with abdominal issues. For instance, a trial of water exercise for pregnant women revealed that the performance of organized physical exercises resulted in enhanced body image, alleviated discomfort, and enhanced mobility (Smith et al., 2002). Also, weight control and body composition have prime significance to the health of the abdomen; an overall exercise regime is demonstrated to reduce the risk of heart disease and enhance overall cardiovascular well-being (Streng, 2006). Eating a well-balanced diet with high fiber intake, greens, and low-fat protein sources along with adequate hydration can assist in maintaining function in the gastrointestinal system and reducing bloating. By making these lifestyle modifications, individuals can build healthier abdomens and feel better overall (Cohen, 2015).

10.4.9. Role of Education in Promoting Abdominal Wellness

Education plays a key role in ensuring abdominal health by empowering people with the information they need to make appropriate health decisions. Information about physical activity and how it influences abdominal health is crucial, particularly in the wake of rising statistics in diseases brought about by sedentary lifestyles. As emphasized in recent studies, public health interventions that make communities aware of the benefits of physical exercise can most enhance participation in health-enhancing behaviors (Longhurst et al., 2018). Furthermore, awareness of risk factors associated with hypertension and obesity, the two entities most impacting abdominal health, is required for prevention and management. The prevalence of hypertension among developing nations, as reported by a cross-sectional study, reflects the need to integrate education programs that enlighten individuals on cardiovascular risk related to abdominal well-being (Ayele et al., 2016). Integrating education into public health is essential so that communities can embrace an improved lifestyle, hence improving abdominal health and mitigating the disease burden.

Test Your Knowledge

1. Differentiate between intraperitoneal and retroperitoneal organs with examples.
2. What is the clinical significance of McBurney's point in the abdomen?

SUMMARY

In summary, the complexity of the abdominal region requires a deep appreciation of its anatomy and physiology, highlighting its role at the center stage of health and disease. The investigation of pathologies such as spontaneous intraperitoneal bladder rupture helps to underscore the importance of identifying abdominal abnormalities, particularly in those with specific medical backgrounds such as having undergone pelvic radiotherapy. As noted, spontaneous rupture of the bladder is to emphasize that occurs years after radiation therapy is to be taken into consideration (Başer et al., 2016). Additionally, the interplay between environmental and genetic factors can exert a potent influence on abdominal traits as well as on disorders, noting that the evolutionary pathways are biased to a specific CRE, which can have implications in abdominal variations (Kopp et al., 2013). These results not only enhance our knowledge of abdominal issues but also point to the need for individualized medical practices in diagnosis and treatment planning.

The discussion of the abdominal region shows significant advancement in medical technology and understanding of the numerous disorders associated with this area. One of the main concerns presented is the new approach of Natural Orifice Transluminal Endoscopic Surgery (NOTES), in which a flexible endoscope is inserted through natural orifices, avoiding external scarring but with challenges in training and execution (Barrow et al., 2016). This emphasizes the necessity of having good simulation technologies, such as NOViSE, which facilitate the learning of surgical skills without posing a patient risk. Additionally, the approval of the active compression abdominal band is another critical advancement, as it is precisely for orthostatic hypotension (OH) prevalent in stroke patients. As per the research, nylon-6,6 actuators can maintain the necessary levels of tension, and as such, they offer better prospects for treating patients (Tamma, 2018). Cumulatively, these findings underscore the forefront position of the abdominal region in contemporary surgery developments and patient care innovations (Schavelzon et al., 2011).

KEY TERMS FROM THIS CHAPTER

- Abdominal anatomical variations
- Abdominal structures
- Cadaveric prosection techniques
- Computed tomography (CT)
- Detoxification
- Diagnostic imaging technology
- Digestive processes
- Electrolyte levels
- Epstein-Barr Virus (EBV)
- Abdominal complexity
- Blood pressure
- Chronic infection
- Deep Inferior Epigastric Artery (DIEA)
- Diagnostic accuracy
- Digestive mechanisms
- Drug metabolism
- Endocrine systems
- Fetal growth assessment

CRITICAL THINKING QUESTIONS

1. **Which of the following is an intraperitoneal organ?**
   a. Kidney
   b. Pancreas
   c. Liver
   D. Aorta
2. **The inguinal canal in males transmits which of the following structures?**
   a. Ureter
   b. Vas deferens
   C. Femoral artery
   d. Pudendal nerve
3. **Which structure forms the posterior boundary of the rectus sheath below the arcuate line?**
   a. Internal oblique aponeurosis
   b. Transversalis fascia
   c. External oblique aponeurosis
   d. Peritoneum
4. **The foregut is supplied by which artery?**
   a. Superior mesenteric artery
   b. Celiac trunk
   c. Inferior mesenteric artery
   D. Renal artery
5. **McBurney's point is located:**
   a. At the midline of the umbilicus
   b. Between the umbilicus and the anterior superior iliac spine
   c. On the costal margin
   d. Below the pubic symphysis

Short Answer Questions

1. What are the boundaries of the abdominal cavity?
2. What is the function and anatomical location of the greater omentum?
3. Describe the course and branches of the abdominal aorta.
4. Explain the role of the mesentery in the abdominal cavity.
5. What structures pass through the inguinal canal in males and females?
6. Define the portal triad and state its components.

Answers to Critical Thinking Questions

1. (c) 2. (b) 3. (b) 4. (b) 5. (b)

REFERENCES

1. Ala-Mattinen, K., Heikinheimo, M., Tuominen, K., & Kainulainen, K. (2023). Anatomy of Real Intermediate State-Subtraction Scheme. Phys. Rev. D 108, 096034 – Publi*shed 29 November, 2023*
2. *Arend*t-*Ni*elsen, L., Morlion, B., Perrot, S., Dahan, A., Dickenson, A. H., Kress, H. G., Wells, C., Bouhassira, D., & Drewes, A. M. (2017). Assessment and manifestation of central sensitization across different chronic pain conditions. European Journal of Pain, 22, 216–241. https://doi.org/10.1002/ejp.1140 (accessed on 8th May 2025).
3. Ayele, G., Girum, T., Kalssa*, A., & Tamiso, A. (2016). P*revalence and associated factors of hypertension among civil servants working in Arba Minch Town, South Ethiopia. International Journal of Public Health Science (IJPHS), 5(4), 375–383 Institute of Advanced Engineering and Science. https://core*.ac.uk/download/480549425.pdf (accessed on 8th May 2025).*
4. Bains KNS, Kashyap S, Lappin SL. Anatomy, Thorax: Diaphragm. [Updated 2023 Jul 24]. In: StatPearls [Internet]. Treasure Island (FL): StatPearls Publishing; 2025 Jan-. Available from: https://www.ncbi.nlm.nih.gov/books/NBK519558/(accessed on 8th May 2025).
5. Baker, R. L., Brock, G. L., Newsome, E. L., & Zhao, M. (2024). Polyploidy and the evolution of phenotypic integration: Network analysis reveals relationships among anatomy, morphology, and physiology. Applications in plant sciences, 12(4), e11605. https://doi.org/10.1002/aps3.11605(accessed on 8th May 2025).
6. Bordoni B, Sugumar K, Leslie SW. Anatomy, Abdomen and Pelvis, Pelvic Floor. [Updated 2023 Jul 17]. In: StatPearls [Internet]. Treasure Island (FL): StatPearls Publishing; 2025 Jan-. Available from: https://www.ncbi.nlm.nih.gov/books/NBK482200/ (accessed on 8th May 2025).
7. Breit, S., Kupferberg, A., Rogler, G., & Hasler, *G. (2018). Vagus nerve as modulat*or of the brain–gut axis in psychiatric and inflammatory disorders. Frontiers in Psychiatry, 9. https://doi.org/10.3389/fpsyt.2018.00044 (accessed on 8th May 2025).
8. Catani, G., Chighine, A., Conte, C., Corona, A., Demontis, R., & Nioi, M. (2022). A Fatal Case of Metastatic Pulmonary Calcification During the Puerperium. MDPI Publishing. https://www.zora.uzh.ch/id/eprint/237527/1/ZORA_pdf_version_1670228279.pdf (accessed on 8th May 2025).
9. Celicanin, Z. (2014). Respiratory Organ Motion in Interventional MRI: Tracking, Guiding and Modeling. 0.5451/unibas-006622037. https://core.ac.uk/download/46605059.pdf (accessed on 8th May 2025).
10. Ciosi, M., Gitau, J., Masiga, D., Mugasa, C. M., Ndungu, N., & Villinger, J. (2018). Morphological Re-Descript*ion and Molecular Identifi*cation of Tabanidae (Diptera) in East Africa. Pensoft Publishers. https://core.ac.uk/download/201756320.pdf (accessed on 8th May 2025).
11. Cohen, E (2015) T*he Hold and Release Practice: A New Way into Meditation and Mindfulness.* Transpersonal Psychology Review, 17 (1). ISSN 1366-6991(accessed on 8th May 2025).
12. Corniani, G., & Saal, H. P. (2020). Tactile innervation densities across the whole body. Journal of Neurophysiology, 124, 1229–1240. https://doi.org/10.1152/jn.00313.2020 (accessed on 8th May 2025).

13. Dakwar, G. R., Shariati, M., Willaert, W., *Ceelen, W., De Smedt, S. C., &* Remaut, K. (2017). Nanomedicine-based intraperitoneal therapy for the treatment of peritoneal carcinomatos*is - Mission possible?. Advanced drug delivery reviews, 108, 13–24. https://do*i.org/10.1016/j. addr.2016.07.001 (accessed on 8th May 2025).

14. Dheenathayalan, P. S. (2019). A Descriptive Study of Naadi Thervu and Its Clinical Features Based on the text "Sadhaga N*aadi." https://core.ac.uk/download/288215845.pdf (accessed on 8th May 2025).*

15. Dogra, J. R. (1930). The Faucial Tonsil: Its Relation to Focal Infection with Particular Reference to Cholecystitis. The University of Edinburgh. https://core.ac.uk/download/429713855.pdf (accessed on 8th May 2025).

16. DOI:https://doi.org/10.1103/PhysRevD.108.096034. https://www.semanticscholar.org/paper/d291774e2001cd5f482d318f639d526cb8ec42b7 (accessed on 8th May 2025).

*17. Engineering Honors. The Univers*ity of Texas at Austin. https://core.ac.uk/download/211333050.pdf (accessed on 8th May 2025).

18. F Freer, G Ail, *T Chan, M Jones, J Broad, G P Canale, P Elston, J Leeney, P Vickerton, 1017 Out With the Old, i*n With the New? Virtual Reality vs. Cadaveric Based Teaching Materials for Anatomy Education*, British Journal of Surgery, Volume 111, Issue Supplement_6, July 2024, znae163.315, https://*doi.org/10.1093/bjs/znae163.315 (accessed on 8th May 2025).

19. Francis, S., Jayaraj, P., Pournami, P., & Puzhakkal, N. (2023). ContourGAN: Auto-Contouring of Organs at *Risk in Abdomen Computed Tomography Images Using Generative Adversarial Network, 33, 1494–1504. https://www.semanticscho*lar.org/paper/a62dab4bd1ec8751921ee04c73f4d1c4bc583c67 (accessed on 8th May 2025).

20. Franco-López, J., Berdejo, J. C., & Ferreira-Bogado, M. (2021). Laparoscopic Cholecystectomy in Situs Inv*ersus Totalis. https://www.semanticscholar.org/paper/2*4a87f8c766d88b9e48ec127c3283819b2c49163 (accessed on 8th May 2025).

21. Georgakopoulos B, Lasrado S. Anatomy, Head and Neck: Inter-scalene Triangle. [Updated 2022 Nov 9]. In: StatPearls [Internet]. Treasure Island (FL): StatPearls Publishing; 2025 Jan-. Available from: https://www.*ncbi.nlm.nih.gov/books/*NB*K*544222/

22. Ghazeeri, G., Hmedeh, C., & Tewfik, I. (2021). Nutritional Management in Polycystic Ovary Syndrome: Challenges and Opportunities. Inderscience Publishers. https://core.ac.uk/download/161103740.pdf (accessed on 8th May 2025).

23. Goyal, H., Singla, U., Gupta, U., & May, E. (2016). Role of cannabis in digestive disorders. Medical Education and Gastroenterology, 29, 135–143. https://doi.org/10.1097/meg.0000000000000779 (accessed on 8th May 2025).

24. Gupta, S., Gupta, G., Sharda, P., & Mittal, K. (2017). Study evaluating chronic abdominal pain and functional abdominal pain syndrome. International Journal of Research in Medical Sciences, 3(9), 2290–2298. https://doi.org/10.18203/2320-6012.ijrms20150619 (accessed on 8th *May 2025).*

*25. Indahswari, N. W., Indrayani, A. W., Thanaya, S. A., & Wibawa, A. (20*19). The Correlation Between Body Fat Percentage and Peak Expiratory Flow in Children Aged 10–12 Years at SD Negeri 8 Dauh Puri. Faculty of Engineering, Diponegoro University. https://core.a*c.uk/download/234033578.pdf (accessed on 8*th May 2025).

26. Koreyba, L., Hlebeniuk, V., & Plys, V. (2024). Infections of reproductive organs in female rabbits. Scientific Messenger of LNU of Veterinary Medicine and Biotechnologies. Series: Veterinary Sciences, 26(1*14), 70-77. https://doi.org/10.32718/nvlvet11411(accesse*d on 8th May 2025).

27. Langford, E. (2019). Physiological Profile of Rural Structural Firefighters in Southeast Georgia. Digital Commons@Georgia Southern. https://core.ac.*uk/download/229335038.pdf (accessed on 8th May 2025).*

28. *Li, D., & Wu, M. (2021). Pattern Recognition Receptors in Health an*d Diseases, 6. https://doi.org/10.1038/s41392-021-00687-0 (accessed on 8th May 2025).

29. Li, R., Frasch, M. G., & Wu, H. T. (2017). Efficient Fetal-Maternal ECG Signal Separation from Two Channel Maternal Abdominal ECG via *Diffusion-Based Channel Selection. Frontiers in physiology, 8, 277. https://doi.org/10.3389/fphys.*2017.00277 (accessed on 8th May 2025).

30. Lieberman, Z. E., Billen, J., van de Kamp, T., & Boudinot, B. (2*022). The ant abdomen: The skeletomuscular and soft tissue anatomy of Ambly*opone australis workers (Hymenoptera: Formicidae). Journal of Morphology, 283, 693–770. https://www.semanticscholar.org/paper/bf265*df709df5a975b632ad2dea8c856a008a778 (accessed on 8th* May 2025).

31. Longhurst, G. (2018). Project ViTAL ViTAL (Vitality Through Active Living) Fijian Project. Wintec. https://core.ac.uk/download/187724706.pdf (accessed on 8th May 2025).

32. Lyu, F. J., Cui, H., Pan, H., *Cheung, K. M. C., C*ao, X., Iatridis, J. C., & Zheng, Z. *(2021). Painful Inter***v***ert*ebral Disc Degeneration and Inflammation: From Laboratory Evidence to Clinical Interventions, 9. https://doi.org/10.1038/s41413-020-00125-x (accessed on 8th May 2025).

33. Löfgren E, Lindfors P, Nilsson K, Wannstedt J, Bonnert M, Uusijärvi A. Gastrointestinal Group Education for Children and Adolescents with Functional Abdominal Pain Disorders—A Feasibility Study of a Brief Intervention. Gastrointestinal Disorders. 2024; 6(1):1-12. https://doi.org/10.3390/gidisord6010001*(accessed on 8th May 2025).*

34. *Malvy, D., McElroy, A. K., De Clerck, H., Günther, S., & van G*riensven, J. (2019). Ebola virus disease. The Lancet, 393, 936–948. https://doi.org/10.1016/s0140-6736(18)33132-5 (accessed on 8th May 2025).

35. Nikolaeva, E. A. (2024). Specialization of Literature by Means of Interdisciplinary Inte*gration. Pedagogy Theory & Practic*e, том 9, издание 8, страницы 740-746 DOI: 10.30853/ped20240094

36. Patel, S. M., Venkatesan, V., Barras, A. A., & Pacheco, L. L. (2024). Ileo-ileal intussusception secondary to ne*uroendocrine tu*mor in adult patient. Am J Case Rep., 25, 944872-1–944872-4. https://www.semanticscholar.org/paper/b95d2eae20f*6330f1c2751ddc3ff11a3945bbfc6 (accessed on 8th May 2025).*

37. *Sayyaf, D. B.*, Pironi, F., Rossetti, E., & Herlyn, H. (2024). New Insights on the Male and Female Reproductive Organs of Centrorhynchus Globocaudatus (Acanthocephala), Intestinal Parasite of Birds of Prey. 13. https://www.semanticscholar.org/paper/f4751b7cb427ca77627868a86ca49cf9*d231eaeb (accessed* on 8th May 2025).

38. Schavelzon, D., Habbema, L., Rapprich, S., Lisborg, P., Blugerman, G., A., J., ... Sigue, M. (2011). Application of the Liposuction Techniques and Principles in Specific Bod*y Areas and Pathologies. InTech. doi: 10.5772/24809(accessed on 8th May 2025).*

39. *Sharma, V., & Panchal, P. (2024). Hiding Beaver Tail Liver: A Rare* Anatomical Variant of the Liver, 16. https://www.semanticscholar.org/paper/9734fa7c007d244dbe74723685c0ced0fae8ce3c (accessed on 8th May 2025).

40. *Singo, T. P. P. (2016). Abdominal CT Findings in HIV-Infected Pati*ents Presenting with Acute Abdomen. A research report submitted to the Faculty of Health Sciences, University of the Witwatersrand, Jo*hannesburg, in partial fulfillment of the requirements for the degree of Mas*ter of Medicine in Diagnostic Radiology. Johannesburg, 2016. URI: https://hdl.handle.net/10539/25786 (accessed on 8th May 2025).

41. Slavu I, Filipoiu F, Tulin R, Dima I, Dogaru A, Socea B, Tomescu L, Badea T, Oprescu Macovei A, Tulin A. Arterial Vascularization of the Colon; A Guide to Surgical Resection. Journal of Mind and Medical Scien*ces. 2024; 11(1):203-209. https://doi.org/10.22543/2392-7674.1498(accessed on 8th May 2025).*

42. *Smith, M., & Storey, P. (2008). Methods and Approaches to Improving* the Emotional Health and Well-Being of Children: A Briefing Paper Concerning Interventions to Prevent Internalizing Disorders. Institute of Education, University of London. https://core.ac.uk/download/pdf/82102.pdf (accessed on 8th May 2025).

43. Song Q, He Y, Chen L, Xia X, Wang N, Song Q and Liu A (2024) Feasibility of the application of frequency modulated continuous wave radar trigger technique in abdominal m*agnetic resonance imaging. Front. Phys. 12:1319678. doi: 10.3389/fphy.2024.1319678(acces*sed on 8th May 2025).

44. Streng, Vicki. CORONARY HEA*RT DISEASE RISK STRATIFICATION IN FULL-TIME MIAMI V*ALLEY HOSPITAL EMPLOYEES. 2006. Wright State University, Master›s thesis. OhioLINK Electronic Theses and Dissertations Center, http://rave.ohiolink.edu/etdc/view?acc_num=wright1165604997.(accessed on 8th May 2025).

45. Sumadewi K T, Embryology, anatomy and physiology of the liver: *Review. Indian J Clin Anat Physiol 2023;10(3):138-144 (*accessed on 8th May 2025).

46. Sun, J., Tanaka, J., & Valenti, L. (2022). The Changing Epidemiology of Liver Diseases in Asia, 42. *https://www.semanticscholar.org/paper/540b03dd9e42a31b1359*a7e37b2a563d6af835ab (accessed on 8th May 2025).

47. Tamma, P. (2018). Quantifying Viscoelastic Properties of Nylon-6,6 Actuators. BME 679H | May 2018

48. Truitt, R. V. (1939). *Our Water Resources and Their Conservation.* Chesapeake Biological Laboratory. https://core.ac.uk/download/11018274.pdf (accessed on 8th May 2025).

49. Western University. (1959). *UWOMJ,* 29(3). Scholarship@Western. https://core.ac.uk/download/61662876.pdf (accessed on 8th May 2025).

50. Yabut, K. C. B., Martynova, A., Nath, A., Zercher, B. P., Bush, M. F., & Isoherranen, N. (2024). Drugs Form Ternary Complexes with Human Liver Fatty Acid Binding Protein (FABP1) and FABP1 Binding Alters Drug Metabolism. *bioRxiv : the preprint server for biology*, 2024.01.17.576032. https://doi.org/10.1101/2024.01.17.576032(accessed on 8th May 2025).

PELVIS AND PERINEUM

11

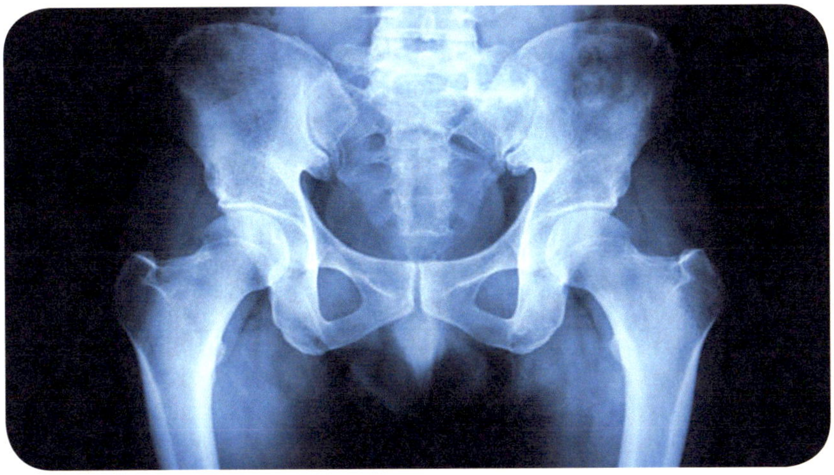

LEARNING OBJECTIVES

After studying this chapter, you will be able to:

1. Discuss the anatomy of the pelvis
2. Explain the functions of the pelvis
3. Know clinical significance of the pelvis and perineum
4. Focus on cultural and social perspectives on the pelvis and perineum

Introduction

The human body is highly complicated, particularly in regions that are both structural and functional by nature. Among these, the pelvis and perineum stand out for their significance in a variety of physiological processes, including locomotion, reproduction, and the elimination of waste products. This anatomical space, which is often glossed over in general accounts of human anatomy, offers critical support for the weight of the torso and facilitates a number of vital functions. The interaction of muscle, bone, and soft tissue here is complex and critical and affects not only individual well-being but also overall health. Both the pelvis and perineum can only be grasped by adopting a multi-faceted approach, both in their anatomy and clinical importance. In the course of this discussion, we will unveil how these structures form part of human anatomy and how vital they are in medical practice, emphasizing the need for extensive training in this important field of human health.

Definition of the Pelvis and Perineum

The pelvis functions as a vital anatomical structure that not only supports the weight of the upper body but also forms a protective shield over the pelvic organs. It consists of a complex arrangement of bones, ligaments, and muscles and is also in charge of many of the functions of the body, including movement and giving birth. Found beneath the pelvis, the perineum can usually be described as a diamond-shaped region which cushions the pelvic organs and is circumscribed by the pubic symphysis anteriorly and posteriorly by the coccyx. In the postpartum environment, understanding the anatomy of the pelvis and perineum is essential since physical changes and dysfunctions that may occur after childbirth can have an immense impact on women's health. An information brochure designed for new mothers has the priority of providing this information by introducing potential complications such as pelvic floor dysfunctions and the various treatment methods, thus ensuring early detection and early intervention (Olson et al., 2001) (Figure 11.1).

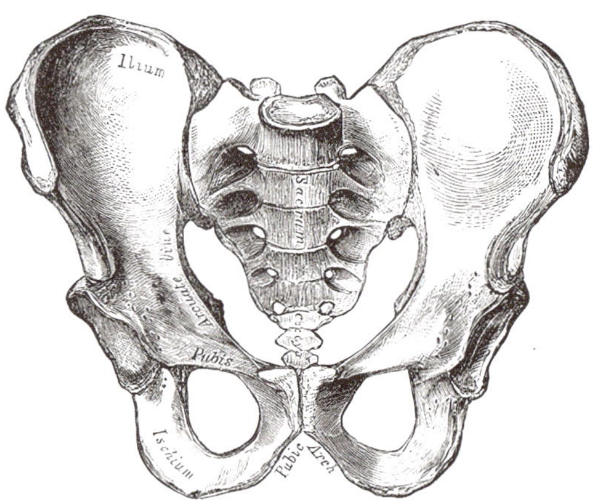

Figure 11.1. The pelvis and perineum.

Source: By Henry Vandyke Carter - Henry Gray (1918) Anatomy of the Human Body (See "Book" section below)Bartleby.com: Gray's Anatomy, Plate 241, Public Domain, https://commons.wikimedia.org/w/index.php?curid=323668

Importance of the Pelvis and Perineum in Human Anatomy

Perineum and pelvis are the essential structures of human anatomy, possessing both structural integrity and functional significance. Not only do they contain various organs, but they are also central to the most critical of human functions, such as urination, defecation, and delivery. Pelvic floor injury, particularly during delivery, can lead to enormous complications and emphasize the need for a more in-depth appreciation of such anatomical structures. A more current research incorporating magnetic resonance diffusion tensor imaging (MR-DTI) has noted the architecture of the pelvic floor muscles (PFMs), showing their complex connections and formation. For instance, studies indicate that external anal sphincter muscle fibers cross midline in the perineal body, further contributing to the purse string effect of the muscles, which in turn highlights the complexity of this region (Cory et al., 2018). Furthermore, the production of 3D anatomical models enhances the understanding of pelvic anatomy, gaining students valuable insights to enhance understanding of relations among structures (Imielinska et al., 2004).

Overview of the Functions of the Pelvic Region

The pelvic region has important functions beyond the mere structural support of the body. Primarily, it is a pathway for the urinary and reproductive systems, containing important structures such as the bladder and uterus, both useful in elimination of waste and reproductive health. The pelvic floor also provides muscular support as an integral part of the mechanism of urination and defecation, as well as sexuality. As highlighted by more recent research, the anatomy of the perineum comprises dynamic interactions among various organs and tissues that determine the overall functioning of the perineum, especially in pelvic organ prolapse

(POP) and incontinence (Aijaz et al., 2022). Moreover, the surgical operations, such as pelvic exenteration, emphasize the importance of the pelvic anatomy and the subsequent reconstruction, thereby reinforcing how pelvic integrity impacts the quality of life (QoL) of the patient (Arcieri et al., 2024). Thus, the pelvic region is crucial not just for its anatomical roles but also for maintaining body functions and general health.

Historical Perspective on the Study of the Pelvis

With time, the pelvis has been at the forefront in clinical practice and anatomical investigations due to shifting paradigms of medical science. In the past, the pelvis was first investigated mainly from the descriptive perspective as influenced by existing cultural beliefs regarding childbirth and anatomy. Vesalius and other ancient anatomists set the stage by describing the structure of the pelvis very accurately, but the evidence for the observations did not hold up to empirical standards of today. With advances in imaging technology and methodology, including ultrasound, visualization of pelvic anatomy and pathology has come a long way. Such progress allows for a better understanding of conditions of the pelvis, including complications of penetrating abdominal trauma, especially in settings such as urban violence in South Africa, where the research in penetrating abdominal trauma shows the importance of pelvic evaluations in trauma care (Sander et al., 2020). These advances underscore the crucial role that the pelvis plays in reproductive as well as general health, its prominence in medical education in general (Figure 11.2).

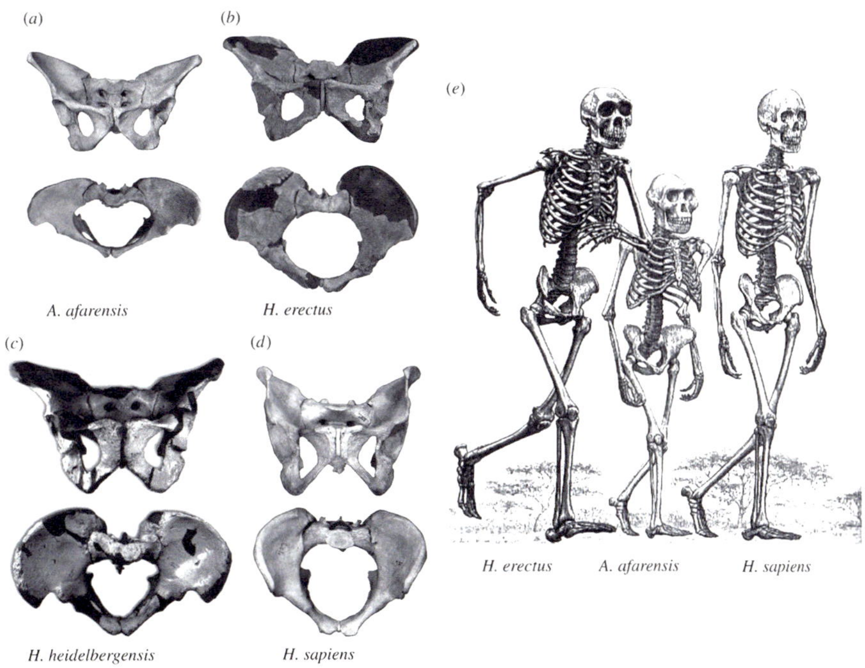

Figure 11.2. Historical perspective on the study of the pelvis.

Source: Royal Society Publishing. (2014). *Pelvic morphology and full-body skeleton comparison among A. afarensis, H. erectus, H. heidelbergensis, and H. sapiens.*

Relevance in Medical and Health Sciences

The understanding of the perineum and pelvis is most important for doctors due to its central role in various physiological as well as pathological processes. As the foundation of the reproductive and urinary apparatus, detailed knowledge of this region is required for proper diagnosis and surgical skill. As evidenced by the addition of cadaveric dissection modules into medical curricula, as presented in Nova Medical School, the hands-on experience enhances students' comprehension and makes it easier to relate theory to clinical practice (Arora et al., 2017). Secondly, a more evolved core syllabus that addresses 156 learning outcomes illustrates the significance of a structured paradigm in studying anatomy to secure that medical students comprehend body system complexities pertinent to their subsequent practice (Smith et al., 2015). As such, pelvic region learning not only improves anatomical education but indeed impacts effective healthcare delivery and patient outcomes.

Significance of Understanding the Pelvis and Perineum

It is more valuable than gold to have a good knowledge of the pelvis and perineum, particularly in anatomy and medicine, because these are the sites of many physiological processes and operations. Looking at problems such as endometriosis provides a hint on how complex these sites are. The relationship between the pelvic organs and initiation of disease is an excellent example of the need for extensive anatomical knowledge; retrograde menstruation, as a cause of endometriosis formation, is an exemplification of pelvic anatomy's capability to complicate health (Carmichael & Mills, 2022). Furthermore, advancements in technology regarding surgical techniques, especially for low-lying rectal cancer, are also examples of the need for a sophisticated understanding of pelvic anatomy to have optimal surgical outcomes. Intersphincteric resection as a method of preserving anal function with oncological security requires sensitive appreciation of the pelvic anatomical barriers and relationships (Guglielmo et al., 2021). It is therefore important to have mastered the technical aspects of the pelvis and perineum in a bid to improve patients' health and maximally enhance surgical efficacy.

11.1. Anatomy of the Pelvis

Learning Outcome

1. Give an Overview of Pelvic Bones
2. Describe the Structure of the Pelvic Girdle
3. Differences Between Male and Female Pelvis
4. Explain the Pelvic Inlet and Outlet
5. Understand Ligaments Associated with the Pelvis
6. Focus on Muscles of the Pelvic Floor
7. Learn about Neurovascular Supply to the Pelvis
8. Discuss the Anatomical Landmarks of the Pelvis
9. Explain the Imaging Techniques for Pelvic Assessment

Knowing about the pelvis anatomy is relevant in relation to comprehending the complex role played by it in human function and biology. There are vital structures within this region, like the reproductive system, and pelvic floor muscles (PFMs) whose role in supporting and maintaining stability is important. The pelvis also has critical anatomical relationships that are difficult to visualize, and therefore the need for advanced tools in learning, like 3D models that successfully represent pelvic anatomy from multiple dimensions (Imielinska et al., 2004). Besides, the healthy function of the pelvic region is strongly linked with practices like Moola Bandha, which activates the floor of the pelvis by contracting the levator ani muscles (LAMs) and thereby shielding pelvic organs and promoting general well-being (Bhatnagar et al., 2016). Therefore, a thorough examination of the pelvic anatomy not only expands our understanding of physiological interactions but also informs clinical practice for pelvic health and dysfunction (Figure 11.3).

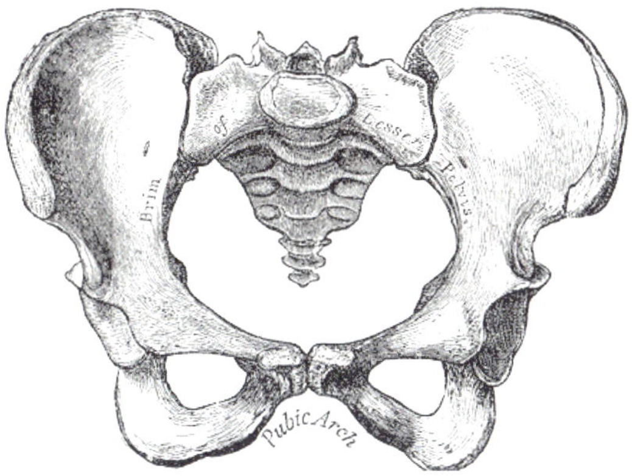

Figure 11.3. Pelvis anatomy.

Source: By Henry Vandyke Carter - Henry Gray (1918) Anatomy of the Human Body (See "Book" section below)Bartleby.com: Gray's Anatomy, Plate 242, Public Domain, https://commons.wikimedia.org/w/index.php?curid=323669

11.1.1. Overview of Pelvic Bones

The pelvic bones form a complex structure that plays a vital role in weight-bearing and the shielding of internal organs. The pelvis, composed of the ilium, ischium, pubis, sacrum, and coccyx, facilitates a multitude of functions, particularly relating to childbirth. In addition to serving as a foundation for the lower limbs, this structure also provides attachment points for the various muscles and ligaments necessary for movement and stability. Because of its significance, the pelvic region is susceptible to damage during delivery, which could lead to severe injuries such as obstetric anal sphincter injuries (OASIS) and LAM injuries, with implications for long-term maternal health and quality of life (QoL) (Kimmich et al., 2024). The pelvic bones need to be comprehended to grasp the pelvic floor dysfunctions often endured following childbirth, as explained in literature reviews covering this period (Olson et al., 2001). These findings stress the importance of anatomical knowledge in the successful management of pelvic health issues.

11.1.2. Structure of the Pelvic Girdle

The pelvic girdle is a critical structure that connects the axial skeleton and lower limbs to support and provide mobility. Composed of the ilium, ischium, and pubis, they conjoin at the acetabulum to provide for femoral articulation. It not only provides a firm base of support for the spine but is also crucial for bearing weight during bipedal support.

Moreover, the human pelvis has evolved from the quadruped ancestors to become more specialized in their function, adapting to support the abdominal viscera and accommodate childbirth, which demands a broader and more consistent structure than in any other mammal (Aggarwal et al., 2020). This complex architecture is required for maintaining pelvic floor function, a region that is central to gynecologic health, as it supports the pelvic organs and provides the foundation for urinary and fecal continence (Parente et al., 2008) (Figure 11.4).

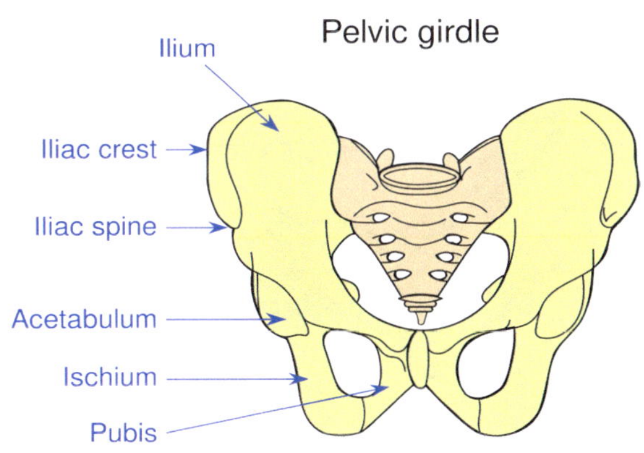

Figure 11.4. Pelvic girdle structure.

Source: Wikipedia. (n.d.). *Pelvic Girdle Illustration.*

11.1.3. Differences Between Male and Female Pelvis

These anatomical differences between the male and female pelvis have significant implications for both biological processes and surgery. Females have a more circular and broader pelvic inlet compared to males, who possess a narrower heart-shaped pelvis. This is largely determined by evolution and facilitates childbirth by providing a larger birth canal. Studies indicate that the distribution pattern of perforator vessels (PV) of the internal pudendal artery (IPA), needed for pelvic reconstruction procedures, is also gender-specific; females exhibit a predominance of perforators in the anterior-central region, while males show a concentration in the central-posterior region (Bassetto et al., 2020). These anatomic variations are crucial in formulating gender-specific surgical techniques because they lead to better understanding of male and female vascular pedicle supply. Lastly, these variations aid in identifying them for preoperative planning and achieving the highest outcome in reconstructive surgery, underlining the importance of gender-based anatomical insight (Parente et al., 2008) (Figure 11.5).

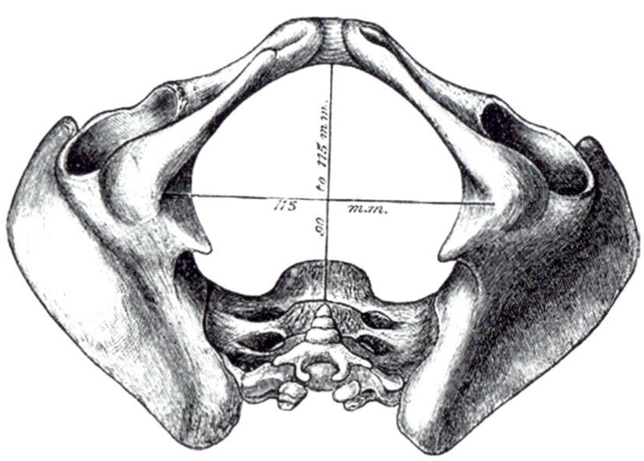

Figure 11.5. Male vs female pelvic bones.

Source: By Henry Vandyke Carter - Henry Gray (1918) Anatomy of the Human Body (See "Book" section below)Bartleby.com: Gray's Anatomy, Plate 239, Public Domain, https://commons.wikimedia.org/w/index.php?curid=792152

11.1.4. Pelvic Inlet and Outlet

The pelvic inlet and outlet are significant anatomical planes that facilitate various physiological functions, particularly during delivery. The pelvic inlet, being the superior opening of the true pelvis, is an inverted heart-shaped structure that will accommodate passage of the fetus during delivery. Its size and shape may affect labor progress and mode of delivery significantly. Conversely, the pelvic outlet—the inferior opening—is most critical in the final stages of labor. Its dimensions and contours are relevant because they dictate the potential vaginal delivery and influence the mother's comfort during delivery. Clinicians must take these anatomical characteristics into consideration since intervention may vary based on the evaluation of these regions during pregnancy. For instance, sonographic guidance during labor assessment can help enable better decision-making regarding the management of delivery (Ghi et al., 2018), obtaining the best possible outcomes for both mother and child while handling complicated clinical cases (Carmichael & Mills, 2022).

11.1.5. Ligaments Associated with the Pelvis

The integrity and stability of the pelvis are provided mainly by a ligamentous system that provides much-needed support to pelvic organs. These ligaments, including the sacroiliac ligaments, sacrospinous ligament, and the uterosacral ligaments, play very significant roles in securing the bony elements of the pelvis and offering resistance to excessive movement. This interconnectivity is especially important in the case of the pelvic floor, which must be able to support not just the bladder and the rectum but also the uterus in females, thus maintaining urinary and fecal continence, along with overall pelvic organ function. A solid understanding of pelvic floor dynamics is a necessity for any gynecologist since the integrity of the ligaments influences not just the anatomical position but also the mechanical forces in the course of different activities like pregnancy and childbearing (Aggarwal et al., 2020). It becomes even more relevant when one considers the effects of any ligamentous dysfunction or injury on pelvic health (Parente et al., 2008).

11.1.6. Muscles of the Pelvic Floor

PFMs are tasked with guaranteeing not only the structural integrity of the pelvis but also the working well-being of the lower organs of the body. The group of muscles stabilizes the pelvic organs, including the bladder and intestines, and guarantees urinary and fecal continence and thus becomes a vital component in gynecological well-being (Aggarwal et al., 2020). Moreover, understanding their complex musculature is important, especially since they can be injured in childbirth and other forms of physical stress. It is through recent studies using magnetic resonance diffusion tensor imaging (MR-DTI) that precise information about the configuration of such muscles has been disclosed, a discovery that sheds light on their functional dynamics (Carmichael & Mills, 2022). This new imaging technique illustrates how muscle fibers interconnect to form a supportive network crossing the midline in the perineal area, an element critical to both functional and aesthetic surgical planning in pelvic health.

11.1.7. Neurovascular Supply to the Pelvis

The pelvic region is richly supplied with an elaborate and complex network of blood vessels and nerves needed for its function and overall health. The main arteries like the internal iliac artery branch and divide to provide oxygen to the pelvic organs, and the lumbar and sacral plexuses form a highly complex network of nerves that are tasked with innervating the pelvic floor musculature. These neurovascular structures are necessary to maintain pelvic organ function and to facilitate activities such as urination, defecation, and sexual health. In addition, conditions such as pelvic floor disorders (PFDs) and organ prolapse are brought about by disruption in the supply, thus emphasizing the importance of studying its anatomy. Surgery, like pelvic exenteration, necessitates adequate consideration of such neurovascular routes to ensure a lack of complications and the best recovery outcomes, as evidenced by the need for reconstructive surgeries following surgery to restore pelvic stability and function (Arcieri et al., 2024). As such, a thorough knowledge of the pelvis's neurovascular supply is necessary for effective clinical practice and maximum patient care (Figure 11.6).

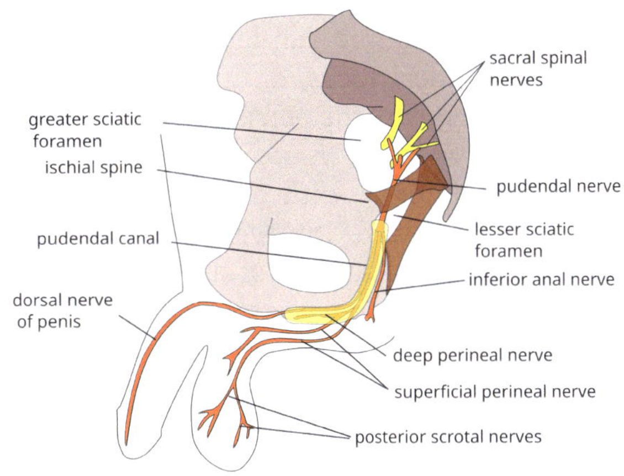

Figure 11.6. Neurovascular supply to the pelvis.

Source: By Mikael Häggström.When using this image in external works, it may be cited as:Häggström, Mikael (2014). "Medical gallery of Mikael Häggström 2014". WikiJournal of Medicine 1 (2). DOI:10.15347/wjm/2014.008. ISSN 2002-4436. Public Domain.orBy Mikael Häggström, used with permission.Cleanup by User:CFCF - Essential Clinical Anatomy. K.L. Moore & A.M. Agur. Lippincott, 2 ed. 2002. Page 263, Public Domain, https://commons.wikimedia.org/w/index.php?curid=3457065

11.1.8. Anatomical Landmarks of the Pelvis

Anatomy students and medical professionals must be aware of the complex anatomical landmarks of the pelvis. The bony structure provides an essential background with the ilium, ischium, and pubis making up the pelvic girdle. Not only do the organs of reproduction and the urinary system find protection from the pelvis, but the upper half of the body's weight is also supported by it. Interestingly, the vasculature of the region, particularly the IPA, becomes a deciding factor in reconstructive surgery, as seen in research comparing PV based on gender (Bassetto et al., 2020). Not only do these vessels differ in their distribution but also in their caliber, which can have a significant influence on planning surgery. With its most salient anatomical focus, an understanding of the characteristics of the pelvis enhances clinical practice, particularly reconstructive surgery in which familiarity with gendered anatomy could guide effective interventions (Bassetto et al., 2020). Identification of these landmarks thus not only enhances anatomical knowledge but also plays a fundamental part in surgical practice and effective patient outcomes.

11.1.9. Imaging Techniques for Pelvic Assessment

There are a number of imaging techniques that play an important role in the assessment of pelvic health, providing clinicians with vital information that aids diagnosis and treatment. Techniques such as ultrasound, magnetic resonance imaging (MRI), and computed tomography (CT) scans are employed to visualize the complex anatomy of the pelvic region to identify dysfunctions or abnormalities. Specifically, MRI is highly beneficial in the assessment of soft tissue structures and can highlight effectively conditions such as myofascial pelvic pain (MFPP). The detection of the presence of myofascial trigger points with the use of imaging can justify intervention that involves both physical therapy and minimally invasive interventions (Katzman et al., 2012). Furthermore, the creation of a consensus on nomenclature for pelvic floor dysfunction highlights the benefit of standard imaging assessment. Transparency allows for interdisciplinary collaboration, facilitating clinicians sharing results and treatment plans to optimize patient care (Abramov et al., 2016). Ultimately, the addition of advanced imaging methods adds depth to our understanding of the perineum and pelvic region, providing new opportunities for more effective care.

Test Your Knowledge

1. What are the key bony landmarks used to identify the pelvic inlet and outlet?
2. Which imaging modality is commonly used to evaluate soft tissue structures in the pelvis?

11.2. Functions of the Pelvis

Learning Outcome

1. Discuss the Support for the Abdominal Organs
2. Explain the Role in Locomotion and Posture
3. Understand Contribution to Reproductive Functions
4. Discuss the Involvement in Childbirth
5. Know Function in Urinary Control
6. How to Impact on Sexual Health
7. Know Role in the Digestive System
8. Evaluate Pelvic Floor Dynamics During Physical Activity
9. Learn about Importance in Maintaining Pelvic Stability

The pelvis serves many important functions that extend far beyond structural support. It is first and foremost a base component of the skeleton that supports the upper half of the body while allowing for functional mobility of the lower extremities. The pelvis is also an essential component of both the reproductive and urinary systems, providing shelter and protection for organs such as the bladder, uterus, and rectum.

In complex surgical contexts, particularly trauma, the integrity of the pelvis has to be restored to facilitate important functions. For example, the application of a composite pedicled fasciocutaneous anterolateral thigh flap can reconstruct pelvic defects effectively, further emphasizing the multi-functionality of the pelvis in human anatomy by not only supporting important organs but also facilitating independent ambulation and maintaining urinary and anal continence (Hansen et al., 2015). Further, ongoing research into pelvic mechanics continues to provide data relevant to engineering and rehabilitation, as in recent studies (Parente et al., 2008) (Figure 11.7).

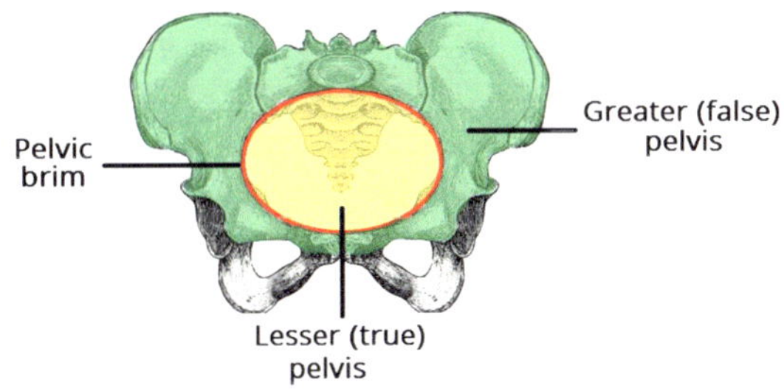

Figure 11.7. The pelvis serves multiple critical functions.

Source: TeachMeAnatomy. (n.d.). *Greater and Lesser Pelvis Divided by the Pelvic Brim.*

11.2.1. Support for the Abdominal Organs

The human pelvis is also important in supporting the abdominal organs, acting as a support base for different structures that provide stability for the body. This anatomical region has been significantly changed due to the evolution from quadrupedal to bipedal movement and has led to some adaptations of the pelvic structure. The pelvic girdle and a complex arrangement of fascia and muscle provide vital support for the abdominal viscera to counteract the force of gravity when erect. As the literature has described, the bony pelvis is inferiorly uncovered, a testament to the importance of the pelvic floor in the continuation of this support system. The pelvic floor not only holds the pelvic organs but also ensures the appropriate function of urinary and fecal continence mechanisms, a fundamental aspect of health and QoL (Aggarwal et al., 2020). Such relations are essential to understand for gynecology specialists and the related fields because they directly correlate with treatment outcomes and patient management (Parente et al., 2008).

11.2.2. Role in Locomotion and Posture

The evolution of the pelvis has been at the core of much of the progress of bipedal gait and its related implications for posture. When humans left quadruped posture and began walking on two legs, the pelvis adapted to stabilize a vertically aligned spine that would allow for a more efficient gait and greater stability. This change in posture significantly altered the relationship between the urethro and vesical, leading to pressure dynamics changes within the abdominal cavity, with relevance to conditions like stress urinary incontinence (SUI) (Hodgkinson, 1969).

Furthermore, the evolutionary changes noted in Australopithecines illustrate the delicately balanced coexistence between bipedalism and brain development, enabling relatively immature infant delivery and promoting cooperative breeding behavior (Fornai et al., 2022). As a result, the pelvis is not just a locomotion platform but also influences a lot of our physiological activities, thus underlining its important role in our complete evolutionary success and adaptative approach.

11.2.3. Contribution to Reproductive Functions

The perineum and pelvic area focal points for the reproductive mechanisms, being a complex anatomical structures that support varied physiological activities. The accurate structure of muscles, connective tissue, and nerves of this location not only facilitates the mechanical activity of reproduction, i.e., parturition but also provides for the hormonal and neural interactions required for fertility and sexual function. Understanding the anatomy and physiology of the PFMs, particularly the pubo-coccygeus, is significant as this muscle group is responsible for controlling the pelvic organs like the bladder and reproductive organs (Wilson et al., 2020). Additionally, the absence of clear limits among these muscles complicates surgical intervention and anatomy training, highlighting the imperativeness of proper identification of their functions in normal activity as well as diseases (Anaston et al., 1952). Accordingly, the functions of this region are diversified in terms of reproductive processes and thus necessitate a thorough investigation of its anatomy and dynamics.

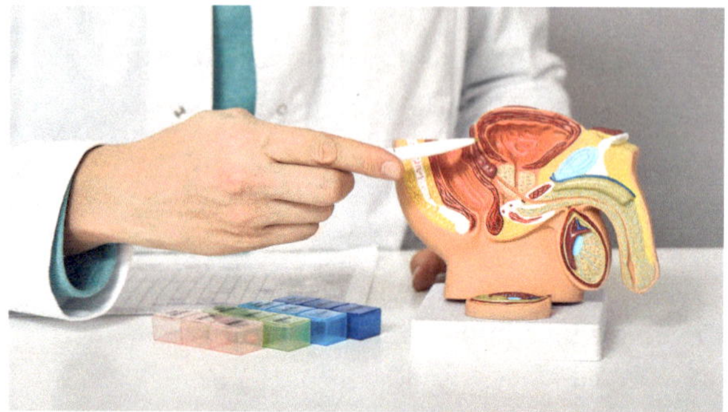

Source: Verywell Health. (n.d.). *Doctor Explaining Male Reproductive Anatomy Using Anatomical Model.*

11.2.4. Involvement in Childbirth

Childbirth is not only a physical process but one with extensive emotional and social implications for women. During this life-changing experience, the quality and degree of interaction and support from health caregivers can significantly impact their overall well-being. Evidence shows that dyspareunia and vulvodynia can follow parturition, having a considerable impact on a woman's QoL since many suffer in silence due to the lack of active inquiry on the part of healthcare providers (Carmichael & Mills, 2022). This underscores the need for providers to establish an environment of open communication and support in prenatal and postnatal care. Further, growing awareness of women's health complications, including urinary incontinence, identifies the necessity of a holistic approach to women's health (Carmichael & Mills, 2022). Such advocacy is called for in the empowerment of women and improved childbirth experiences, emphasizing the need for comprehensive support systems spanning physical as well as emotional aspects of maternal health.

11.2.5. Function in Urinary Control

The delicate balance of the structures within the pelvis is an essential function in the control of urine, which is a very important function in obtaining body health and social living. The PFMs, that encircle the bladder and urethra, control this management to a large extent. It works normally depending on the coordination of these muscles, and any dysfunction may lead to symptoms such as incontinence or pelvic pain. MFPP, a significant player in chronic pelvic pain (CPP) syndromes, demonstrates how dysfunction here can manifest with urinary symptoms, with myofascial trigger points producing referral pain to adjacent areas (Katzman et al., 2012).

Moreover, the introduction of consensus terms for conservative treatments for pelvic floor disorder emphasizes understanding these conditions thoroughly to help healthcare workers accurately diagnose and treat urinary control disturbances (Abramov et al., 2016). In general, identification of the cause of urinary function is essential to enhance therapeutic as well as diagnostic techniques.

11.2.6. Impact on Sexual Health

The complex connection between sexual conduct and pelvic wellbeing highlights the remarkable power that sexual disorder can yield over sexual wellness. CPP, particularly MFPP, not merely affects physical comfort but also psychological intimacy and sensual pleasure. Highlighted in newer studies, MFPP is the major etiology of CPP and often results through myofascial trigger points, which can suppress sexual function (Katzman et al., 2012).

Moreover, how pelvic floor dysfunction intrudes upon regular body experiences is of greatest importance. Developing the coverage of a broad terminology around conservative management of related symptoms has aimed to build clinicians' knowledge and help in treating such dysfunctions in the best manner possible (Abramov et al., 2016). Accordingly, the treatment and management of these pelvic disorders holistically are critical for enhancing sexual health and overall QoL, exemplifying the imperative of multidisciplinary methods of approach and treatment in this delicate field.

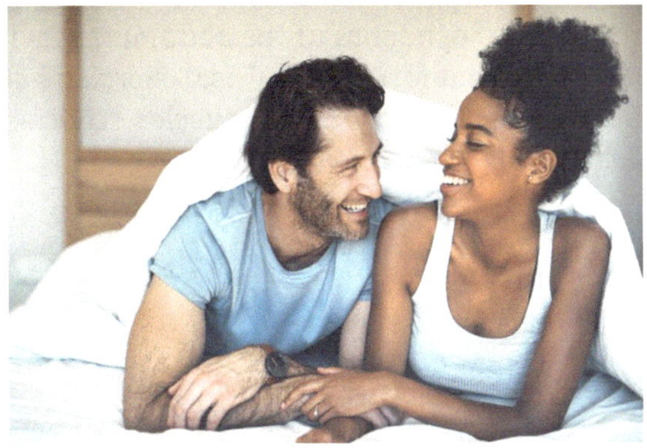

Source: International Society for Sexual Medicine. (2024). *Happy Couple Relaxing Together in Bed*.

11.2.7. Role in the Digestive System

Situated in the pelvis, the digestive system plays a core role in the processing and absorption of nutrients and directly affects overall health. Within this region, there are specific anatomical adaptations that enable the efficient digestion of complex foods. The avian digestive tract, for instance, as noted by Diyar et al. (2023), exhibits significant morphological variation based on dietary requirements, highlighting the importance of organ size and function in nutrient uptake. Moreover, the complex relationship between the microbacteria and digestive organs allows for the uptake of nutrients while maintaining gut health. As part of the fermentation of undigested nutrients, the caeca also acts as a reservoir for beneficial bacteria that can similarly aid in nutrient breakdown and gut function. This complex relationship emphasizes the pelvic area's essential role in digestion, demonstrating how anatomical and microbiota variation can influence dietary effectiveness and overall health outcomes.

11.2.8. Pelvic Floor Dynamics During Physical Activity

Understanding the function of the pelvic floor during physical exercise is vital to both functional and clinical understanding. The PFMs, apart from supporting the pelvic organs, are crucial in stabilizing the core on movement. The pressure dynamics of the abdominal cavity during different forms of physical exercise have a bearing on the way these muscles relax and contract.

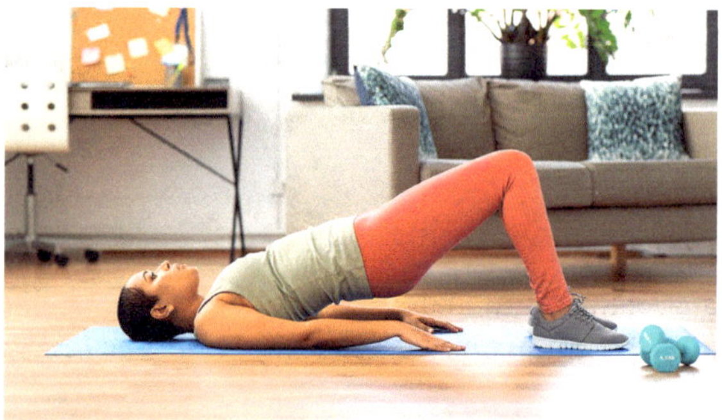

Figure 11.8. Pelvic floor, exercise to strengthen a weak pelvic floor.

Source: Livi. (n.d.). *Woman Doing Pelvic Floor Strengthening Exercise at Home.*

Consequently, improper activation can lead to conditions such as incontinence or pelvic pain. For example, excessive stress is potentially placed on the pelvic floor during high-impact activity, and intense training and rehab strategies need to be employed to develop strength in this area. In addition, habitual pelvic floor exercise can minimize adverse effects, promoting overall pelvic health. Hence, a detailed analysis of such dynamics becomes unavoidable, particularly for participants of sport or intense physical exercises, as the integrity of the pelvis is of utmost relevance for performance as well as health (Denis, 2024) (Figure 11.8).

11.2.9. Importance in Maintaining Pelvic Stability

Pelvic stability is paramount to general health, particularly in childbearing-aged women when the body is dynamically changing. The pelvic floor supports organs that are essential to life and plays a role in maintaining bladder function and sexual health. After giving birth, the majority of women are unlucky enough to endure MSK dysfunctions like low back pain (LBP) and stress urinary incontinence (SUI), and their QoL is compromised. For instance, in a study, 61% of women said they had SUI after an episiotomy but received little or no treatment, demonstrating an appalling gap between knowledge and treatment (Parker et al., 2001). Moreover, appropriate rehabilitation of pelvic dysfunctions by appropriate physical therapy might lead to improved outcomes and prevention of long-term issues since most women accept their condition as a part of normal motherhood (Olson et al., 2001). Therefore, prioritizing stability in the pelvis via education and intervention is paramount to maintain long-term health and well-being.

Test Your Knowledge

1. Discuss the Contribution to Reproductive Functions.
2. Explain the Pelvic Floor Dynamics During Physical Activity.

11.3. Clinical Significance of the Pelvis and Perineum

Learning Outcome

1. Discuss the Common Pelvic Disorders
2. Explain the Pelvic Pain Syndromes
3. Describe the Impact of Pelvic Floor Dysfunction (PFD)
4. Explain the Role of the Pelvis in Urological Health
5. Focus on Gynecological Conditions Related to the Pelvis
6. Understand Pelvic Fractures and their Implications
7. Know Surgical Interventions in the Pelvic Region
8. Evaluate Rehabilitation Strategies for Pelvic Health
9. Learn about Importance of Pelvic Health Education

Both pelvis and perineum are significant when it comes to structural support and functional capacity within the body. Such regions support vital internal organs and support vital physiological functions such as childbirth, sexual activity, and urination. Besides, MFPP often arises because of a dysfunction within these regions, which significantly affects QoL. Specifically, MFPP, a major cause of CPP, can be the manifestation of myofascial trigger points of the pelvic floor muscles and, therefore, needs accurate evaluation and interdisciplinary treatment techniques like myofascial trigger point release and biofeedback (Katzman et al., 2012). Familiarity with the anatomy of the PFMs is also indispensable in the creation of optimal treatment, particularly in the case of perineal trauma resulting from childbearing (Cory et al., 2018). In general, appreciation of the clinical importance of the pelvis and perineum is crucial to improve health outcomes and treat pelvic-related diseases.

11.3.1. Common Pelvic Disorders

Abnormalities in the pelvis are a serious issue for the majority of individuals, particularly females who are affected by the condition due to various phases in their lives such as pregnancy and childbirth. The primary condition is PFD, which can be brought about by birth trauma or physical stress during pregnancy. The conditions tend to lead to complications such as incontinence and pelvic organ prolapse (POP), affecting global QoL. The PFM is vulnerable to trauma during birth and this contributes to sagging of the pelvic floor and may lead to PFD (Chye et al., 2017). The effects of these disorders extend beyond the provision of instant physical relief; they may also affect mental wellbeing and social well-being. Hence, it is imperative to foster pelvic health with prevention and rehabilitation. One of the novel techniques uses noninvasive mechanical devices that provide support during pregnancy, thereby highlighting the significance of preventive management in managing these widespread pelvic disorders (Parente et al., 2008).

11.3.2. Pelvic Pain Syndromes

Multidimensional and multifactorial, pelvic pain syndromes plague numerous individuals, often leading to chronic pain and disruption of activities of daily living. A frequent component of CPP, MFPP is induced by trigger points within the musculature of the pelvic floor, leading to referred pain in adjacent zones (Katzman et al., 2012). Identification and diagnosis of MFPP are crucial as it tends to remain hidden from health care providers. Interdisciplinary management plays a key role in effective management, and it involves techniques like myofascial trigger point release, biofeedback, and electrical stimulation. Moreover, an integrated nomenclature is essential in clinical management of pelvic floor dysfunctions. The International Urogynecological Association (IUGA) and the International Continence Society (ICS) have been tasked with a comprehensive terminology report, providing accuracy to the treatment and symptoms of these disorders (Abramov et al., 2016). This team work is designed to improve diagnosis and treatment algorithms and ultimately the care of patients (Figure 11.9).

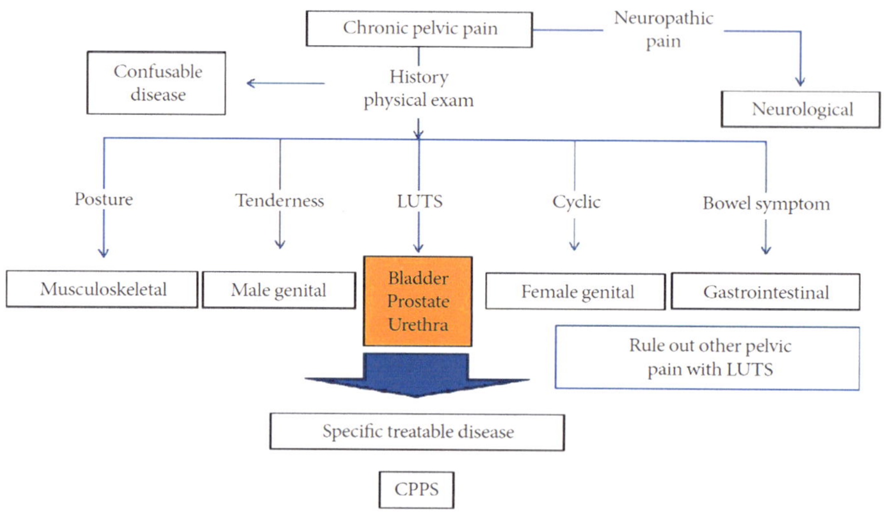

Figure 11.9. Localization of chronic pelvic pain. LUTS, lower urinary tract symptoms; CPPS, chronic pelvic pain syndrome.

Source: Zhang, Y., Li, Q., & Deng, H. (2023). *Localization of Chronic Pelvic Pain (LUTS: Lower Urinary Tract Symptoms; CPPS: Chronic Pelvic Pain Syndrome).*

11.3.3. Impact of Pelvic Floor Dysfunction (PFD)

PFD has a profound impact on QoL, and it is behind an overwhelming host of physical and psychological challenges. Women are particularly tormented by the consequences of chronic pain and infertility because endometriosis, or the growth of endometrial tissue outside of the uterine cavity, is a classic example. The condition triggers incapacitating symptoms that not only jeopardize the physical condition but also emotional condition, leading to a substantial financial input into healthcare systems globally (Carmichael & Mills, 2022). In addition, the terminology of PFM assessment has also evolved to emphasize the growing recognition of this disorder's complexity. The systematic documentation of ICSs on PFM function underscores the use of standardized assessment protocols to improve diagnosis and treatment in optimizing outcomes (Carmichael & Mills, 2022). In general, therapy of PFD requires an integrated approach toward gaining insight into the convergence of physical health, emotional support, and ready access to the proper healthcare interventions, underscoring its profound influence on women's lives.

11.3.4. Role of the Pelvis in Urological Health

The pelvic region serves as a critical foundation for urological health, housing essential organs and structures that support urinary and reproductive functions. Its complex anatomy directly influences the functionality of the bladder, urethra, and lower urinary tract. Dysfunction in pelvic muscles can lead to conditions such as MFPP, significantly impacting QoL and often complicating diagnoses

(Katzman et al., 2012). Moreover, the pelvis plays a pivotal role during surgical interventions for urological emergencies, where exposure and experience can vary among healthcare providers. For instance, a study found that a cadaveric simulation course significantly boosts trainees' confidence in managing urgent urological procedures, highlighting the pelvis's relevance in both education and practice (Armitage et al., 2020). Therefore, understanding the intricacies of pelvic health is paramount for both preventive care and effective intervention in urological disorders, underscoring the need for specialized training and comprehensive management options.

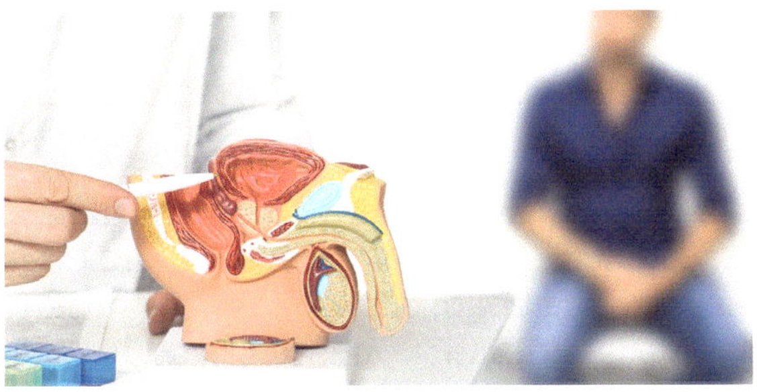

Source: Healix Hospitals. (n.d.). *Doctor Explaining Male Urogenital Anatomy Using Anatomical Model, with Patient in Background.*

11.3.5. Gynecological Conditions Related to the Pelvis

Pelvic morbidity can significantly influence the QoL of women and therefore it is important to understand the numerous gynecological pathologies of the pelvis. Aggressive angiomyxoma is an uncommon benign soft tissue neoplasm that typically occurs in the female pelvis, and it highlights the significance of precise evaluation and early treatment of the gynecological abnormality. For instance, a 1-year history of vaginal protrusion in a young woman emphasizes the diagnostic difficulty of such tumors (Adoke et al., 2018). Dynamic MRI studies also show a good correlation between perineal position and POP symptoms, where symptom expression is most pronounced at rest (Fauconnier et al., 2010). These findings underscore the correlation between anatomical changes and functional symptoms, keeper of the place of careful pelvic assessment in diagnosing and treating gynecological illness effectively. Last but not least, an integrative understanding of these diseases is indispensable for fostering pelvic health and enhancing QoL among patients with them.

11.3.6. Pelvic Fractures and their Implications

Pelvic fractures are a serious form of injury often resulting from high-energy trauma, such as car accidents or bomb blasts. Pelvic fractures are not solitary events; they are almost always followed by significant associated injuries, including neurologic impairment and pelvic ring instability. Indeed, neurologic injury is seen in as many as 50% of patients who have sacral fractures (Bellabarba et al., 2017). Further, combat studies have also recognized pelvic vascular injuries as a significant cause of death among wounded persons, particularly if the fracture is compounded by traumatic amputation or displaced fractures (Rankin et al., 2021). Treatment and management of a pelvic fracture must therefore involve a complex process that addresses not only the fracture, but also the very wide spectrum of injuries that are concomitant. Failure to diagnose and treat these related injuries can significantly alter patient outcomes, emphasizing the severity and emergency nature of the treatment of pelvic fractures in the clinical setting.

11.3.7. Surgical Interventions in the Pelvic Region

The complexity of pelvic surgeries highlights the need for precise vocabulary and detailed understanding of associated anatomical structures. PFDs, such as POP, are typically problematic for surgeons, where various surgical methods need to be adopted to achieve restoration of function and symptom relief. IUGA and the ICS have collaborated to produce an extremely extensive Terminology Report that explains these conditions and their surgical management possibilities (Bernard et al., 2016). The report is comprised of over 230 definitions and categorizes common diagnoses, facilitating communication more clearly among clinicians and improving patient outcomes (Bernard et al., 2016). Through the development of a shared lexicon of pelvic surgery procedures, experts are able to ensure that technique and method are effectively passed on, eventually resulting in enhanced clinical practice and research avenues in pelvic care. Such innovations are a reflection of the pursuit of relentless progress in pelvic disorder management.

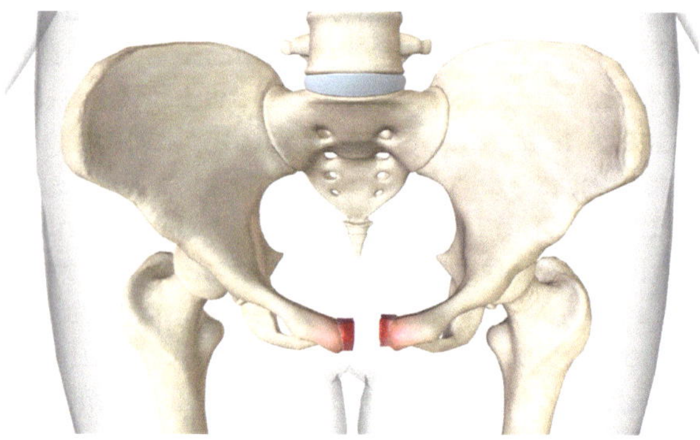

Source: Vitality Tulsa. (2024). *Pelvic Fracture Illustration Highlighting Affected Areas.* Vitality Wellness and Aesthetics.

11.3.8. Rehabilitation Strategies for Pelvic Health

The pelvic health rehabilitation plans play a very crucial role in enhancing the QoL of patients experiencing pelvic dysfunctions, e.g., diseases such as endometriosis and neurogenic bowel. The improvement is attained primarily through a multi-disciplinary approach that integrates physical therapy, dietary management, and psychotherapy. For instance, neurogenic bowel disorders due to spinal injury patients may be assisted through tailored programs of bowel management that involve pharmacological as well as mechanical interventions, as recent guidelines stress (Carmichael & Mills, 2022). Similarly, endometriosis patients can be treated by pelvic floor rehabilitation, where muscle impairment and pelvic pain are addressed to aid better functional outcomes (Carmichael & Mills, 2022). These rehabilitation strategies not only aim to minimize symptoms but also allow patients to be responsible participants in their own recovery process, eventually resulting in a sustained QoL. A comprehensive approach to rehabilitation of pelvic health is thus important in an effort to tackle the multi-dimensional issues of these conditions.

11.3.9. Importance of Pelvic Health Education

Education in pelvic health provides a significant foundation for the development of overall well-being and the treatment of an array of medical conditions. Education and information about PFDs, particularly in women, are imperative for enabling earlier intervention as well as reducing stigmatization of these disorders. Recent developments in terminology and standardization, as reported in IUGA and ICS reports, highlight the importance of linguistic consistency when discussing female sexuality and pelvic dysfunction (Carmichael & Mills, 2022). Furthermore, the Anatomical Society's perception highlights the importance of anatomical knowledge among nursing graduates, referencing that good knowledge of the pelvic region is a component of good clinical practice (Sparenberg, 2024). By offering individuals accurate information and resources, pelvic health education has the ability to empower both patients and practitioners, ultimately creating a more informed way of treating and enhancing overall quality care for individuals with pelvic floor-related issues.

Test Your Knowledge

1. What do you understand Gynecological Conditions Related to the Pelvis?
2. Understand Rehabilitation Strategies for Pelvic Health

11.4. Cultural and Social Perspectives on the Pelvis and Perineum

Learning Outcome

1. Describe the Historical Views on Pelvic Anatomy
2. Explain the Cultural Significance of the Pelvis in Different Societies
3. Understand Gender Differences in Pelvic Health Perceptions
4. How to Impact of Societal Norms on Pelvic Health
5. Evaluate Representation of the Pelvis in Art and Literature
6. Know Education and Awareness Campaigns
7. Explain the Stigmas Associated with Pelvic Health Issues
8. Discuss the Role of Healthcare Providers in Pelvic Education
9. Learn about Future Directions in Cultural Understanding of the Pelvis

Perineum and pelvic examination reveals significant cultural and social meaning regarding body experience and birth. In the majority of cultures, birth has shifted from a natural and collective process towards being a clinical intervention most often driven by medical protocols, as described in the study addressing episiotomy and its impact on women's physical health (Filho et al., 2016). The shift towards gynecological practice has altered the experience of giving birth as much as it has impacted the general views of the female body and its natural talents. Moreover, because artists and performers train methods that emphasize psycho-physical connectivity, they draw attention to breath and body awareness about speech and action (Bryon et al., 2012). This intersection of performance and embodied consciousness facilitates a broader cultural narrative one that disrupts traditional means of seeing the pelvis and perineum, one that facilitates an embodied understanding of their role within both personal identity and the socialized experience of childbearing (Figure 11.10).

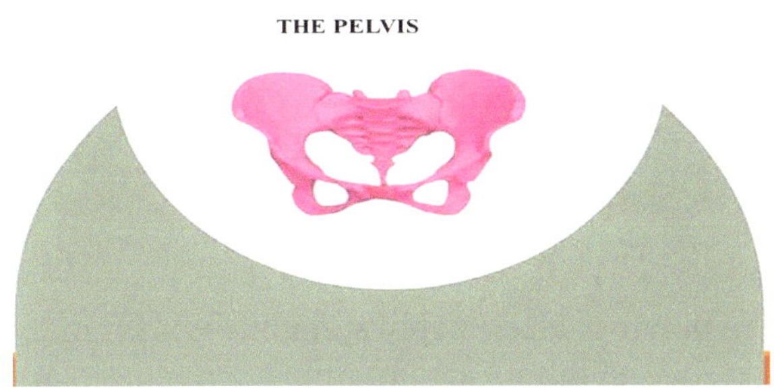

Figure 11.10. Exploration of the pelvis and perineum reveals significant cultural and social implications regarding childbirth and bodily perception.

Source: https://cdn.slidesharecdn.com/ss_thumbnails/maternalpelvis-241212043254-e62b88dd-thumbnail.jpg?width=560&fit=bounds.

11.4.1. Historical Views on Pelvic Anatomy

An appreciation of the evolution of understanding of pelvic anatomy shows a significant transformation from ancient times right up to contemporary medical practice.

Anteriorly, pelvic anatomy was widely accepted unexamined on the basis of limited empirical observation and led to mistakes in the functional importance of anatomical structure. For example, the early studies did not consider the aftermath of LAM injuries during birth, which recent studies indicate can lead to long-term negative impacts, e.g., pelvic floor dysfunction (Rotstein, 2022). A recognition of the levator ani's role in pelvic function and stability has caused a change in present-day surgical interventions and rehabilitative procedures. Furthermore, advancements in the imaging sciences and biomechanical evaluation have enhanced understanding of pelvic injuries obtained from trauma, prioritizing preventive treatments under combat conditions to negate life-threatening situations arising from injury, particularly of lower limbs (Webster et al., 2018). This has followed heightened awareness of pelvic anatomy complexity and its major implications for treatment as well as care of patients.

11.4.2. Cultural Significance of the Pelvis in Different Societies

The pelvis is also deeply symbolic within many societies, symbolizing not only womanhood and fertility but also strength and societal roles. Across many societies, the shape and size of the pelvis are related to one's reproductive wellbeing, which dictates societal views of womanhood. For instance, in many traditional societies, it is desirable to have a wider pelvis because it signifies the capability to bear children and nurture future generations. This illustrates a consistent theme of relating anatomical structures to basic societally important functions, as demonstrated by the anatomical understanding developed in physiotherapy, where comprehension of body functions in relation to health results is prioritized (Carmichael & Mills, 2022). Secondly, the pelvis is a crucial cultural object within rituals, symbolizing the interrelatedness of life, motherhood, and womanhood transition stages. Therefore, variations in pelvis perception across cultures reveal deep psychological and social forms that shape identities and traditional assumptions.

11.4.3. Gender Differences in Pelvic Health Perceptions

Knowledge of attitudes towards pelvic health reveals significant gender differences, particularly in the experience and coping with conditions involving the pelvis. Women have unique challenges, as evidenced by the occurrence of OASIS following childbirth, possibly leading to physical and psychological consequences, such as anal incontinence and sexual dysfunction (Ankarcrona et al., 2022). The degree of awareness and knowledge about pelvic health issues also differs significantly by sex; for instance, the advanced level of women's knowledge about their reproductive organs determines their actions towards their health.

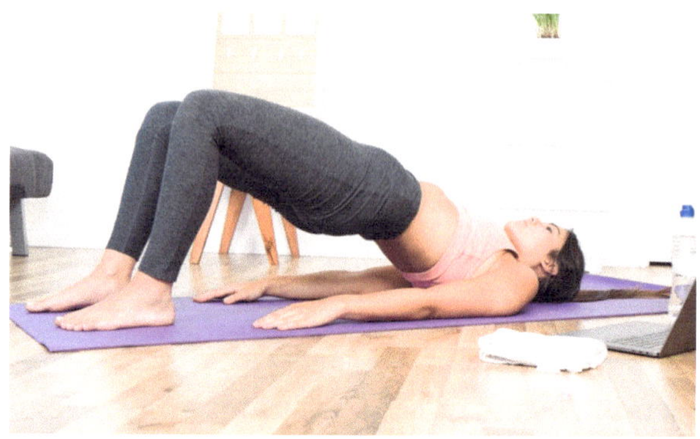

Source: RG Hospitals. (n.d.). *Woman Performing Pelvic Bridge Exercise.*

In contrast, men may minimize or ignore pelvic health issues because of societal stigmatization. Such inequality is further fortified by the lack of broad education of physicians on pelvic health during medical schooling, as seen through studies where medical staff lacked proper comprehension of the preventive measures required to avoid complications like

OASIS (Abrams et al., 2016). Such disparities are critical to understand for the development of gender-specific interventions that meet the specific requirements of each gender.

11.4.4. Impact of Societal Norms on Pelvic Health

Social convention contributes so much to shape the perception and practice of pelvic health, skewing the life of individuals during reproduction and after. In the U.S., the commonality of semi-recumbency during labor is a prime example of how institutional practice indexes the overall attitudes toward birth in society, tending to subtract from maternal preference and choice for other positions that have the potential to enhance comfort and outcomes. Research indicates that other cultures' practices, such as squatting or side-lie positions, can lead to faster deliveries and improved maternal and fetal health, necessitating a reconsideration of current birthing practices (Heskett, 2022). Furthermore, cultural fear of the time pregnant represents to be able to discuss sexual health may perpetuate myths and fear of sexual intimacy, which may undermine relational interactions during this time of susceptibility (Geuens et al., 2023). Thus, it is crucial to critically assess how deeply rooted societal norms can harm both pelvic health and overall well-being, necessitating a shift towards more open-minded and supportive healthcare practices.

11.4.5. Representation of the Pelvis in Art and Literature

Art and literature have a long history of dealing with the pelvis as an emblem of human connection, identity, and even vulnerability. Throughout the different forms of art, the pelvis is frequently used as a center of themes dealing with childbirth and femininity, expressing how society views gender and motherhood. For instance, the description of pelvic injury in fiction is not only depicting the physical result of trauma but also the psychological impacts that emerge due to such traumas, parallel to the clinical presentation in books like Sparenberg, (2024), where the emphasis is on the healing process after damage to the pelvic region.

Additionally, the evolving depiction of obstetric procedures in art as well as in scientific literature mirrors the evolving comprehension of child birth, the interaction between physical machinery for delivery and profound human feelings. This dualism resonates with the issues raised in scientific studies on vacuum-assisted birth, where technology intersecting with natural processes exposes to a broader discussion regarding the human experience of birth, echoing the sentiments of Goordyal et al. (2020). Lastly, such literary and artistic representations illustrate the complexity of scientific descriptions of the pelvis alongside its significance in scientific descriptions of human existence.

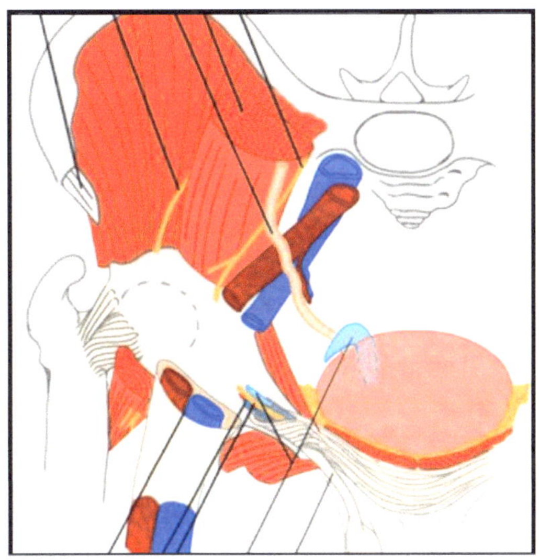

Source: Edward, J. T., et al. (2022). Genitourinary complications in orthopedic surgery. *European Journal of Orthopedic Surgery & Traumatology, 32*(5).

11.4.6. Education and Awareness Campaigns

Educational campaigns and awareness programs play an important role in enhancing understanding and health awareness in the pelvis and perineum region, particularly in the context of midwifery and maternity care. Such campaigns introduce information on the process of labor and potential complications thereof, giving empowerment to both the expectant mothers and the medical practitioners. Besides, successful campaigns can dispel myths and stigma for women's health issues and establish a welcoming community where one will not be shy to open up regarding one's concerns.

For instance, the transformation of midwifery organizations over the past is embodied in the transformation of The Alliance of Nurse-Midwives' newsletters to those of the Association of Midwives of Newfoundland and Labrador, which indicate the necessity of ongoing communication and education in the practice (Carmichael & Mills, 2022). By the training that includes workshops, public service announcements, and outreach, the critical information regarding pelvic health will enhance awareness, which will result in improved maternal and neonatal health outcomes (Matthews et al., 2009).

11.4.7. Stigmas Associated with Pelvic Health Issues

Pelvic disorders are often plagued with severe social stigmas that can prevent individuals from receiving necessary medical attention or support. For most, shame related to disorders such as incontinence, pelvic pain, or sexual dysfunction encourages secrecy and isolation. This stigma is particularly acute when discussing sexual intimacy and health, something that is rarely venturously encountered during healthcare professional training, the growing literature on midwifery and sexuality suggests (Geuens et al., 2023). The avoidance by omission of frank discussion has the potential to reinforce shame, something that may in turn deter patients from raising such matters with their healthcare practitioners. Besides this, a better understanding of anatomy and how it can relate to health is quite crucial for clinicians; without good communication between patients and providers, individuals can feel stigmatized and disrespected, thus affecting their QoL (Rodriguez & Gater, 2022)). Removing these barriers is quite crucial in establishing a supportive culture that encourages individuals to place their pelvic health first.

11.4.8. Role of Healthcare Providers in Pelvic Education

Health professionals are an important part of pelvic education. They offer support and advice where necessary to help those with pelvic floor dysfunction. During their childbearing years, many women endure MSK problems, such as LBP and SUI, as highlighted in recent studies (Parker et al., 2001). Despite its prevalence, however, a majority of women will not seek treatment due to a lack of information or knowledge about available facilities.

Patient education and intervention by healthcare professionals can fill this knowledge gap, educating patients about their health status as well as the importance of pelvic care. Moreover, the development of standardized pelvic care terminology, as outlined in a consensus document by IUGA and ICS, enhances communication among practitioners, so that patients hear the same message from all healthcare professionals regarding their pelvic health requirements (Legleiter, 2023). Thus, by paying attention to pelvic education, healthcare providers can empower the patients, facilitate early intervention, and significantly improve QoL (Figure 11.11).

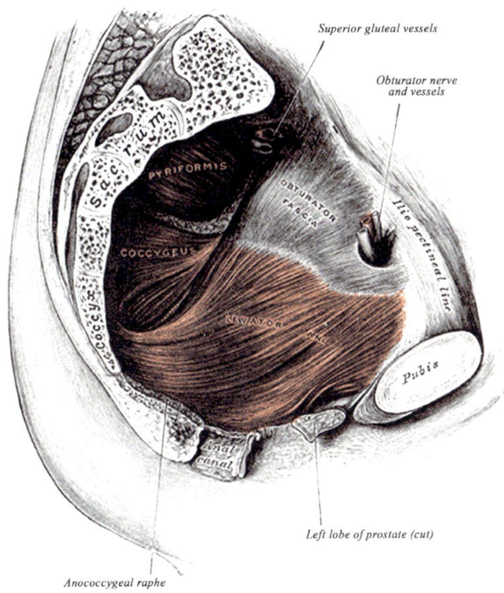

Figure 11.11. Stress urinary incontinence (SUI).

Source: By Henry Vandyke Carter - Henry Gray (1918) Anatomy of the Human Body (See "Book" section below)Bartleby.com: Gray's Anatomy, Plate 404, Public Domain, https://commons.wikimedia.org/w/index.php?curid=158672

11.4.9. Future Directions in Cultural Understanding of the Pelvis

As society itself moves forward, the cultural significance of the pelvis is on the verge of significant expansion and transition. Long understood from an exclusively anatomical perspective, emerging knowledge emphasizes the pelvis's complex role in both physical health and cultural identity. For instance, the now-present focus on avoiding injury in combat settings underscores the vulnerability of the pelvis and its required structural stability, as evidence from studies exist that broken pelvic rings will have devastating effects (Webster et al., 2018). This can be applied to the more broader societal conversation when discussing awareness within bodies and the ramifications of pelvic health in different populations. Moreover, a review of the narratives on the pelvis in maternal health and midwifery, as documented in community newsletters, illustrates the importance of cultural competence and shared knowledge among healthcare practitioners (Carmichael & Mills, 2022). Operating from these intersections produces a broader view for understanding how cultural perceptions affect, and are affected by, our knowledge regarding the pelvis and perineum region.

Test Your Knowledge

1. List the components of the pelvic diaphragm and state their function.
2. What are the contents of the pelvic cavity in males and females?

SUMMARY

In looking at the applicability of the perineum and pelvis area, it is clear that the complex blend of anatomy, surgical procedures, and rehabilitative protocols must be adhered to in the interest of ensuring pelvic health. Complications with reconstructive procedures, like how one compares VRAM, gluteal, and gracilis flaps, act to illustrate the need for choosing the most superior method of surgery so that there are fewer complications during such procedures as abdominoperineal excision of the rectum. As noted, the VRAM flap can be improved regarding perineal wound and flap complication rates (Johnstone, 2017). Also paramount is an understanding of the PFMs' anatomical architecture, as placed into context by innovative techniques like MR-DTI, which can reveal significant muscle interactions during delivery and consequent damage (Johnson, 2022). Ultimately, a clear understanding of these factors promotes better management techniques and patient outcomes within surgical and rehabilitative settings.

The relationship among anatomical structures and their functions within the pelvis and perineum is essential to an understanding of both common dysfunctions and conservative management methods. One key aspect is standardization of nomenclature, facilitating simple communication among medical professionals. The joint collaboration of the IUGA and the ICS has resulted in the development of a terminology report with special reference to the conservative management of female pelvic floor dysfunction. This report defines over two hundred symptom, assessment, and treatment terms, thereby making clinical relevance and usage more straightforward (Abramov et al., 2016). The sheer size of such an undertaking is of paramount importance to facilitating interdisciplinary collaboration and guiding research agendas in the direction of better patient outcomes. Further, the comingling of perspectives among various medical specialties, as shown in the process of constructing the report, highlights the multidisciplinary nature of pelvic health management and the necessity for ongoing updates to remain relevant in practice (Parente et al., 2008).

KEY TERMS FROM THIS CHAPTER

- Cadaveric dissection modules
- Internal pudendal artery (IPA)
- Medical education
- Obstetric anal sphincter injuries (OASIS)
- Pelvic anatomy
- Pelvic floor disorders (PFDs)
- Pelvic floor injury
- Defecation
- Levator ani muscles (LAMs)
- Myofascial pelvic pain (MFPP)
- Pelvic anatomical barriers
- Pelvic bones
- Pelvic floor dysfunctions
- Pelvic floor muscles (PFMs)

CRITICAL THINKING QUESTIONS

1. **Which of the following bones does NOT contribute to the formation of the pelvis?**
   a. Ilium
   b. Ischium
   c. Femur
   d. Pubis
2. **The pelvic diaphragm is primarily composed of which muscles?**
   a. Piriformis and obturator internus
   b. Levator ani and coccygeus
   c. Gluteus maximus and minimus
   d. Rectus abdominis and transversus abdominis
3. **Which structure passes through the greater sciatic foramen?**
   a. Femoral nerve
   b. Pudendal nerve
   c. Sciatic nerve
   d. Inferior epigastric artery
4. **The perineum is divided into two triangles by a line connecting the:**
   a. Pubic symphysis and coccyx
   b. Ischial tuberosities
   c. Iliac crests
   d. Sacroiliac joints
5. **Which of the following is a content of the deep perineal pouch in males?**
   a. Bulb of the penis
   b. Crus of the penis
   c. Membranous urethra
   d. Testes

Short Answer Questions

1. Describe the course and function of the pudendal nerve.
2. Differentiate between the true pelvis and the false pelvis.
3. Understand the location and function of the ischioanal fossa.
4. Describe the structure and function of the pelvic diaphragm.
5. Explain the course and function of the pudendal nerve.

Answers to Critical Thinking Questions

1. (c) 2. (b) 3. (c) 4. (b) 5. (c)

REFERENCES

1. Aijaz, S., Chughtai, N. G., Kash*if, U., & Malik, S. (2022). Functional* Anatomy of Female Perineum. IntechOpen. https://core.ac.uk/download/539672649.pdf (accessed on 8th May 2025).
2. Almeida, T., Comber, R., Balaam, M. (2016)
3. Bryon, E. (2012). From Walking and Talking to Cartwheels and High Cs: An Examination of Practice-Based Laboratory Work into Physio-Vocal Integration. Informa UK Limited. https://core.ac.uk/download/11337858.pdf (accessed on 8th May 2025).
4. Carmichael, J., & Mills, S. (2022). Anatomy and Embryology of the Colon, Rectum, and Anus. In The ASCRS Textbook of Colon and Rectal Surgery. http://dx.doi.org/10.1007/978-3-030-66049-9_1 Retrieved from https://escholarship.org/uc/item/8gj3b19f(accessed o*n 8th May 2025).*
5. *DOI: h*ttps://doi.org/10.33015/dominican.edu/2022.NURS.ST.21
6. Filho, M. F. da C., Guimarães da Sil*va, D. S., Lemos, C. I. L., Rodrigues, C. N. C., & Serrão, C. C. A. (2016). Relation Between Episiotomy and Osteomioarticular Symp*toms. European Scientific Institute (ESI). https://core.ac.uk/download/328025651.pdf (accessed on 8th May 2025).
7. Fornai, C., Frémondière, P., Haeusler, M., Marchal, F., Thollon, L., & Webb, N. M. (2022). Dynamic Finite-Element Simulations Reveal Early Origin of Complex Human Birth Pattern. Springer Science and Business Media LLC. https://www.zora.uzh.ch/id/eprint/225970/1/ZORA_s42003_022_03321_z.pdf (accessed on 8th May 2025).
8. from Societal Norms" (2022). Nursing | Senio*r Theses. 65.*
9. *Gangata, H., Porter, S., Artz, N., & Major,* K. (2023). A proposed anatomy syllabus for entry-level physiotherapists in the United Kingdom: A modified Delphi methodology by physiotherapists who teach anatomy. Clinical Anatomy, 36, 503–526. http*s://doi.org/10.1002/ca.24001 (accessed on 8th May 2025).*
10. *Geuens, S., Gianotten, W. L., & Mivšek, A. P. (2023). Midwifery and Sex*uality. Springer International Publishing AG. https://core.ac.uk/download/588747178.pdf (accessed on 8th May 2025).
11. Goordyal, B. D. (2020). Design and Development of Atraumatic Vacuum Assisted Delivery Devices. University of Leeds. https://core.ac.uk/download/327079153.pdf (accessed on 8th May 2025).
12. Hansen*, E., Jami, M., Much*iri, A., Nthumba, P., & Nyoro, P. (2015). Reconstruction of complex post-traumatic perineal/pelvic defects using a pedicled an*terolateral thigh flap* in a child. African Journals Online (AJOL). https://core.ac.uk/download/478421225.pdf (accessed on 8th May 2025).
13. Haylen, B. T., Maher*, C., Barber, M. D., et al. (2016). Erratum to: An International Urog*ynecological Association (IUGA) / International Continence Society (ICS) joint report on the terminology for female pelvic organ prolapse (POP). International Urogynecology Journal, 27, 655–684. https://doi.org/10.1007/s00192-016-3003-y (accessed on 8th May 2025).
14. HCI and Intima*te Care as an Agenda for Chang*e in Women's Health
15. Heskett, Amberlyn, "Effects and Outcomes of Different Laboring Positions and the Influence
16. Hodgkinson, C. P. (1969). Stress Urinary Incontinence in the Human Female: Gravity and Ecomorphologic Influences on Bladder and Urethral Function of the Human Female. Henry

Ford Health System Scholarly Commons. https://core.ac.uk/download/287196166.pdf (accessed on 8th May 2025).

17. https://doi.org/10.1145/2858036.2858187 (accessed on 8th May 2025).
18. In: 34TH ANNUAL CHI CONFERENCE ON HUMAN FACTORS IN COMPUTING
19. Johnson, R. A. (2022). Promoting Alternative and Evidence-Supported Birthing Options in Healthcare Facilities. Digital Commons @ Gardner-Webb University. https://core.ac.uk/download/564024319.pdf (accessed on 8th May 2025).
20. Johnstone, M. S. (2017). Vertical Rectus Abdominis Myocutaneous Versus Alternative Flaps for Perineal Repair After Abdominoperineal Excision of the Rectum in the Era of Laparoscopic Surgery. Ovid Technologies (Wolters Kluwer Health). https://core.ac.uk/download/84148290.pdf (accessed on 8th May 2025).
21. Legleiter, K. (2023). Occupational Therapy Graduate Students,' Recent Graduates,' and Educators' Perceptions of the Value of Anatomy Knowledge. Journal of Occupational Therapy Education, v7 n2 Article 10 2023 (accessed on 8th May 2025).
22. Matthews, T. (2009). An Investigation of Firearm-Related Injuries and Fatalities Amongst Children in the Cape Metropolitan Area (2001–2006). Department of Medicine. https://core.ac.uk/download/185433817.pdf (accessed on 8th May 2025).
23. McDonald, C., Scott, E., Ruderman, G., Schildmeyer, K., Gill, S., & Ashdown, S. (2023). Landmarking for Improved Digital Product Creation. TU Dresden. https://core.ac.uk/download/597918438.pdf (accessed on 8th May 2025).
24. Mohammed, Y. (n.d.). Analysis of Immediate Birth–Related Morbidity in Omdurman Maternity Hospital. UOFK. https://core.ac.uk/download/pdf/71668982.pdf (accessed on 8th May 2025).
25. Osborne, K. (2010). Pushing Techniques Used by Midwives When Providing Second Stage LABOR CARE. e-Publications@Marquette. https://core.ac.uk/download/67759133.pdf (accessed on 8th May 2025).
26. Parker, T. K. (2001). Determining the Need for Program Development for Women in Their Childbearing Years. UND Scholarly Commons. https://core.ac.uk/download/235074312.pdf (accessed on 8th May 2025).
27. Piozzi, G. N., Baek, S. J., Kwak, J. M., Kim, J., & Kim, S. H. (2021). Anus-preserving surgery in advanced low-lying rectal cancer: A perspective on oncological safety of intersphincteric resection. Cancers, 13, 4793. https://doi.org/10.3390/cancers13194793 (accessed on 8th May 2025).
28. Rankin, I. A. (2021). Dismounted Pelvic Blast Injury: Mechanisms of Injury, Associated Injuries and Mitigation Strategies. Bioengineering, Imperial College London. https://core.ac.uk/download/564418517.pdf (accessed on 8th May 2025).
29. Rodriguez, G. M., & Gater, D. R. (2022). Neurogenic bowel and management after spinal cord injury: A narrative review. Journal of Personalized Medicine, 12, 1141. https://doi.org/10.3390/jpm12071141 (accessed on 8th May 2025).
30. Rossoff, M. R. (2017). Align and Crumble: Internally Falling Towards Authentic Behavior in Acting and an Investigation of Anton Chekhov's Three Sisters. https://core.ac.uk/download/84743901.pdf (accessed on 8th May 2025).

31. *Rotstein, Emilia Simone (2022). Pelvic floor dys*function after childbirth : symptoms, diagnosis, treatment. Karolinska Institutet. Thesis. https://hdl.handle.net/10616/48302(accessed on 8th May 2025).
32. Sander, A. (2020). Penetrating Abdominal Trauma: Spectrum of Disease in a Level *1 Trauma Center. Basrah Medical Col*lege – Department of Surgery. https://core.ac.uk/download/288496604.pdf (accessed on 8th May 202*5).*
33. *Smith, C. F., Finn, G. M., Stewart, J., Atkinson, M. A., Davies, D. C., Dyball, R., Morris, J., Ockleford, C., Parkin, I., S*tandring, S., Whiten, S., Wilton, J., & McHanwell, S. (2016). The Anatomical Society core regional anatomy syllabus for undergraduate medicine. Journal of anatomy, 228(1), 15–23. https://doi.org/10.1111/joa.12405(accessed on 8th May 2025).
34. Sparenberg, S. (2024). Reconstructive Surgery: Risk *Factors, Outcomes and Advanced Indications. Doctoral thesis, University of* Amsterdam, the Netherlands © Sebastian Sparenberg, 2024 ISBN: 9789090385136 (accessed on 8th May 2025).
35. SYSTEMS, CHI 2016 (pp. 2599-2611). ASSO*C COMPUTING MACHINERY*
36. *Østborg, T. B. (2023). Maternal and Iatrogenic Fa*ctors Influencing the Duration of Labor. The University of Bergen. https://core.ac.uk/download/580972092.pdf (accessed on 8th May 2025).

HEAD AND SKULL

12

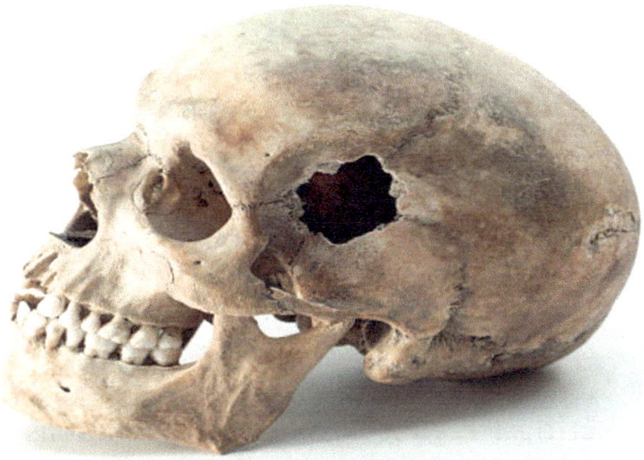

Introduction

The intricacies of the skull and head anatomy have always fascinated medical professionals and researchers due to their complex nature as well as critical functions. The evolution of technologies in surgical procedures, especially in procedures such as endoscopic sinus and skull base surgery, has raised the need for an in-depth understanding of these regions. Methods such as the nasoseptal flap and inferior turbinate flap have expanded reconstructive options for central skull base lesions, enhancing clinical success while reducing morbidity (Lee et al., 2025). Concurrently, the issue of practicing physicians in mincing operations has triggered studies into alternative anatomical models. For instance, the ovine model, being anatomically similar to the human head, presents a valid alternative to cadaveric dissection for surgery training, resolving ethical and practical limitations while gaining valuable hands-on experience (Surov et al., 2020). Taken together, these innovations illuminate the transformed landscape of head and

LEARNING OBJECTIVES

After studying this chapter, you will be able to:

1. Explain the anatomy of the head and neck
2. Discuss the common disorders and diseases
3. Focus on diagnostic techniques
4. Know treatment and management

skull science, merging anatomical data with practical surgical procedure.

Definition of the Head and Skull

It is necessary to differentiate between the head and the skull, two closely related but distinct structures, to comprehend the general anatomy of the head. The head is described as the entire upper part of the body, including the brain and face, since it encompasses the site of the body's most vital sensory organs and neural activity. The skull, the bony structure that stabilizes the head, is concerned with protection of the brain and support of the facial structure. It is made up of various bones such as the frontal, parietal, temporal, occipital, maxillary, and mandibular bones that have varied functions including housing sensory organs and enabling mastication.

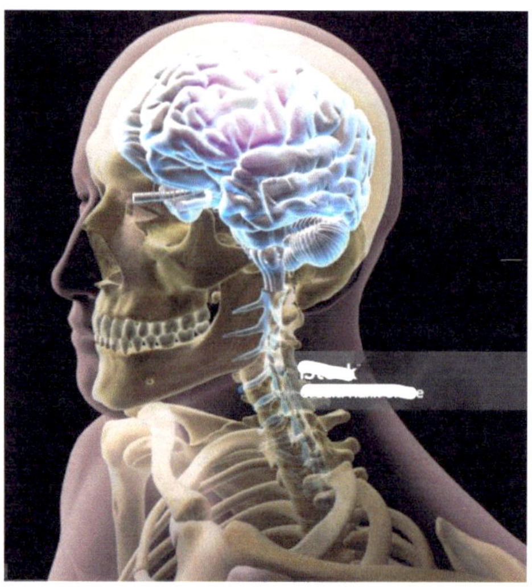

Figure 12.1. The fundamental anatomy of the head necessitates distinguishing between the head itself and the skull.

Source: iStock. (n.d.). Male Head, Skull, and Brain on Black Background.

For example, mandible plays a crucial role in food processing by supporting teeth for grinding, thereby illustrating the multidimensional function of the skull in physiology and survival (Mothé et al., 2024). Anatomical and surgical studies, particularly of the complex regions of the skull like the temporal bone and jugular foramen, emphasize the critical correlation between skull morphology and protective and functional capabilities of the head (Surov et al., 2020) (Figure 12.1).

Importance of the Head in Human Anatomy

The complex architecture of the head plays a key role in sheltering and housing the brain, eyes, ears, and other sensory organs for human shape and perception. Its bony casing, the skull, not only shelters these life-supporting features but also forms the foundation for facial features and oral machinery for communication and nourishment. Anatomical education innovations, such as virtual and AR, have made understanding the complex relationships in the skull possible, enabling more active involvement and more effective learning in terms of this critical region despite the limitations of the traditional cadaveric study (Sellés, 2019). Apart from this, its significance also extends to clinical environments like transcranial electric stimulation, a technique that relies on the correct understanding of head anatomy and electrical conductivity to target brain regions effectively (Huang et al., 2017). Thus, the head anatomy plays a vital role in both protecting essential neurological function as well as enhancing medical therapies.

Overview of the Skull's Structure

The human skull is the tough framework supporting the brain but also providing structural support for the face. The 22-bone skull consists of two main components: the neurocranium, the compartment in which the brain resides, and the viscerocranium, the facial skeleton. The bones are all closely interlocked through sutures, allowing little movement at birth and growth. Primarily, the skull protects important sensory organs housed in cavities such as the eyes, ears, and nostrils. Its complex form accommodates the embedding of muscles used in facial expressions and chewing. Because it is responsible for the protection of neurological structures and the formation of the contour of the head, the analysis of skull morphology becomes significant. Advances in technology in imaging have raised the potential for evaluating skull integrity in a clinical setting, especially for head and neck diseases (Surov et al., 2020). Additionally, interdisciplinary practice in diagnosis and treatment of skull disorders accentuates the functional and clinical significance of the skull (David et al., 2020) (Figure 12.2).

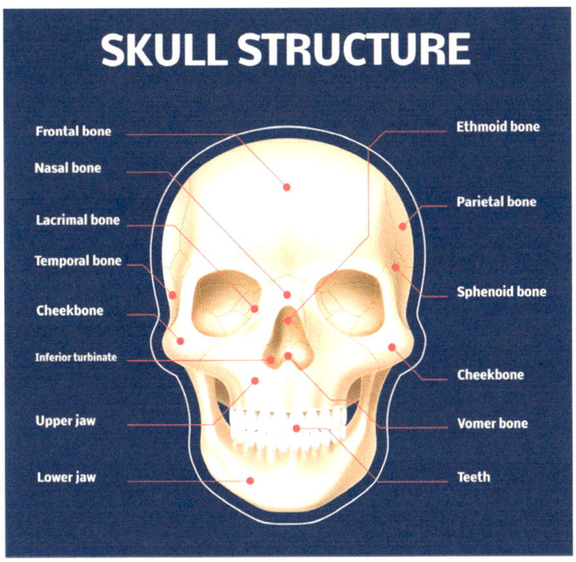

Figure 12.2. Overview of the skull's structure.

Source: VectorStock. (n.d.). Human Skull Anatomy: Realistic Head and Face Bones.

Historical Significance of Skull Studies

Skull studies have long provided key data on human history, migration, and cultural contact, and they give a physical link to the past population. From a study of cranial form and the genetic data contained in ancient bones, scientists can reconstruct ancestry and patterns of movement and illuminate the complex tapestry of human evolution. For example, genome analyses of several ancient populations show how migrations such as those linked with the Yamnaya culture positioned human groups across Eurasia but with mixed genetic influence, suggesting different European and Asian historical pathways (Surov et al., 2020). Moreover, mummy studies have eroded population continuity assumptions by affirming genetic linkages between ancient Egyptians and Near Easterners rather than modern Egyptians, who show greater amounts of sub-Saharan ancestry, thus transforming the view of regional identity changes spanning thousands of years (Verena et al., 2017). Therefore, skull studies not only document bodily characteristics but also complement historical accounts by interpreting the biological heritages etched in the human cranium (Figure 12.3).

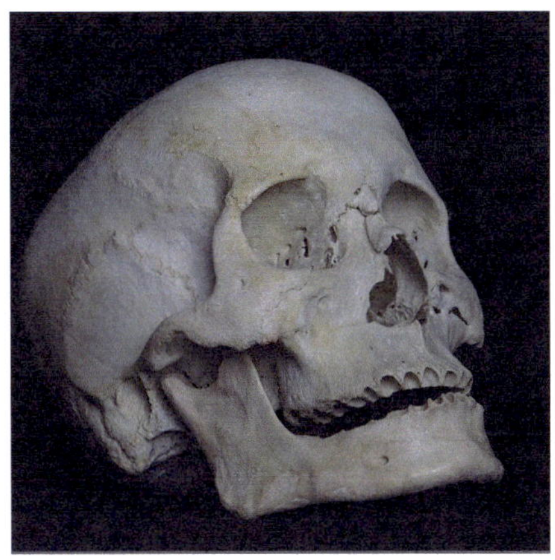

Figure 12.3. Historical significance of skull studies.

Source: By Wasiul Bahar - Own work, CC BY-SA 4.0, https://commons.wikimedia.org/w/index.php?curid=152379258

Brief Outline of Main Topics

The complex anatomy of the skull and head includes several regions to be investigated to understand fully their intricacy and clinical relevance. Core anatomy first learns the bony structure and soft tissues covering it, which is necessary to understand spatial relationships in the region.

This is followed by knowledge about pathologies, such as tumors, trauma, and congenital abnormalities, which highlight the vast array of clinical problems encountered. Surgical intervention is another key focus, particularly endoscopic and minimally invasive surgery, which has made significant strides in recent years and underscores the intersection of otolaryngology with neurosurgery. Devices and navigation systems critical to precise operative management also show advancements in this field. Lastly, the specialized topics, including temporal bone anatomy and neurotological considerations, present functional aspects related to hearing and balance, with emphasis on the multi-disciplinary nature of head and skull study and management (Sperling, 2011; Zaidi et al., 2014).

Relevance to Medical and Biological Sciences

Advances in imaging technologies through technology have significantly enhanced understanding of the head and skull in medical and biological sciences. Recent biomedical imaging modalities such as photoacoustic imaging enable high-resolution visualization of the cranial structures through the combination of optical resolution and deep penetration with sound.

This multi-disciplinary approach allows clinicians to obtain structure, function, and molecular information of great significance to the diagnosis and treatment of an array of disorders that affect the head and brain, including vascular malformations and tumor formation (Attia et al., 2019). Moreover, precise fetal growth evaluation through ultrasound biometric measurements, such as biparietal diameter and head circumference, plays a vital role in assessment of neurological maturation and congenital anomaly detection.

The establishment of standard fetal growth charts emphasizes the significance of these measurements in global health settings, providing a point of reference for normal cranial development and the identification of deviations that can impact long-term neurological outcome (Kiserud et al., 2017). Together, these technological and clinical discoveries advance the understanding of head and skull morphogenesis and pathology.

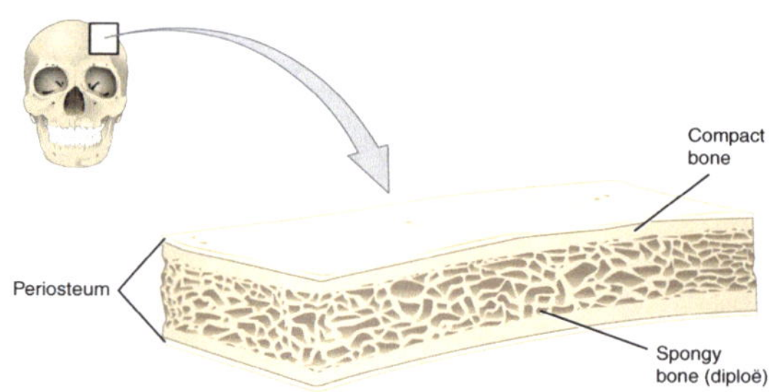

Source: By OpenStax College - Anatomy & Physiology, Connexions Web site. http://cnx.org/content/col11496/1.6/, Jun 19, 2013., CC BY 3.0, https://commons.wikimedia.org/w/index.php?curid=30131423

Cultural Perspectives on the Head and Skull

In many cultures, the skull and head have symbolic and deeper meanings that transcend their biological functions, representing the values and identity of a culture. In Afro-diasporic and indigenous societies, these sites of anatomy are repositories of memory of ancestors and sacred as well as religious significance, in most instances being linked with race, ethnicity, and cultural identity. The sensory and communicative functions of the head, particularly via voice and hearing, have been explored on the basis of such paradigms as acousmatic blackness, highlighting the complex relationship between race and auditory experience in cultural contexts (Baatenburg et al., 2024).

In addition, earlier and more current studies reveal the manner in which perceptions of the skull overlap with social stratifications and common memory, especially among Black and Indigenous populations subjected to postcolonial identity and social movements (Wade, 2015). These perceptions resist only scientific comprehension, requiring a holistic understanding comprising cultural, racial, and historical factors embedded in the head and skull.

12.1. Anatomy of the Head and Neck

Learning Outcome

1. Discuss the Major Bones of the Skull
2. Explain the Muscles of Facial Expression
3. Focus on Muscles of Mastication
4. How to Major Blood Vessels in the Region
5. Know Nerves of the Head and Neck
6. Learn about Lymphatic Drainage
7. Explain the Organs of the Head (e.g., Eyes, Ears, Nose)
8. More details Salivary Glands and their Functions
9. Focus on Anatomical Landmarks and their Significance

Head and neck are a complex interaction of structures essential both to form and function. The region includes essential structures such as the skull, facial bones, and soft tissue that comprise the complex architecture necessary to house the brain, provide speech, and facilitate breathing. Anatomically, the head and neck are divided into various subsites like the oral cavity, pharynx, larynx, and musculature that encircles them, and each subsite has a specific function to perform. For example, in laryngeal and hypopharyngeal surgeries, obtaining satisfactory resection margins more than 5 mm has usually been a problem with anatomical limitations; this is a phenomenon that clearly occurs since varying resection surfaces have specific restrictions as outlined in recent research (Baatenburg et al., 2024).

Understanding such anatomical complexities is a condition precedent to effective medical intervention and is the basis for our knowledge of potential complications, especially in relation to adaptive therapies used to reverse treatment side effects, as seen with head and neck cancers (HNCs) (Schwartz & Dong, 2011).

12.1.1. Major Bones of the Skull

The human skull is an extremely complex structure consisting of many major bones, each playing a vital role in brain protection and facial feature support. Among these, the frontal bone forms the forehead and upper portion of the eye sockets, while the parietal bones form the top and sides of the cranium. The occipital bone at the back houses the foramen magnum, through which the spinal cord will be attached to the brain.

Again, the temporal bones, situated behind the ears, play a critical role in hearing by housing the apparatus necessary for hearing. The maxilla and mandible form the upper and lower jaw, respectively, and are essential for mastication as well as articulation. The complex bone structure of such bones is also demonstrated in reptiles, where patent sutures of the skull provide more uniform strain distribution, thus enabled balanced craniofacial growth (Curtis et al., 2013). This functional and structural interdependence emphasizes the significance of each bone in providing the integrity and functionality of the head and neck region (Figures 12.4 and 12.5).

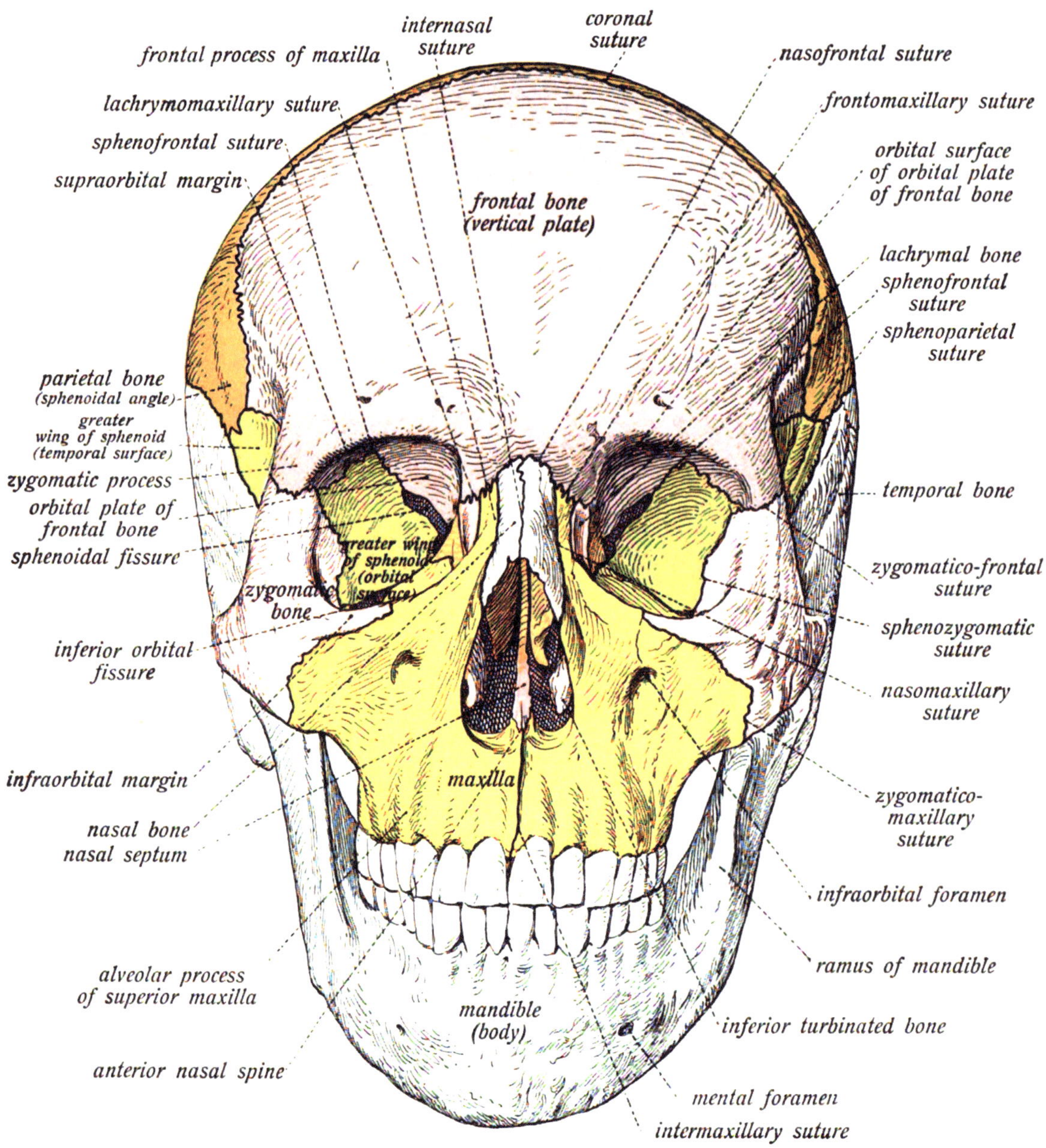

Figure 12.4. The bones of the skull, left lateral view.

Source: By Dr. Johannes Sobotta - Sobotta Atlas and Text-book of Human Anatomy 1909, Public Domain, https://commons.wikimedia.org/w/index.php?curid=29760948

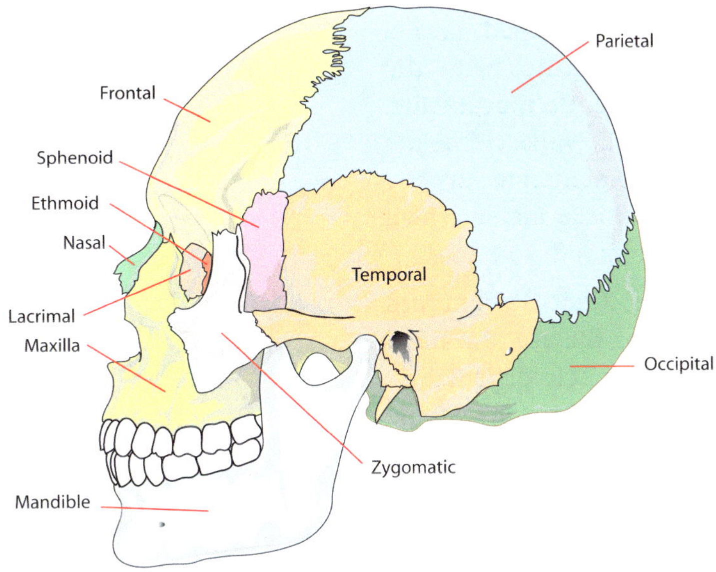

Figure 12.5. Nursing Hero. (n.d.). Anterior(anterolateral) View of the Bones of the Skull.

Source: By LadyofHats Mariana Ruiz Villarreal - made it myself, Public Domain, https://commons.wikimedia.org/w/index.php?curid=1524860

12.1.2. Muscles of Facial Expression

Facial expression is a significant component of human communication, allowing humans to convey emotions and intention without language.

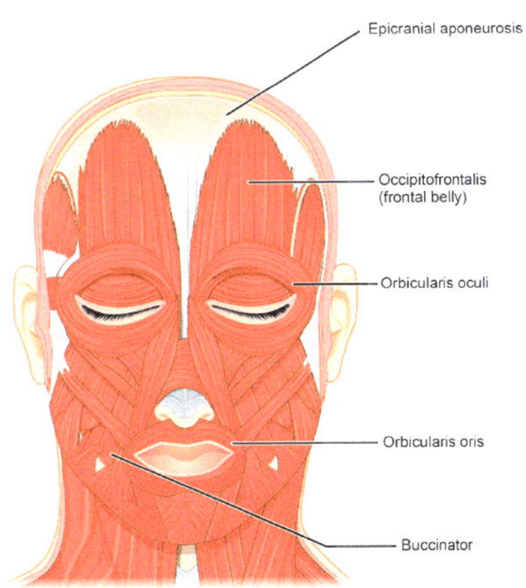

Figure 12.6. Front views of the muscles of facial expressions.

Source: OpenStax. (n.d.). *Front View of the Muscles of Facial Expressions.*

Facial muscles used in these expressions are beneath the face skin, grouped into a complicated system that integrates with the nervous system to achieve subtle movements. These are the orbicularis oculi, which closes the eyelids and is employed to demonstrate surprise or sadness, and the zygomaticus major, which elevates the corners of the mouth to smile.

As demonstrated by advanced techniques in facial animation, including the use of trained models like FLAME, facial muscle articulation supports rich expressions that closely mimic natural humans, enhancing emotional realism in communication (Sellés, 2019). Knowledge about the anatomy and function of such muscles significantly aid areas like psychology, art, and medicine, reflecting their significance in both social interaction and aesthetic depiction (Sellés, 2019) (Figure 12.6).

12.1.3. Muscles of Mastication

The complex mastication muscle mechanism forms part of the processes that make efficient eating possible, thus playing a large role in global health and quality of life (QoL). Muscles involved, which are primarily the masseter, temporalis, medial pterygoid, and the lateral pterygoid, work together to facilitate jaw movement that makes grinding and tearing of food possible.

This complex interaction ensures that food is well chewed before swallowing, a function that is controlled by the anatomical structures of the head and neck. Dysfunction of these muscles can cause problems such as dysphagia, where swallowing dysfunction affects nutrition and hydration (Ayodele et al., 2017). Thus, understanding of the muscles of mastication is crucial, not only for their role in mechanical digestion but also for their broader implications in overall health, well-being, and QoL (Figure 12.7).

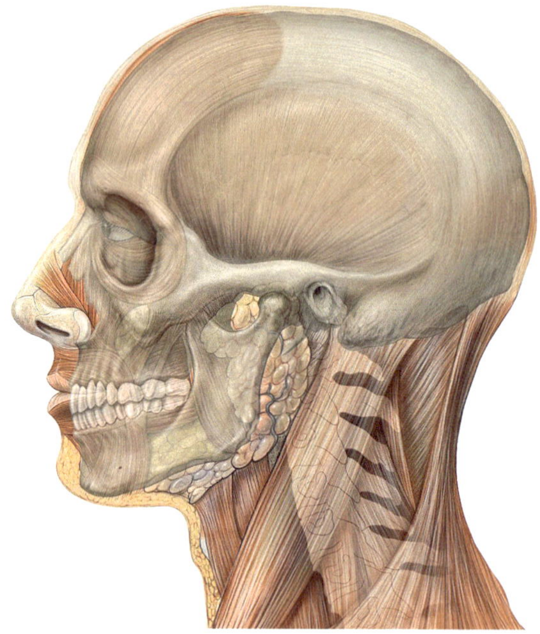

Figure 12.7. Muscles of mastication.

Source: By Patrick J. Lynch, medical illustrator - Patrick J. Lynch, medical illustrator, CC BY 2.5, https://commons.wikimedia.org/w/index.php?curid=1498166

12.1.4. Major Blood Vessels in the Region

In the head and neck, the vascular system is extremely complex and required for numerous physiologic processes. The major vessels are the common carotid arteries, which bifurcate into the internal and external carotid arteries, supplying oxygenated blood to the brain, face, and neck. The jugular veins are also significant in returning deoxygenated blood from the head and neck to the heart. The general understanding of these ships is also relevant in surgical conditions; for instance, in surgical procedures such as hip resurfacing arthroplasty, where the posterior approach compromises vascularity and thereby impacts recovery as seen also in relevant studies (Amarasekera et al., 2012). It is thus relevant to understand the impact of surgery on blood flow both for recovery and for preserving vascular integrity of neck and head region. Proper management of these blood vessels is of pivotal importance in both medical and surgical procedures.

12.1.5. Nerves of the Head and Neck

The neck and head contain a delicate collection of nerves that are meant to supply the sensations and movement. The nervous system is broadly divided into the cranial and cervical nerves that originate from the brain and the spinal cord to supply the varied structures. The facial and the trigeminal nerves belong to the cranial nerves and they supply the sensations and movements on the face which create expressions and sensory feedback. In particular, the three branches of trigeminal nerves facilitate sensation to the forehead, cheeks, and jaw, indicative of its essential roles in daily activities like chewing and facial recognition. Moreover, advances in neuroanatomy highlight the relationship between ancient models of acupuncture with modern neuroscience, suggesting that acupuncture channels may be a reflection of the neurological anatomy of the head and neck (Sellés, 2019). Collectively, these nerves not only enhance our understanding of the facial anatomy but also give significant insights into the therapeutic potential of nerve stimulation and repair in the region (Chou et al., 2013).

12.1.6. Lymphatic Drainage

A network of complex lymph vessels is necessary to maintain fluid balance and permit immune response in the neck and head region. Lymph drainage provides a pathway for distribution of lymph, a fluid filled with immune cells, nutrients, and wastes. An interference with such a system can lead to complications, for instance, localized infection or swelling, particularly in the case of deep neck space infections, which can present serious clinical challenges to clinicians. Conditions like peritonsillar abscesses (PTAs) or retropharyngeal abscesses reflect the complexity of such a lymphatic system, as they present the dissemination of infection along the lymphatic vessels, which treatment might involve surgical intervention to drain and cure the condition (Bălălău et al., 2018). Also, lymphatic drainage specific paths knowledge is important in clinical application like radiation therapy planning where the precise anatomical information can limit the therapy and minimize damage to the surrounding structures (Brinkley et al., 2009). Thus, comprehensive knowledge of head and neck lymphatic drainage is essential for effective medical practice and improved patient results (Figure 12.8).

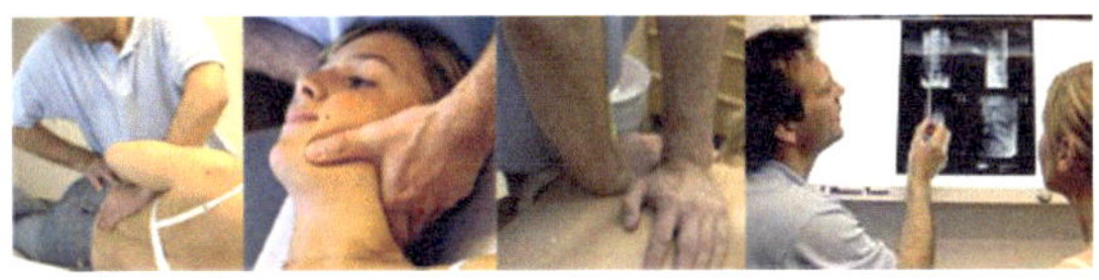

Figure 12.8. Lymphatic drainage.

Source: By Espen Mathisen - Own work, Public Domain, https://commons.wikimedia.org/w/index.php?curid=2148410

12.1.7. Organs of the Head (e.g., Eyes, Ears, Nose)

The elaborate head organs, including the eyes, ears, and nose, play a significant role in sensory perception and communication with the world. The organs are specialized, with the eyes enabling vision through a complex interaction between light and nerve paths to allow us to perceive color, shape, and movement. The ears not only facilitate hearing but also play a crucial role in balance through their physical structure, which, in combination with the brain, interprets auditory information. In addition to this, the nose allows for an entrance for olfactory sensations, which powerfully connects us to memory and feeling through scent. Getting to know the function of these organs demonstrates how they are all interconnected; for instance, vision and sound can influence one's perception of a location simultaneously. Overall, the functions of these head organs highlight their importance not only as individual systems but also as part of an integrated network that shapes our sensory experiences daily.

12.1.8. Salivary Glands and their Functions

Integrated within the complex head and neck structures, salivary glands are an essential part of oral health and digestion. Salivary glands secrete saliva, which has a number of significant roles, including being an aid to the initial processes of digestion, lubricating food so it may be swallowed easily, and maintaining oral cleanliness through the removal of food debris and bacteria from the mouth. Anatomical differences in salivary glands can lead to disorders like xerostomia, wherein reduced secretion of saliva has a significant effect on QoL (Steenbakkers et al., 2021). Furthermore, developmental pathologies like aplasia of salivary glands or masses of ectopic tissues can be involved in such functions (Lucrezia et al., 2019). Recognition of the varied functions of salivary glands adds to their value not just to digestion, but to overall oral health, confirming the need for ongoing research and clinical practices to preserve and restore gland function.

12.1.9. Anatomical Landmarks and their Significance

Anatomical references within the complex realm of the head and neck region serve as important reference points for medical, surgical, and diagnostic treatment. Anatomical landmarks enable targeted interventions, minimizing the risk of complications and maximizing the precision of surgery. For instance, a study demonstrates how the understanding of anatomical relationships among the most important landmarks in craniomaxillofacial (CMF) bones can greatly improve surgery planning and deformation analysis, as in the development of the relational reasoning network (RRN) which identifies landmark positions with high accuracy, even in extreme pathologies (Sellés, 2019). In addition, comparative analysis of Göttingen Minipigs mandible and human anatomy has revealed significant differences, implying that an efficient understanding of such landmarks is essential in ensuring successful surgery and experimentation (Corte et al., 2019). It is thus imperative to have thorough knowledge of anatomical landmarks for the realization of the best patient outcomes and improving surgical practices in the head and neck region.

Test Your Knowledge

1. What do you understand Lymphatic Drainage?
2. Understand Anatomical Landmarks and their Significance

12.2. Common Disorders and Diseases

Learning Outcome

1. Discuss the Headaches and Migraines
2. Explain the Sinusitis and Nasal Disorders
3. Focus on Oral Health Issues (e.g., Cavities, Gum Disease)
4. Understand Throat Infections (e.g., Tonsillitis)
5. Know Neck Pain and Cervical Spine Disorders
6. Describe the Tumors and Cancers of the Head and Neck
7. What do you understand Congenital Anomalies
8. Define the Traumatic Injuries (e.g., Fractures, Lacerations)
9. How to Impact of Systemic Diseases (e.g., Diabetes, Hypertension)

The incidence of disorders in the head and neck region is a topic of significant clinical concern, particularly due to their impact on critical functions like swallowing, speech, and respiration. The ailments can be as disparate as benign tumors to debilitating diseases like cancers, each of which provokes the clinician to diagnose and treat in its own unique manner. For example, HNCs are extremely prevalent in Asia, and according to evidence, India contributes 30% of the total cases globally. The cancers tend to manifest as squamous cell carcinoma, primarily in patients older than 40 years, showing the age-related vulnerability of the cancers (Indranil et al., 2019). Furthermore, dysphagia or the inability to swallow usually associated with such pathologies, because of anatomical distortion or tumor and intervention-related pathologies secondary to pain (Schindler et al., 2014). Knowledge of these common diseases is thus extremely critical for clinicians, as it ensures a multidisciplinary therapy and patient management approach in such complex anatomy (Figure 12.9).

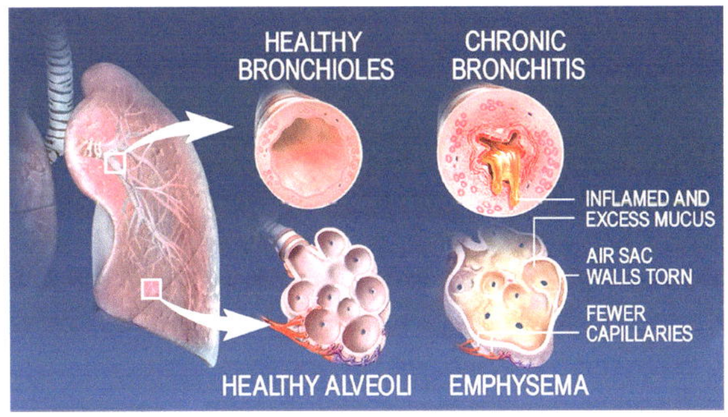

Figure 12.9. Common disorders and diseases.

Source: https://regencyhealthcare.in/wp-content/uploads/2019/09/12_09_Sept.jpg.

12.2.1. Headaches and Migraines

The subjective perception of headaches and migraines is a significant aspect of health, often linked to a multitude of physiological and psychological factors. Classical migraines, characterized by frequent, incapacitating headaches, typically comprise a range of symptoms including nausea, photophobia and phonophobia. Such incapacitating attacks can have a profound effect on the QoL of individuals, affecting social and occupational functioning. Additionally, studies show an alarming connection between migraines and increased suicidal behaviors, especially among women, who indicate headaches at twice the frequency of men (Nazem et al., 2011). This underlines the importance of healthcare providers employing a holistic approach to their treatment procedures, attending to both the physical conditions and psychological impacts of migraine patients. Finally, an awareness of the complexities of headaches is vital in developing practical prevention and management methods in the medical field.

12.2.2. Sinusitis and Nasal Disorders

Affecting individuals of various socio-economic backgrounds routinely, conditions like sinusitis and nasal conditions result from both infectious and non-infectious etiology, causing significant distress and complications if left untreated. They are usually routine conditions resulting from inflammation of the sinuses due to conditions such as allergies, polyps, or infections, causing symptoms such as nasal congestion, pain, and olfactory dysfunction. In Tanzania, for instance, disorder prevalence levels of conditions like epistaxis highlight the importance of nasal health management because trauma and hypertension become the leading causes of such disorders (Sellés, 2019). Additionally, varying diagnostic techniques like computed tomography (CT) become central in identifying underlying pathologies of the head and neck region, thus improving treatment outcomes. Better imaging not only provides clear views of normal and abnormal sinus anatomy but also allows for timely intervention, congruent with the need for overall management plans in the treatment of sinusitis and similar nasal conditions (Crijns et al., 2016) (Figure 12.10).

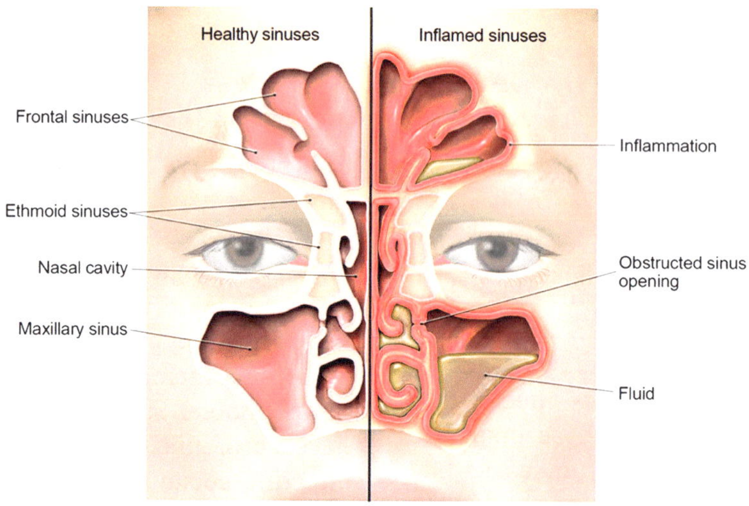

Figure 12.10. Sinusitis.

Source: By Centers for Disease Control and Prevention - https://www.cdc.gov/sinus-infection/about/, Public Domain, https://commons.wikimedia.org/w/index.php?curid=155109646

12.2.3. Oral Health Issues (e.g., Cavities, Gum Disease)

Having the best oral health possible is the key to avoiding a variety of problems, both cavities and gum disease, and both can greatly affect the overall state of one's health. Cavities due to tooth enamel decay are usually brought about by inadequate oral hygiene practices and heavy intake of sugars. Likewise, gum disease, from gingivitis to periodontitis, is due to the build-up of plaque and can result in the loss of one's teeth if not addressed. According to a paper presented in an extensive manual for dental students, the importance of preventive oral care, like regular check-ups and proper hygiene practices, cannot be undermined. Along with this, the employment of modern technology in the form of products like an oral health database can make individuals more effective in taking care of their oral health, thus reducing the prevalence of such issues (Sellés, 2019). So, curing cavities and gum disease is vital to enhancing dental health, as well as overall health.

12.2.4. Throat Infections (e.g., Tonsillitis)

The incidence and management of throat infection, particularly tonsillitis, is a serious issue in the health industry, especially in the context of surgical interventions like tonsillectomy. Tonsillitis often takes the form of a recurring but severe medical condition, often resulting in complications like PTA, reported to be the most common deep neck infection. Acute tonsillitis is shown to predispose to PTA; however, the two are not always correlated with some examples of PTA taking place in the absence of previous tonsillitis (Sanmark et al., 2019). Moreover, striking regional variations in surgery volumes, such as the extremely high tonsillectomy rates in South Africa compared with international rates, point toward the necessity of a review of patient outcomes and healthcare practice (Douglas-Jones et al., 2017). This difference suggests that training, socio-cultural, and environmental concerns are likely to substantially affect treatment practices, hence the necessity for more discriminative clinical guidelines when treating throat infections.

12.2.5. Neck Pain and Cervical Spine Disorders

There is a complex interaction of neurological and musculoskeletal (MSK) conditions in the incidence of cervical spine disorders and neck pain that exerts a significant impact on QoL. The disorders can be due to varied etiologies like improper posture, repetitive stress, or traumatic injury, leading to symptoms that range from mild stiffness to disabling pain. The intricacy of cervical anatomy makes it particularly susceptible to disorders that can also affect swallowing mechanisms, as seen in the interlink between dysphagia and cervical spine disorders (Schindler et al., 2014). Furthermore, recent research indicates the way somatic modulation can influence symptoms like tinnitus, particularly when there are cervical spine disorders alongside auditory disorders (Cialente et al., 2017). Management of neck pain has to be a multidisciplinary affair in both diagnosis and treatment, considering both MSK rehabilitation and neurological aspects. Lastly, appreciation of the interrelationship of cervical disorders with other health situations is essential for effective patient management and improved outcomes (Figure 12.11).

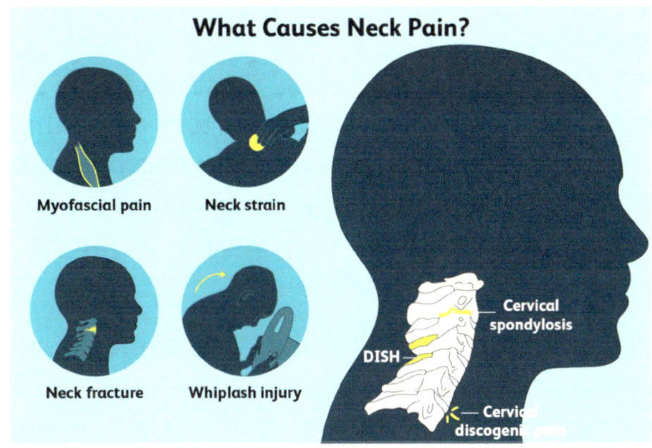

Figure 12.11. Neck pain and cervical spine disorders.

Source: Verywell Health. (n.d.). *What Causes Neck Pain?*

12.2.6. Tumors and Cancers of the Head and Neck

The occurrence of head and neck cancers and tumors is becoming more of a global concern, necessitating greater awareness and research. HNCs present substantial geographic variation in incidence and types; Epstein-Barr virus (EBV), for instance, is closely associated with nasopharyngeal carcinoma, particularly in areas with high incidences (Sellés, 2019). The strong link of human papillomavirus (HPV) to head and neck squamous cell carcinoma also underscores the infectious cause of such cancers, with type 16 HPV implicated in the majority of cases (Sellés, 2019). Furthermore, cancer registry statistics showed that HNC, along with lymphomas, comprises a large proportion of cancers among men diagnosed, pointing to a contrasting trend with Western populations. It is essential to learn these trends to guide targeted prevention and treatment approaches in the fight against HNCs.

12.2.7. Congenital Anomalies

Congenital head and neck malformations are a heterogenous collection of conditions that are not well realized until later in life, despite their impact on the health of patients. They can manifest as changes in blood vessel anatomy, for instance, the internal carotid artery anomalies such as unilateral hypoplasia or agenesis, which can affect cerebral circulation and are most commonly discovered incidentally in imaging studies (Aktaş et al., 2020).

Similarly, branchial anomalies, for instance, cysts and fistulas, are the most common congenital lesions within the region and can lead to infection or cosmetic concerns (Termedia, 2018). Recognition of these differences is crucial not only to provide proper surgical interventions but also to decide on the treatment of future possible complications, such as thromboembolic events or the risk of aneurysm formation in the brain. Diagnosis and knowledge of congenital defects significantly enhance patient prognosis and can guide future clinical intervention.

12.2.8. Traumatic Injuries (e.g., Fractures, Lacerations)

Injuries to the head and neck region can result from various traumatic events, leading to complex medical challenges. Fractures and lacerations frequently occur as a consequence of road traffic accidents, a prevalent source of trauma. For instance, a study conducted at Muhimbili National Hospital revealed that road traffic accidents accounted for a staggering 64.2% of oral and maxillofacial injuries, with a significant percentage of patients suffering from fractures and soft tissue injuries such as lacerations and bruises (Kileo et al., 2012). Similarly, another investigation highlighted that traumatic brain injuries were particularly common among pedestrians and cyclists involved in accidents, emphasizing the vulnerability of these groups compared to motor vehicle occupants who typically sustained thoracic and abdominal injuries (Surov et al., 2020). Collectively, these findings underscore the need for targeted interventions to mitigate the risks associated with road traffic accidents and improve safety measures for all road users.

12.2.9. Impact of Systemic Diseases (e.g., Diabetes, Hypertension)

System illnesses play a significant role in determining the health outcomes of patients, particularly in head and neck illnesses. Diabetic and hypertensive complications during HNC treatment are enhanced. For instance, diabetic patients are more likely to have a higher incidence of thyroid disorders, which is likely to inhibit reproductive potential and complicate treatment approaches in general, as exhibited in recent studies (Farzana et al., 2020).

In addition, hypertension can increase the risk of adverse cardiovascular events in the context of surgical procedures and slow recovery following treatment. Such systemic disease can alter the response to therapy and necessitate even more customized care approaches. For head and neck oncology practice, knowledge about how these diseases interact with therapy is essential because it can inform critical decisions regarding how to modify therapy, thus highlighting the necessity for a thorough, multimodal assessment of the patient. Optimal management of systemic illness must be achieved to maximize outcomes in head and neck disease.

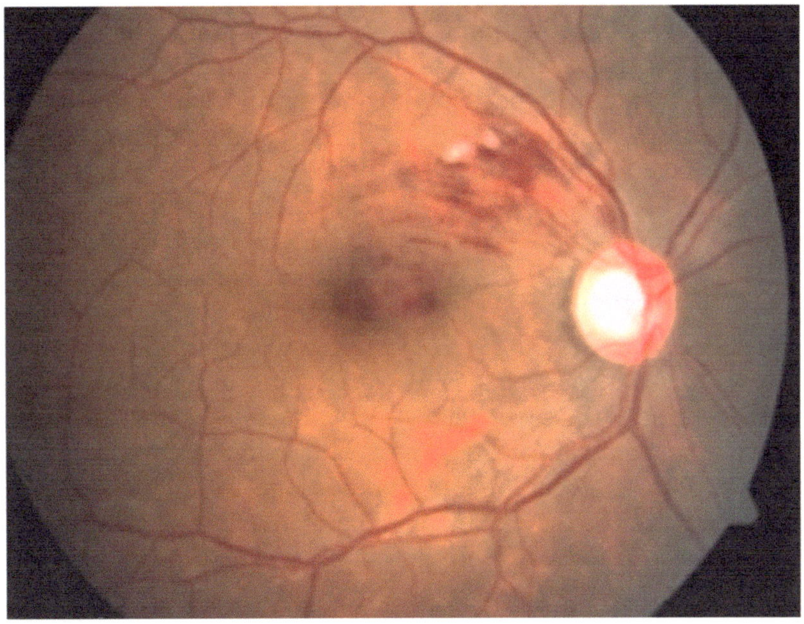

Source: Best Practice Eyecare. (2023). *Retinal Hemorrhage Image.*

Test Your Knowledge

1. What do you understand Tumors and Cancers of the Head and Neck?
2. How to Impact of Systemic Diseases (e.g., Diabetes, Hypertension)

12.3. Diagnostic Techniques

Learning Outcome

1. Discuss the Physical Examination Methods
2. Explain the Imaging Techniques (e.g., X-Rays, CT Scans)
3. Focus on MRI in Head and Neck Diagnostics
4. Know Endoscopy Procedures
5. Discuss the Biopsy Techniques and their Importance
6. Focus on Laboratory Tests Relevant to Head and Neck Conditions
7. Understand the Role of Ultrasound in Diagnosis

85. More details Emerging Technologies in Diagnostics
9. Evaluate Challenges in Diagnosing Head and Neck Disorders

Proper diagnostic techniques are crucial for the accurate assessment of medical disorders, particularly in anatomically complex regions like the head and neck. Traditional techniques such as clinical palpation are often poor in sensitivity and specificity, leading to misdiagnosis and inappropriate treatment planning (Baatenburg et al., 1990). With advances in imaging, there have been modalities like high-frequency ultrasound, which have been non-invasive methods improving the detection of both cervical lymph nodes and head and neck masses. These are highlighted by recent reports that have stressed the poor accuracy of conventional diagnostic tests (Baatenburg et al., 1990). Furthermore, integrating molecular imaging modalities, through the administration of targeted contrast agents, enhances the detection and characterization of tumors, resulting in better diagnostic outcomes and treatment planning. As these diagnostic technologies are further refined, their potential to increase patient management, reduce morbidity, and facilitate timely interventions becomes increasingly apparent.

12.3.1. Physical Examination Methods

In head and neck examination, various physical examination methods are crucial for diagnosis and management. Visual and manual inspection is typically done by clinicians, focusing on lesions, swellings, and abnormalities of the oral cavity and surrounding structures. This careful examination is particularly necessary given the fact that early detection of diseases such as HNC significantly influences patient prognosis. For instance, a national screening program in Oman emphasized the importance of clinical examinations, recognizing that approximately 12.8% of the screened population were positive, highlighting the utility of thorough physical examination (Al-Dhahli et al., 2020). Additionally, ultrasonography has emerged as an adjunct, bringing sensitivity to the detection of metastasis to lymph nodes, especially in melanoma. Integrating both methods allows for adequate appreciation of potential malignancies and enables early interventions (Sellés, 2019). The combination of traditional examination and contemporary imaging modalities, therefore, offers a very robust platform for the assessment of head and neck status.

12.3.2. Imaging Techniques (e.g., X-Rays, CT Scans)

Imaging techniques are a major part in the head and neck pathology diagnosis, providing dense information about intrinsic pathologies. CT scans and X-rays, for instance, allow physicians to visualize bones and tissues, necessary when it comes to identifying injuries, tumors, or congenital defects. These modalities enhance a doctor's ability to make informed decisions about treatment plans, as evidenced by recent findings that patients who have reviewed their imaging scans are more likely to be aware of their diagnoses (Blaxter et al., 2014). Moreover, the limitations of conventional imaging modalities like CT and PET to permit patient exposure to radiation indicate the necessity for a breakthrough in imaging technology. Innovative technologies, such as Near Infrared Chemical Imaging, offer promising alternatives through the ability to provide low-cost, high-resolution diagnostics while minimizing the risks associated with traditional techniques (Sellés, 2019). Integrating these imaging modalities thus enables timely interventions and improved patient outcomes in the head and neck region.

12.3.3. MRI in Head and Neck Diagnostics

In contemporary medical diagnosis, particularly in the complex head and neck region, MRI plays a critical role in enhanced visualization and examination of anatomical structures. MRI is better at differentiating soft tissues and is thus especially valuable for tumor evaluation, inflammatory diseases, and other pathology assessments. MRI accuracy is imperative since a number of pathologies in this area are subtle and challenging to diagnose using standard imaging. For instance, certain malignancies, such as oral squamous cell carcinoma (OSCC), have a predilection to metastasize to cervical lymph nodes, where detection of metastatic involvement can be particularly difficult. In a research evaluation of the effectiveness of pre-operative imaging, the detection sensitivity for pathological lymph nodes was as low as 44.8%, underscoring the need for advanced diagnostic modalities like MRI to supplement outcomes (Pakkanen et al., 2022). In general, the inclusion of MRI in head and neck diagnosis is a cornerstone for proper disease assessment and management (Figure 12.12).

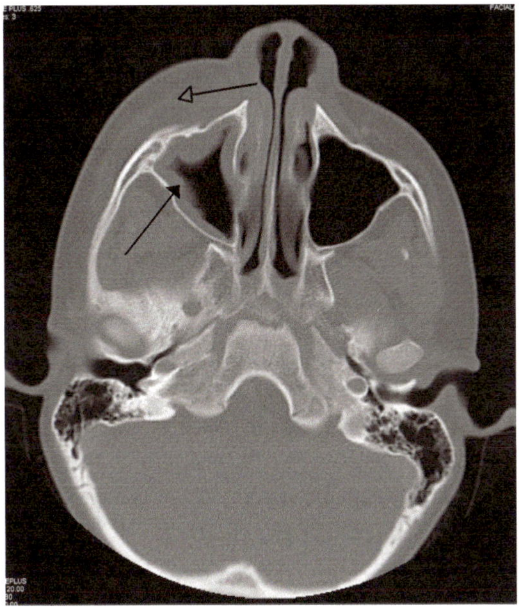

Figure 12.12. Magnetic resonance imaging (MRI) of the head and neck region.

Source: By James Heilman, MD - Own work, CC BY-SA 3.0, https://commons.wikimedia.org/w/index.php?curid=16263221

12.3.4. Endoscopy Procedures

The use of endoscopy methods in the head and neck region is of extreme significance in the diagnosis and treatment of various conditions, particularly chronic rhinosinusitis. Due to the ability of direct visualization of inner structures, endoscopy enhances accuracy in clinical assessment and modalities of treatment. For example, in one study of adult patients presenting with suspected chronic rhinosinusitis, it was found that the conventional diagnostic criteria might overestimate the prevalence of the disease, highlighting the need to improve diagnostic measures. By dropping some of the pain symptoms from the diagnostic criteria, scientists were able to determine that diagnostic specificity grew significantly, assisting physicians in making more informed choices and reducing unnecessary interventions, such as incorrect antibiotic prescriptions (DiNardo et al., 2017). Moreover, most endoscopic procedures allow not only diagnosis but also therapeutic intervention, thereby broadening patient treatment in otolaryngology. Thus, endoscopic evaluation plays a pivotal role in calibrating our approach towards head and neck disorders.

12.3.5. Biopsy Techniques and their Importance

The deployment of effective biopsy techniques is vital in the diagnosis and treatment of head and neck diseases, particularly malignancies. Biopsies allow physicians to obtain tissue samples that may furnish critical information about the nature of lesions, recently distinguishing between malignant and benign processes. For instance, thyroid fine needle aspiration cytology (FNAC) is widely employed in thyroid nodule evaluation, in which precision may sometimes be hindered by non-diagnostic yields. Even though the total malignancy rate is as low as 4.5% in non-diagnostic FNAC, the risk factors that determine such results highlight the requirement for appropriate evaluation via multimodal approaches, including imaging (Bakshi et al., 2012). Similarly, hybrid molecular imaging, such as FDG PET/CT, has played a significant role in assessing head and neck sarcoidosis because it aids in identifying active disease and assessing response to therapy (Artiko et al., 2019). Together, these biopsies underscore the importance of correct diagnosis in directing therapy and ultimately enhancing patient outcomes.

12.3.6. Laboratory Tests Relevant to Head and Neck Conditions

Laboratory studies are valuable in the diagnosis and management of head and neck diseases, providing vital information that is useful in clinical evaluation. Among the many tests, serum concentrations of angiotensin-converting enzyme (ACE) are of special value in the evaluation of sarcoidosis, an inflammatory condition that can happen in the head and neck regions. In a study of patients with chronic sarcoidosis, it was found that subsequent ACE levels after therapy adjustments on the basis of FDG PET/CT scans were not indicative of treatment response, implying that while ACE testing is useful, it is not necessarily a reliable indicator of disease activity (Sellés, 2019). Furthermore, imaging modalities such as FDG PET/CT are also crucial in imaging the head and neck involvement, allowing physicians to adjust therapeutic strategies in turn. Thus, utilization of both laboratory and imaging exams can provide a global perspective of head and neck pathology, guiding treatment and follow-up management (Figure 12.13).

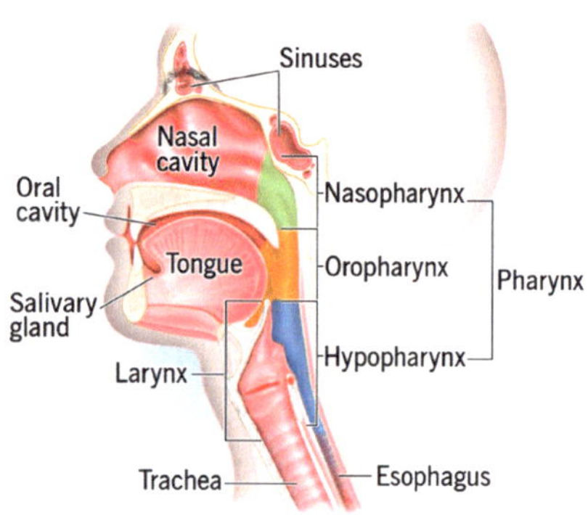

Figure 12.13. Laboratory tests relevant to head and neck conditions.

Source: Cleveland Clinic. (n.d.). *Head and Neck Cancer Anatomy Illustration*.

12.3.7. Role of Ultrasound in Diagnosis

During the last few decades, ultrasound has evolved as an important diagnostic tool in the diagnosis of numerous diseases located in the head and neck region. Its ability to provide real-time images helps in the evaluation of soft tissues structures, thus making it particularly useful in the identification of abnormalities such as cysts, tumors, and vascular diseases. The non-invasiveness of ultrasound, added to its accessibility and affordability, renders it a first choice imaging modality for the majority of cases. Significantly, ultrasound can be employed to guide interventions, conferring both therapeutic and diagnostic benefit. For instance, in the assessment of congenital anomalies, ultrasound might initially identify problems requiring further assessment using MRI, as attested in recent reviews (Sellés, 2019). In addition to this, ultrasound is able to demonstrate metastatic disease in the parotid gland, commonly secondary to a remote primary tumor, demonstrating its crucial role in early and accurate diagnosis in the neck and head region (Sellés, 2019).

12.3.8. Emerging Technologies in Diagnostics

The future of medical evaluation, particularly of the neck and head, is being fueled by dramatic advancements in diagnostic technology. Non-surgical technologies such as optical techniques are being explored for the potential to identify early malignancies and to reflect biochemical changes in tissues before cancerous transformation. They offer a low-cost and real-time method of diagnosis, as indicated by the findings given at the Third Scientific Meeting of the Head and Neck Optical Diagnostics Society, which underscore the need for interdisciplinary methods in diagnostics (Amelink et al., 2011). Also emphasized is the X-ray and optical modalities synergy, representative of their complementary functions; while X-rays provide deep penetration of tissues, optical modalities deliver molecular specificity important for precise diagnostics. The synergy enhances therapeutic monitoring and can lead to personalized treatment intervention, emphasizing the transformative impact of emerging technologies on head and neck pathology outcomes (Pogue et al., 2018).

12.3.9. Challenges in Diagnosing Head and Neck Disorders

The complex anatomy and multifarious symptomatology of neck and head disease present a daunting task of making an accurate diagnosis. The patient will only report nonspecific complaints of headache or nasal obstruction, which may be caused by many diseases, and hence an uphill task in making a diagnosis. For instance, nasopharyngeal carcinoma cancers tend to go undetected until the condition has progressed, mainly due to the ambiguous early symptoms that have a high tendency of being overlooked by both practitioners and patients (Sellés, 2019).

Moreover, the similarity between the symptoms of malignant and benign diseases tends to mislead practitioners since the first onset of such diseases usually presents in the manner of more common conditions, hindering intervention at an early stage. In acute settings, a lack of standardized protocols for the treatment of headache is typical of the broader issue of inconsistency in the diagnosis of head and neck disorders, highlighting the critical necessity for educational programs that will improve the diagnostic capabilities of healthcare professionals (Arocha et al., 2024). Thus, addressing these issues becomes necessary to improve patient outcomes within this complex field of medicine.

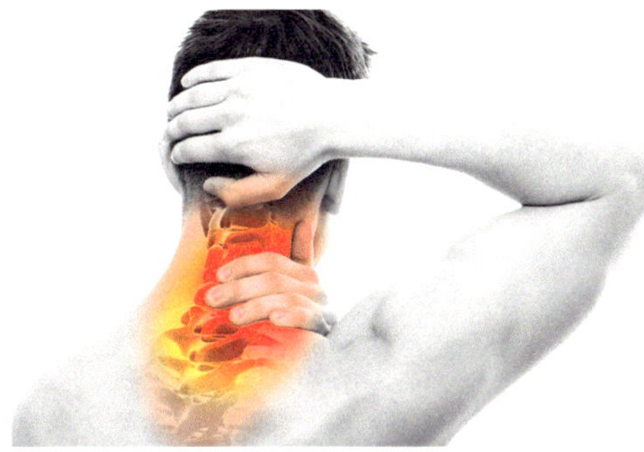

Source: The Advanced Spine Center. (2018). *Understanding Cervicogenic Headaches.*

Test Your Knowledge

1. Which blood tests are commonly ordered to assess infections in the head and neck region?
2. What challenges are posed by overlapping symptoms between ENT, neurological, and dental conditions?

12.4. Treatment and Management

Learning Outcome

1. Discuss the Pharmacological Treatments
2. Explain the Surgical Interventions
3. Focus on Physical Therapy Options
4. Understand Dental Treatments and Oral Care
5. More details Radiation Therapy for Cancers
6. Know Nutritional Considerations in Treatment
7. Evaluate Psychological Support and Counseling
8. Describe the Rehabilitation Strategies
9. Learn about Preventive Measures and Public Health Initiatives

Ideal management and treatment of head and neck disorders, such as oropharyngeal squamous cell carcinoma (OPSCC) and potentially life-threatening infections such as necrotizing fasciitis, require thoughtful consideration that attempts to weigh aggressive therapy against patient survival. For HPV-related OPSCC, data inform us that patients tolerate high-dose cisplatin-based chemoradiotherapy well, further highlighting the potential for deintensification strategies that may minimize treatment-related toxicities without compromising efficacy (Brugnoletti et al., 2019). In contrast to this, pathologies such as cervical necrotizing fasciitis, prevalent in immunocompromised individuals, involve immediate surgical intervention to overcome high risks of morbidity and mortality with delayed diagnosis and treatment (Abramo et al., 2012). Thus, the management of such diverse head and neck pathologies focuses on the adaptation of treatment guidelines to the case-specific considerations with incorporation of advances in medical science and imaging modalities (Figure 12.14).

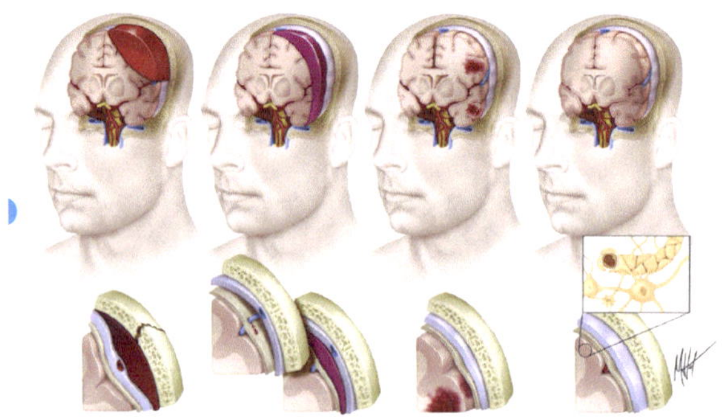

Figure 12.14. The treatment and management of head and neck conditions.

Source: Pascual, J. M. (n.d.). *Types of Intracranial Post-Traumatic Lesions: Epidural Hematoma, subdural Hematoma, Contusion, and Diffuse Axonal Injury* [Image]. ResearchGate.

12.4.1. Pharmacological Treatments

In the treatment of disorders of the head and neck area, pharmacologic therapies have emerged as a key role to play as valuable adjuncts to surgery. Among these are the use of monoclonal antibodies and targeted therapy, which have proven to be highly effective in managing most cancers of the region, such as head and neck squamous cell carcinoma. The advancements in antibody engineering have produced therapeutic products that selectively destroy cancer cells with minimal side effects, and therefore they are the preferred drug in the majority of patients. As attested by reports that therapeutic monoclonal antibodies are the global best-selling drugs, with a market size forecasted to reach $300 billion in 2025, their uses in oncology are increasingly becoming frontline issues (Ruei-Min et al., 2020). Also, new strategies for targeting dependencies typical of oncogenic pathways, such as HRAS mutations, show the potential value of pharmacologic therapies in inducing selective vulnerabilities in cancer cells, with the promise of more effective and tailored treatments (Sellés, 2019).

12.4.2. Surgical Interventions

Among the essential components of the treatment of disorders in the head and neck region is the application of surgery, which may vary significantly in terms of technique and complexity. Simple procedures to very complex reconstructive operations are performed, generally necessitating expert knowledge of the unique anatomical difficulty associated with this region. For instance, dental, maxillo-facial, and ear-nose-throat (ENT) surgeries carry intrinsic risks, including the risk of surgical site infections (SSIs) due to the natural bacterial colonization of the respiratory and mouth tracts. As an expert consensus document has emphasized, proper antimicrobial prophylaxis needs to be ensured in such pediatric groups, and it underscores the significance of interventions with a particular emphasis in this context (Rigotti et al., 2022). Moreover, the rarity of diagnoses such as intramuscular hemangioma (IMH) necessitates more complexity; the definitive management remains surgical resection despite other possibilities (Il-Kyu et al., 2017). Therefore, surgical planning and execution are paramount to optimal patient outcome in the head and neck.

12.4.3. Physical Therapy Options

In head and neck rehabilitation, there are a number of physical therapy procedures that are central in enhancing patient rehabilitation and QoL. In aftermaths such as total laryngectomy, the following can afflict patients, including voice loss and swallowing. Successful physical therapy interventions can significantly aid in solving such issues, focusing on restoration of normal function and improving emotional status. As mentioned, women are able to experience heightened emotional responses to physical constraints like tracheostomy, which means individualized therapy measures are essential (Popescu et al., 2015). Patient participation also matters; research mentions that individuals' views of therapy have a key role to play in determining adherence to exercise regimens (Sellés, 2019). By understanding each patient's unique experience and rehabilitation situation, physical therapists are able to tailor programs that not only facilitate the physical recovery but also psychological resilience.

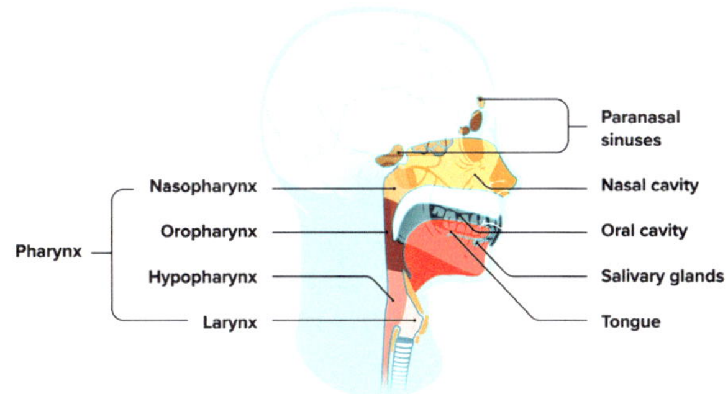

Figure 12.15. Location of head and neck cancers (HNCs).

Source: Healthline. (2022). *Anatomy of the Head and Neck Related to Cancers.*

12.4.4. Dental Treatments and Oral Care

Oral treatment and dental care access are required, particularly for patients with specific medical conditions like HNC. HNC patients experience severe changes in their oral status due to treatments like surgery and radiotherapy that have the tendency to produce greater infection, caries, and periodontal disease risk (Lexomboon et al., 2017).

Consequently, frequency of dental procedures goes up upon diagnosis, with the patient needing preventive and restorative dental therapies to manage such complications. For individuals undergoing radiotherapy, frequent oral hygiene becomes even more imperative since they may have higher dental care costs and differently effective treatments (Lexomboon et al., 2017). Moreover, when metal artifacts obstruct imaging during treatment planning, they can impede accurate tumor delineation, which in turn influences the general accuracy of radiation therapy. Therefore, incorporating thorough dental care within oncologic treatment planning is essential for enhancing patient outcomes in this high-risk group (Figure 12.15).

12.4.5. Radiation Therapy for Cancers

Among various treatment modalities of cancer, radiation therapy is a key in the case of HNCs. Radiation therapy serves more than a single purpose, including curative intent, organ preservation, and symptom relief. As highlighted in various studies, radiation therapy can go a long way in patient outcomes when combined with surgery and chemotherapy, which has been referred to as chemoradiation in many instances. In the instance of HNCs, where preservation of the essential functions is paramount, including speech and swallowing, advanced approaches like 3D conformal radiation therapy (3DCIIT) have been introduced. These technologies enable clinicians to deliver high doses of radiation with increased accuracy while sparing the overlying normal tissues and structures (Wijers et al., 2002). In addition, while some interventions like the bioadhesive chlorhexidine gel have been evaluated for their effectiveness in preventing treatment-related complications like oral mucositis, studies show that they are not likely to improve patients' QoL (Díaz et al., 2015). This ongoing evolution of radiation therapy validates its place in comprehensive cancer care.

12.4.6. Nutritional Considerations in Treatment

In the context of treatment strategies for head and neck region conditions, a very important factor that does not get taken into account frequently is nutritional planning. Nutritional support forms an integral part of the recovery process, particularly after surgeries or therapies disrupting the ability to consume normal diets. For instance, patients undergoing radiation therapy may suffer from mucositis, and this can severely disrupt their ability to eat and be administered adequate nutrition (Bernasconi et al., 2019). Thus, personalized nutritional treatment becomes imperative in such situations. Nutritional requirements should encompass not only macronutrient but also specific micronutrient uptake that is known to facilitate healing and immune function. As discussed in Copeland et al. (2019), integrating nutritional intervention into the treatment regime can greatly enhance patient outcomes and accelerate recovery. Therefore, clinicians need to place priority on nutrition as an integral component of treatment so that patients are given holistic care that caters to both their medical and nutritional requirements.

12.4.7. Psychological Support and Counseling

The psychological effect of HNCs transcends physical symptoms, with serious effects on the psychological well-being of patients. Owing to the high incidence of communication and self-esteem issues that arise post-surgery, such as laryngectomy, mental health is the primary issue to be dealt with. For instance, the depression may occur among patients by reason of the feelings of loneliness and loss of vocal capabilities, as reported with the argument that the psychological profile shifts are common in such patients (Popescu et al., 2016). The effects may be overcome through psychological counseling and support by providing coping strategies. Empirical research indicates that structured interventions, like the eating as treatment (EAT) program, not only improve nutrition but also build emotional resilience in radiation therapy patients (Baker et al., 2019). Therefore, integrating intensive psychological support into treatment plans is vital to supporting mental as well as physical recovery in individuals battling HNCs.

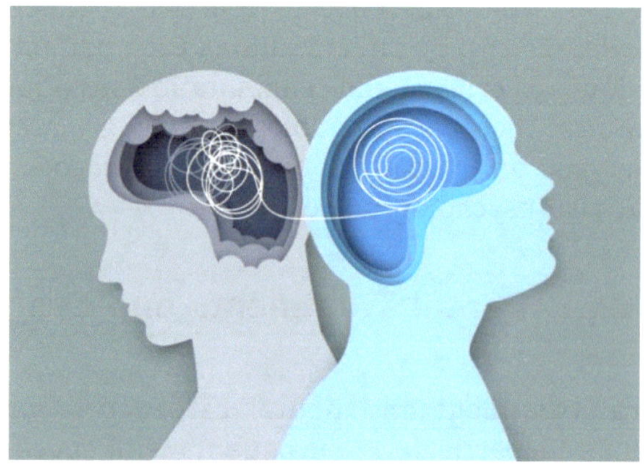

Source: iStock. (n.d.). *Psychological Help Vector Illustration: Two Human Heads, Paper Cut Design.*

12.4.8. Rehabilitation Strategies

Effective rehabilitation activities are responsible for the healing process of HNC patients because they are likely to develop chronic post-treatment swallowing and voice difficulties. The intervention of targeted management, such as swallowing maneuvers and exercises, proves to be influential in the effectiveness of swallowing behavior and quality improvement of the patient's life (Sellés, 2019). In addition, treatment of psychological conditions like anxiety and depression, which are prevalent among this patient population, is crucial in establishing treatment adherence. Scientific evidence indicates that reduced QoL and heightened anxiety can have a detrimental impact on patients' compliance with therapy (Lenich et al., 2012). Thus, an interdisciplinary rehabilitation program combining physical therapies with psychological interventions is critical to promoting enhanced outcomes. Finally, by treating both the physical and emotional aspects of recovery, health professionals can also improve the overall health of patients that face the challenges of HNC treatment and rehabilitation.

12.4.9. Preventive Measures and Public Health Initiatives

Effective public health intervention is necessary in controlling the prevalence of injury, particularly in such high-risk pursuits as horse riding and other sports activities. The high hospitalization and death rates from the same indicate the requirement for intervention through targeted preventive methods. For instance, studies on traumatic injuries caused by horse riding accidents indicate that these injuries are likely to be hospitalizing compared to those sustained while participating in other sports, such as football and skiing, and therefore justify additional safety precautions (Fofana et al., 2021). Additionally, Irish injury mortality statistics verify extensive inequalities in the prevention of injury and the pressing need for additional surveillance to identify policy intervention (Fitzpatrick et al., 2001). By utilizing this evidence, public health professionals can implement evidence-based interventions like educational programs on protective equipment and safety protocols, thereby striving toward a safe environment and reducing the burden of injury among vulnerable populations.

Test Your Knowledge

1. What is the role of the temporomandibular joint (TMJ), and which bones are involved?
2. What are the clinical implications of a fracture to the base of the skull?

SUMMARY

The complex function and anatomy of the skull and head is a critical pursuit in scientific and medical research. With enhanced imaging and modeling technologies, as seen through current studies in the segmentation of brain tumors, the precision to which cranial anatomy can be measured has progressed significantly, and the complexities in the protection and support roles of the skull have been accentuated (Menze et al., 2014). In addition, emerging technologies such as 3D printing offer captivating ways of supplementing both learning content and practical application in this topic through offering actual physical models that depict the complex nature of the cranial bones and tissues (Bethany et al., 2014). These developments in aggregate point to the dynamic interplay between technologic progress and anatomical insight, with prospects for a future in which our capacity to diagnose, teach, and treat cranial well-being will be vastly enhanced. Ongoing interdisciplinary collaboration will thus be required in an effort to further comprehend and treat the head and skull (Dorsher, 1999).

The complex nature of the skull and head anatomy further emphasizes the importance of acquiring extensive knowledge for medical staff, particularly for otolaryngologists and neurosurgeons. Complex textbooks promote a methodical learning style with a focus on extensive anatomical knowledge combined with clinical correlation. Key topics are the complex skull base anatomy, physiology of hearing and balance, and the surgical correction of congenital craniofacial deformities, all necessitating precision in both diagnosis and surgical treatment. Integrating newer imaging modalities and surgical tools such as 3D reconstruction and endoscopic techniques further maximizes treatment efficacy and patient outcomes. These study materials not only consolidate fundamental science but also guide professionals through complex operative procedures with clear, step-by-step instructions and brilliant pictures. Mastering these key points is thus imperative to enhance head and skull pathology and surgery care (Faris, 2015; Stamm, 2011).

KEY TERMS FROM THIS CHAPTER

- Carotid arteries
- Cervical nerves
- Craniomaxillofacial (CMF)
- Deoxygenated blood
- Endoscopic sinus
- Facial expression
- Facial skeleton
- Fetal growth
- Head organs
- Hip resurfacing arthroplasty
- Human skull
- Hypopharyngeal surgeries
- Inferior turbinate flap
- Larynx
- Medial pterygoid
- Nasoseptal flap

CRITICAL THINKING QUESTIONS

1. **Which of the following bones is unpaired in the skull?**
   a. Parietal
   b. Temporal
   c. Occipital
   d. Zygomatic
2. **The pterion is the junction of which bones?**
   a. Frontal, parietal, temporal, sphenoid
   b. Temporal, occipital, zygomatic, sphenoid
   c. Parietal, temporal, nasal, sphenoid
   d. Frontal, nasal, ethmoid, zygomatic
3. **Which bone contains the foramen magnum?**
   a. Sphenoid
   b. Temporal
   c. Occipital
   d. Ethmoid
4. **Which of the following is part of the viscerocranium?**
   a. Parietal
   b. Temporal
   c. Maxilla
   d. Occipital
5. **The temporomandibular joint (TMJ) is formed between the mandible and which bone?**
   a. Frontal
   b. Maxilla
   c. Temporal
   d. Sphenoid

Short Answer Questions

1. What is the anatomical significance of the pterion?
2. Describe the major sutures of the skull and the bones they connect.
3. What is the function of the paranasal sinuses, and where are they located?
4. Differentiate between the neurocranium and the viscerocranium.
5. Describe the development and closure of the fontanelles in infants.
6. Explain the role of the mandible in mastication and speech.

Answers to Critical Thinking Questions

1. (c) 2. (a) 3. (c) 4. (c) 5. (c)

REFERENCES

1. Akdemir Aktaş, H., Farımaz, M., Fırat, A., & Göçmen, R. (2020). Rare congenital anomalies of the internal *carotid artery: anatomic* and radiologic aspects of three cases and review of the literature. Surgical and radiologic anatomy : SRA, 42(11), 1363–1370. https://doi.org/10.1007/s00276-020-02549-w (accessed on 8th May 2025).
2. Akram, M., Iqbal, M., Daniyal, M., & Khan, A. U. (2017). Awareness and *current knowledge of breast cancer. Bio*logical Research, 50. https://doi.org/10.1186/s40659-017-0140-9 (accessed on 8th May 2025).
3. Arocha, C. (2024). An Educational Intervention Regarding Headache Management to Increase the Knowledge of Emergency Department Providers in a Tertiary Care Facility – A Quality Improvement Project. FIU *Digital Commons. https://core.ac.uk/download/*622984266.pdf (accessed on 8th May 2025).
4. Baianu, I. C. (2011). Early Diagnosis of Alzheimer's Disease by *NIRF Spectroscopy and Nuclear Medicine. https://core.ac.uk/download/pdf/290230.pdf (accessed on 8th May 2025).*
5. *Balalau, C., Balalau, O. D., Bertesteanu, S. V., Dumitrache, P.,* Paun, A. O., Popescu, B., Popescu, C. R., & Scaunasu, R. V. (2015). Differences Between Men and Women with Total Laryngectomy. JMMS 2015, 2(2): 100- 107. https://core.ac.uk/download/144552340.pdf (accessed on 8th May 2025).
6. Blum, A., Dill-Muller, D., Eberle, J. Y., Kuchelmeister, C., *Mauss-Kiefer, V., & Schmid-Wendtner, M. H. (2006).* Ultrasound Mapping of Lymph Node and Subcutaneous Metastases in Patients with Cutaneous Melanoma: Results of a Prospective Multicenter Study. S. Karger AG. https://core.ac.uk/download/16432788.pdf (accessed on 8th May 2025).
7. Brinkley, J. F., Kalet, I., Mejino, J. L. V., Wang, V., & Whipple, M. (2*009). Content-Specific* Auditing of a Large-Scale Anatomy Ontology. https://core.ac.uk/download/pdf/9412368.pdf (accessed on *8th May 2025).*
8. *Brugnoletti, O., De Felice, F., de Vincentiis, M., Mezi, S., Poli*meni, A., Tombolini, V., & Valentini, V. (2019). Advances in the Management of HPV-Related Oropharyngeal Cancer. Hindawi Limited. https://core.ac.uk/download/196295509.pdf (accessed on 8th May 2025).
9. Carmi*chael, J., David, A., Davidson, J. R., et al. (2021). Feta*l Body MRI and Its Application to Fetal and Neonatal Treatment: An Illustrative Review. Elsevier Sci Ltd. https://core.ac.uk/download/477686545.pdf (accessed on 8th May 2025).
10. Chengoden, *R., Victor, N., Huynh-The, T., et al. (2023). Me*taverse for healthcare: A survey on potential applications, challenges and future directions. IEEE Access, 11, 12765–12795. https://doi.org/10.1109/access.2023.3241628 (accessed on 8th May 2025).
11. Chou, S., Osman, S., Ros*ing, J., & Sahar, D. E. (2013). Total Posterior Leg Open Wound Management with Free Anterolateral Thigh Flap: Case and Literature Review. e*Scholarship, University of California. https://core.ac.uk/download/323068446.pdf (accessed on 8th May 2025).
12. Chowdhury, A., & Landgraf, S. (2015). Factoring Emergin*g Markets Into the Relationship Between Global Liquidity an*d Commodities. e-Publications@Marquette. https://core.ac.uk/download/213086817.pdf (accessed on 8th May 2025).
13. Cook, A., Jenkins, L. M., & Plant, P. (1999). A Casemix Analysis of Hospital *Admissions in Six Specialties for Barking & Havering Health Au*thority. South East Institute of Public Health.

https://core.ac.uk/download/10631591.pdf (accessed on 8th May 2025).

14. Corte, G. M., Hünigen, H., Niehu*es, S. M., Plendl, J., & Richardson, K. C. (2019). Cephalometric studies of the mandible,* its masticatory muscles and vasculature of growing Göttingen minipigs—A comparative anatomical study to refine experimental mandibular surgery. PLoS ONE, 14(4), e0215875. https://core.ac.uk/download/222573931.pdf (accessed on 8th May 2025).

15. C*rijns, C. P., B*aeumlin, Y., De Rycke, L., Broeckx, B. J., Vlaminck, L., Bergman, E. H., van Bree, H., & Gielen, I. (2016). Intra-arterial versus intra venous *contrast-enhanced computed tomography of the equine head. BMC veterinary research, 12, 6. https://doi.or*g/10.1186/s12917-016-0632-9 (accessed on 8th May 2025).

16. Curtis, N., Evans, S. E., Fagan, M. J., Jones, M. E. H., & O'Higgins, P. (2013). Cranial Sutur*es Work Collectively to Distribute Strain Throughout the Reptile Skull. J. R. Soc. Interf*ace.1020130442http://doi.org/10.1098/rsif.2013.0442(accessed on 8th May 2025).

17. Deaton, A., & Cartwright, N. (2017). Understanding and misunderst*anding randomized controlled trials. Social Science & Medicine, 210, 2–21. https://doi.org/10.1016/j*.socscimed.2017.12.005 (accessed on 8th May 2025).

18. DiNardo, L. J., Hirsch, S. D., Reiter, E. R., Schuman, T. A., & Wan, W. (2017). Elimination of Pain Improves Specificity of Clinical Diagnostic Criteria for Adult Chronic Rhinosinusitis. VCU Scholars Compass. https://core.ac.uk/download/130355229.pdf (accessed on 8th May 2025).

19. Dorsher, P. The Neuroanatomic Basis of the Acu*puncture* Principal Meridians. Nat Prec (2009). https://doi.org/10.1038/npre.2009.3795.1 (accessed on 8th May 2025).

20. Douglas-Jones, P., & Fagan, J. J. (2017). Tonsillectomy Rates *in the South African Private Healthcare Sector. Health and Medical Publishing Group. https://core.ac.uk/do***wn**load/478309602.pdf (accessed on 8th May 2025).

21. Fofana, D., Lim, J., Mutore, K., Skubic, J., & Torres-Reveron, A. (2021). Hearing Hoofbeats? Think Head and Neck Trauma: A 10-Ye*ar NTDB Analysis of Equestrian*-Related Trauma in the USA. ScholarWorks @ UTRGV. https://core.ac.uk/download/358281093.pdf (accessed on 8th May 2025).

22. Ginat, D. T., & Neilio, J. M. (2024). Emergi*ng Head and Neck Tumor Targeting Contrast Agents for the Purpose of CT, MRI, and Multimodal Diagnostic Ima*ging: A Molecular Review. https://core.ac.uk/download/614775487.pdf (accessed on 8th May 2025).

23. Hansen, C., Christiansen, R., Lorenzen, E., Bertelsen, A., Asmussen, J., Gyldenkerne, N., Eriksen, J., Johansen, J., & Brink, C. *(2017). Contouring a*nd *Dos*e Calculation in Head and Neck Cancer Radiotherapy After Reduction of metal Artifacts in CT Images, 56, 874–878. https://www.semanticscholar.org/paper/*d651e7a*6feada6d1896fb4b0de1ecde8b9a89dc2 (accessed on 8th May 2025).

24. Hosny, A., Parmar, C., Quackenbush, J., Schwartz, L. H., & *Aerts, H. J. W. L. (2018). Artificial intelligence in radiology.* Nature Reviews Cancer, 18, 500–510. https://doi.org/10.1038/s41568-018-0016-5 (accessed on 8th May 2025).

25. Impey, A. (2013). Keeping in Touch Via Cassette: Tracing Dinka Songs from Cat*tle Camp to Transnational Audio-Letter. Taylor and Francis. https://core.ac.uk/download/17184732.pdf (accessed* on 8th May 2025).

26. Jung, J., Cho, K. J., Naji, A., et al. (2019). HRAS-driven cancer cells are vulnerable to TRPML1 inhibition. EMBO *Reports, 20. https://doi.org/10.15252/embr.201846685.*

27. *Khan, W. A., Khan, Z. K., & Malik, I. A. (1998). Pattern of Malignant Tumors Obse*rved in a University Hospital: A Retrospective Analysis. eCommons@AKU. https://core.ac.uk/download/212884238.pdf (accessed on 8th May 2025).

28. Kileo, B. F. (2012). The Pattern of Oral and Maxillofacial Injuries *Among Patients Attending Muhimbili National Hospital, Dar es Salaam, Tanzania. https://core.ac.uk/download/pdf/11307821*.pdf (accessed on 8th May 2025).

29. Kim, I. K., Seo, J. H., Cho, H. Y., Lee, D. H., Jang, J. M., Kim, J. M., & Park, I. S. (2017). Intramuscular Hemangiomas on the Masseter Muscle and Orbicularis Oris muscle: A Report of Two Cases, 43, 125–133. https:*//www.semanticschola*r.org/paper/8693488b3cbd0e7a81760b24bd4393425f84db3b (accessed on 8th May 2025).

30. Korenevskaya, N. A., *Sakharuk, N. A., & Volkova, M. N. (2016). Guideline on Therapeutic Dentistry for the 5th Term.* VSMU N. N. Burdenko. https://core.ac.uk/download/80150453.pdf (accessed on 8th May 2025).

31. LeBoff, M. S., Greenspan, S. L., Insogna, K., Lewiecki, E. M., Saag, K. G., Singer, A., & Siris, E. S. (2022)*. The clinician's* guide to prevention and treatment of osteoporosis. Osteoporosis International, 33, 2049–21*02. https://doi.org/10.1007/s00198-021-05900-y (accessed on 8th May 2025).*

32. *Lenich, A.,* Bachmeier, S., Dendorfer, S., Mayr, E., Nerlich, M., & Füchtmeier, B. (2012). Development of a test system *to analyze different hip fracture osteosyntheses under simulated walking. Biomedizinische Technik. Biomedical engineering, 5*7(2), 113–119. https://doi.org/10.1515/bmt-2011-0999 (accessed on 8th May 2025).

33. Lexomboon, D., Karlsson, P., Adolfsson, J., Ekbom, A., Naimi-Akbar, A., Bahmanyar, S., Mo*ntgomery, S., & Sandborgh-Englund, G. (2017). Consumption and Direct Costs of Dental Care for Patien*ts with Head and Neck Cancer: A 16-year Cohort Study, 12. https://www.semanticscholar.org/paper/03c08bf1868308e746e7577cd2ca87890758b739 (accessed on 8th May 2025).

34. Li, T., Bolkart, T.*, Black, M. J., Li, H., & Romero, J. (2017). Learni*ng a model of facial shape and expression from 4D scans. ACM Transactions on Graphics, 36, 1–17. https://doi.org/10.1145/3130800.3130813 (accessed on 8th May 2025).

35. Lu, R. M., Hwang, Y. C., Liu, I. J., Lee, C. C., Tsai, H. Z., Li, H. J., & Wu, H. C. (2020). Development *of therapeutic antibodies for* the treatment of diseases. Journal of Biomedical Science, 27. https://doi.org/10.1186/s12929-019-0592-z (accessed on 8th May 2025).

36. Mathew, R. T. (2017). The prognostic role of VEGF in head and neck squamous cell carcin*oma. https://open.bu.edu/bitstream/2144/23808/5/Mathew_bu_0017N_12667.pdf (accessed on 8th May 2025).*

37. *Muzaffar*, R., Osman, M. M., Raslan, O. A., & Shetty, V. (2015). Image Findings of Cranial Nerve Pathology on [18F]-2-Deoxy-D-Glucose (FDG) Positron Emission Tomography with Computerized Tomography (PET/CT): A Pictorial Essay. eScholarship, Univ*ersity of California. https://co*re.ac.uk/download/323068802.pdf (accessed on 8th May 2025).

38. Nazem, S. (2011). Pain and Suicide in a Population-Based Sample. The Research Repository @ WVU. https://core.ac.uk/download/230486284.pdf (accessed on 8th May 2025).

39. Pakkanen, A. *L., Marttila, E., Apajalahti, S.,* Snäll, J., & Wilkman, T. (2022). Reliability of the pre-operative imaging to assess neck nod*al involvement in oral cancer patients, a single-center study. Medi*cina oral, patologia oral y cirugia bucal, 27(2), e191–e197. https://doi.org/10.4317/medoral.25228 (accessed on 8th May 2025).

40. Park, J., Nam, I. C., Kim, C. S., et al. (2022). Sex differences in the prevalence of head and neck cancers: A 10-year follow-up study of 10 million healthy people. Cancers, 1*4(10), 2521. https:*//www.semanticscholar.org/paper/c726d36e21873bcf9e625acefa40baf9c3c2541d (accessed on 8th May 2025).

41. Pogue, B. W., & Wilson, B. C. (2018). Optica*l and X-Ray Technology Synergies Enabling Diagnostic and Therapeutic Applications in Medicine. Dartmouth Digital Commons. https://core.ac.uk/download/231149083.*pdf (accessed on 8th May 2025).

42. Popescu, B.,, Balalau, C., Bertesteanu, S. V., Paun, O. A., & Scaunasu, R. V. (2016). Psychologic*al Profile of Laryngectomized Patients. J Min*d Med Sci. 2016; 3(1): 31-38.. https://core.ac.uk/download/144552425.pdf (accessed on 8th May 2025).

43. Pullon, B. M. (2014). Relationship of the Cricothyroid Space with Vocal Range in Female Singers. University of Waikato. https://core.ac.uk/download/29202383.pdf (acce*ssed on* 8t*h* May 2025).

44. Sahiner, B., Pezeshk, A., Hadjiiski, L. M., Wang, X., Drukker, K., Kenny, H., Summers, R. M., & Giger, M. L. (2018). Deep learning in medical imag*ing and radiation therapy. Medical Physics, 46. https://doi.org/10.1002/mp.13264 (accessed on 8th* May 2025).

45. Sanmark, E. (2019). Etiology of Peritonsillar Abscess: Role of Minor Salivary Glands. University of Helsinki Li*braries. https://core.ac.uk/download/228181126.pdf (accessed on 8th May* 2025).

46. Sasegbon, A., & Hamdy, S. (2017). The anatomy and physiology of normal and abnormal swallowing in oropharyngeal dysphagia. Neurogastroenterology & Motility, 29. https://doi.org/10.1111/nmo.13100 (accessed on 8th May 2025).

47. Schindler, A., Ginocchio, D., Mozzanic*a, F., Roncoroni, L.*, Pizzorni, N., & Letizia, S. (2014). Head and Neck Diseases and Disorders Causing *Oropharyngeal Dysphagia. ACT Publishing. https://core.ac.uk/dow*nload/187975939.pdf (accessed on 8th May 2025).

48. Schwartz, D. L., & Dong, L. (2011). Adaptive radiation therapy for head and neck cancer-can an old goal evolve into a new standard?. Journal of oncology, 2011, 690595. https://doi.*org/10.1155/2011/690595 (accessed on* 8th May 2025).

49. Sellés de Lucas, V. The role of soft tissues and minor osseous structures in cranial biomechanics. (Thesis). University of Hull. https://hull-rep*ository.worktribe.com/output/4222601 (accessed on 8th May 2025).*

50. Sen, I., Ghosh, S., & Saha, T. N. (2019). Epidemiological Profile of the Head-Neck Pathologies in a Peripheral Referral Institute. The Association of Otolaryngologists of India, West Bengal. https://core.ac.uk/download/440931012.pdf (accessed on 8th May 2025).

51. Surov, A., Meyer, H. J., & Wienke, A. (2020). Apparent Diffusion Coefficient for *Distinguishing Between Malignant and Benign Lesions in the Head and Neck Region: A Syst*ematic Review and Meta-Analysis. Frontiers in oncology, 9, 1362. https://doi.org/10.3389/fonc.2019.01362 (accessed on 8th May 2025).

52. Togni, L., Mascitti, M., Santarelli, A., Contaldo, M., Romano, A., Serpico, R., & Rubini, C. (2019). Unusual conditions impairing saliva secretion: Developmental anomalies of salivary glands. *Frontiers in Physiology, 10*. https://doi.org/10.3389/fphys.2019.00855 (accessed on 8th May 2025).

53. Zhao, H., Wu, L., Yan, G., Chen, Y., Zhou, M., Wu, Y., & Li, Y. (2021). Inflammation and tumor progression: Signaling pathways and targeted intervention. *Signal Transduction and Targeted Therapy,* 6. https://doi.org/10.1038/s41392-021-00658-5 (accessed on 8th May 2025).

BRAIN AND CRANIAL NERVES

13

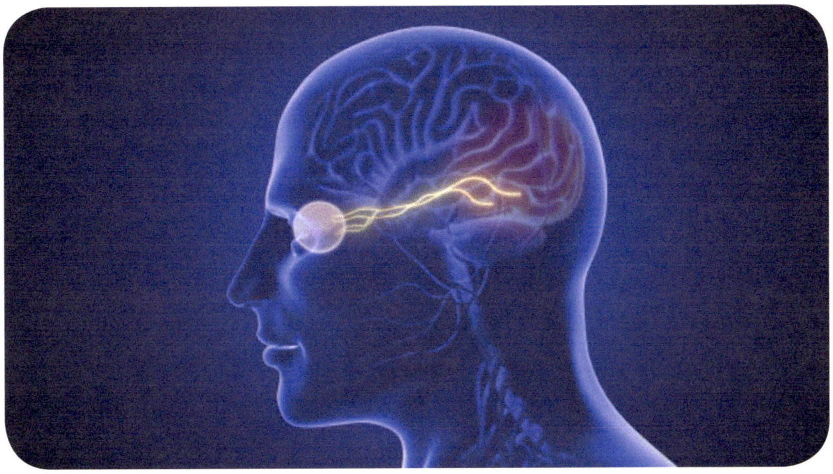

LEARNING OBJECTIVES

After studying this chapter, you will be able to:

1. Focus on the anatomy of the brain
2. Explain the functions of the brain
3. Give an overview of cranial nerves
4. Give a detailed examination of cranial nerves
5. Know disorders related to the brain
6. Learn about research and advances in neuroscience

Introduction

The complexity of the human nervous system has intrigued scientists and physicians for centuries, particularly the complex relationship between the brain and cranial nerves. An understanding of this relationship is at the heart of the understanding of how sensory and motor functions integrate to produce coordinated behavior. The brain, protected within the skull cavity, serves as the processing unit, interpreting information and sending instructions through a series of cranial nerves. These nerves directly exit the brain and control such fundamental activities as facial movement, vision, hearing, and taste. Further, the anatomical variations of the brain and its nerve pathways illustrate evolutionary changes that have optimized survival mechanisms. The close scrutiny of these connections offers both the complexity and simplicity of neurological function, enabling advancements in the diagnosis and treatment of cranial and brain disorders. When learning about the anatomy and function of the cranial nerves and brain, it is important to learn about both their anatomical structure and clinical application. The brain, which is divided into the forebrain, midbrain, and hindbrain, has regions that are accountable for different cognitive and physiological processes. The cranial nerves, 12 pairs of which emanate from these regions, innervate muscles and organs to allow sensory input and motor function. Anatomical studies with advanced imaging and cadaveric dissections have raised knowledge of how these nerves relate to structures within the brain. Endoscopic neurosurgical procedures, for example, have clarified trajectories that minimize brain tissue manipulation in reaching areas like the suprasellar area, demonstrating the clinical relevance of precise anatomical knowledge (Cappabianca et al., 2008). These findings are significant not only for the understanding of normal physiology but also for the development of surgical techniques that will preserve neural function.

More recent advances in paleoneurology contribute to the understanding of brain and cranial nerve development, yielding information on neural development from the fossil record. Analysis of endocranial casts of fossil animals, such as the Upper Cretaceous snake Dinilysia patagonica, provides evidence of the primitive structure of the brain and nerve pathways (Triviño et al., 2017). The findings indicate simplicity of brain structure and secondary acquisition of complexity, reflecting functional adaptations like enhanced sensory function and locomotor activity. These evolutionary viewpoints emphasize the dynamic nature of the brain-nerve interaction and its role in the interface of the organism with the environment. The incorporation of fossil data completes the anatomical blueprint, tying modern neuroanatomy to its history and guiding an integrated approach to brain and cranial nerve study (Figure 13.1).

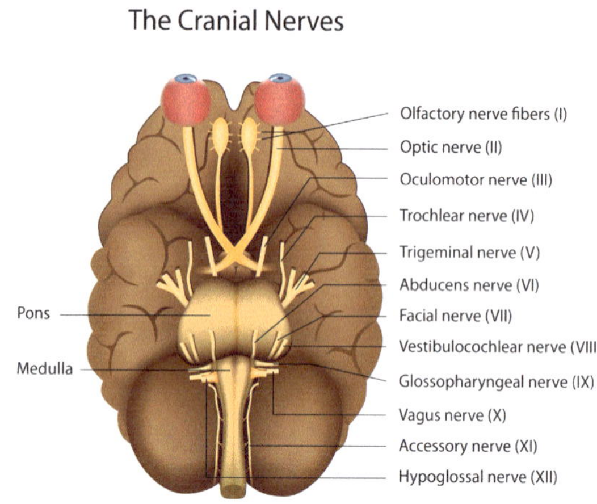

Figure 13.1. Brain and cranial nerves.

Source: CogniFit. (2019). The Cranial Nerves.

Definition of the Brain and Cranial Nerves

Understanding of the complex design of the human nervous system requires an exploration of its central components, the brain and cranial nerves. The brain serves as the body's operation control center, cognition, and processing of sensation, integrating information from various sources to maintain homeostasis and coordinate responses. It is composed of various structural areas with specific functions, the cerebrum, cerebellum, and brainstem. The 12 pairs of cranial nerves, which emerge from the brainstem, are the principal means for transmitting sensory and motor information between the brain and the specialized regions of the head and neck. The cranial nerves provide for essential functions like vision, hearing, taste, and facial movement. Their direct connection to the brain underscores their role in the rapid communication required for survival and interaction with the environment, making them essential components of the nervous system structure. The intricacy of the anatomical structure of the brain is mirrored in the refined courses and roles of the cranial nerves, a testament to the evolutionary precision of sensory and motor integration. As opposed to spinal nerves, cranial nerves originate directly from various segments of the brainstem, reflecting a median rather than bilaterally symmetrical origin. This arrangement enables them to provide specialized structures such as the eyes, ears, and facial muscles with specific innervation. Furthermore, advancements in surgical techniques, as exemplified in the extended endoscopic endonasal transplanum sphenoidale approach, illustrate how the function of complex neurovascular knowledge is necessary in working with brain regions proximal to the origin of these nerves, illustrating the multiangled, close-up view needed for surgical precision (Cappabianca et al., 2008). Understanding of the spatial and functional relationships of these structures enhances clinical procedures and allows targeted treatment of pathologies of the suprasellar and other critical brain regions. Comparative anatomy of the cranial nerves and associated structures may also explain their developmental and functional properties between species, and illustrate adaptive responses to ecological and physiological stresses. Inspections of marsupial chondrocrania demonstrate conserved bony and neural configurations of the cranial nerves with exacting histological variation mirroring evolutionary history and different neonatal functional requirements (Sánchez-Villagra & Forasiepi, 2017). For instance, anterior nasal stoutness and highly developed sensory anatomy in marsupial neonates underscore the interplay of cranial nerve development and environment-imposed survival specializations. This comparative context strengthens our definition of the brain and cranial nerves by showing them not as isolated anatomic structures, but rather as evolved, dynamic systems shaped to specific organismal needs, with a deeper appreciation of their core functions in human and general mammalian neurobiology (Figure 13.2).

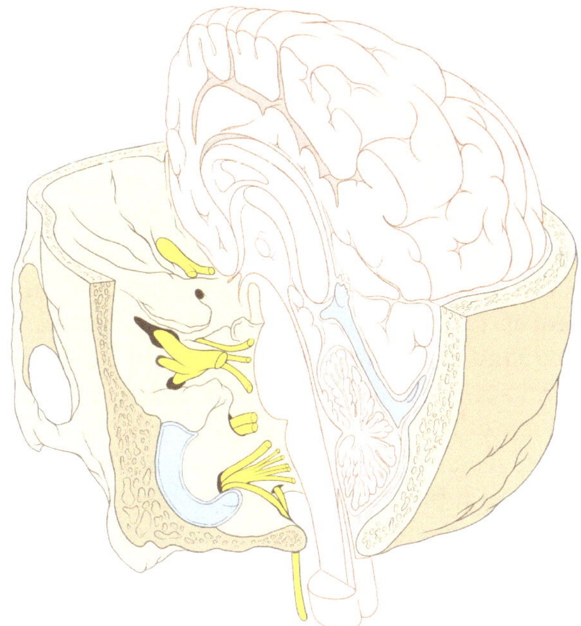

Figure 13.2. The complex architecture of the human nervous system requires an exploration of its central components.

Source: By Patrick J. Lynch, medical illustrator - Patrick J. Lynch, medical illustrator, CC BY 2.5, https://commons.wikimedia.org/w/index.php?curid=1496709

Importance of Studying the Brain and Cranial Nerves

Understanding of the complex interaction between brain function and human behavior is becoming more significant in a variety of scientific and forensic uses. Brain functions are complex and include profound subcortical and superficial cortical structures, which are required for functions like decision making and the expression of free will. Improvements in recent years in the methods of neuroimaging and electrophysiology have made it possible for researchers to examine these processes with greater precision, revealing the critical roles played by neurotransmitters like dopamine in reward behavior and motivation. Brain and cranial nerve research is thus required not just to outline such networks but also to understand how impairment may lead to neurological disease. Through knowledge of these mechanisms, we can design targeted therapies as well as improve diagnostic methods, which highlights the need for a multidisciplinary framework with which we can integrate functional anatomy and cognitive neuroscience. Brain and cranial nerve investigation is not merely anatomy and neuroscience; it also intersects with law and medicine, most prominently. Human behavior, personality, and cognitive function are the outcome of coordinated activity among many organ systems, with the nervous system playing a critical interface role. Legal professionals and clinicians stand to benefit immensely from in-depth understanding of brain organization because changes in neurological function can influence personality and behavior, with a direct impact on forensic and medical evaluations. Appreciation of the fact that injuries or disabilities impact both anatomical structures and psychological states provides a foundation for scientific practice in medico-legal environments. The knowledge enables appropriate diagnoses, effective treatment strategies, and knowledgeable legal decisions, pointing to the need for studies on the brain and cranial nerves to address complex issues that cross over between biology and social responsibility (Bradford & Smith, 1953). Furthermore, the applications in real life of what is learned about the brain and cranial nerves illustrate the importance of them in today's medicine. Neurological impairment generally manifests as manifestations of cranial nerve dysfunction, which impact sensory and motor functions that are vital to daily functions. With a good appreciation of these nerves, medical practitioners are also well equipped to treat diseases like Parkinson's disease, cranial neuropathies, and other neurodegenerative illnesses. Precise and timely diagnosis relies on this understanding, enabling interventions that improve patient outcome and quality of life (QoL). In addition, the intersection of neuroanatomical understanding with clinical expertise offers motivation for the development of new treatment modalities, including neuromodulation and rehabilitation protocols. Truly, scientific study of these structures is not esoteric but is utilitarian in its relationship to improvement in patient treatment and effectiveness.

13.1. Anatomy of the Brain

Learning Outcome

1. Discuss the Major Regions of the Brain
2. Focus on Brain Structure and Function
3. Explain the Protective Layers of the Brain

The complex architecture of the brain forms the basis for its multifaceted functions, from simple sensory processing to highly complex cognitive processes. The bases of this architecture are the different nuclei and regions that are connected through sophisticated neural pathways, most of which have the cranial nerves involved. These nerves are conduits that transmit sensory information from the external environment to the brain itself to enable perception and cognition. Relative to other forms of neuromodulation, cranial nerve stimulation directly stimulates specific neural axon pathways with the potential to precisely recruit brain circuits like thalamo-cortical networks. Such a potential emphasizes the central role of cranial nerves not only in sensation but also in modulation of higher-order brain function. Modern methods leverage computational simulation to optimize stimulation parameters, optimizing therapeutic effects in clinical and behavioral use by shaping neural activity in specific brain regions (Adair et al., 2020). The evolution and brain development heavily influence its complex anatomy and functional specialization. Vertebrate head development, including brain, face, and their respective sensory organs, took place through dynamic interaction among neural crest cells, placodes, and cardiopharyngeal field, which all work in unison towards concerted morphogenesis. The cerebral contribution toward the development of protective skull structures, sensory organs, and muscles has its explanation in this integration, which further forms pathways and functions for cranial nerves. Furthermore, cerebral developmental diseases are inclined to be coupled with craniofacial deformities and malformations of cranial nerves, emphasizing their anatomical and functional relationship. Such complex ontogeny accounts for the variability and multiforphism of cranial nerves, which is problematic in embarking on surgical procedures and regenerative medicine (José, 2019). Apart from their classical sensory and motor functions, cranial nerves also contribute to developmental signaling and regeneration in the adult brain and craniofacial tissues. Existing research suggests that migrating Schwann cell precursors along axons of cranial nerves are responsible for producing postganglionic neurons and neural crest-derived stem cells that act on organogenesis and repair. These nerve-associated progenitors carry out interactions that are required for craniofacial patterning and maintenance and regeneration of adult neuronal populations. This neurobiological plasticity gives an additional level of complexity to brain anatomy, with cranial nerves acting as channels for both cell transport and neural communication. These findings hold promising directions for treating neurological diseases and injuries by taking advantage of the inherent regenerative potential carried with the cranial nerve system (José, 2019) (Figure 13.3).

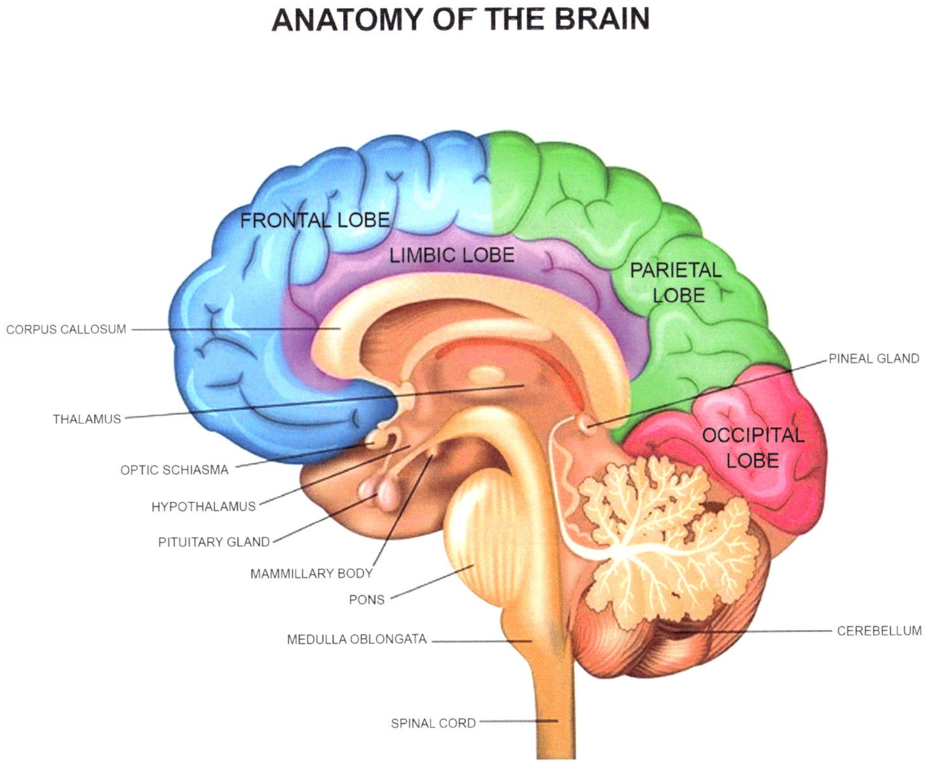

Figure 13.3. Anatomy of the brain.

Source: Shutterstock. (2020). *Anatomy of the Brain.*

13.1.1. Major Regions of the Brain

The very complex nature of the human brain is reflected in its division into large areas, each performing specialized tasks critical to overall neurological health and thinking. These are the cerebrum, cerebellum, brainstem, and diencephalon, and they all work together to integrate sensory input, motor function, and autonomic functions. The largest part, the cerebrum, processes higher-order functions such as reasoning, emotion, and memory, and the cerebellum coordinates voluntary movement and balance. The brainstem functions as an essential passageway for signals between the spinal cord and the brain and regulates automatic functions such as heartbeat and breathing. The delicate regulation of cerebral blood flow via these regions facilitates metabolic demands and homeostasis maintenance, emphasizing the brain's dependency on vascular support mechanisms to maintain maximum function and waste removal (Claassen et al., 2021). Awareness of these regions provides crucial insight into the manner in which cranial nerves interact with specific brain regions to facilitate complex physiological processes. A comprehension of brain areas requires considering the brain's own mechanisms for maintaining a healthy internal environment, specifically waste clearance and nutrient delivery. The glymphatic system is a prime example of a key physiological process committed to clearing metabolic waste from the brain's extracellular space. Unlike the peripheral organs with lymph vessels, the brain does not have access to conventional lymphatics but depends on this glial-dependent route to support efficient drainage of soluble proteins and metabolites. This pathway is strongly linked with dural lymphatic networks surrounding large cerebral arteries and cranial nerves, highlighting the interconnectedness between cranial structures and brain regions. The activity of this waste removal pathway has important implications for neural health, affecting regions involved in cognitive processes and neurovascular control throughout the brain (Benveniste et al., 2018). Such physiological integration serves to underscore the significance of primary brain areas not only for neural function but also for the long-term health of the brain. Primary brain areas are also central to the question of neural connectivity, and especially in regard to how cranial nerves carry sensory and motor information with these specialized areas. Each cranial nerve is predisposed to develop from specific locations in the brainstem or diencephalon to come into direct contact with peripheral targets influencing vision, hearing, facial expression, and autonomic control. The diencephalon, with its content of the thalamus and hypothalamus, serves as a relay station and center of control and regulates sensory inputs and maintains homeostasis through endocrine control. The particular vascular anatomy of these regions supplies that perfusion fluctuations adapt to metabolic needs dynamically, thereby preserving neural function and waste removal mechanisms of high fidelity (Claassen et al., 2021). This complex ballet between the large brain regions and cranial nerves guides the integration of sensory data and motor responses needed for life and thinking.

13.1.2. Brain Structure and Function

The complex structure of the brain underpins its diverse and complicated functions. Enclosed within the cranial cavity, the brain is surrounded by several layers of protection, including the meninges and cerebrospinal fluid (CSF), that work together to cushion and maintain homeostasis. A critical component in this protection is the subarachnoid space between the arachnoid and pia mater, where the trabeculae structures play a significant part. They mechanically support through the decrease of brain displacement, thereby restricting strain under physical loads. With advanced modeling and finite element analysis, a hierarchy of the five identified trabecular structures has been determined by their ability to minimize strain on brain tissue. This protective mechanism is crucial to the preservation of neural integrity and function under mechanically stressful states, illustrating the highly developed interplay between brain structure and its protection mechanisms (Brady et al., 2024). At the center of the operation of the brain is the integration and relay of neural signals, processes that are very dependent on the cranial nerves. These 12 pairs of nerves directly arise from the brain and serve essential sensory and motor functions. Advances in biomedical engineering have generated new approaches to restore impairment within these neural pathways. Electrical stimulation, brain-computer interfaces, and bio-mimetic scaffold-based tissue engineering have shown promise in recovering motor function and cognition compromised by neurological disease. Cranial nerve electrical stimulation, in particular, has been found to improve neurological function and modulate neural activity, thereby exerting direct therapeutic effects. These multidimensional therapies underscore the dynamic interplay of brain structure and function and point to the promise of technology in augmenting neural repair and recovery (Brady et al., 2024). Also, understanding of the functional organization of the brain extends from protection and repair but also encompasses regulation of the higher motor and cognitive functions. The structural composition of the brain, the cortical and subcortical regions, coupled with the cranial nerves, work in synergy to generate sensory perception, motor coordination, and sophisticated cognitive processes. Pathology of these interconnected networks can lead to catastrophic disabilities, and hence the study of brain structure-function relationships is of paramount interest to develop targeted treatments. Integrating neuromodulation techniques, such as those based on brain-computer interfaces, has been found to enhance recovery potential by enabling neuroplasticity and replacement of impaired neural pathways. Collectively, these advances illustrate an evolving appreciation for how the structural components of the brain operate together with cranial nerve function to maintain and restore neurological health (Xi, 2024) (Figure 13.4).

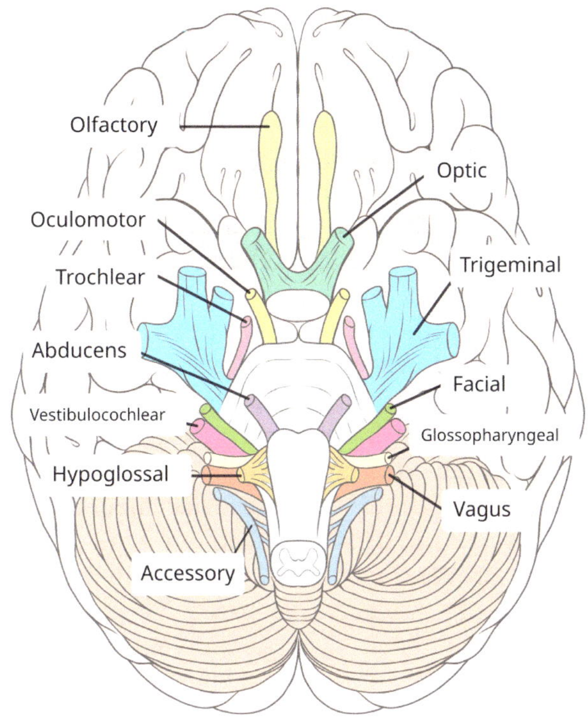

Figure 13.4. Brain structure and function.

Source: By Brain_human_normal_inferior_view_with_labels_en.svg: *Brain_human_normal_inferior_view.svg: Patrick J. Lynch, medical illustratorderivative work: Beaoderivative work: Dwstultz (talk) - Brain_human_normal_inferior_view_with_labels_en.svg, CC BY 2.5, https://commons.wikimedia.org/w/index.php?curid=15108118

13.1.3. Protective Layers of the Brain

The complex structure of the human brain not only reflects its complexity but also the necessity for robust protection against physical and biochemical attacks. Three distinct layers encircle the brain, which collectively are known as the meninges, providing mechanical support and a barrier against pathogens. The outermost covering, the dura mater, is thick and hard, firmly fixed against the inner wall of the skull to restrain excessive brain movement upon sudden impacts. Beneath it lies the arachnoid mater, a web-like fibrous layer, which cushions the brain by an intermediate space known as the subarachnoid space containing CSF. The fluid acts as a shock absorber and provides an avenue for the exchange of nutrients and waste. The deepest pia mater wraps the brain surface tightly, closely embracing the brain shape, thus protecting delicate neural tissue. All these layers collectively conserve the brain's microenvironment crucial to cranial nerve function and overall neural integrity (Cozart et al., 2017). In addition to meningeal layers, CSF also protects the brain by acting as a fluid buffer between the brain and the skull. This colorless, transparent fluid also absorbs mechanical shocks and reduces the effective weight of the brain, preventing blood vessels and nerves from being subjected to excessive pressure. The CSF circulates through the ventricles and the subarachnoid space, being continuously produced and absorbed to maintain equilibrium. Its flow also removes metabolic waste from the central nervous system (CNS), thereby maintaining neural health. The protective function of CSF is of particular importance in the clinical environment, such as concussion treatment, where disturbance of such layers or fluid dynamics exacerbates neural injury and affects recovery rates (Persoage, 2014). An understanding of such equilibrium is essential to appreciating how the protective layers of the brain are not only involved in mechanical protection but also physiological homeostasis. Apart from the meninges and CSF, the osseous structure of the skull provides an external case of protection necessary to safeguard the brain and corresponding cranial nerves against external trauma. The bones of the cranium are tightly connected to each other, forming a firm case resistant to penetration trauma and also acting as points of attachment for muscles and membranes. The foramina of these bones are passageways along which cranial nerves travel, offering communication between the brain and peripheral structures without compromising the integrity of the protective casing of the brain. Because cranial nerves have sensitive functions in sensory and motor pathways, the triple protection by bone, meninges, and fluid must be had to prevent damage that would ruin neural signaling. Together, these protective coverings form a multi-level system that preserves brain function and underscores the complexity of neural anatomy (Persoage, 2014; Cozart et al., 2017).

Test Your Knowledge

1. How does the cerebral cortex contribute to higher-order functions like reasoning and memory?
2. What is the function of cerebrospinal fluid (CSF) in brain protection?

13.2. Functions of the Brain

Learning Outcome

1. Explain the Cognitive Functions
2. Focus on Emotional Regulation
3. Understand Motor Control

The complex integration of bodily processes depends on coordination and integration performed by the brain, a remarkable organ at the very heart of human existence. Though in the past viewed as where consciousness and free will resided, the activities of the brain extend very much into regulating autonomic activity that sustains life. Sensory information from the various regions of the brain makes perception, cognition, and motor response possible, and the cranial nerves offer significant routes for the transfer of information between the peripheral sense organs and the brain. These routes enable not only voluntary response but also involuntary reflexes, which protect and assist in the maintenance of homeostasis. Also, recent research identifies how neuropeptides such as PACAP-38 structure cranial nerve-mediated circuits to include both neurological disorders and typical brain behavior, highlighting the complexity of brain signaling circuits in disease and health (Waschek et al., 2018). The brain's ability to process and integrate diverse signals is also evidenced by its complex structural organization with specialized regions dedicated to single yet interactive functions. For example, the brainstem governs life-sustaining processes such as respiration and cardiovascular function, in an intimate relationship with cranial nerves that regulate the sensory perception of the head and neck. This coordination allows for reflex and voluntary responses essential to survival and engagement with the world. Further, the characterization of educational programs in neurological surgery indicates the significance of the understanding of such a complex function as a prerequisite for surgical intervention and treatment of neurological diseases. Such a thorough knowledge allows for guarding the multifunctionality of the brain during clinical procedures, which accentuates the clinical relevance of neural anatomy and physiology (Traynelis et al., 2000). Besides ordinary physiological regulation, the brain is also charged with governance processes like cognition, emotion, and memory, testaments to its broad functional range. Specific cortical and subcortical regions collaborate to facilitate these different operations, and the cranial nerves provide sensory and motor integration to assist in communication and perception of the senses.

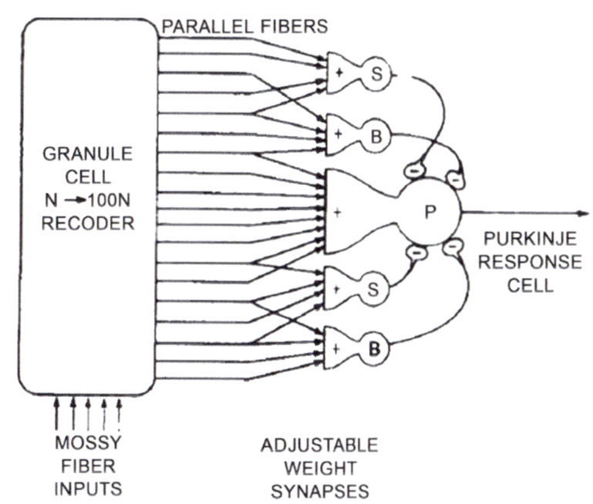

Figure 13.5. Functions of the brain.

Source: By Albus, J.S., NIST - Theory of Cerebellar Function, Public Domain, https://commons.wikimedia.org/w/index.php?curid=7470709

Notably, research into molecules like PACAP-38 has determined that their role extends beyond vasodilation and holds implications in the neurochemical modulation of pain pathways associated with migraines and other neurological conditions. This characterization of the molecular influence on brain function opens up new avenues for therapeutic strategies to target cranial nerve circuits and alleviate neurological symptoms. To date, the understanding of brain functions, both macroscopic structure and molecular communication, remains crucial in advancing neurological treatment and health (Waschek et al., 2018) (Figure 13.5).

13.2.1. Cognitive Functions

The complex interdependence among brain structures and cognitive operations underlies knowing how people think, reason, and adapt to the environment. Executive functions of the brain, found predominantly in the frontal lobes, control such key abilities as inhibition, attention, and adaptive thinking. Research on people with Chiari Type I malformation indicates that structural abnormalities in the brain can lead to some forms of impairments in such cognitive functions. Studies have shown that impaired patients show considerable defect on inhibitory control and sustained attention tasks, and it is inferred that dysfunction in neural circuits has the potential to impair higher-order processes that are essential for goal-directed action and self-regulation (Gonz et al., 2018). These findings reveal the importance of intact neural pathways and show how cranial nerve pathology could influence integrated brain functions as well by having faulty signaling or altered brainstem dynamics that impinge on global cognitive potential. In addition to structural damage, the effects of chronic inflammatory conditions on higher-order brain function are being appreciated ever more in neurosciences. Periodontal disease, with chronic bacterial infection and inflammation, is a superb illustration of a systemic condition that exerts its effects through indirect means on CNS dysfunction. The spread of pathogenic bacteria and pro-inflammatory mediators from peripheral locations to the brain will likely trigger resident immune cells such as microglia and lead to persistent neuroinflammation. These inflammatory chronic diseases compromise neuronal integrity and synaptic function, processes that underlie cognitive impairment, namely memory loss in Alzheimer's disease and related neurodegenerative disorders (Singhrao et al., 2014). This evidence relates peripheral pathology with cerebral consequences, illustrating that cranial nerves and their coverings are pathways for injurious agents, thereby influencing cognitive well-being through complex neuroimmune mechanisms. Cognitive function can be appreciated only through an integrated view of neuroanatomy, immune mechanisms, and environmental factors influencing the brain and cranial nerves. Cognitive impairments often reflect not only focal brain injury but also generalized pathologic mechanisms influencing cerebral homeostasis and neural transmission. The function of cranial nerves as critical channels of communication between peripheral organs and the brain exposes them to mechanical injury and infection-induced inflammation, which aggravate cognitive impairments. For this reason, cognitive testing must include multifactorial causes like structural malformations, chronic infection, and neuroinflammation for the development of comprehensive diagnostic and therapeutic strategies (Singhrao et al., 2014). This is an integrative strategy that enhances comprehension of brain function and guides interventions toward the maintenance of cognitive integrity in neurological disorders.

13.2.2. Emotional Regulation

The complex relationship between the brain and emotion regulation is reflected in complex neural circuitry of cortical and subcortical structures. The autonomic nervous system, as used in Japanese sources typically referred to as jiritsu shinkei-kei, plays a role in modulating the physiological component of emotional response. Understanding how this system works is important because disturbance of the autonomic pathways can lead to what is clinically known as jiritsu-shinkei shiccho-sho, or vegetative disorders, that affect emotional stability and control (Alkatout et al., 2021). These disorders demonstrate how the autonomic nervous system controlled by the brain dictates direct emotional response and physiological processes such as heart rate, sweating, and hormonal secretion, which are crucial in the attainment of emotional homeostasis. Research on such pathways deepens our knowledge of how brain areas coordinate in a bid to create emotional homeostasis under various environmental and social contexts. Production and regulation of emotional expressions, most importantly, weeping, unveil unique aspects of the human neurobiological infrastructure for emotional regulation.

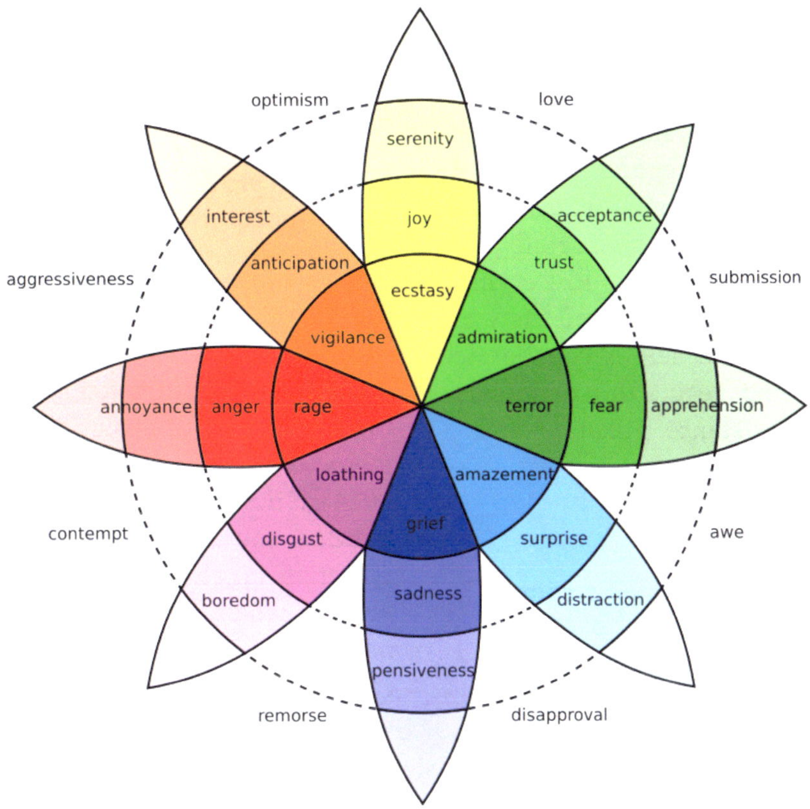

Figure 13.6. Emotional regulation.

Source: By Machine Elf 1735 - Own work, Public Domain, https://commons.wikimedia.org/w/index.php?curid=13285286

Emotional tears, a behavior categorically unique to Homo sapiens, are an interesting overlap of neural, autonomic, and psychosocial processes (Bylsma et al., 2019). Studies of the neuroanatomical and neurochemical bases of crying tears show that complex interactions between the brainstem, limbic structures, and autonomic nervous system are responsible for this affective behavior. The participation of the cranial nerves in controlling facial musculature and tear glands serves to highlight the importance of these neural circuits in regulating emotional expression and social communication. This complex mechanism demonstrates that emotional regulation is not just internally controlled by the brain but also externally conveyed through action mediated by cranial nerves to consequently influence interpersonal relations. Emotion regulation exceeds mere expression and physiology and involves higher cortical control processes governing emotional experience and adaptive behavior. Cortical areas such as the prefrontal cortex exercise executive control over subcortical areas such as the amygdala, which is prominently involved in the perception and generation of emotional responses. The cranial nerves, especially the facial nerve, transmit the somatic components of emotional expression, interfacing the brain's internal regulation with outward behavioral expression. This complex neural coordination allows humans to regulate emotions in context, shifting responses depending on social norms and individual aims. Integrating evidence from studies of the autonomic nervous system and neurobiological research into emotional behaviors like crying, it is possible to achieve an integrated view of how the brain and cranial nerves collaborate to organize emotional regulation processes essential to human existence (Alkatout et al., 2021) (Figure 13.6).

13.2.3. Motor Control

The complex coordination of motor control is central to the brain in the control of voluntary and involuntary movements, achieved through an intricate set of neural pathways. In the brainstem, crucial to the integration of sensory input and motor output, cranial nerves are presented as integral pathways to facilitate communication between head and neck muscles and the CNS. The brainstem integrates afferent input and elicits efferent responses that modulate reflexive motor activity, such as eye movement and facial expression. Dysfunctions in brainstem circuitry governing these outputs have the potential to elicit profound impairments, given their function in the regulation of life-critical motor processes. Furthermore, brainstem modulation of sensory input impacts motor response, i.e., motor control is not a completely hierarchical process but involves continuous feedback loops essential to the performance of fine motor skills and coordinated movement (Cuomo-Granston & Drummond, 2010). Evolutionary developments have shaped the brain's organization to facilitate improved motor control and sensorimotor integration, namely in the contralateral mapping of the forebrain. This adaptive transformation results in cross-wired projections from the neural tissue, such as in the optic chiasm and some cranial nerve tracts, to allow for precise motor coordination and spatial awareness. The axial twist hypothesis provides this phenomenon an explanation by suggesting that compensatory developmental migrations establish a crossed state of the forebrain and spinal cord structures which can provide complex control of lateralized motor functions.

This crossed architecture is required for the coordinated activation of muscles and coordination of movement, particularly in cranial nerve-controlled muscles, confirming the importance of evolutionary morphology in motor control mechanisms (de Lussanet et al., 2014). It describes how evolutionary constraints molded the brain's motor architecture to optimize function. Motor control by cranial nerves involves complex integration at various neural levels encompassing reflex and voluntary control. Cranial nerves such as the trochlear nerve have characteristic decussations that function to provide the precise motor function of the eye, pointing towards the unique adaptations in motor coordination of the cranial nerve system. Additionally, brainstem nuclei also interact with higher cortical structures to control the initiation and execution of movement and hence are an integrative but hierarchical control system. Neurotransmitters in these systems fine-tune the motor output, and pathology can manifest as motor impairments or disorders. The understanding of motor control within the context of brain and cranial nerve anatomy acknowledges the complex net required to facilitate coordinated and adaptive movement that is a part of survival and interaction with the environment (Cuomo-Granston & Drummond, 2010).

Test Your Knowledge

1. Which brain regions are primarily involved in memory, attention, and language?
2. How does the prefrontal cortex contribute to decision-making and problem-solving?
3. What is the role of the hippocampus in learning and memory formation?

13.3. Overview of Cranial Nerves

Learning Outcome

1. Definition and Classification of Cranial Nerves
2. Focus on Number and Names of Cranial Nerves
3. Know Importance of Cranial Nerves in the Nervous System

The multiheterogeneity of cranial nerve formation mirrors the multiheterogeneity of the embryonic head, in which multipotent heterotypic populations of progenitor cells develop into differentiated tissues. Peripheral nerves not only serve as conduits for neural impulses but are also crucial niches for multipotent glial cells of neural crest origin. These nerve association glial cells are extremely plastic, differentiating into various cell types that are implicated in craniofacial growth and regeneration, including dental tissue. Their ability to transform and travel along developing nerves reflects an adaptive developmental plan by which the nervous system organizes the development of other organ systems in the head. This concept challenges traditional notions of neural development and implies novel directions for the regenerative treatment of craniofacial malformations. These findings underscore the intimate association between the peripheral nervous system (PNS) and embryogenesis tissue morphogenesis (Shahidi et al., 2015). The functional diversity of the cranial nerves results from their motor, sensory, and autonomic components that allow for the specific control of facial and oral mechanisms required to survive. For instance, the hypoglossal nerve or cranial nerve XII is used for motor innervation of the tongue muscles and controls vital functions such as mastication, swallowing, and vocalization. The ontogeny of the hypoglossal nerve nuclei illustrates the dynamic process of cellular progression from the primitive migrating neuroblasts to mature differentiated neurons ensuring the fine coordination of the movements of the tongue. Abnormalities in this nerve lead to serious motor deficits, highlighting the importance of this nerve in elementary survival processes as well as sophisticated behaviors. Histological studies have investigated the developmental trends of hypoglossal neurons during gestation, providing fresh insights into structural development and the windows of critical periods necessary to prepare to function (Sreeja et al., 2018). Apart from motor control, cranial nerves also contain autonomic fibers responsible for homeostatic activity involved in day-to-day functions. The parasympathetic nervous system within cranial nerve tracts governs functions like salivation and lacrimation, performing activity primarily during rest and digestion. Paradoxically, parasympathetic neurons arise from glial progenitors of peripheral nerves, which migrate and differentiate later to form ganglia in target tissues. This process of development demonstrates a very sophisticated bidirectional interaction in which nerves not only transmit signals but even contribute cellular material toward constructing post-synaptic structures. An understanding of this cellular and molecular organization enhances knowledge of cranial nerve physiology and perhaps even future treatment of congenital abnormalities or trauma of craniofacial innervation (Shahidi et al., 2015).

13.3.1. Definition and Classification of Cranial Nerves

The complex anatomy of the human nervous system involves a special group of nerves that primarily coordinate sensory and motor functions of the head and neck. These nerves, known as cranial nerves, directly emerge from the brain and brainstem, in contrast to spinal nerves which come from the spinal cord. The cranial nerves play primary roles in vision, hearing, taste, facial movement, and autonomic functions, indicating their complexity and clinical significance. Their definition is discerned by the realization that these nerves represent significant conduits of sensory input and motor control and serve as an interface between the CNS and peripheral targets. Their unique origin and role distinguish them from the other peripheral nerves, making them a focal point of neurological research and clinical practice dealing with brain activity and cranial pathologies. Cranial nerve classification is traditionally done according to their function—sensory or motor, or both, and to their anatomical course. There are 12 pairs of cranial nerves, each designated by a Roman numeral and a specific name derived from their primary function or distribution. Sensory nerves, e.g., the optic and olfactory nerves, carry sensory information to the brain. Motor nerves, e.g., the oculomotor and hypoglossal nerves, control muscle movements. Mixed nerves, e.g., the trigeminal and facial nerves, have both sensory and motor fibers. This functional difference is extremely significant clinically where dysfunctions result in diagnostic information. Also, an advanced classification proposes the division of cranial nerves into intraneural, perineural, and extraneural types based on their anatomical relationship to lesions such as cavernous malformations, with prognostic value for neurosurgical treatment planning (Li et al., 2024).

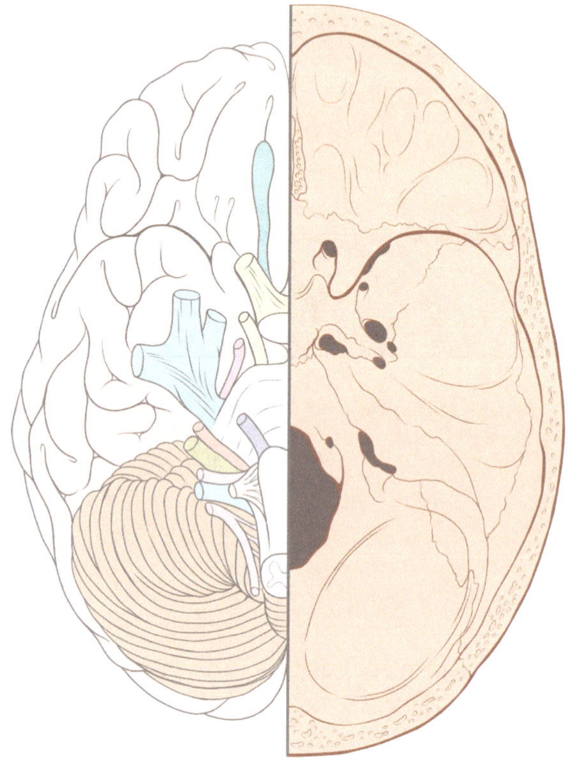

Source: By Patrick J. Lynch, medical illustrator - Patrick J. Lynch, medical illustrator, CC BY 2.5, https://commons.wikimedia.org/w/index.php?curid=1496715

Recent technological advances have moved the classification and therapeutic approaches regarding cranial nerves well beyond traditional anatomical and functional frameworks. Biomedical engineering innovations, including electrical stimulation and tissue-engineered scaffolds, have introduced a multidisciplinary methodology for cranial nerve function restoration and understanding. These modalities promote selective neuromodulation and regeneration with increasing specificity for motor and sensory defects. In parallel, brain-computer interfaces are emerging as innovative tools for the restoration of lost motor abilities by utilizing neurofeedback and motor imagery strategies. These approaches underscore the active interplay of fundamental neuroanatomical classes and novel clinical therapies, emphasizing the need for ongoing research to optimize the therapeutic potential of cranial nerve repair and regeneration (Xi, 2024).

13.3.2. Number and Names of Cranial Nerves

The complex system that connects the brain to various areas of the head, neck, and body is dependent mainly on a set of specialized nerves. The cranial nerves play a critical role in sensory and motor functions by carrying signals critical to vision, hearing, taste, and facial movement. There are 12 pairs of cranial nerves in total, with each possessing distinct functions and pathways. Their orderly nomenclature, either according to function or developmental sequence from the brainstem, provides valuable information on their specific roles. The standard sequence begins with the Olfactory nerve, sense of smell, and the Optic nerve, sight, and then continues up to the Hypoglossal nerve, which controls tongue movement. An awareness of these names and their numbers is the foundation for an appreciation of the delicate coordination of the nervous system, which underlies both simple activity and complex mental processes (Xi, 2024). In addition to numbering, the range of functions of the cranial nerves is evidence of specialized development that enables the brain to regulate diverse areas of physiology. For instance, cranial nerves III (Oculomotor), IV (Trochlear), and VI (Abducens) predominantly are responsible for eye movement, a critical parameter in visual stability and concentration. Any dysfunction in any of the nerves, as observed in clinical studies, can result in measurable motor impairment such as palsy, reflecting the fine balance required in motor coordination. The fifth cranial nerve, the Trigeminal nerve, is the largest and double sensory and motor, carrying facial sensation and mastication. Research into palsies of cranial nerves III, IV, and VI has provided informative prognostic data, demonstrating that the onset of symptoms and single nerve involvement are important determinants of recovery, and thereby the clinical interest in information about individual nerve anatomy and function (Srimanan et al., 2024). Clinical advancements have also enhanced the curative advantages associated with cranial nerve repair and rehabilitation. New treatments currently utilize technologies such as electrical stimulation and brain-computer interfaces designed to promote functional recovery following nerve injury. Such multimodal interventions not only emphasize the significance of comprehensive anatomical knowledge of cranial nerve numbering and nomenclature but also facilitate the tailoring of the creation of particular treatments in neurological disease. Tissue engineering and neurofeedback techniques also exhibit high rates of rehabilitation improvement in motor function, demonstrating synergy between clinical neuroscience and bioengineering for the treatment of cranial nerve pathologies. The precision in their identification and understanding therefore becomes priceless, as these 12 nerves play functions that extend beyond simple sensory and motor functions to become a center for advanced therapeutic regimens (Xi, 2024).

13.3.3. Importance of Cranial Nerves in the Nervous System

The sophistication of the nervous system is delicately supported by specialized anatomy that enables precise communication between the brain and the rest of the body. Within these anatomy, cranial nerves are pivotal in enabling vital sensory and motor functions to survive and enhance QoL. They integrate a wide range of physiological functions such as vision, hearing, taste, smell, facial movements, and swallowing. Their privileged direct access to brainstem allows speed and economy of transmission without relay through spinal cord, underscoring their functional significance. It is particularly remarkable that dysfunction of cranial nerves can lead to severe neurological impairment, not merely of simple senses but also of complex behaviors and autonomic control. Prevalence of involvement of cranial nerves in illness, including illness that is the result of viral infection like COVID-19, highlights their crucial function in maintaining neural integrity and overall homeostasis (Melamed et al., 2023). Beyond their critical sensory and motor duties, cranial nerves subtly contribute to the immune and defense mechanisms of the nervous system. The olfactory nerve, a cranial nerve, provides a pathway which links the external world directly to brain structures and thus is engaged both in sensing and immune surveillance. This pathway is not only dedicated to smell detection but also provides a route for CSF movement and immune cell interaction at the brain-nose interface. These functions suggest that cranial nerves are not only just channels of neurological signals but are also involved in clearing metabolic waste and potentially toxic substances from the CNS. Understanding such pathways allows for an understanding of their broader functions in neuroprotection and insights into the pathogenesis of neurodegenerative disorders where clearance of toxic substances is impaired (Neel et al., 2022). Clinically, their importance is also underscored by their linkage with a variety of neurological sequelae encountered in individuals with systemic illnesses. For instance, post-viral syndromes, i.e., post-acute sequelae of SARS-CoV-2 infection, may have cranial nerve dysfunctions such as facial palsy, smell impairment, and neuropathic pain, which testify to their vulnerability in systemic illness (Melamed et al., 2023). Such conditions highlight the necessity for careful neurological examination of cranial nerve status in the treatment and diagnosis of complicated disorders. Further, such intervention highlights the necessity for treatment strategies that are multifaceted, reflecting the widespread impact of the cranial nerves on both somatic and autonomic functions. This clinical feature integrates the cranial nerves as key components of the nervous system anatomy, whose preservation is vital to neurological health and patient QoL (Figure 13.7).

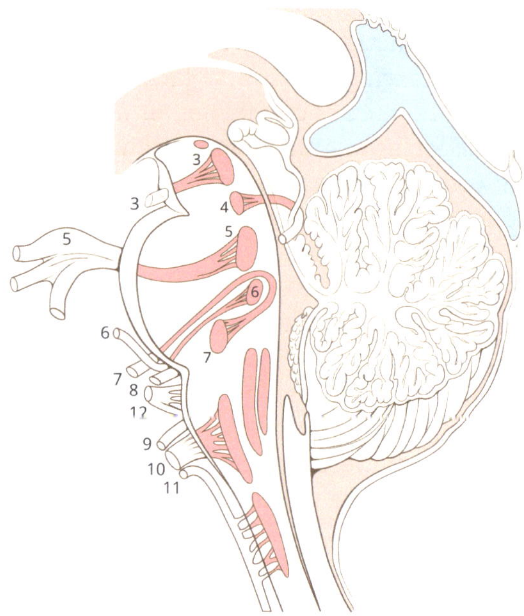

Figure 13.7. Importance of cranial nerves in the nervous system.

Source: By CFCF - Own work, CC BY-SA 3.0, https://commons.wikimedia.org/w/index.php?curid=31097174

Test Your Knowledge

1. Which cranial nerves are primarily motor, sensory, or mixed in function?
2. What roles do cranial nerves play in sensory and motor control of the head and neck?

13.4. Detailed Examination of Cranial Nerves

Learning Outcome

1. Describe the Functions of the Olfactory Nerve (CN I)
2. Define the Functions of the Optic Nerve (CN II)
3. Learn about Functions of the Vagus Nerve (CN X)

The complex functional operations of cranial nerves necessitate a full comprehension greater than mere anatomical identification. These 12 sets of nerves that directly originate from the brain and brainstem are essential to the facilitation of a wide variety of sensory and motor activities, ranging from facial feeling and eye movement to taste and swallowing. More recent developments in biomedical engineering have significantly improved this knowledge by the addition of electrical stimulation techniques and neuroimaging in clinical applications. Multidisciplinary methods like these not only illuminate the physiological intricacies of such nerves but also hold potential to repair damaged functioning. For instance, electrical neuromodulation can reduce neurological disease symptoms through enhanced neural plasticity and facilitating particular neural activation, underpinning the requirement for subtle analyses in both clinical and research scenarios (Xi, 2024). Cranial nerve function is significant for diagnostic accuracy as well as for the creation of therapeutic applications. Embryological development is critical for knowing the growth and maturity of cranial nerves, forming basic foundations for both congenital disease pathogenesis and normal neurological function. Reconstructive 3D human embryo studies have revealed certain timelines to the development and target organ innervation of the nerves, primarily occurring between Carnegie stages 12 and 18, equating to development days 26 to 46. This morphogenetic development, with maximum relative growth close to stage 17, underscores the developmental critical windows at which abnormalities of development are possible. Quantitative volumetric measurements of nerves at these stages offer unparalleled information, enabling researchers and clinicians to put observed disease abnormalities such as in Duane syndrome or Pierre Robin sequence into spatial and temporal perspective (Johannes et al., 2022). These comprehensive embryological researches support the anatomical and developmental foundation needed to advance diagnostic and interventional techniques. Along with developmental information, comprehensive examination of cranial nerves includes new therapies towards the reconstitution of nervous system function following damage or disease. Bioengineered scaffolds, autologous nerve grafts, and brain-computer interfaces are just a few of the excursions between tissue engineering and neurotechnology for repair of cranial nerves. These multidisciplinary treatments are not without difficulties in the guise of axonal misdirection but offer hopeful possibilities for recovery of function, particularly when combined with neurofeedback training and motor imagery. The brain-computer interface has been found to be promising in improving motor outcome through volitional activation of paralyzed muscles by decoding neural activity. This blending of anatomical information with new technology signals a promising new frontier in neurorehabilitation, bringing attention to the imperative for accurate, integrated investigations of cranial nerve biology and treatment (Xi, 2024). Additional investigation is required to optimize these interventions and enhance their versatility.

13.4.1. Functions of the Olfactory Nerve (CN I)

Integration of sensory information is central to the brain's ability to perceive and respond to the world. One of the most ancient, most immediate processes this does is through the olfactory nerve, or cranial nerve I, as its primary pathway for olfactory sensory information. This nerve is unique among cranial nerves in that it bypasses the thalamus, projecting directly to the olfactory bulb and on to the limbic system, a brain region involved with emotion and memory. Direct projections like this underscore the preeminence of smell in survival behaviors such as locating food, predators, and mates during the course of evolution. This intimate connection facilitates rapid processing of odor stimuli, influencing conscious perception as well as subconscious responses crucial for adaptive behavior in complicated situations (Bumeister et al., 2017). Besides its intrinsic sensory role, the olfactory nerve also has a significant role in higher-order cognitive processes through widespread neural connections. It contributes to the modulation of emotional states and memory retrieval by connecting the sensory input of the nasal epithelium directly with the hippocampus and amygdala in the limbic system. This neurological setup is the reason why particular odors have the ability to retrieve vivid memories or trigger emotional responses. Moreover, the function of olfactory nerve in neurogenesis and plasticity is under research focus with respect to its potential as a monitor for neurodegenerative processes or recovery following brain damage. The understanding of such functions is indicative of the broader function of the nerve in maintaining sensory perception alongside neurocognitive health and behavioral adaptation (Bumeister et al., 2017). The study of olfactory nerve function extends beyond the realm of humans and provides insight into evolutionary biology and behavioral ecology. Comparative neuroanatomy studies, as well as studies on extinct animals, demonstrate the relationship between olfactory ability and survival strategies and social activity. As a case in point, studies of dinosaur endocranial anatomy suggest varied olfactory acuity in concert with ecological shifts and social complexity, indicating the key sensory role of the olfactory system throughout taxa. These findings contribute to our knowledge of the olfactory nerve's capacity to impact behavior due to sensory input, enabling environmental acclimatization in diverse taxa. These comparative studies provide contextual depth to our present knowledge regarding CN I's function in the vertebrate clade and its sensory evolutionary significance (Figure 13.8).

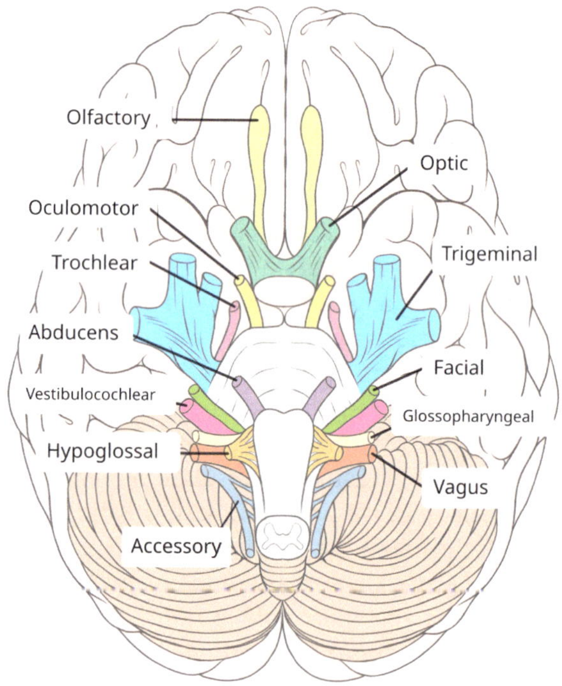

Figure 13.8. Functions of the olfactory nerve (CN I).

Source: By Brain_human_normal_inferior_view_with_labels_en.svg: *Brain_human_normal_inferior_view.svg: Patrick J. Lynch, medical illustratorderivative work: Beaoderivative work: Dwstultz (talk) - Brain_human_normal_inferior_view_with_labels_en.svg, CC BY 2.5, https://commons.wikimedia.org/w/index.php?curid=15108118

13.4.2. Functions of the Optic Nerve (CN II)

The human brain relies on an exceedingly complex network of cranial nerves for interpreting sensory input and coordinating motor functions with the crucial optic nerve (CN II) playing the major role for visual perception. The nerve is the critical conduit in and through which vision information is transferred to the visual cortex of the brain from the retina, enabling perception of light, color, and spatial information. In contrast to other cranial nerves with the principal role of executing motor commands or transmitting a large amount of sensory inputs, the optic nerve has only the role of transmitting afferent visual information. The process begins as electrical signals are generated by retinal ganglion cells when they are exposed to light stimuli, which are transmitted via the optic nerve to central processing systems. Integrity of CN II is critical as damage or dysfunction could lead to severe visual impairments or blindness, reinforcing its non-substitutable position in the neurological system in sensory processing. Optic nerve functionality extends beyond primitive sight to include coordination of reflex actions necessary for ocular health and vision stability. These are the pupillary light reflex, where the optic nerve transmits light intensity information to the midbrain, causing the constriction of the pupils that regulates the amount of light entering. Through this, visual acuity is enhanced and retinal photoreceptors are spared from injury caused by excess light exposure. The optic nerve also has communication with other cranial nerves to allow complex eye movement to support binocular vision and depth perception. The vulnerability of the nerve in traumatic brain injuries underscores the value of comprehensive neurological assessment, as studies have found that optic nerve injury, though less frequent than in some of the other cranial nerves, significantly impacts patient outcomes in head trauma situations (Khantal et al., 2024). Recent research further elucidates the vulnerability of the optic nerves to abnormal pathological conditions that can impair its function. Such as, cavernous malformations of the optic nerve are a unique form of vascular anomalies that can disrupt normal optic nerve transmission by causing localized hemorrhage or compression. These lesions have clinical significance since they possess the potential for progressive visual deterioration, pointing out the delicate interaction between anatomical integrity and functional ability in CN II. As the quality of classification and therapeutic protocols for such malformations continues to improve, preoperative nerve function status is a reliable predictor of postoperative outcomes and thus plays a role in guiding clinical decision-making. An understanding of the optic nerve's diverse functions, from basic signal transduction to its involvement in disease processes, helps better appreciate its place within the grand scheme of cranial nerve function and neurologic health (Li et al., 2024).

13.4.3. Functions of the Vagus Nerve (CN X)

The extremely complex structure of the brainstem is utilized as a point of convergence for a set of cranial nerves, the vagus nerve (cranial nerve X) being a primary element utilized in autonomic control. Unlike other cranial nerves that are primarily sensory or motor, the vagus nerve has a complex combination of both, regulating parasympathetic output to a wide system of visceral organs. Its diffuse innervation to the heart, lungs, and GI tract is implicated in the regulation of cardiac rate, bronchial constriction, and digestion. This function positions the vagus nerve as a primary transmitter of autonomic information in homeostatic regulation. Furthermore, its sensory fibers are components of reflex arcs, such as the gag and cough reflexes, which demonstrate its function in defensive processes. More recent neurophysiological monitoring techniques have better informed us of the roles played by such nerves during surgery (Singh et al., 2016). In addition to autonomic function, the vagus nerve plays a role in somatic motor function, particularly in the control of muscles utilized in phonation and swallowing. Its branchial motor fibers innervate laryngeal, pharyngeal, and soft palate muscles, encoding complex movements required for speech and protective deglutition. Damage or dysfunction of the vagus nerve can result in hoarseness of the voice, dysphagia, or even aspiration pneumonia, and this serves to highlight the clinical importance of its motor fibers. These somatic motor activities serve to underscore the dual role of the vagus nerves, balancing involuntary autonomic function with voluntary motor activity ensuring airway patency. The knowledge of these diverse modalities also provides further insights into the singular and converging pathways between the cranial nerves, emphasizing the significance of fine anatomical and physiological understanding in operative and diagnostic procedures (Benninger & McNeil, 2010). In addition, the engagement of the vagus nerves also enters the higher neural interaction concerning inflammation and mood regulation, highlighting its significance above usual autonomic and motor roles. Recent work has demonstrated that the vagus nerve controls inflammatory processes through the cholinergic anti-inflammatory pathway, a mechanism of interest for therapeutic intervention in chronic inflammatory disorders. In addition, its afferent fibers convey sensory input from the viscera to brain centers responsible for mood and stress regulation, the nucleus tractus solitarius and the limbic system. These findings position the vagus nerve at the convergence of neuroimmune communication and neuropsychiatric health, expanding the domain of cranial nerve function beyond purely physical regulation to psychosomatic integration. These multifunctional behaviors continue to challenge innovation in neurophysiology and clinical use, revealing the vagus nerve's profound impact on human health (Singh et al., 2016) (Figure 13.9).

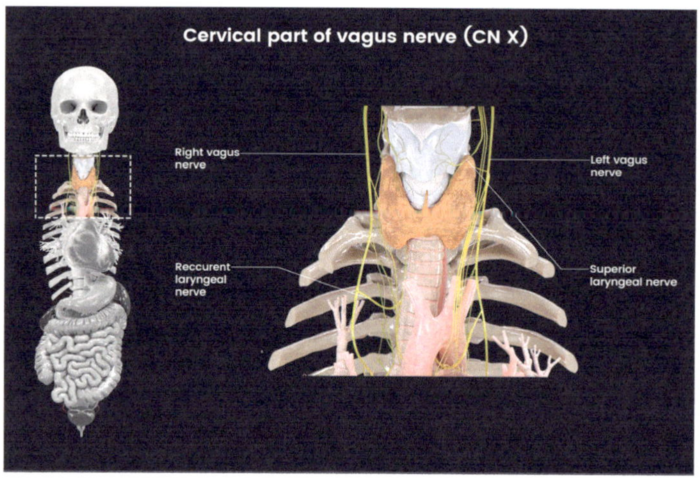

Figure 13.9. Functions of the vagus nerve (CN X).

Source: Anatomy.app. (n.d.). *Cervical Part of Vagus Nerve (CN X).*

Test Your Knowledge

1. Where are the olfactory receptors located, and how do they contribute to the sense of smell?
2. Which major organs receive parasympathetic innervation from the vagus nerve?

13.5. Disorders Related to the Brain

Learning Outcome

1. Discuss the Common Neurological Disorders
2. How to Impact of Brain Disorders on Cranial Nerve Function
3. Explain the Treatment Options for Brain Disorders

The brain's complex structure and function make it susceptible to an extensive variety of disorders, many of which involve disruptions in neural communication or tissue damage. Among these are viral pathogens, which can have a significant effect on neurological health, often producing a constellation of symptoms that make diagnosis and treatment more challenging. Notably, the COVID-19 pandemic has also demonstrated how respiratory viruses can exert neurotropic effects, with subsequent neurological findings of acute cerebrovascular events, altered mental status, and cranial neuropathies. These symptoms can result either from direct viral invasion of neural tissue or indirectly via immune-mediated processes, an intersection of infectious disease and neurology that mandates vigilant clinical attention. Such a complicated effect obscures results, especially with the limited availability of antiviral vaccines and therapeutics against these types of neurological impacts. The prolonged impacts of these CNS complications are a major subject of ongoing research and clinical surveillance (Boon et al., 2020). Another prevalent form of brain disorder is migraines, which entail periodic yet debilitating headaches with related neurological symptoms such as aura and sensory distortions. Recent research has pointed to the role of neuropeptides like PACAP-38 in the pathophysiology of migraine; intravenous administration of this peptide can induce delayed migraine-like headache in susceptible individuals. The initial hypothesis that migraine pain is due to vascular dilatation has been superseded, and attention is now being given to PACAP-38's potential to modulate nociceptive neural pathways and cause inflammation of cranial tissues. Knowledge of the receptor subtypes and pathways activated by PACAP-38 provides critical insight into the mechanisms initiating migraine attacks, moving closer to therapeutic targets.

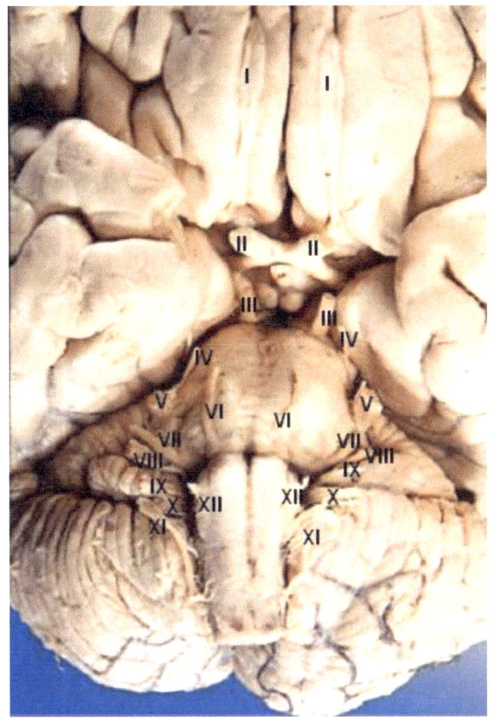

Figure 13.10. Disorders related to the brain.

Source: By John A Beal, PhDDep't. of Cellular Biology & Anatomy, Louisiana State University Health Sciences Center Shreveport - http://www.healcentral.org/healapp/showMetadata?metadataId=40566 (Internet Archive of file description page), CC BY 2.5, https://commons.wikimedia.org/w/index.php?curid=891480

Not only does this study illuminate migraine pathogenesis, but it also illustrates the complex interaction between the neurovascular system and cranial nerve activity in brain disease (Waschek et al., 2018). Cranial nerve disorders in themselves are responsible for a significant proportion of neurological morbidity with often sensory or motor deficits and catastrophic functional consequences. Guillain-Barré syndrome, described not infrequently after infections like COVID-19, is one example of how autoimmune processes may target peripheral nerves, including cranial nerves, to produce paralysis or deranged sensation. The ability of the brain to coordinate complex motor and sensory functions through these cranial nerves underscores their importance in maintaining everyday activities like swallowing, facial expression, and vision. Compromise of these nerves, as a result of infectious, inflammatory, or degenerative processes, often requires a multidisciplinary approach to diagnosis and management. The intersection of neuroanatomy and neuroimmunology is thus responsible for developing effective interventions that can be utilized in preserving cranial nerve function and, by that, brain health (Boon et al., 2020) (Figure 13.10).

13.5.1. Common Neurological Disorders

Neurological disorders manifest with a broad variety of clinical presentations and elementary pathologies affecting the brain and cranial nerves, their sensory, motor, and cognitive functions. They generally arise from multifaceted etiologies such as genetic predispositions, traumatic injuries, infections, and autoimmune processes. The complex anatomy of cranial nerves, which run directly between the brain and disparate facial and cervical regions, makes these nerves incredibly susceptible to both systemic and focal neurological disorders. For instance, viral illnesses such as COVID-19 have attested to being able to instigate neurological symptoms, including damage to cranial nerves like anosmia or ageusia, indicative of either direct viral invasion or immunologically mediated neural destruction. Understanding such complex interactions is of the highest relevance in clinical practice to identify and address neurological impairment resulting from infectious processes or other common neurological disorders that affect brain and cranial nerve function (Boon et al., 2020). Certain neurological disorders selectively affect the cranial nerves, leading to impairments in sensory perception and motor control. Conditions such as trigeminal neuralgia, Bell's palsy, and glossopharyngeal neuralgia illustrate how damage or failure of specific cranial nerves results in extremely severe, often incapacitating pain or paralysis of the face and head regions. The pathophysiology in these entities is varied, ranging from inflammatory and vascular compression mechanisms to demyelinating diseases such as multiple sclerosis. Modern intraoperative neurophysiological monitoring (IONM) plays a crucial role in diagnosis and prevention of further neurological injury during brain and cranial nerve tract surgeries. Techniques such as electromyography (EMG) and a variety of evoked potentials allow for ongoing assessment of nerve function, with immediate correction that lessens postoperative neurological defect (Ali et al., 2016). Apart from structural damage and infection, the majority of neurological diseases also possess vascular and autoimmune components that account for cranial nerve and brain dysfunction. Stroke, which is the primary source of neurological morbidity, can hurt brain regions responsible for processing sensory data or controlling motor output via cranial nerves and cause deficits such as facial weakness or dysphagia. Autoimmune diseases such as Guillain-Barré syndrome also illustrate mechanisms of neurological diseases by immune-mediated attacks on peripheral nerves, including cranial nerves, with resulting rapidly progressive paralysis. These diseases need to be treated by multidisciplinary teams of neurologists, neurosurgeons, and rehabilitative specialists to achieve maximum functional recovery. Continual advances in neurodiagnostic technology and therapy strategies are essential for improved outcomes in patients with such complicated neurological diseases (Boon et al., 2020).

13.5.2. Impact of Brain Disorders on Cranial Nerve Function

Neurological integrity is required for uncompromised function of the cranial nerves, which are essential conduits between the brain and other sensory and motor elements of the neck and head. Abnormalities of the brain such as tumor, stroke, and degenerative diseases can compromise these conduits, leading to extreme compromise of cranial nerve functions. For instance, brainstem lesions containing most of the cranial nerve nuclei could disrupt the process of transmission of neural impulses and create defects such as paralysis of the face, altered sensation, or defective movement of the eyes. These not only affect simple processes like vision and swallowing but also decrease the QoL. Appreciation of the impact on cranial nerve function of such disorders necessitates clear comprehension of CNS as well as PNS anatomy, which is the subject of the majority of neurosurgical educational paradigms presently impinging on clinical practice (Traynelis et al., 2000). Beyond gross disruption of structure, brain disorders may impact horrifically on cranial nerve function by inducing subtle disorganization of autonomic control. The autonomic fibers of certain cranial nerves also control vital physiological reflexes, including salivation, lacrimation, and pupil constriction. Brain pathologies can impair these autonomic tracts to cause such problems as dry eyes or the lack of ability to regulate blood supply to the head and neck. Such interactions demonstrate the importance of knowing the detailed topography and function of cranial nerves beyond motor and sensory levels to encompass autonomic regulation. Recent advances in the mapping of pelvic and cranial nerves further underscore the complexity of such connections, allowing for improved diagnosis and treatment of dysfunction due to CNS disease (Alkatout et al., 2021). Secondary inflammatory, ischemic, and intracranial pressure changes, as a complicating factor, further enhance nerve dysfunction. Diseases such as encephalitis or multiple sclerosis include inflammatory mechanisms that injure axons and myelin sheaths and disrupt conductance of signals in cranial nerves. In turn, elevated intracranial pressure due to hemorrhage or hydrocephalus may compress nerve fibers, reducing blood flow and resulting in ischemic damage. These secondary insults highlight the precarious balance required for optimal cranial nerve function and stress the need for integrated management strategies that address both the primary brain pathology and its downstream impact on cranial nerves. This combined strategy is core to neurosurgical management and neurorehabilitation (Traynelis et al., 2000; Alkatout et al., 2021;) (Figure 13.11).

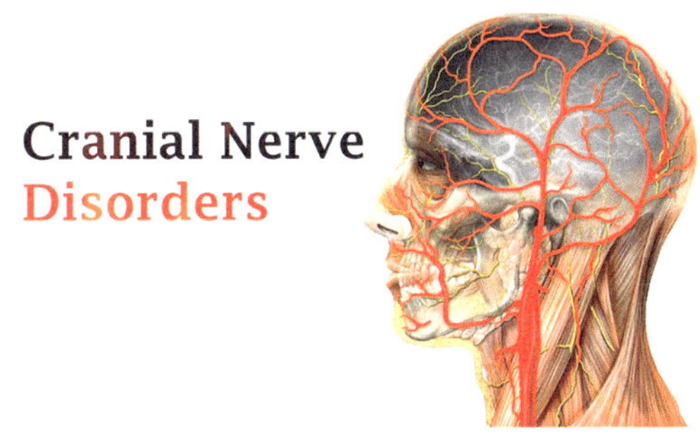

Figure 13.11. Impact of brain disorders on cranial nerve function.

Source: https://i.ytimg.com/vi/GrGtzWnn0D4/maxresdefault.jpg.

13.5.3. Treatment Options for Brain Disorders

Progress in understanding how the complex interaction of different body systems works has begun to shape new approaches to treating brain diseases. Recent research highlights the function of the microbiota-gut-brain axis as a powerful driver of neurological and psychiatric illness. This axis facilitates communication between gut microbiota and the brain via immune mechanisms, metabolic end-products, and neural connections such as the vagus nerve. Consequently, current treatments extend beyond the traditional pharmacologic strategies to include intervention against the gut microbiota, such as probiotics, dietary modification, and fecal microbiota transplantation. These treatments are aimed at restoration of microbial balance and enhancement in neurological function and can potentially offer therapeutic benefit in conditions like anxiety, autism, and neurodegenerative diseases. As empirical evidence mounts, these therapy with microbiota may complement existing treatments to provide more complete and efficacious outcomes for brain disorders (John et al., 2019). Such an integrated strategy is a paradigm shift in personalized medicine for brain wellness. Despite the progress thus far in understanding brain disorders, many conventional treatment strategies remain inadequate, especially when addressing neuropathic perceptions that accompany brain diseases. Chemotherapy-induced peripheral neuropathy (CIPN), for example, is a classic instance of treatment side effect making care for patients with cranial nerve cancers and brain tumors more difficult. Clinical manifestations of CIPN ranging from sensory to motor to autonomic dysfunction illustrate the challenge in achieving the balance between aggressive cancer treatments with the maintenance of QoL. To date, no effective preventive or therapeutic interventions for CIPN exist, and treatment is mainly based on symptom alleviation and dose adjustment of neurotoxic drugs. Direct investigation of the mechanisms of neurotoxicity of chemotherapeutic drugs is required to develop new protective drugs or less toxic therapeutic agents. In this context, specific neuroprotective therapies remain a current urgent unmet need among brain disorder treatments, as it indicates the complexity of multidisciplinary applications (Zaj et al., 2019). New modalities of treatment for brain disorders increasingly integrate multidisciplinary approaches that are sensitive to the heterogeneity of underlying etiologies. Pharmacologic treatments, including antiepileptic drugs, neuroleptics, and antidepressants, remain the mainstay for symptom control related to impairment of cranial nerves and CNS disease. However, progressive neuromodulation therapies such as deep brain stimulation, transcranial magnetic stimulation, and vagus nerve stimulation (VNS) break with tradition by offering focal, non-pharmacologic intervention. These modalities have the ability to modulate the neural circuits that mediate movement disorders, epilepsy, and mood changes and provide alternative therapy when medication is ineffective or produces unacceptable side effects. At the same time, cognitive and motor training rehabilitation therapies also ensure neurologic recovery and autonomy. With the further evolution of personalized medicine, integrating genetic, microbiome, and neurophysiologic data will make these treatment paradigms more efficient and less toxic. All of these developments constitute a more holistic and responsive system for the treatment of brain and cranial nerve disease.

Test Your Knowledge

1. Which cranial nerve is commonly affected in multiple sclerosis, and what symptom does it cause?
2. What are two common treatment approaches for brain disorders that affect cranial nerves?

13.6. Research and Advances in Neuroscience

Learning Outcome

1. Focus on Current Research Trends in Brain Studies
2. Explain the Technological Advancements in Studying Cranial Nerves
3. Learn about Future Directions in Neuroscience Research

Newer findings in neuroscience have profoundly enriched the understanding of the complex mechanisms of the brain, particularly in relation to the cranial nerves. One of the most significant developments is the work on the neuropeptide PACAP-38, which, when administered intravenously, has been shown to induce migraine-like headaches. This observation not only justifies the therapeutic targeting of PACAP pathways but also illuminates the complex sequence of migraine, from aura through headache. Interestingly, while PACAP-38 and related peptides were initially implicated in the dilation of vessels, later research suggests that migraine headache is the result of mechanisms that are neural but not pure vascular. In agreement with this, insights into the receptor subtypes and neural pathways involved in PACAP signaling offer avenues for further clarification of migraine pathophysiology as well as new directions for treatment development of cranial nerve pain disorders (Waschek et al., 2018). Neuroscientific research has moved beyond pain mechanisms to examine cognitive and executive function impairments secondary to structural brain defects. For instance, studies have established that patients with Chiari Type I malformation exhibit large executive function impairments in regulation of attention, mental flexibility, and inhibitory control. By the application of neuropsychological tests like the Stroop Test, Continuous Performance Test (CPT), and Wisconsin Card Sorting Test (WCST), researchers have detected alterations in processes necessary for the maintenance of cognitive control and adaptive behavior. Such findings suggest that the brainstem and cerebellar region structural malformations could be accountable for more pervasive neuropsychological dysfunctions, suggesting complicated relations between cranial nerve pathology and executive defects (Gonz et al., 2018).

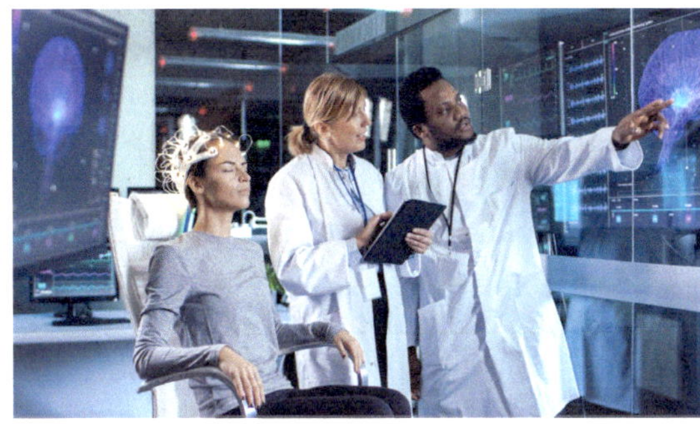

Source: Neuroscience 2020. (n.d.). *Researchers Analyzing brain Activity in Neuroscience Lab.*

Together, these advances constitute a paradigm shift in the field of neuroscience in which molecular, structural, and cognitive methods take center stage in arriving at a comprehension of cranial nerve and brain functions as an entity. The discussion of neuropeptide roles in migraine and neuropsychological impacts in Chiari malformations speaks to the complexity of neurological diseases.

This unifying paradigm is crucial for more precise diagnostic tools and interventions, which address not only focal cranial nerve disease but also systemic impact on sensory and cognitive processing. Interdisciplinary investigation remains capable of revolutionizing clinical practice, improving patient outcomes through focal neural pathway modulation and enhanced understanding of brain network activity.

13.6.1. Current Research Trends in Brain Studies

Recent advances in brain research symbolize an increasing desire to bridge the gap between technological innovation and biological complication. Previous methods for curing nervous tissue injury have been of limited success, particularly since neural tissue operates within the background of an extremely complicated biochemical and topological environment. Current developments in neural tissue engineering (NTE) have witnessed the introduction of biomaterial scaffolds that replicate this sophistication to direct cell migration and tissue regeneration at injury sites. These scaffolds are meticulously designed with controlled topographies and biochemical signals that influence neuronal activity, indicating the multidisciplinary orientation of current trends. Besides, NTE strategies have been used for purposes outside therapy, such as creating *in vitro* models of neurodegenerative diseases, especially those difficult to model in animal models. Breakthroughs in fabrication techniques such as additive manufacturing and soft lithography have led the field forward, but the complication of optimizing scaffold design for full functional recovery and disease modeling is still an issue (Papadimitriou et al., 2020). Concurrently with regenerative approaches, brain imaging technologies have become pivotal in advancing our understanding of brain function and disease. Magnetoencephalography (MEG), a non-invasive technique for recording weak magnetic fields evoked by neurons, is an example of this breakthrough in providing real-time data at millisecond resolution. MEG compliments electroencephalography (EEG) to give a dynamic snapshot of brain networks in health and disease. While its medical application is primarily limited to the diagnosis of epilepsy and preoperative assessment, recent research is expanding MEG's potential application in such psychiatric and developmental disorders, and stroke rehabilitation. This development aligns with the overall trend towards integrating neuroimaging and functional mapping to enable patient-specific treatments and improve the specificity of neurological diagnostics (Hari et al., 2018). The marriage of tissue engineering and advanced neuroimaging is representative of a transformative age in brain science with emphasis on structural rehabilitation as much as functional assessment. Research is shifting increasingly toward the creation of platforms that not only support neuronal regeneration but also allow for accurate monitoring of brain activity changes in the process of recovery or disease development. Lab-on-a-chip platforms are a prime example of this by offering microenvironments for the examination of neural networks *in vitro* with unmatched control and relevance. Not only do these technologies enable the exploration of basic neurobiological mechanisms, but they also enable the growth of personalized medicine strategies that target the complex interaction of brain and cranial nerve function. As the technology continues to improve, overcoming current limitations in scaffold biocompatibility and imaging resolution will be crucial to taking these directions of research to the clinic (Hari et al., 2018; Papadimitriou et al., 2020).

13.6.2. Technological Advancements in Studying Cranial Nerves

During the last several decades, there has been a shift in the practice of neuroanatomical research and clinical practice due to the advancement of technology, particularly the evaluation of cranial nerves. High-resolution imaging modalities such as magnetic resonance imaging (MRI) and diffusion tensor imaging (DTI) provide an unmatched view of nerve fiber tracts to enable precise characterization of nerve tracts and lesions. These improvements significantly enhance diagnostic accuracy and surgical planning with less damage to delicate neural structures. In addition, integrating stereotactic radiosurgery (SRS) has revolutionized the therapy of cranial nerve tumors like vestibular schwannomas, making possible precise, minimally invasive therapy. Multidisciplinary and including neurosurgery, radiation oncology, and radiation physics, the collaboration ensures optimal treatment effect with minimal morbidity, reflecting the evolving interface between technology and cranial nerve research and treatment (Braunstein & Ma, 2018). These developments mirror the manner innovations continue to drive knowledge and treatment strategies in neuroanatomy. Acquisition of microsurgical skills relevant to cranial nerve surgery has also progressed through simulation models of technologically enhanced sophistication. Owing to the complexity of neurosurgical interventions and the paucity of human cadaveric material, animal models have been significantly focused in the neurosurgeon's training. Bovine, ovine, and porcine cranial models provide a true anatomical and haptic simulation equal to that of human anatomy, allowing trainees to develop surgical finesse and competency in procedures for cranial nerves. Models developed in the lab simulate various techniques such as the retrosigmoid and interhemispheric transcalosal pathways, which are important to provide secure passage through critical neurovascular zones around cranial nerves. By providing repeated, risk-free practice, learning technology aids reduce the learning curve and are returned as better operating outcomes in the clinical environment (Morosanu et al., 2019). This amalgamation of animal models and neurosurgical education represents a giant stride in understanding cranial nerve anatomy and function. Moreover, the advancements in simulation technologies and minimally invasive surgery equipment have changed the landscape of cranial nerve therapy and research. Virtual reality (VR) and augmented reality (AR) environments allow for experiential visualization of anatomy and simulation rehearsal of surgery, allowing trainees and clinicians to gain a dynamic appreciation of spatial relationships between cranial nerves. Used in conjunction with advances in robotics and endoscopy, these technologies allow for precision and safety in surgical intervention, particularly in smaller cranial compartments. All of this equipment also facilitates better assessment of nerve integrity and functional outcome following intervention to facilitate more advanced comprehension of nerve repair and regeneration mechanisms. With ever-advancing technology, it will possibly enhance scientific understanding of cranial nerve pathology and enhance patient care, marking a new generation of technological innovation in neuroscience and neurosurgery (Figure 13.12).

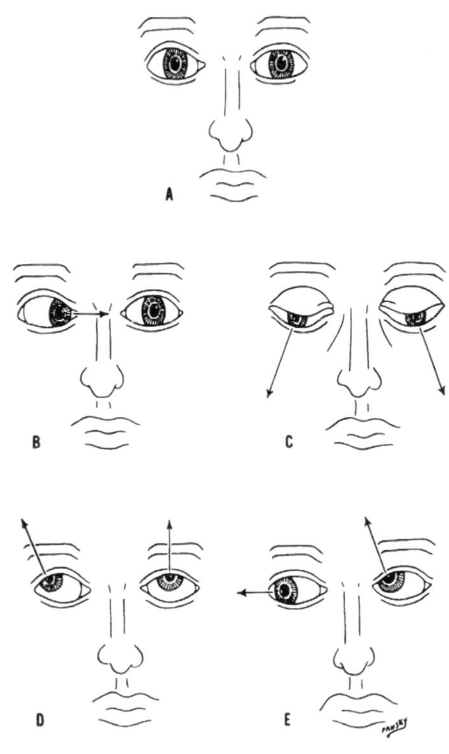

Figure 13.12. Technological advancements in studying cranial nerves.

Source: By House, Earl Lawrence. Pansky, Ben. - A functional approach to neuroanatomy 1960, Public Domain, https://commons.wikimedia.org/w/index.php?curid=30833881

13.6.3. Future Directions in Neuroscience Research

The complex complexity of the brain and its cranial nerves continues to pose a challenge to scientific understanding, calling for new approaches to research. Advances in neuroimaging and molecular biology have provided new windows of opportunity to examine neural pathways and synaptic functions with greater precision. Future research in neuroscience will likely be aimed at integrating various multi-modal approaches that combine genetic, electrophysiological, and computational methodologies in an effort to discern the mechanisms of cranial nerve function and dysfunction. This integrative strategy is the linchpin to deciphering the subtle variability in nerve pathology observed across disorders such as trochlear nerve palsy, which has heterogeneous etiologies spanning trauma to microvascular (Puetz, 2024). Additionally, the innovation of highly sensitive non-invasive neural recording devices can revolutionize diagnostics and selective treatments by enabling interventions predicated on personal neural signatures. As we push these boundaries, however, the objective remains to unite clinical neurology and fundamental science, creating a translational continuum that boils down to increased therapeutic advantage for patients with cranial nerve deficiency. Technological innovation will also be key in the future in setting the course of neuroscience research, particularly in addressing the complexity of cranial nerve disorders. Emerging techniques such as high-resolution DTI and optogenetics hold promising potential for *in vivo* neural circuitry mapping with relevance to neural plasticity and regeneration. These are complemented by advances in artificial intelligence (AI) and machine learning algorithms capable of parsing big data to elucidate patterns and predictive markers of disease progression. This multidisciplinary approach is necessary as research attempts to unravel multifactorial etiologies of cranial nerve pathology, including idiopathic and congenital cases reported in clinical research (Puetz, 2024). Advances in biomaterials and nanotechnology can also facilitate targeted drug delivery systems, which may enhance treatment outcomes by crossing the blood-brain barrier. Such potential future directions highlight an integrative and comprehensive understanding of brain and cranial nerve interactions that can transform patient care with earlier diagnosis and precision medicine strategies.

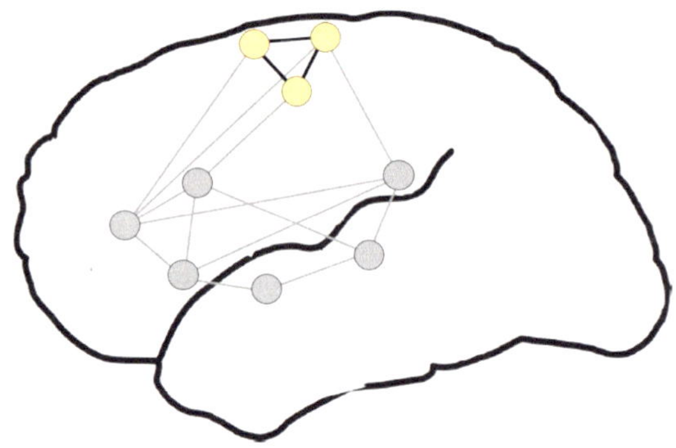

Figure 13.13. Future directions in neuroscience research.

Source: By Novasdid - Own work, CC BY-SA 4.0, https://commons.wikimedia.org/w/index.php?curid=58421153

Ethical considerations and global collaborations will become a component of neuroscience research in the future, especially with the greater possibilities of neural modulation and enhancement technologies. The ability to intervene in neural circuits is of paramount importance in terms of consent, privacy, and long-term effects and necessitates robust responsible research frameworks. Moreover, open data and international partnerships can accelerate discovery by facilitating data sharing and standardization of research protocols for cranial nerve disorders, as demonstrated by diverse epidemiological findings (Kadrija et al., 2025). Multidisciplinary collaboration between clinicians, neuroscientists, engineers, and ethicists will assist in translating bench-side studies to bedside advantages, such that the technological innovation is aligned with patient well-being. Ultimately, the way forward for neuroscience is not just to decipher the secrets of the brain and cranial nerves but also to improve the QoL of patients with neurological illness (Figure 13.13).

Test Your Knowledge

1.

SUMMARY

The complex coordination between the cranial nerves and brain underscores the character of highly complex neurological function, which represents a subtle relationship essential to motor and sensory integration. The developments in neuropathology in the recent past, particularly studies involving proteinopathies such as tauopathies, have illuminated knowledge regarding neurodegenerative pathology caused by both central and PNSs. Of note, progressive supranuclear palsy studies identify the presence of phosphorylated tau in cranial nerves, describing an emergent pathological process that may play a role in diagnostic specificity and development of targeted therapies (Tanaka et al., 2023). The correlation suggests that cranial nerve disease reflects and may even precede CNS disease, emphasizing convergent approaches in neurologic assessment and therapy. New treatments also illustrate the dynamic neuroplasticity between cranial nerve functions and brain structures, particularly in psychiatric disease where neural networks show altered connectivity. Contrastive comparisons of standard pharmacological treatments and neuromodulation techniques, such as transcutaneous auricular VNS, indicate the potential for modulating interactions between brain networks to effectively treat (Liao et al., 2023). These findings are the basis for the concept that cranial nerves, besides their peripheral roles, deeply influence central neural circuits, and hence offer new horizons to understand and cure brain disorders. The differential modulation of the brain networks also attaches greater importance to individualized medicine to select appropriate therapeutic approaches based on the connectivity pattern of the patient's neural network. As a whole, the analysis of brain and cranial nerves offers a integrated system for examination of neurological well-being and ailment. Together with structural pathology, as seen in tau protein deposits within cranial nerves, and functional neuromodulation of brain circuits through innovative interventions, the difficulty of neurobiology lies. Pathological and clinical application integration could enhance diagnostic specificity and therapeutic outcome in numerous neurological illnesses. Continued interdisciplinary research is essential to unravel the complex mechanisms of brain-cranial nerve interactions, ultimately resulting in improved treatment of neurodegenerative and neuropsychiatric diseases (Liao et al., 2023; Tanaka et al., 2023).

The sophistication of brain functioning is evinced by its highly complex cellular and molecular processes, as borne out by reactions to stressors like cranial irradiation. Research has observed how radiation-induced neuroinflammation evolves in various steps, with the microglia being a key player in coordinating these inflammatory responses. First, cell death of neural progenitor cells triggers a brief inflammation followed by a temporally delayed phase with changes in microglial phenotypes and cytokine production that correlate with cognitive impairment. This biphasic response accounts for the time-course development of neuroinflammatory processes in key brain regions like the hippocampus and emphasizes the need for timely therapeutic intervention to these dynamic processes. Peripheral macrophage invasion and the long-term effects on neuronal circuitry further complicate brain response to injury, suggesting the interconnectivity of immune and neural repair mechanisms in guaranteeing cognitive functions (Puetz, 2024). Aging further complicates brain function by altering neurogenesis, synapse kinetics, and neurometabolism, and neuroinflammation exacerbation. Experimental paradigms such as the senescence-accelerated mouse-prone 8 (SAMP8) provide valuable insight into physiological as well as accelerated processes of brain cortex aging. Using whole-genome transcriptomics, researchers have delineated age-related declines in cognitive capacities and the respective gene-expression alterations involved. This has enabled them to identify important genes and regulatory modules governing functional changes arising in the aging brain, with valid molecular targets for therapeutic interventions. These findings advance our understanding of how neurobiological mechanisms worsen with age and inform the development of interventions to reverse cognitive aging effects (Fujiwara et al., 2023). Overall, advances in molecular profiling and transcriptional analysis have greatly enhanced our comprehension of brain and cranial nerve function, particularly under conditions of injury and aging. The results underscore the duality of inflammation as response to damage and causative factor in neural dysfunction and the requirement of complex strategies with temporal and cellular specificity. Further, the establishment of major molecular pathways in brain aging models points toward new drug development and clinical strategies against neurodegenerative pathologies. Collectively, these researches provide a conceptual model for what processes neuroinflammatory and aging pathways utilize to impair brain integrity and for what interventions may be applied to uphold cognitive health and neural connections.

KEY TERMS FROM THIS CHAPTER

- Autonomic control
- Coordinated behavior
- Cranial nerve system
- Electrophysiology
- Human nervous system
- Brain-nerve interaction
- Cranial nerve development
- Craniofacial patterning
- Facial movement
- Cerebrospinal fluid (CSF)
- Cranial nerve stimulation
- Craniofacial tissues
- Facial muscles

CRITICAL THINKING QUESTIONS

1. **Which part of the brain is primarily responsible for coordination and balance?**
   a. Cerebrum
   b. Brainstem
   c. Cerebellum
   d. Thalamus
2. **Which cranial nerve is responsible for vision?**
   a. Optic nerve (II)
   b. Oculomotor nerve (III)
   c. Trochlear nerve (IV)
   d. Trigeminal nerve (V)
3. **The medulla oblongata is part of which region of the brain?**
   a. Forebrain
   b. Midbrain
   C. Hindbrain
   D. Cerebrum
4. **Which cranial nerve controls facial expression?**
   a. Trigeminal (V)
   b. Facial (VII)
   c. Glossopharyngeal (IX)
   d. Accessory (XI)
5. **The olfactory nerve (I) exits the skull through which foramen?**
   a. Jugular foramen
   b. Optic canal
   c. Cribriform plate
   d. Superior orbital fissure

Short Answer Questions

1. What is the role of the cerebellum in motor coordination?
2. Describe the anatomical location and function of the medulla oblongata.
3. What is the blood-brain barrier, and why is it important?
4. Define the function of the thalamus in sensory processing.
5. Differentiate between the sensory and motor functions of the trigeminal nerve (CN V).
6. Which cranial nerves carry parasympathetic fibers, and what are their general functions?
7. How is cerebrospinal fluid (CSF) produced, and what is its function?
8. Briefly describe the pathway of the facial nerve (CN VII) and its main functions.

Answers to Critical Thinking Questions

1. (c) 2. (a) 3. (c) 4. (b) 5. (c)

REFERENCES

1. Waschek, J. A., Baca, S. M., & Akerman, S. (2018). PACAP and migraine headache: immunomodulation of neural circuits in autonomic ganglia and brain parenchyma. *The journal of headache and pain*, *19*(1), 23. https://doi.org/10.1186/s10194-018-0850-6 (accessed on 8th May 2025).
2. Triviño, L. N., Albino, A. M., Dozo, M. T., & Williams, J. D. (2018). First Natural Endocranial Cast of a Fossil Snake (Cretaceous of Patagonia, Argentina). *Anatomical record (Hoboken, N.J. : 2007)*, *301*(1), 9–20. https://doi.org/10.1002/ar.23686(accessed on 8th May 2025).
3. Ali, Liaquat; Iqrar, Ambreen; and Asumal Khealani, Bhojo (2016) "Review of various intraoperative neurophysiologic monitoring techniques," Pakistan Journal of Neurological Sciences (PJNS): Vol. 11: Iss. 2, Article 10. Available at: https://ecommons.aku.edu/pjns/vol11/iss2/10(accessed on 8th May 2025).
4. Alkatout, I., Wedel, T., Pape, J., Possover, M., & Dhanawat, J. (2021). Review: Pelvic nerves - from anatomy and physiology to clinical applications. *Translational neuroscience*, *12*(1), 362–378. https://doi.org/10.1515/tnsci-2020-0184(accessed on 8th May 2025).
5. Benninger, B., & McNeil, J. (2010). Transitional Nerve: A New and Original Classification of a Peripheral Nerve Supported by the Nature of the Accessory Nerve (CN XI). *Neurology research international*, *2010*, 476018. https://doi.org/10.1155/2010/476018(accessed on 8th May 2025).
6. Benveniste, H., Liu, X., Koundal, S., Sanggaard, S., Lee, H., & Wardlaw, J. M. (2018). The glymphatic system and waste clearance with brain aging: A review. *Gerontology, 65*, 106–119. https://doi.org/10.1159/000490349 (accessed on 8th May 2025).
7. Besteiro González, J. L., & Torres Campa-Santamarina, J. M. (2018). Anomalies in the cognitive-executive functions in patients with Chiari Malformation Type I. *Psicothema*, *30*(3), 316–321. https://doi.org/10.7334/psicothema2017.401 (accessed on 8th May 2025).
8. F. Keith Bradford and Hubert W. Smith, Medico-Legal Aspects of the Nervous System as a Functioning Unit of the Body, 6 Vanderbilt Law Review 815 (1953) Available at: https://scholarship.law.vanderbilt.edu/vlr/vol6/iss4/1 (accessed on 8th May 2025).
9. Braunstein, S., & Ma, L. (2018). Stereotactic radiosurgery for vestibular schwannomas. *Cancer management and research*, *10*, 3733–3740. https://doi.org/10.2147/CMAR.S140764(accessed on 8th May 2025).
10. Bylsma, L. M., Gračanin, A., & Vingerhoets, A. J. J. M. (2019). The neurobiology of human crying. *Clinical autonomic research : official journal of the Clinical Autonomic Research Society*, *29*(1), 63–73. https://doi.org/10.1007/s10286-018-0526-y (accessed on 8th May 2025).
11. Claassen, J. A. H. 5., Thijssen, D. H. J., Panerai, R. B., & Faraci, F. M. (2021). Regulation of cerebral blood flow in humans: Physiology and clinical implications of autoregulation. *Physiological Reviews, 101*, 1487–1559. https://doi.org/10.1152/physrev.00022.2020 (accessed on 8th May 2025).
12. Traynelis, V. C., Andrews, B. T., Awad, I. A., Batjer, H. H., Belzberg, A., Leibrock, L., Couldwell, W., Follett, K., Friedman, A., Loftus, C. M., Maniker, A., Mapstone, T., Pollock, B. E., Schochet, S. S., Jr, Valadka, A., & Wolfla, C. (2000). Resident curriculum guidelines for neurosurgery.

Congress of Neurological Surgeons Education Committee. *Clinical neurosurgery*, *47*, 589–681. (accessed on 8th May 2025).

13. Cozart, D., Hesse, D., Nichols, R., & Szymik, J. (2017). *UGA Anatomy and Physiology 1 Lab Manual* (3rd ed.). https://core.ac.uk/download/217306564.pdf (accessed on 8th May 2025).
14. Singhrao, S. K., Harding, A., Simmons, T., Robinson, S., Kesavalu, L., & Crean, S. (2014). Oral inflammation, tooth loss, risk factors, and association with progression of Alzheimer's disease. *Journal of Alzheimer's disease : JAD*, *42*(3), 723–737. https://doi.org/10.3233/JAD-140387 (accessed on 8th May 2025).
15. Cryan, J. F., O'Riordan, K. J., Cowan, C. S. M., Sandhu, K. V., Bastiaanssen, T. F. S., Boehme, M., Codagnone, M. G., et al. (2019). The microbiota-gut-brain axis. *Physiological Reviews, 99*, 1877–2013. https://doi.org/10.1152/physrev.00018.2018 (accessed on 8th May 2025).
16. Cuomo-Granston, A., & Drummond, P. D. (2010). Migraine and motion sickness: what is the link?. *Progress in neurobiology*, *91*(4), 300–312. https://doi.org/10.1016/j.pneurobio.2010.04.001(accessed on 8th May 2025).
17. Singh, H., Vogel, R. W., Lober, R. M., Doan, A. T., Matsumoto, C. I., Kenning, T. J., & Evans, J. J. (2016). Intraoperative Neurophysiological Monitoring for Endoscopic Endonasal Approaches to the Skull Base: A Technical Guide. *Scientifica*, *2016*, 1751245. https://doi.org/10.1155/2016/1751245 (accessed on 8th May 2025).
18. Morosanu, C. O., Nicolae, L., Moldovan, R., Farcasanu, A. S., Filip, G. A., & Florian, I. S. (2019). Neurosurgical cadaveric and in vivo large animal training models for cranial and spinal approaches and techniques - a systematic review of the current literature. *Neurologia i neurochirurgia polska*, *53*(1), 8–17. https://doi.org/10.5603/PJNNS.a2019.0001 (accessed on 8th May 2025).
19. Sánchez-Villagra, M. R., & Forasiepi, A. M. (2017). On the development of the chondrocranium and the histological anatomy of the head in perinatal stages of marsupial mammals. *Zoological letters*, *3*, 1. https://doi.org/10.1186/s40851-017-0062-y (accessed on 8th May 2025).
20. Hari, R., Baillet, S., Barnes, G. R., Burgess, R. C., Forss, N., Groß, J., Hämäläinen, M., et al. (2018). IFCN-endorsed practical guidelines for clinical magnetoencephalography (MEG). *Clinical Neurophysiology, 129*, 1720–1747. https://doi.org/10.1016/j.clinph.2018.03.042 (accessed on 8th May 2025).
21. Kadrija, M., & Rudi, G. (2025). *Understanding Trochlear Nerve Palsy: Etiological Perspectives from the Literature.* https://core.ac.uk/download/640070670.pdf (accessed on 8th May 2025).
22. Khantal, N., Kankane, V., & Sharma, A. (2024). A prospective study on the incidence and outcome of cranial nerve injuries in patients with traumatic brain injuries. *Asian Journal of Medical Sciences.* https://www.semanticscholar.org/paper/18bb6620d80cd16316f46fa4c343ec39a1974182 (accessed on 8th May 2025).
23. Khatibi, S. M. (2015). *Peripheral Nerve Glia as Multipotent Progenitors in Craniofacial Development.* https://core.ac.uk/download/70341260.pdf (accessed on 8th May 2025).
24. Li, Z., Chen, L., Wang, J., Dong, G., Jia, G., Jia, W., & Li, D. (2024). Cavernous Malformation From Cranial Nerves: A Systematic Review With a Novel Classification and Patient-Level Analysis. *Neurosurgery*, *95*(6), 1274–1284. https://doi.org/10.1227/neu.0000000000003011 (accessed on 8th May 2025).

25. Mehta, N. H., Sherbansky, J., Kamer, A. R., Carare, R. O., Butler, T., Rusinek, H., Chiang, G., et al. (2022). The brain-nose interface: A potential cerebrospinal fluid clearance site in humans. *Frontiers in Physiology, 12*. https://doi.org/10.3389/fphys.2021.769948 (accessed on 8th May 2025).
26. Papadimitriou, L., Manganas, P., Ranella, A., & Stratakis, E. (2020). Biofabrication for neural tissue engineering applications. *Materials Today Bio., 6*, 100043–100043. https://doi.org/10.1016/j.mtbio.2020.100043 (accessed on 8th May 2025).
27. Persoage, Katelyn, "Current Trends in Concussion Management among Athletic Trainers in Different Workplace Settings" (2014). Theses and Dissertations. 123. https://ir.library.illinoisstate.edu/etd/123 (accessed on 8th May 2025).
28. Puetz, Emma, "Ontogenetically Driven Changes in the Endocranial Anatomy of Maiasaura Peeblesorum and its Implications for Sensory Functions" (2024). Masters Theses. 8208. https://scholarsmine.mst.edu/masters_theses/8208 (accessed on 8th May 2025).
29. Sreeja MT, Vatsalaswamy P, Leo Rathinaraj AS. Morphometric study of the neurons in human hypoglossal nerve nucleus during early gestation. Anatomy Journal of Africa. 7 (2): 1274 - 1280.(accessed on 8th May 2025).
30. Trejo, J. L. (2019). Cranial nerves: Mind your head. *The Anatomical Record, 302*, 374–377. https://doi.org/10.1002/ar.24071 (accessed on 8th May 2025).
31. Zajączkowska, R., Kocot-Kępska, M., Leppert, W., Wrzosek, A., Mika, J., & Wordliczek, J. (2019). Mechanisms of chemotherapy-induced peripheral neuropathy. *International Journal of Molecular Sciences, 20*, 1451. https://doi.org/10.3390/ijms20061451 (accessed on 8th May 2025).

NECK AND CERVICAL VISCERA

14

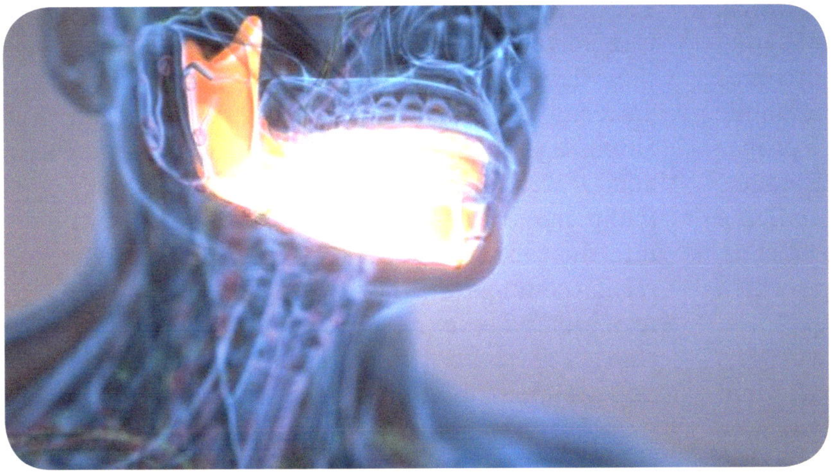

Introduction

An understanding of the complex human body anatomy forms the foundation for clinical practice and medical education. Among the essential anatomical regions is the neck, which has a variety of vital structures known as the cervical viscera. The neck's organs, muscles, vessels, and nerves coordinate crucial physiological processes such as respiration, swallowing, and endocrine regulation. The complex interdependency and organizational sophistication of these structures require extensive study by both students and practitioners. The course-curricular has evolved to address foundational learning outcomes that allow graduates to acquire accurate knowledge needed for safe and effective patient care, with the focus of acquiring expertise in this field in any medical program (Claire et al., 2015). The cervical viscera include salient structures such as the thyroid and parathyroid glands, larynx, pharynx, and neurovascular bundles. Their intimate relationship with one another necessitates reflective consideration, especially

LEARNING OBJECTIVES

After studying this chapter, you will be able to:

1. Discuss the anatomy of the neck
2. Focus on muscles of the neck
3. Explain the vascular structures
4. Understand nervous system components
5. Know cervical viscera overview
6. Learn about the pharynx
7. Explain the larynx
8. Focus on the esophagus
9. Learn about the thyroid gland
10. Discuss the parathyroid glands

in clinical diagnoses and surgeries. This compartmentalization of the neck's organs and soft tissues reflects an evolutionary adaptation to support crucial human functions such as voice production and metabolism. Extensive awareness of these interactions is crucial for the treatment of diseases like thyroid disease, obstruction of the airway, or vascular disease. Anatomical proficiency in this regard is thus paramount, predilection for diagnostic thinking as well as for planning treatments in head and neck medicine (Smith et al., 2015). Clinical relevance extends to cervical viscera beyond anatomy, dictating treatments and outcomes for many diseases. For instance, the metabolic function of the thyroid gland necessitates proper identification and management of pathologies such as cancer or goiter. Modern medicine also resorts to interdisciplinary approaches, in which ancient-world practices, among which herbal drugs feature prominently, are explored as treatments for cervical structure disorders. While primarily associated with hepatic and systemic interventions, such integrated practice reinforces the overall state of patient care that may indirectly affect cervical organ health. Thus, studying the neck and cervical viscera blends anatomical data with advancing clinical application, maintaining its relevance within holistic medical education.

Definition of Neck and Cervical Viscera

The anatomical complexity of the region between the base of the skull and the thoracic inlet is a vital juncture between the head and the rest of the body. Within the compartment are found various vital structures that are essential as a group and referred to as the cervical viscera. These include the respiratory airways of the trachea and larynx, components of the digestive tract like the pharynx and esophagus, and vital endocrine organs like the thyroid and parathyroid glands. This group of organs is covered with fascial layers that provide both protection and compartmentalization to enable organized functioning as well as to contain any potential pathological process. The musculoskeletal (MSK) framework, vascular, and nervous components of the neck work together with these viscera to offer homeostasis and protect essential physiological processes. An appreciation of how structural anatomy interfaces with function in the comprehension of this region highlights the significance of cervical viscera to the overall human health (Clark et al., 1906). When demarcating the cervical viscera, it is important to appreciate the interface between their developmental, physiological, and clinical patterns. For example, the larynx is not only an air passage but also a critical organ for phonation and protection of the airway. The trachea is found anteriorly in the neck, curving downward into the thorax to provide a passage for air to reach the lungs. Further, the thyroid gland with its lobulated lobes situated on either side of the trachea plays a critical role in hormone control and metabolism. Alongside the thyroid lie the parathyroid glands, responsible for calcium homeostasis. The pharynx, located behind the others, acts as a channel both for food and for air to allow respiration and digestion. These viscera show not only anatomical closeness but also functional interdependence, thus exact anatomical knowledge is vital for therapeutic as well as diagnostic maneuvers (Clark et al., 1906). Neck and cervical viscera examination also comprises pathological anomalies and deviations that reveal their scientific and clinical relevance. Developmental anomalies and atypical presentations, as rare as they are, generate additional interest in cervical anatomy and physiology. Studies of antenatal pathology and congenital malformations, including teratological malformations, provide insight into the complexity of this region's development and potential dysfunctions. Access to rarefied collections and facilities has enhanced awareness and demonstrated that structural deviations are often accompanied by extreme disturbances in function, reinforcing the fundamental osteopathic idea that structural changes are responsible for the majority of diseases. This way of thinking also reinforces the necessity for meticulous examination of the viscera of the neck in health and disease (Figure 14.1).

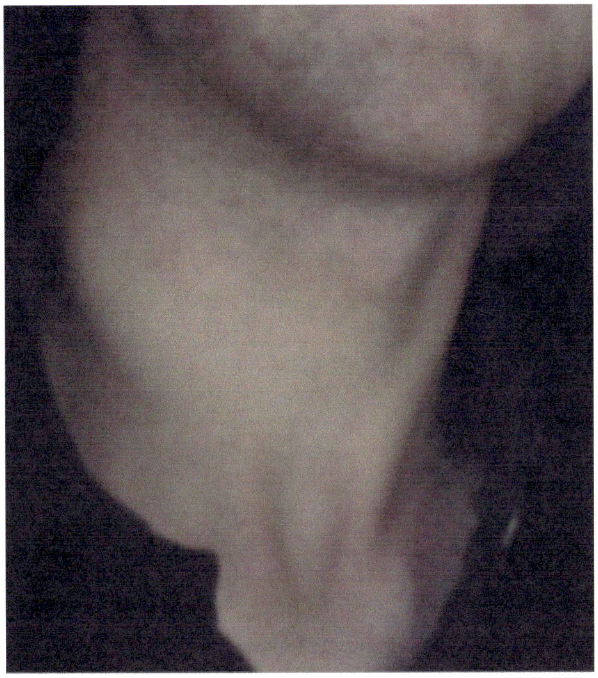

Figure 14.1. Definition of neck and cervical viscera.

Source: CC BY-SA 3.0, https://commons.wikimedia.org/w/index.php?curid=1428562

Importance of the Neck in Human Anatomy

The complex nerve network that passes through the neck is responsible for coordinating essential body processes, indicative of the region's complex anatomical function. Among them is the longest nerve in the human body, the vagus, which plays an important role in the parasympathetic nervous system. This nerve finely tunes physiological functions by allowing communication between the brain and organs such as the heart and gastrointestinal tract, thus ensuring homeostasis. The ability of the vagus nerve to modulate the immune response through its anti-inflammatory action highlights the role of the neck beyond structural support. Therapeutic interventions such as vagus nerve stimulation (VNS) have demonstrated effective results, particularly in the control of diseases showing chronic inflammation and systemic disorders, highlighting the critical function of the neck in neuroimmune regulation (Johnson et al., 2018). This expands the theory of the neck as a critical passageway for autonomic regulation and immunologic balance. Apart from its neurological importance, the anatomical structures of the neck hold vital cervical viscera for survival and health. The thyroid gland in the anterior part of the neck controls metabolism, growth, and development through hormone secretion, while parathyroid glands control calcium homeostasis. Additionally, the trachea and esophagus pass through this region, functioning as the primary airway for respiration and the major vessel for digestion, respectively. The close relationship and interdependency of these organs in a confined anatomical space underscore the importance of the neck in integrating multiple physiological systems. Disruptions in this area, such as trauma or disease of the cervical viscera, have the potential to profoundly impact respiratory, endocrine, and digestive function. The neck is therefore not merely a structural pathway but also a convergence center that integrates heterogeneous organ systems critical for adaptive physiology. In addition, parasympathetic and sympathetic divisions of the autonomic nervous system, both of which exist in the cervical region, balance to regulate health and disease. Anti-inflammatory effects of the vagus nerve coordinate with the sympathetic nervous system to manage immune response through the reduction of pro-inflammatory cytokines such as tumor necrosis factor alpha (TNFα) through signaling involving the splenic nerve. This neuro-immune cross-talk, present in the cervical region, forms a significant axis with influence on inflammatory bowel disease and postoperative ileus, which manifest as autonomic imbalance. Pharmacological means to stimulate this vagal pathway have been introduced by medical research, which is a possible non-pharmacological treatment for chronic inflammatory conditions with emphasis in the cervical and viscerally related regions (Bonaz et al., 2017). Thus, the anatomical and physiological complexity of necks is inherent in the maintenance of systemic homeostasis and the development of therapeutic approaches (Figure 14.2).

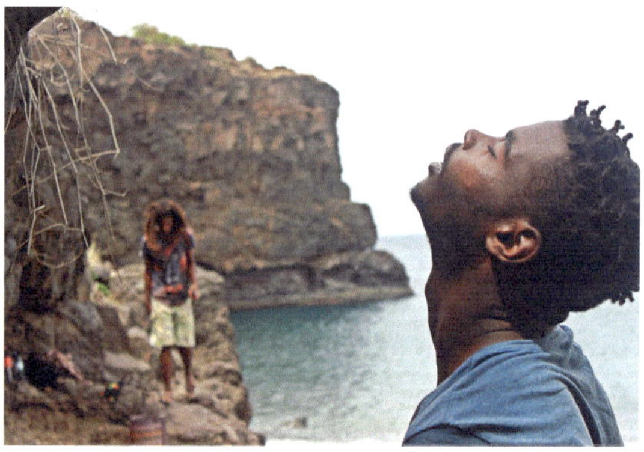

Figure 14.2. Importance of the neck in human anatomy.

Source: By Kriolog - Own work, CC BY-SA 4.0, https://commons.wikimedia.org/w/index.php?curid=63147954

14.1. Anatomy of the Neck

Learning Outcome

1. Discuss the Major Regions of the Neck
2. Explain the Key Anatomical Landmarks
3. Focus on Relationship to Surrounding Structures

An understanding of the complex anatomy of the neck is necessary because it contains an immense network of fascial layers, muscles, blood vessels, and nerves that contain vital functions. One of the most critical fascial structures, the alar fascia, lies deep in the cervical space and plays an important role in compartmentalizing spaces around the cervical viscera. It extends from the skull base to the superior thoracic vertebrae, between the carotid sheaths to between the retropharyngeal space and the danger space. Morphologically different from the prevertebral fascia, alar fascia contains neurovascular components and can prevent infection spread downward and thus is clinically important. Such structural design not only allows for the protection function of the fascia but also allows for the physiological movements and protections necessary for the cervical viscera integrity (Snosek et al., 2020). Deep within the neck is innervated by the vagus nerve, a critical element of the cervical viscus anatomy, that captures the neurological richness of the neck. As a powerful parasympathetic nerve, the vagus runs along the whole neck, providing innervation to several organs and governing autonomic function. Besides its basic functions in governing heart rate, digestion, and reflexes, recent studies have shed light on its therapeutic potential through VNS (VNS). Already approved for drug resistant epilepsy and depression, VNS is being investigated for its anti-inflammatory properties in the treatment of chronic inflammatory diseases like rheumatoid arthritis and sepsis. This expands the understanding of cervical neural anatomy not just in physiological mechanisms but also in emerging medical procedures that are relevant in neck and cervical viscera (Johnson et al., 2018). The anatomy of the neck also reveals a clear interrelationship between vascular, muscular, and fascial structures to ensure the function and protection of the cervicothoracic region. The cervical fascia, except for the alar part, consists of superficial and prevertebral layers that envelop the neck and make space for visceromotor interactions. The juxtaposition of such significant structures as carotid arteries, jugular veins, trachea, esophagus, and thyroid gland reflects the tight, functional organization of the neck. Spatial relationships and fascial boundaries are very important to know in surgical procedures as well as treating pathological processes such as retropharyngeal infections or tumors whose development is restricted or supported by fascial planes. Anatomical information thus not only supports diagnostics but also improves the clinical effects of diseases related to the neck (Snosek et al., 2020).

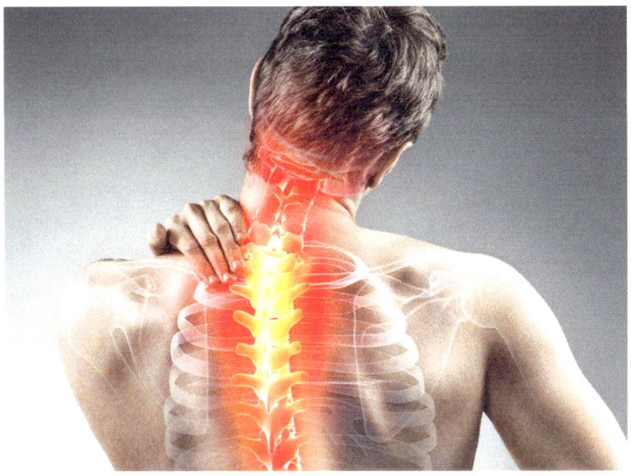

Source: Chirp. (n.d.). *The Anatomy of Your Neck*.

14.1.1. Major Regions of the Neck

The complex neck anatomy is segmented into several major regions, each with critical structures that cater to the neurovascular, respiratory, and digestive requirements. The anterior triangle, bordered by sternocleidomastoid muscle, mandible, and midline of the neck, harbors critical cervical viscera such as the thyroid gland, larynx, trachea, and pharynx. This region is also home to major vessels like the common carotid artery and internal jugular vein and vagus nerve, which are in charge of autonomic control of thoracic and abdominal organs, indicating the integrated functioning of the cervical viscera in systemic homeostasis. Understanding the spatial relationship of this triangle is important for the clinical management of airway and vascular system procedures and detection of pathology that can impact these structures. Hiding behind the anterior triangle is the posterior triangle, which is defined by the sternocleidomastoid, trapezius muscle, and clavicle. This space is primarily utilized to enable the passage of neurovascular structures providing supply to the upper limb and neck, including the brachial plexus and subclavian vessels. The cervical plexus also originates from the area, supplying sensory innervation to the neck and shoulder skin through somatosensory neurons, as discussed in current reviews explaining the double origin of cranial sensory ganglia and their involvement in relaying somatosensory and visceral sensory information to the central nervous system (CNS) (Vermeiren et al., 2020). These complex neural networks illustrate the highly complex embryological and functional plan of cervical innervation, its critical role in sensory and motor function. Recognition of disease in these areas of the neck requires understanding of the osseous and soft tissue structures involved. For example, bony growths such as osteochondromas—benign bone tumors—may appear on cervical vertebrae, which may compress adjacent vessels or nerves and cause clinical symptoms even though they are usually asymptomatic (Tepelenis et al., 2021). The anterior and posterior triangles are prone to such compressions due to the small spaces within them. Surgical interventions are likely to necessitate complete resection not to recur, once more illustrating the fine interrelation between anatomy and pathology in the major areas of the neck. Such detailed anatomical knowledge of the neck and its visceraoffers the basis for effective diagnosis and treatment of vascular, neck, and head diseases.

14.1.2. Key Anatomical Landmarks

Understanding the complex anatomy of the neck is essential and requires accurate identification of several important landmarks that serve as clinical assessment and operative intervention guides. The sternocleidomastoid muscle is one landmark that is an easily identifiable surface landmark employed to divide the neck into anterior and posterior triangles so that intra-compartmental life-critical structures become locatable. The hyoid bone, at the level of the third cervical vertebra, is another significant landmark that provides attachment for muscles involved in swallowing and speech. Furthermore, the thyroid cartilage, palpated by most as the "Adam's apple," indicates the location of the larynx and provides a covering to the vocal cords housed within. Correct identification of these landmarks not only plays a crucial role in diagnosing cervical viscera pathologies but also helps in avoiding injury to surrounding neurovascular bundles during surgery. Underlying the surface landmarks are deeper structures within the anatomy that are essential to cervical viscera functioning. Bifurcation of the carotid artery lies at the level of superior border of thyroid cartilage, and it is an important landmark for vascular assessment and treatment. Alongside it is the internal jugular vein, which lies within the carotid sheath along with the common carotid artery and vagus nerve, invested in the deep cervical fascia which partitions the neck. Superiorly, the larynx, lying between the thyroid cartilage and cricoid cartilage, houses the vocal apparatus, whereas the trachea goes on inferiorly, starting below the cricoid cartilage. The identification and knowledge of these landmarks enable clinicians to transcend the complexity of neck anatomy, make directed laryngoscopic exams, and carry out tracheostomies safely. While an appreciation for stationary landmarks provides structure, variations in anatomical features among persons necessitate a dynamic approach to their study. Differences in the lymph node morphology, for example, between men and women have been described (Damineni et al., 2022), emphasizing gender variation in clinical use and surgical planning. Although this research focuses on lymph nodes in regions other than the neck, the general principle underscores the significance of detailed regional observations of lymph nodes within cervical compartments to properly appreciate their size, number, and distribution. Similarly, comparisons of avian cervical anatomy reveal morphological and positional differences in respiratory and skeletal components (Echols et al., 2024), which are broader biological insights that can be applied to human cervical anatomy based on evolutionary factors. This comparative and individualized insight deepens knowledge of anatomical landmarks of the neck, improving diagnostic accuracy and therapeutic outcomes (Figure 14.3).

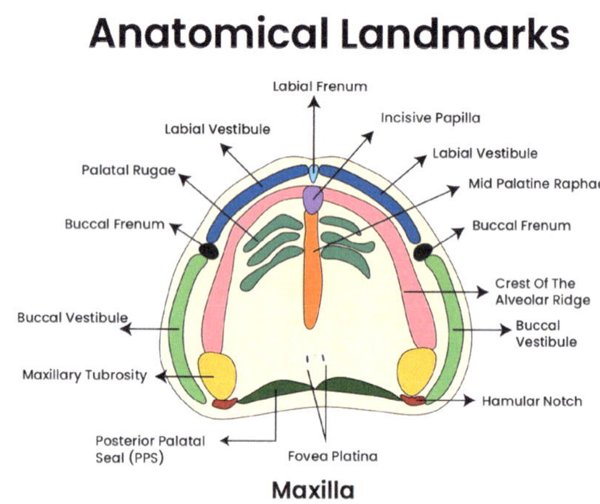

Figure 14.3. Key anatomical landmarks.

Source: Dental Anatomy Source. (n.d.). *Anatomical Landmarks of the Maxilla.*

14.1.3. Relationship to Surrounding Structures

The complex anatomy of the neck demands an adequate appreciation of the interaction of the cervical viscera with the overlying and underlying structures. The thyroid gland, for example, has an intimate association with important vasculature such as the carotid arteries and jugular veins, and the recurrent laryngeal nerve, which follows the tracheoesophageal groove closely. This topographic relationship emphasizes the importance of meticulous technique while performing surgery lest vocal cord paralysis follows. Moreover, the esophagus is located posterior to the trachea andthe thyroid gland is found anterolateral to the trachea , producing a stratified configuration that is both protective as well as functional in nature. It is these intimate relationships that make it possible for multiple physiological processes like respiration, swallowing, and endocrine regulation to occur simultaneously, marking the necks complex structural symphony. Awareness of the planes of connective tissue and fascial layers that invest the cervical viscera deepens information regarding their organization in space and motion. Deep cervical fascia separates the neck into areas, each with specific structures that protect against infection spread and improve functional independence. For instance, the pretracheal fascia encloses the trachea and thyroid gland, marking their association with the strap muscles in the front and the carotid sheath on the side. This compartmentalization assists in illuminating pathways for potential pathological processes and for surgical procedures. Furthermore, overlying fat is not only protective for these necessary structures but is also involved in metabolic regulation of the cervical region, illustrating how the viscera's relation to the surrounding tissues facilitates systemic homeostasis (Chait et al., 2020). This organization reflects both anatomical precision and physiological necessity. Adjacent to the cervical viscera, the vulnerability of surrounding tissues to pathological processes is extensive and necessitates their relationships to be understood to prevent and manage complications. Heterotopic ossification, for example, as much as it has occurred within soft tissues and muscles, can affect the functional mobility of the neck and surrounding visceral organs by way of abnormal bone formation (Carolyn et al., 2019). The cervical viscera are closely related to muscular and osseous elements, which means that inflammation, trauma, or surgery in one area can have sequelae on neighboring organs. The proximity of the trachea and esophagus to neurovascular groups presents hazards in disease or iatrogenic trauma capable of compromising critical functions like airway patency or perfusion. Therefore, the viscerally connected relationship of cervical viscera with nearby anatomical structures demands careful consideration during the process of clinical diagnosis and treatment (Figure 14.4).

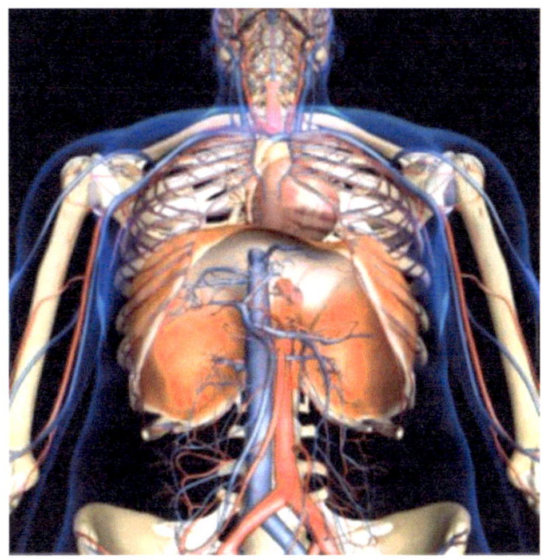

Figure 14.4. Relationship to surrounding structures.

Source: https://beachealth.com/wp-content/uploads/2023/03/Untitled-design-17-300x300.jpg.

Test Your Knowledge

1. What is the anatomical significance of the sternal angle (Angle of Louis)?
2. What is the relationship of the diaphragm to surrounding thoracic and abdominal structures?

14.2. Muscles of the Neck

Learning Outcome

1. Discuss the Superficial Muscles
2. Understand Deep Muscles
3. Know Functions of Neck Muscles

An understanding of the complex anatomy of the neck requires an understanding of the muscular components that facilitate its compound motion range and maintain essential functions. The muscles of the neck are generally divided into superficial, prevertebral, and infrahyoid muscles, each playing a different role to the mobility and stability of the neck. Superficial muscles such as the sternocleidomastoid participate in head rotation and flexion but deeper prevertebral muscles stabilize the cervical spine and offer fine motor movement.

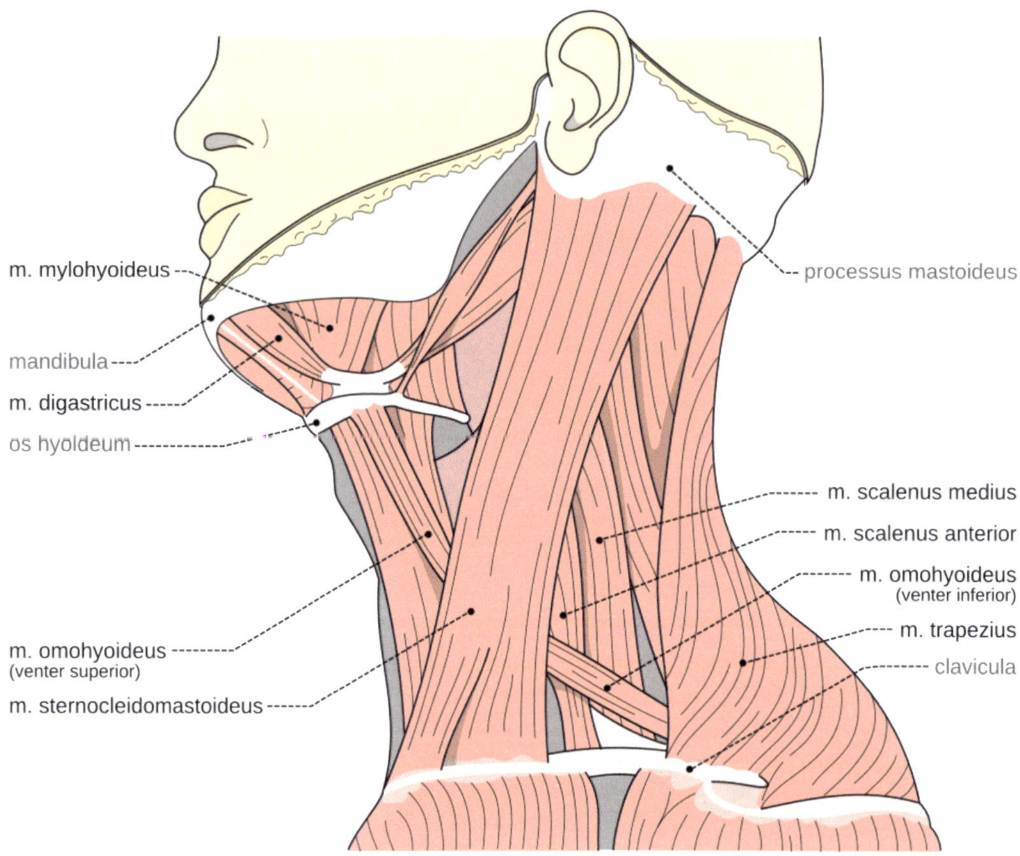

Figure 14.5. Muscles of the neck.

Source: By Olek Remesz (wiki-pl: Orem, commons: Orem) - Own work, based on this picture from Gray's Anatomy., CC BY-SA 2.5, https://commons.wikimedia.org/w/index.php?curid=2339732

The muscles not only permit movement but also cover and protect the integrity of the cervical viscera, including the trachea, esophagus, and neurovascular bundles. Functional defects of these muscles usually present as pain or limited movement, highlighting their clinical relevance in disorders of the cervical spine and neck, particularly in diseases such as radiculopathy where intervention needs to take into account muscular endurance and rehabilitation procedures (Peolsson et al., 2013). Physiological and pathological relationships of neck muscles go beyond simple biomechanics to affect neurological and endocrine functions of the cervical region. Some genetic mutations, such as those occurring in the LHX3 gene, have been linked to development abnormalities in the form of restricted rotation of the neck because of muscular and vertebral column structural malformations. The molecular observations show how musculature malformations may occur at the same time as hormone-secreting gland and sensory system deficiencies, such as hearing loss. These findings highlight the importance of muscular integrity in the maintenance of not just mechanical function but also neurological health and cervical stability. High-resolution imaging tests have supported that malformation of joint and muscle at the occipito-atlanto-axial complex has the potential to severely impair neck mobility, which demonstrates the interdependence of muscular anatomy with cervical viscera and neuroendocrine tissue (Kriström et al., 2009). Therapeutic treatments for dysfunction of the neck muscles emphasize conservative and surgical treatments, more recently with a greater interest in physiotherapy as a first line. Randomized controlled trials comparing anterior cervical decompression and fusion (ACDF) with directed physiotherapy demonstrate no clinically significant differences in improving neck muscle endurance and active range of motion, suggesting that non-surgical treatment appropriately augments muscular function and motor control of the hand. This underlines the potential of focused neck muscle exercises and cognitive-behavioral approaches in the rehabilitation of radiculopathy patients without risking surgery. The best performance by muscles is hence of paramount significance to ensure cervical viscera well-being, since compromised musculature might exacerbate spinal cord or nerve root compression, reflecting neurologic outcomes and general QoL (Peolsson et al., 2013) (Figure 14.5).

14.2.1. Superficial Muscles

An appreciation of the anatomy of the neck requires an understanding of the layering intricacy held within this region. Deep to the skin is a system of superficial musculature that serves crucial roles in protection and function. These muscles are fundamentally responsible for providing movement of the head and neck, including rotation, flexion, and extension, thereby facilitating a variety of critical daily activities like communication and airway protection. Trapezius and sternocleidomastoid are superficial muscles that are prominent with postural as well as dynamic actions over the cervical area. This strategic position not only reflects their mechanical importance but also their function of regulating the protection as well as the exposure of the cervical visceras. The intimate relationship between these surface structures and internal anatomical components underscores the manner in which dysfunction or abnormality of these muscles' shape or function can have far-reaching clinical ramifications (Clark et al., 1906). Functional architecture of superficial muscle is more than mere motion; in certain mammals, these muscles contribute directly to respiratory mechanics, towards an evolutionary window on their importance. Experiments on such animals as the bottlenose dolphin indicate that superficial and cervical muscles play an active part in modulating thoracic cavity volume during episodes of rapid ventilation. For example, muscles like the sternomastoid and scalene group of muscles retract the sternum and ribs cranio-dorsally to assist inspiration, where there is a high-level coupling between cervical musculature and breathing function. This biomechanical relationship suggests that superficial neck muscles may have significant functions in respiratory economy, adapting to the organism's locomotor activity and environmental demands.

The fast-twitch composition of these species' muscle fibers suggests the ability for rapid forceful contractions necessary for survival processes, providing information transferable by analogy to human cervical muscle function (Cotten et al., 2009). Clinically, superficial cervical muscles serve as landmarks and functional structures in the complex cervico-visceral scheme. Their anatomical arrangement forms a surface map in recognizing deeper structures like carotid arteries, jugular veins, and thyroid gland that are located beneath the muscular layers. Damage or dysfunction of these superficial muscles, either through trauma, overuse, or neurologic deficit may lead to secondary complications of the vascular or visceral structures they overlay. Muscle derangement may generate abnormal posture, restricted cervical motion, or even compromise of neurovascular circulation, underscoring the value of a clear understanding of their anatomy and physiology in diagnosing and treating them. Thus, anatomy of such superficial muscles offers necessary knowledge not only for anatomy education but also for complementing clinical treatments in the area of the neck and cervical viscera (Clark et al., 1906).

14.2.2. Deep Muscles

The complex anatomy of the neck includes several layers of muscle that contribute to its functional complexity. Deep to the superficial muscles are the deep neck muscles, which play an important role in maintaining cervical stability and facilitating fine motor function. The deep muscles are precisely positioned about the cervical vertebrae and can perform subtle movements such as segmental flexion, extension, and rotation. Their single direction and attachment points allow them to support the weight of the head and aid in posture and to protect the important cervical viscera and neurovascular structures. Understanding their deeper musculature anatomy is required to obtain an understanding of the relationship between cervical musculoskeletal (MSK) integrity and the physiological function of the cervical viscera, representing the need for high-level anatomical data in clinical assessment and surgery (Frias et al., 2016). In this complex anatomy of both deep neck muscles, large muscle groups such as the longus colli and longus capitis are essential in both cervical motion and stability. These muscles, depending on their position relative to the anterior rest of cervical vertebrae, flex the neck but also shear uncontrolled motion, thus preventing injury to structures below them. These include the trachea, esophagus, and carotid sheath. Deep muscles also comprise the biomechanical setting which stabilizes cervical viscera and thereby influences their function and mobility. For instance, the activity and tone of these muscles regulate cervical viscera spatial arrangement, hence such processes as swallowing and respiration. Their sensory functions, e.g., nociceptive feedback from the region, indicate their significance in pain modulation and pathologies of the neck, underlining muscular anatomy-viscerosensory systems correlations (Smith et al., 2015). Their interaction with the nearby viscera is also underscored while elaborating their role in reflexive and protective responses. They contain proprioceptors and nociceptors that belong to the sensory feedback system of the cervical spines, significant for motor coordination and defensive reflexes to harm. Stimulation of transient receptor potential channels within the viscerosensory nociceptive system shows how deep muscles are engaged not merely mechanically but also in integrating sensation. This duality is important in understanding cervical pain syndromes because muscular misalignment or dysfunction will affect the perception of visceral pain from structures such as the pharynx or larynx. Thus, deep neck muscles' anatomical and physiological characteristics reveal their essential function both in the mechanical organization of the neck and in the complex sensory network between cervical muscles and viscera (Smith et al., 2015; Frias et al., 2016) (Figure 14.6).

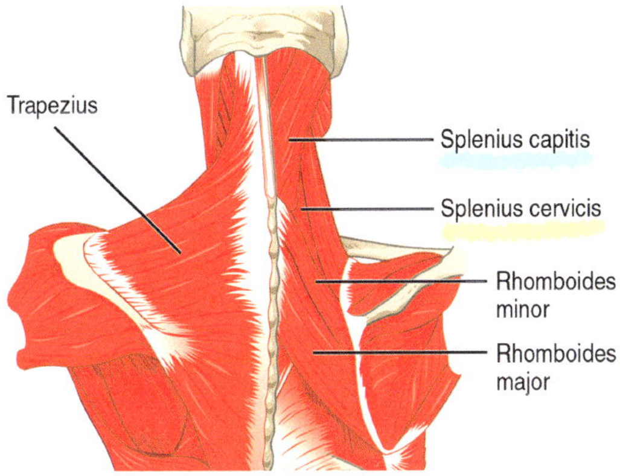

Figure 14.6. Deep muscles.

Source: Geeky Medics. (2019). *Splenius Capitis and Splenius Cervicis Muscles.*

14.2.3. Functions of Neck Muscles

The complex anatomy of the neck enables a range of essential physiological functions, in which the muscular anatomy is the driving force. Neck muscles play an essential part in head stability and movement, such as flexion, extension, rotation, and lateral flexion. All these movements are vital for the ability to perform daily living activities such as visual orientation, communication, and balance in posture. Besides, these muscles protect cervical vital structures by forming a dynamic protective system around the cervical viscera, including the airway and alimentary tract.

The complexity of these functions is supplemented by the fascial layering of the neck, of which alar fascia is a prominent member. This fascial layer offers not only mechanical support but also houses neurovascular structures, which suggests that the associated muscles may have an indirect function in physiological processes such as separation of infection and maintenance of the structural integrity of the spaces of the connective tissue in the neck (Snosek et al., 2020). Neck muscles are more than just mere mechanical movement and engage in critical physiological functions in association with breathing and cardiovascular homeostasis. The coordination between the diaphragm and the neck muscles, extending into the upper thoracic area, reflects a complex network of functional relationships covering the core musculature of the body. Fascial connections between the cervical muscles and the thoracic diaphragm ensure that their simultaneous actions facilitate proper breathing and oxygenation. This integration emphasizes that neck muscles are not isolated entities but contribute to the total operation of the respiratory machinery. Besides, the anatomic and neurologic complexity with which these muscle groups are involved, including their interrelation with the phrenic and vagus nerves, testifies to their role of modulating cardiopulmonary dynamics (Bordoni et al., 2013).

This interaction qualifies them for multi-functionality besides voluntary movement, with a bearing on systemic physiological stability. Functional significance of the muscles of the neck also encompasses their part in guarding cervical viscera against invasion by pathogens and supporting centers of neural control in the neck. The fascial elements, which are specialized to make up the alar fascia, are arranged in compartments that limit the spread of infection, a feature inherently reliant upon the tension and tone of underlying muscles to preserve these barriers. The neurovascular burden in these fascia and muscles also contributes to their role for cervical homeostasis. By modulating vascular resistance and neural conductance pathways of the cervical region, the muscles indirectly contribute to cervical organ function modulation. The muscles of the neck thus function as mechanical effectors of movement and guardians of physiological continuity and protection of cervical viscera defense (Snosek et al., 2020).

Test Your Knowledge

1. Which two muscles are considered major superficial muscles of the anterior neck?
2. What is the primary function of the sternocleidomastoid muscle?

14.3. Vascular Structures

Learning Outcome

1. Explain the Major Arteries of the Neck
2. Discuss the Major Veins of the Neck
3. Know Lymphatic Drainage

The complex neck anatomy houses crucial vascular tissues that are in charge of maintaining cerebral and systemic perfusion. The carotid arteries, including the common, internal, and external branches, form the prominent arterial supply to the head and neck, branching normally to nourish various tissues and organs. Parallel to the arteries are the jugular veins that are accountable for venous outflow from the brain, face, and cervical regions. Their juxtaposition with critical neural pathways underscores the fragility and intricacy of the cervical vascular supply. Pathology and anatomical variations in these vessels can dramatically influence clinical outcome, e.g., compromised blood supply or nerve compression.

Clinicians managing neck trauma, tumor, or vascular disease of the cervical viscera must be aware of this vascular arrangement. Among the vascular components of the cervical region, the lymphatic components have a significant role to play in the maintenance of tissue fluid homeostasis as well as immunoprotection. The recent advances in surgical techniques highlight the critical function of lymph node flaps, especially in the management of lymphedema using vascularized lymph node transfer (VLNT).

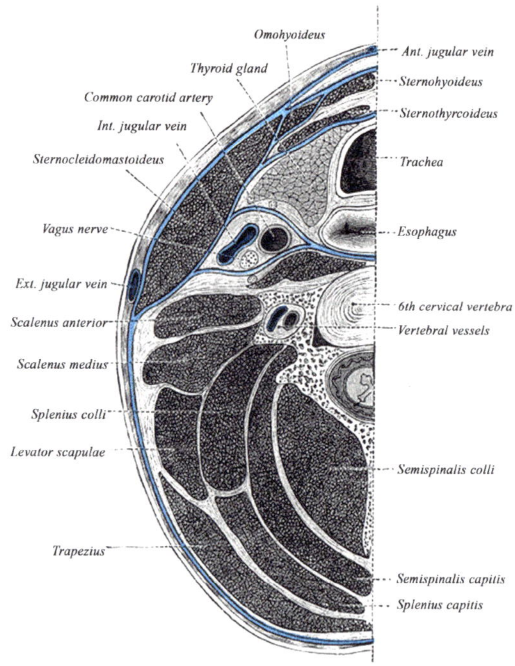

Figure 14.7. Vascular structures.

Source: By Henry Vandyke Carter - Henry Gray (1918) Anatomy of the Human Body (See "Book" section below)Bartleby.com: Gray's Anatomy, Plate 384, Public Domain, https://commons.wikimedia.org/w/index.php?curid=561537

This technique involves microvascular transplantation of healthy lymph nodes that can be harvested from cervical, axillary, or inguinal basins and are all part of the regional lymphatic network. The efficiency of VLNT in the reversal of physiological lymph flow underscores the functional significance of such lymphatic vessels alongside the traditional arterial and venous system. These findings illustrate the way a thorough understanding of vascular as well as lymphatic anatomy can inform meaningful therapeutic interventions to cervical and extremity lymphedema treatment (Mark et al., 2018). Neck vascular anomalies and pathologies can also be caused by neoplastic processes, necessitating meticulous diagnostic and therapeutic measures. Osteochondromas, for example, although primarily bone tumors, can compress adjacent vascular structures with ensuing vessel compression and compromised blood flow. These neoplasms are benign outgrowths but can be symptomatic when they are in close proximity to large cervical veins or arteries. Thickness of cartilaginous cap greater than specific thresholds can suggest malignant transformation, with surgical resection being indicated to prevent persistent vascular compromise or local recurrence. The correlation between bony lesions and overlying vasculature is hence an important consideration in the management of cervical pathologies (Tepelenis et al., 2021) (Figure 14.7).

14.3.1. Major Arteries of the Neck

The blood supply to the neck is significant not just to provide oxygenated blood to the viscera of the cervical area but also to support the vital activities of the head and brain. Among the great arteries, the common carotid artery is in a mid-position by ascending on both sides along the neck before branching off into the internal and external carotid arteries. The internal carotid artery mainly supplies the brain, and the external carotid artery supplies the face and scalp. Their topography and pattern of branching are significant due to their intimate anatomical relationships with important nerves and cervical structures and are therefore susceptible to damage in traumatic disorders of the neck. Understanding these arterial routes is crucial in the clinical environment, particularly during surgical operations and cervical imaging (Clark et al., 1906). The complex arterial arrangement is reflective of the physiological needs as well as evolutionary trade-off within the cervical viscera. Besides the common carotid artery, the vertebral artery is also a conspicuous vessel that traverses the neck, ascending through the transverse foramina of the cervical vertebrae. This artery also makes a significant contribution to posterior cerebral circulation by uniting its counterpart to form the basilar artery at the base of the skull. The course of the vertebral artery highlights the close association between the cervical vertebrae and the vascular system, with very important implications for spinal cord perfusion and neurological health. Injury or compression of the vertebral artery with cervical motion or trauma could lead to clinical syndromes of ischemia or vertebrobasilar insufficiency. Close anatomical relationship underscores the significance of intimate understanding of cervical arterial anatomy in the evaluation of pathologies of the neck and cervical viscera (Prykhodko et al., 2019). In addition to these major arteries, smaller but significant arteries such as the thyrocervical trunk and costocervical trunk arise from the subclavian artery, all of which supply the thyroid gland, muscles of the neck, and structures of the upper thorax. These branches not only support the metabolic needs of the cervical musculature but also supply the thyroid and parathyroid glands, highlighting the neck's vascular structure and glandular function dependency. These branches must be known by clinicians while operating, for instance, thyroidectomy, not to inadvertently produce vascular injury leading to uncontrolled hemorrhage. Also, pathological mechanisms such as arteriosclerosis or trauma to such arteries influence cervical viscera functions, and this makes their anatomical understanding all the more relevant in treatment and diagnosis (Clark et al., 1906).

14.3.2. Major Veins of the Neck

Understanding the venous anatomy of the cervical region is necessary to appreciate the physiological drainage of the neck and head. The great veins of the neck are significant channels that facilitate the return of oxygen-depleted blood towards the heart and maintain intracranial pressure balance. Of these, the internal jugular vein is of most importance due to its direct communication with the dural venous sinuses and its role in draining blood from the brain, face, and superficial neck. The external jugular vein, although smaller but clinically important, drains superficial tissues of the head and neck and is often utilized as an outwardly visible anatomical landmark during surgery. Along with the anterior jugular vein and its tributaries, these veins form a good network for the proper venous drainage, which is essential in healthy physiology and also in pathology of the cervical viscera. The internal jugular vein starts at the jugular foramen, descending with the carotid artery down the carotid sheath. It receives tributaries from thyroid, lingual, and facial veins, incorporating venous drainage of regions such as thyroid gland and oral cavity. Internally, the internal jugular vein is used for central venous catheterization on a routine basis because it is easily accessed and relatively available with ease of recognition, illustrating its procedural importance. The external jugular vein, which lies superficial to the sternocleidomastoid muscle, drains the blood of the face and scalp and empties into the subclavian vein. Being superficial, it is at risk of injury but, conversely, allows non-invasive central venous pressure measurement, an important sign in a number of cardiovascular conditions. Such anatomical associations highlight the importance of knowledge of the venous anatomy of the neck to avoid complications during medical interventions (Smith et al., 2015). While the venous anatomy of the neck is primarily focused on the internal and external jugular veins, care must be taken for the anterior jugular vein due to its involvement in superficial drainage and also due to its anatomical variation. This vein descends inferiorly, typically along the midline, before it drains into the external jugular or its direct connection with the subclavian vein. Plexiform anastomoses with it are of major collateral importance, especially when larger venous channels are obstructed. These venous anastomoses need to be appreciated during neck surgeries, such as tracheostomies or thyroidectomies, to minimize hemorrhagic consequences. In addition, the complex autonomic innervation of such veins, predominantly studied elsewhere, provokes complex interaction between vascular and neural elements still not well elaborated but increasingly relevant to surgical planning and pain relief (Sienkiewicz-Zawilińska et al., 2018). Such interaction underscores the continuing need for wide anatomical and clinical training regarding the major neck veins as part of the general background of cervical viscera (Figure 14.8).

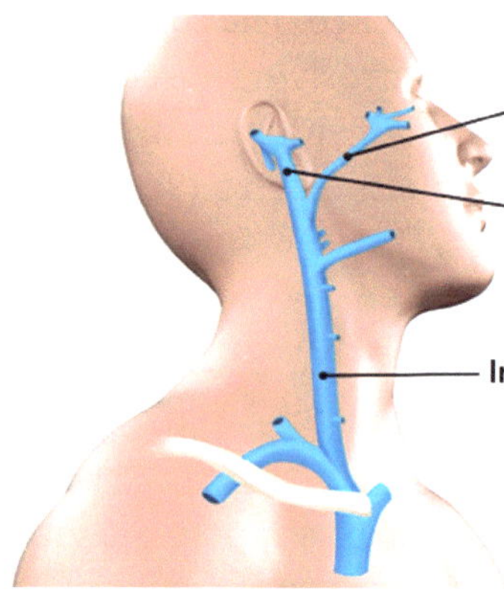

Figure 14.8. Major veins of the neck.

Source: Taweevat A., & Kunlawat, T. (2020). Examination of the neck veins. *N. Engl. J. Med., 383*(24), e132.

14.3.3. Lymphatic Drainage

The complex networks of vessels in the neck and cervical regions are not only important for circulation but also for immune function, notably through lymphatic drainage. The system of drainage is vital for fluid balance and immune cell traffic, a means to clear toxins and pathogens from tissues. Lymph vessels course with veins and arteries in the cervical area, draining lymph to regional lymph nodes. They are biological filters, activating immune response to foreign antigens. In view of the anatomical intricacy of the neck, especially around the viscera of the cervical area, lymphatic drainage is inextricably bound with adjacent structures such as the thyroid gland, trachea, and esophagus. Therefore, the knowledge of the path and role of lymphatic tracts is vital in the diagnosis and treatment of infections, malignancies, or inflammatory illnesses of the neck and associated viscera. The lymphatic system of the thyroid gland illustrates the vital significance of lymphatic drainage of the cervical area. Situated in front of the trachea, lymphatic channels of the gland empty into deep cervical nodes along the carotid sheath, facilitating removal of metabolic waste and cellular debris generated by hormonal activity. This drainage route also explains metastasis of thyroid malignancies to cervical lymph nodes, emphasizing the clinical significance of precise anatomical knowledge for surgical intervention. Proper knowledge of the lymphatic routes around the thyroid is needed to avoid complications such as lymphedema or nerve injury during thyroidectomy. Additionally, the thyroid's association with neural structures such as the recurrent laryngeal nerve reveals the manner in which lymphatic drainage patterns can direct surgical management and assist in delivering effective therapeutic interventions (Samantha et al., 2019). Extrathyroidal meningeal lymphatic network is a novel idea of lymphatic drainage relevant to the cervical area and CNS interaction. Unlike previous postulates that the brain lacked conventional lymph vessels, recent studies confirm meningeal lymphatics assist in cerebrospinal fluid (CSF) clearance to cervical lymph nodes. This increased drainage system is a central regulator of immune surveillance and CNS waste removal and links neurological health with cervical lymphatic function. Dysfunction of this drainage has been linked to neuroinflammatory and neurodegenerative disorders, suggesting that cervical lymphatic pathways establish peripheral as well as central immunity. This new paradigm demands integrating meningeal lymphatic anatomy into the larger context of neck and cervical viscera, underlining its therapeutic potential in the management of neurological disorders (Pal et al., 2020).

Test Your Knowledge

1. Which artery is the main source of blood supply to the head and neck?
2. Which lymph nodes are primarily responsible for draining the head and neck region?

14.4. Nervous System Components

Learning Outcome

1. Discuss the Cranial Nerves in the Neck
2. Explain the Brachial Plexus
3. Focus in Autonomic Nervous System

Within the complex area of the neck and cervical viscera, the nervous system contains a complex interplay of central and peripheral structures that are significant for sensory and motor purposes. Of these, the cranial nerves stand out due to their unique origin and mode of distribution. While 10 of the 12 cranial nerves are derived from the brainstem and are peripheral nerves covered with Schwann cells, olfactory and optic nerves branch out as CNS outgrowths, covered with oligodendrocytes. They develop through foramina at the base of the skull to innervate structures of the head and neck to carry motor commands and sensory stimuli. Their cisternal courses, bathed in CSF within the arachnoid mater, expose them to a wide array of pathological conditions. Imaging methods such as magnetic resonance imaging (MRI) play a significant role in their assessment, allowing for both the structural and functional evaluation necessary for accurate diagnosis and treatment (Rueda-Lopes, 2021). Regulation of involuntary cervical and neck physiological processes requires complex structure of the autonomic nervous system, a subsystem of the peripheral nervous system (PNS) consisting of the sympathetic, parasympathetic, and enteric branches. The sympathetic nervous system is overall influence by a two-neuron efferent system, intensifying cardiovascular activity but depressing digestive motility, consistent with the fight-or-flight response. On the other hand, the parasympathetic nervous system acts particularly on the head, viscera, and genitalia, to allow rest and digestive functions with localized effects such as decreased heart rate and increased gastrointestinal motility. This balance provides homeostatic maintenance of processes essential to survival. Neurotransmitter chemistry between these divisions—presynaptic neurons predominantly acetylcholine and postsynaptic neurons either norepinephrine or acetylcholine—provides another level of sophistication in fine-tuning these physiological reactions (Su et al., 2023). Beyond the cranial and autonomic nerves, peripheral nervous structures containing cervical viscera integrate sensory and motor output in a way to support necessary functions such as respiration, swallowing, and blood vessel maintenance. The accessory nerve, through its singular origin within the brainstem and spinal cord, innervates muscles crucial to movements of the neck, demonstrating the manner in which neural pathways through the cervical spine influence mechanical as well as autonomic functions. The complex network of neural fibers requires precise imaging and anatomical know-how to pick up on pathology, for example, inflammation, neoplasms, or trauma. High-resolution imaging techniques such as neurography enable one to visualize nerve fascicles and integrity so that clinicians can identify structural abnormalities and patterns of denervation relevant to full patient care (Rueda-Lopes, 2021) (Figure 14.9).

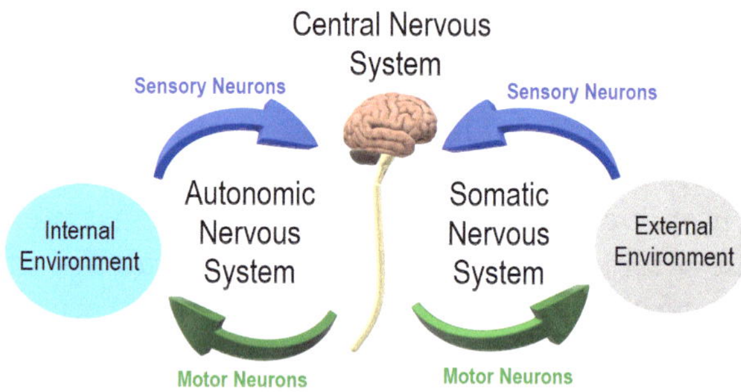

Figure 14.9. Nervous system components.

Source: By Christinelmiller - Own work, CC BY-SA 4.0, https://commons.wikimedia.org/w/index.php?curid=90773326

14.4.1. Cranial Nerves in the Neck

Among the complex neural networks governing the head and neck region, cranial nerves are primary mediators of both sensory and motor functions. These nerves also course through the cervical region, where their interactions with muscular and vascular components orchestrate basic physiological processes. For example, the vagus nerve, or cranial nerve X, courses down to the neck, innervating a number of visceral organs and participating in autonomic regulation, including cardiovascular and respiratory processes. Its complex branching pattern allows for precise control and modulation of these vital systems. An understanding of the course and relationship of such cranial nerves in the neck is necessary to appreciate their integrative roles in homeostasis and their clinical significance in neck diseases and cervical viscera (Ahmed et al., 2022). This anatomical complexity underscores the necessity for precision in mapping and identification of cranial nerve distribution in the clinical context. Somatosensory and visceral sensory components of cranial nerves in the neck are equally complicated, relaying critical information to the CNS. They arise from specific sensory ganglia, each with distinct neurodevelopmental origins from neural crest cells and placodal sources. These two embryonic origins account for the tremendous diversity of neuron types in the cervical region that serve sensory modalities critical for reflexes and homeostatic regulation. Single-cell transcriptomic studies have begun to uncover molecular diversity and transcriptional regulation of cranial sensory ganglia development and function. This emerging appreciation helps to clarify how sensory inputs from the neck region influence broader neural circuits that are responsible for maintaining internal physiological homeostasis (Vermeiren et al., 2020). The convergence of sensory and motor pathways within the neck demonstrates the complexity of cranial nerve function in this anatomical space. Beyond anatomy, the clinical significance of cranial nerve involvement in the neck highlights the importance of specificity in neuromodulatory therapies. The extensive innervation of thoracic and abdominal organs by the vagus nerve makes it an attractive target for therapeutic VNS techniques in managing conditions ranging from epilepsy to cardiovascular and gastrointestinal diseases. Inter-individual variation in nerve anatomy necessitates an approach to stimulate selective discrete nerve fibers or fascicles to exert therapeutic effects with minimal side effects. Emerging technologies that increase targeting of the vagal fibers or branches, along with understanding of neural-electrode interfaces, promise improved efficacy in neuromodulation. Therefore, an in-depth understanding of cranial nerve anatomy and physiology within the neck is at the pinnacle of developing precision medicine at a clinical level (Ahmed et al., 2022). This represents the intersection of anatomical understanding and technological innovation in addressing pathology of the neck and cervical viscera.

14.4.2. Brachial Plexus

The complex network of nerves from the cervical region gives rise to upper limb function, and the brachial plexus is one such fine example of complexity. The brachial plexus, located in the neck and extending into the axilla, is made up of nerve roots of the anterior rami of the spinal nerves C5 to T1. This anatomical organization allows it to function as a vital route for motor and sensory innervation of the hand, arm, and shoulder. Knowledge of the spatial relationships of the brachial plexus to the adjacent cervical viscera is relevant to both its normal physiology and its clinical issues. Its anatomical proximity to the scalene muscles and subclavian vessels explains the importance of this region in most medical procedures and potential compressions or damages to the nerves in trauma or surgery (Smith et al., 2015). The organization of the brachial plexus into roots, trunks, divisions, cords, and branches gives a hint of the complicated neural structure of upper limb function. Each segment is correlated with specific muscle groups and dermatomes, linking cervical nerve roots with peripheral nerve targets. Such organization highlights the plexus as an interface between the central and PNSs incorporated within the cervical viscera. Moreover, the close relationship with neighboring fascial layers and integumentary structures shows how disruption, i.e., fascial scarring or inflammation, can have effects beyond the visible tissue, impacting nerve function and potentially causing complex symptomatology with both motor and sensory deficiency (Bordoni et al., 2013). These interactions emphasize the necessity of a unified knowledge of the brachial plexus in the anatomical context of the neck. The clinical significance of the anatomy of the brachial plexus as it relates to the cervical viscera is profound, particularly with reference to traumatic or iatrogenic injury leading to loss of arm mobility and sensation. Compression syndromes, such as the thoracic outlet syndrome seen when the plexus is compressed between the anatomical structures like scalene muscles and clavicle, are well established. Pathologic processes within the cervical viscera, like inflammation or neoplasms, may also compress these nerves. Detailed anatomical knowledge, as required by fundamental medical competencies, is vital for clinicians who treat these disorders. It enables precise diagnosis and intervention strategies, ranging from physical therapy for fascial disruption to surgical decompression for neural function restoration, to ultimately enhance patient outcomes in the case of brachial plexus compromise (Smith et al., 2015).

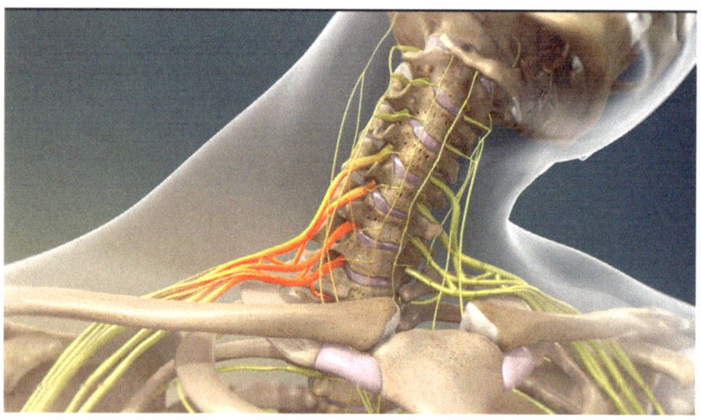

Source: https://d2yjegym0lbr1w.cloudfront.net/thumbs/burnersstingers_1280.jpg?v=20151030.

14.4.3. Autonomic Nervous System

The complex system governing involuntary physiological occurrences in the neck and cervical region is made up of a vital part known as the autonomic nervous system. It is an unconscious system that governs important functions like vascular tone, glandular secretion, and smooth muscle activity in cervical viscera. In particular, sympathetic and parasympathetic divisions of the autonomic nervous system have complementary but opposing effects on such tissues, offering homeostasis as well as adaptive physiological response to environmental stimuli. Sympathetic fibers play a part in vasoconstriction and blood flow regulation, while parasympathetic inputs primarily regulate secretory activities of glands such as salivary and thyroid glands. Identification of these autonomic controls becomes critical to understanding how systemic changes in metabolism can affect cervical function, as the role of faulty adipose tissue in metabolic diseases altering systemic autonomic homeostasis and influencing cervical circulatory mechanisms illustrates (Chait et al., 2020). Beyond its fundamental role in homeostatic regulation, the autonomic nervous system of the cervical region also participates in sophisticated neurophysiological dialogue controlling sensory input and reflex response. For instance, the vagus nerve, a primary parasympathetic pathway, innervates many cervical viscera and conveys afferent inputs to the brainstem, thus integrating central and peripheral autonomic feedback. Newly emerging therapeutic devices such as auricular VNS take advantage of such pathways for autonomic output management, enhancing conditions ranging from inflammatory syndromes to cardiovascular dysfunction. These neuromodulatory approaches underscore the potential of autonomic pathway targeting in the neck for modulation of systemic disease mechanisms and facilitation of physiological homeostasis (Kaniu et al., 2019). Recognition of the physiological and therapeutic significance of these pathways provides key context for their role in the cervical viscera. Further, the functional interplay between autonomic innervation and parasympathetic targets within the cervical region extends to cardiovascular control and metabolic regulation, emphasizing the systemic relevance. The autonomic system's regulatory role maintains vascular tone of cervical veins and arteries, influencing directly cerebral perfusion and systemic arterial blood pressure. Vascular tone changes of autonomic signals in the neck can induce pathologies like hypertension and metabolic syndromes due to adipose tissue dysfunction. These connections reveal the importance of the cervical autonomic network as a composite interface that integrates neurovascular and metabolic signals given that abnormal adipose depots cause inflammatory and cardiovascular pathologies via autonomic dysregulation mechanisms (Chait et al., 2020). Hence, the cervical autonomic nervous system plays a critical role in maintaining local and global well-being, which highlights its importance in clinical research of neck and cervical viscera functions.

Test Your Knowledge

1. What is the function of the external carotid artery in the neck?
2. Which lymph nodes are primarily responsible for draining the head and neck region?

14.5. Cervical Viscera Overview

Learning Outcome

1. Definition and Importance
2. Explain the Types of Cervical Viscera
3. Know Functional Roles

The cervical viscera constitute a multitude of vital organs in the complex neck anatomy, which play significant functions in respiratory, digestive, and endocrine activities. The cervical fascia encloses these structures that lie anterior to the cervical spine and are made up of the pharynx, larynx, trachea, thyroid and parathyroid glands, and esophagus. The three-dimensional configuration accommodates complex neurovascular relationships that are vital for important functions such as phonation, respiration, and swallowing. The larynx, which sits superiorly in the neck, is a conduit to the lower respiratory tract and houses the vocal cords. Inferior to this is the trachea, which is an airway conduit to the lungs. Posterior and lateral to the trachea is the esophagus, the central conduit of alimentary transit. This functional and anatomical complexity is highlighted by the encompassing cervical spine, the stability and alignment of which provide essential protection to such soft tissues and associated neural structures (Kerr, 2000). Endocrine regulation of the cervical viscera is under the predominant control of the parathyroid and thyroid glands, which are heavily invested in the lower anterior neck. The wing-like thyroid gland is closely associated with the trachea and larynx, and plays a vital role in metabolic homeostasis by hormone synthesis. Proper embryological development and vascularization allow it to regulate systemic metabolism, calcium, and growth. The four small posterior nodules on the thyroid lobes, parathyroid glands, regulate calcium and phosphate equilibrium by secretion of parathyroid hormone (PTH). With their intimate association with respiratory and gastrointestinal organs, pathological alteration such as goiter or neoplasm can have a devastating impact on airway patency and on the dynamics of swallowing. Surgical procedures in this area need meticulous knowledge of this anatomy and physiology to prevent complications (Falk, 1998). Cervical viscera are also intimately embedded in the autonomic nervous system, which regulates their functioning and provides homeostasis in the dynamic setting of the neck. Parasympathetic and sympathetic innervations influence such functions as vascular tone, salivary secretion, and glandular activity. The vagus nerve, traveling through the carotid sheath adjacent to the cervical viscera, provides abundant motor supply to the larynx and parasympathetic fibers to thoracic and abdominal viscera. The cervical sympathetic chain also regulates vasomotor control required for local perfusion. This neural coordination provides synchronized respiratory and digestive activity, metabolic demand adjustments, and protective reflexes. Because of the relatively small spaces of the neck, any pathological or traumatic injury to these viscera or their innervations can lead to emergent clinical symptoms, which explains the necessity for extensive knowledge of cervical viscera anatomy and physiology in clinical life (Kerr, 2000) (Figure 14.10).

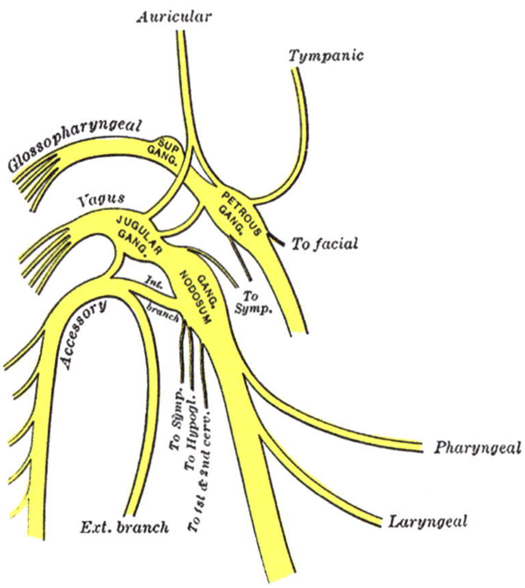

Figure 14.10. Overview of cervical viscera.

Source: By Henry Vandyke Carter - Henry Gray (1918) Anatomy of the Human Body (See "Book" section below)Bartleby.com: Gray's Anatomy, Plate 791, Public Domain, https://commons.wikimedia.org/w/index.php?curid=537001 Osmosis. (n.d.). *Cervical Viscera: Endocrine, Respiratory, and Alimentary Layers.*

14.5.1. Definition and Importance

The complex anatomical structures of the neck are at the center of numerous vital physiological processes, and thus their study is central to the knowledge of human and comparative vertebrate biology. The cervical viscera, such as the larynx, pharynx, thyroid gland, and associated neurovascular structures, are housed in a limited space that enables them to participate significantly in respiration, phonation, digestion, and endocrine regulation. This complex assembly adapts dynamically to permit head movements and perform specialized functions, underscoring the importance of maintaining structural integrity and functional coordination in the cervical spine. Data from multiple species, including avian models, provide insights into how evolutionary pressures and environmental demands shape the morphology and function of neck components, reaffirming their critical function across taxa (Christine et al., 2019). As such, the cervical viscera constitute a basic subject of study for medical, evolutionary, and functional anatomy. The boundaries and importance of the neck and cervical viscera extend beyond gross anatomy into the field of clinical relevance, particularly in diagnosis and surgery. The neck serves as a conduit and guarding chamber for the cervical viscera, which must maintain both mobility and stability against complex biomechanical forces. Pathology or disturbances of this region, including inflammatory, neoplastic, or traumatic diseases, can potentially jeopardize breathing, swallowing, and voice, and thus the significance of correct anatomical knowledge is obvious. Moreover, the sophistication of medical imaging modalities now allows for intimate assessment of the complex cervical anatomy, enabling diagnosis and treatment planning. These interdisciplinary approaches confirm that the neck and cervical viscera definition involve not only static anatomy, but also dynamic functional relationships that are required for the maintenance of homeostasis and QoL. Additionally, the neck and cervical viscera are of paramount importance in the field of interdisciplinary healthcare, where anatomy encounters several medical specialties.

For example, imaging modalities such as MR defecography, although primarily directed at disorders of the pelvis, emphasize the overall clinical need to visualize and evaluate soft tissue integrity and function within anatomically complex regions (João et al., 2019). Similarly, the unique arrangement of the cervical spine demands comprehensive knowledge to prevent surgical complications and optimize patient outcomes, especially given the closeness of critical neurovascular structures. Thus, the definition of cervical viscera encompasses both their anatomical structures and vital physiological functions, as well as the requirement of integrated research and clinical methods in the management of pathological conditions. Such a unified perspective reiterates the neck and cervical viscera as a significant region in both anatomical research and clinical practice.

14.5.2. Types of Cervical Viscera

Anatomy of the neck has a large array of structures vital to the physiology of the body known as the cervical viscera, which all perform a varied range of functions integral to physiological activity. Cervical viscera are broadly categorized into three primary groups: the respiratory, digestive, and endocrine structures. Of these, the respiratory viscera consist mainly of larynx, trachea, and pharynx, which provide passage for air to the lungs and play a role in the production of voice and protection of the lower airways. In the digestive category are the pharynx and upper esophagus, which act as pathways for food and liquids to enter the stomach. The endocrine viscera are mostly the thyroid and parathyroid glands, whose function is to regulate metabolism and calcium levels. Understanding these divisions highlights the close interdependence of structures within the neck required to facilitate essential body functions and thus proves the complexity of cervical viscera. This division is not only anatomical but also functional, as it highlights the central role of the neck in a variety of life-sustaining processes. In addition to conventional cervical viscera taxonomy, recent studies reveal molecular and pathological nuances that add to our understanding of these structures. As one example, epigenetic changes that take place in certain cancers of cervical viscera, such as head and neck squamous cell carcinomas secondary to HPV16 infection, illustrate dynamic interaction between cervical tissue and pathologic mechanisms. These tumors harbor typical methylation signatures encompassing specific genes, not just aiding in tumor categorization but perhaps influencing therapeutic responses and clinical behavior as well. These findings emphasize the value of considering cellular and molecular characteristics alongside anatomical and functional classes when studying cervical viscera. The relevance of this broader perspective is expansive and extends into diagnostic, predictive, and management strategies to cervical pathology, particularly those concerning the upper aerodigestive and neck endocrine organs (Berglund et al., 2022). And while awareness usually is drawn to soft tissue elements, certain bony components intimately interact or affect the cervical viscera and thus influence their clinical assessment. For example, vertebral hemangiomas, since they are not viscera themselves, are common benign vascular lesions of the cervical spine and can impact overlying cervical viscera either via mass effect or via mimicking metastatic disease on imaging studies. Staging of such lesions by MRI-signal patterns adds to the accuracy of diagnosis and aids in differentiation of such benign processes from malignancies involving cervical viscera. Their regular pattern of behavior and sluggish growth afford radiologists a way of monitoring the change without unnecessary intervention, thereby ensuring the structural and functional integrity of cervical viscera they cover. This radiologic data adds a valuable element to the whole concept and clinic management of neck region pathologies (Abul-Kasim et al., 2022) (Figure 14.11).

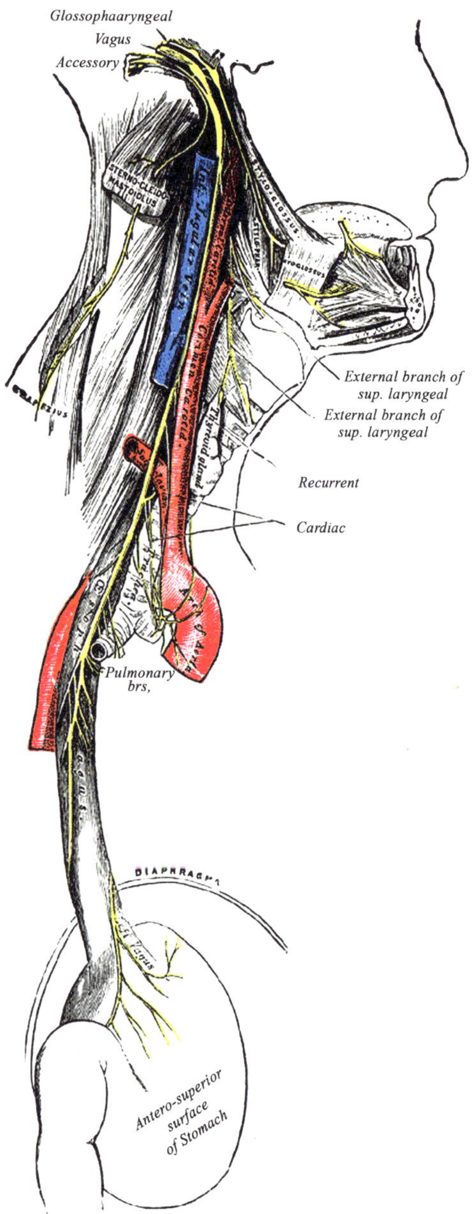

Figure 14.11. Types of cervical viscera.

Source: By Henry Vandyke Carter - Henry Gray (1918) Anatomy of the Human Body (See "Book" section below)Bartleby.com: Gray's Anatomy, Plate 793, Public Domain, https://commons.wikimedia.org/w/index.php?curid=526636

14.5.3. Functional Roles

The complex structures of the neck and cervical viscera account for a multitude of important functions that ensure homeostasis and sustain essential physiological processes. Among these, the vagus nerve function is particularly significant owing to its extensive distribution and parasympathetic regulation control. Through innervation of organs such as the heart, lungs, and digestive system, the vagus nerve modulates autonomic balance and the resulting cardiovascular and respiratory stability. Its ability to modulate organ function in both the afferent and efferent directions reflects the complexity of neuronal control within this anatomical region. Outside of neural pathways, breathing control through specific respiration patterns in the cervical region has been shown to affect the autonomic nervous system, potentially acting as a bridge between behavioral training and physiological improvement (Roderik et al., 2018). This highlights the collaborative functional domains of neural and visceral elements found in the neck region. Apart from neuronal mediation, the cervical viscera have critical roles regarding endocrine and immune system modulation. For example, the vagus nerve possesses anti-inflammatory effects by cytokine modulation of TNFα levels through direct and indirect mechanisms. Such neuroimmune interface is critical in preventing excess inflammatory response and immune homeostasis, such as in Crohn's disease. Modern therapeutic advances using VNS have promise for inflammatory process modulation with the cervical viscera's functional role highlighted to respond and dialogue with systemic immune processes (Bonaz et al., 2017). Therefore, the cervical viscera not only ensure mechanical and metabolic functions but directly contribute to immunological regulation, commenting on overall physiological resilience. In addition, the functional roles of the neck and cervical viscera involve integrative processes with respect to neurophysiology as well as systemic health.

Controlled breathing, often facilitated by the cervical anatomical region, influences vagal tone and also parasympathetic output, which in turn influence mental health and cognitive functioning. Controlled breathing exercises activate the vagus nerve, with neurophysiological benefits that are involved in stress modulation and enhanced autonomic control (Roderik et al., 2018). The cervical viscera are therefore engaged in a feedback loop between respiratory mechanics and neural activation that ultimately works to enhance physical as well as psychological health. This integration of neural, immune, and respiratory function in the neck highlights the multi-functionality of its tissues and offers valuable lessons for the development of therapeutic intervention exploiting these mechanisms.

Test Your Knowledge

1. Which organs are included in the endocrine part of the cervical viscera?
2. What structures make up the respiratory and alimentary parts of the cervical viscera?

14.6. The Pharynx

Learning Outcome

1. Discuss the Anatomy of the Pharynx
2. Know Functions of the Pharynx
3. Understand Clinical Significance

The region of the neck has anatomical refinement demanding careful scrutiny, particularly where it intersects passages integral to the respiratory and digestive systems. The pharynx is a model structure functioning as a vital passage connecting the nasal cavity and oral cavity with the larynx and esophagus. The position of the pharynx ideally within the cervical viscera allows coordinated access and passage of air and food through delicately regulated muscular and neural activities. The pharynx is separated into three regions—the nasopharynx, oropharynx, and laryngopharynx—each having different anatomical boundaries and responsibilities. The separation allows for the bimanual use of the pharynx as a respirator and deglutitor, highlighting its role in airway patency and diversion of ingested substances on swallowing. Understanding spatial relationships and functional integration of the pharynx within the neck is essential to understanding the broader anatomical and physiological context of the cervical viscera (Smith et al., 2015). The pharynx is neurologically controlled in the form of a complex interaction between several cranial nerves that organize swallowing and airway protection. Damage or lesions to these nerves, particularly the lower cranial nerves, often present clinically as signs of dysphagia, alteration in speech, or impairment in cough reflex, showing the dependence of the pharynx on precise neural control. Complex etiologies like vascular, traumatic, infectious, and neoplastic illnesses can affect nerve function, so one must possess broad anatomical and clinical information for diagnosis and treatment. The conduction function of the pharynx also entails it in numerous pathological processes which may incidentally include other adjacent structures of the neck, necessitating complete evaluation of the cervical viscera in cases of cranial nerve dysfunction or of oropharyngeal disease (Loidl et al., 2015). The histological structure of the pharynx also reflects its multivalency with the cervical viscera of the neck. Composed mainly of mucosal, muscular, and connective tissue layers, the pharynx reflects variations in epithelium type based on location exposure and function. The nasopharynx, for example, is covered by ciliated pseudostratified columnar epithelium to permit mucociliary clearance, while the oropharynx and laryngopharynx have stratified squamous epithelium for mechanical abrasion protection from food passage. Circular and longitudinal musculature fibers allow for the synchronized constriction and shortening of the musculature required for effective swallowing. The pharyngeal structural adjustments thus complement the central coordination function of the pharynx in controlling both breathing and digestive processes within the anatomical boundaries of the neck (Smith et al., 2015) (Figure 14.12).

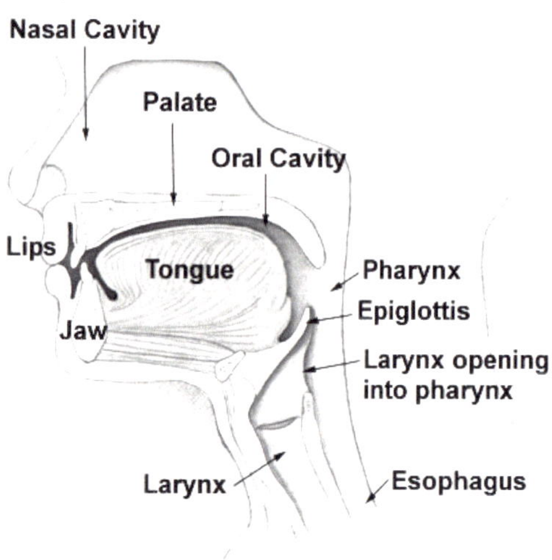

Figure 14.12. The pharynx.

Source: By Arcadian - http://training.seer.cancer.gov/head-neck/anatomy/overview.html, Public Domain, https://commons.wikimedia.org/w/index.php?curid=1678037

14.6.1. Anatomy of the Pharynx

The complex organization of fascial layers in the neck profoundly influences the anatomical structure of the pharynx, which acts as an essential passage in the cervical viscera. Such fascial components, particularly the intercarotid fascia or alar fascia, influence the compartmentalization of the pharyngeal space by forming separate compartments that impact its mobility as well as defense mechanisms. More dissection studies find this fascia as a strap of connective tissue that lies across carotid sheaths over midline structures and usually joins the visceral fascia that invests the pharynx. Its connectedness is where it derives strength but retains pliability to allow for required pharyngeal movement in critical physiological actions like swallowing and respiration. Understanding such fascial interactions is essential to surgical maneuvers and radiologic assessments because improper interpretation of these layers can contaminate clinical interventions in the cervical area (Feigl et al., 2020). The fascia thus serves as both a cover and a facilitator of pharyngeal dynamics in the cervical system. In addition to its anatomical content, the pharynxs functional sophistication is highlighted by its innervation that coordinates the stepwise stages of swallowing critical for nutrition and protection of the airway. Not only is the pharyngeal phase stimulated by mechanical contact but also through pharyngeal distension sensed by advanced neural circuitry. This phase is predominantly served by the pharyngeal plexus, comprising cranial nerves IX, X, and XI, supplemented by contributions from cranial nerves V, VII, IX, and XII. Further convergence with the cervical plexus and connections like the Ansa cervicalis serve MSK dynamics of the hyoid-laryngeal complex. Such neural coordination ensures the pharynx's easy transition from oropharyngeal bolus manipulation to esophageal propulsion, highlighting a complex motor control hierarchy critical in ensuring airway patency and successful swallowing (Melc, 2018). This coordination reflects the pharynxs two roles of feeding and breathing within the viscera of the neck. Morphologically, the pharynx is a fibromuscular tube with components of nasopharynx, oropharynx, and laryngopharynx, each having unique physiological functions that overlap surrounding neck structures. Striated muscular coats of constrictors and longitudinal fibers allow for dynamic diameter and shape changes to facilitate bolus transit and maintenance of resting airway. The fascial envelopes covering these muscles, including the prevertebral and visceral layers, serve to preserve space relations as they accommodate the pharynxs wide range of motion. This finespun anatomical arrangement testifies to evolutionary adaptation that has enhanced the pharynx to service both respiratory and digestive functions concurrently with ease. Moreover, the anatomical complexity needs proper clinical insight, particularly in the treatment of pathologic conditions like tumors or abscesses that exploit fascial spaces, substantiating the pharynxs central role within the network of cervical viscera (Feigl et al., 2020).

14.6.2. Functions of the Pharynx

The rich anatomy of the neck contains diverse vital structures, one of which is the pharynx that has a pivotal role in coordinating complex physiological activities. As a muscular tube, the pharynx is a vital conduit for the respiratory and digestive system along which air moves unimpeded to the larynx and esophagus for food and liquids, respectively. Neural control of these orderly movements involves multiple cranial nerves, including glossopharyngeal, vagus, and accessory nerves, which collectively govern the pharyngeal phase of swallowing. This phase is triggered not just by the presence of a food bolus but also by mechanoreceptive feedback of pharyngeal pressure distension, further establishing the pharynx's role as both motor and sensory center in swallowing. Through complicated muscular contractions, the pharynx enables sufficient bolus propulsion without compromising airway obstruction, emphasizing its functional importance in ensuring airway protection and functional swallowing processes (Melc, 2018). Besides its function in swallowing, the pharynx is involved in other significant physiological processes including phonation and breathing. Although voice production primarly takes place in the larynx,the pharyngeal musculature adjusts dynamically to change the topography and tension of the upper airway, and thus directly influences voice production and sound resonance. This complex adjustment is regulated by the coordination of various cranial nerves and cervical plexus inputs, regulating muscle functions like the motion of the hyoid bone and larynx. Dysfunction or lesions in these neural tracts may result in dysphagia, speech impairment, or impaired airway protection, proving the relevance of pharyngeal integrity to cervical viscera and appropriate neck function. Complete information about the multifunctionality of the pharynx is essential in the identification of disorders resulting from lower cranial nerve dysfunction as well as in treatment modality planning (Loidl et al., 2015). The pharynx is also protective in nature by integrating the reflexes that prevent aspiration and choking during swallow. This protection is regulated by a highly evolved neural complex of cranial nerves and centers of the brainstem to secure timely closure of the laryngeal inlet and opening of the esophagus. The pharyngeal phase of swallowing coordinates the motor output and sensory input to maintain respiratory and gastrointestinal tract separation during swallowing. Consistent with this, the coordination process leads to stimulation of the pharyngeal plexus and other muscles of the neck to raise the hyoid-laryngeal complex and assist in bolus stabilization. These coordinated movements exhibit the role of the pharynx as not only a passage but also as a basic organ to neurophysiologically control the cervical viscera in maintaining airway patency and effective food transmission to the esophagus (Melc, 2018).

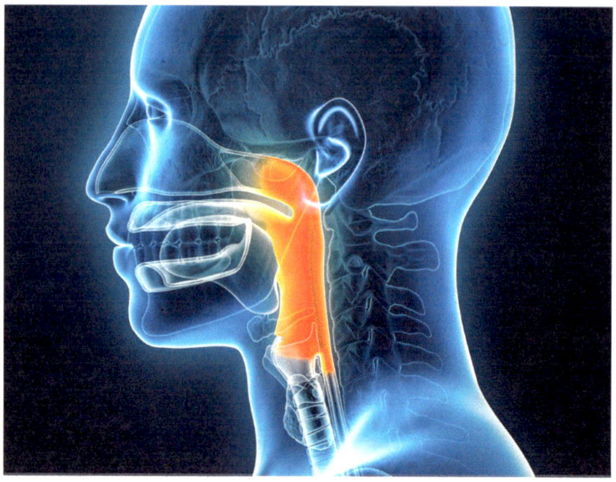

Source: eRemedium. (2024). *Pharynx Meaning in Tamil.*

14.6.3. Clinical Significance

The complex anatomy of the cervical viscera and neck is of tremendous clinical importance due to the vast number of vital structures present in a confined space. Anatomical variations related to the bony structures, such as vertebrae and ribs, can significantly affect diagnostic and therapeutic interventions. For instance, anomalies like supernumerary or subnumerary ribs and vertebrae, or sternum anomalies, may complicate the interpretation of radiological images and mislead clinical procedures like lumbar punctures or thoracic drainage. Such osteological variations, while at times incidental, transform into risks in the course of surgical planning and forensic analysis, making it paramount for clinicians to have proper anatomical know-how to avert operative complications and diagnostic errors (Ochieng & Ibingira, 2016). Understanding these variations is relevant in preoperative planning of individualized patient treatment, thereby reducing procedural complications and improving clinical outcomes in neck and chest intervention. In addition to bony variations, the cervical viscera also play a fundamental role in the maintenance of neurovascular and respiratory functions, where pathologic processes can have profound implications on a patient's health. Cervical radiculopathy secondary to spondylotic foraminal stenosis is one such example of a common clinical problem that necessitates surgical intervention for the relief of nerve root compression. The choice between an anterior or posterior cervical foraminotomy is based on long-term effectiveness and safety, outcomes that remain under investigation. Modern clinical trials attempt to inform best practices by comparing techniques, patient-reported disability indices, radiologic outcomes, and health-related quality of life (HRQOL) measures. Data obtained from such studies is expected to enhance treatment modalities by enabling clinicians to select the optimal surgical approach for an individual patient, thereby optimizing recovery and reducing complications (Hegewald et al., 2014). Additionally, the clinical significance of the cervical viscera is not only in surgery but also in diagnostic imaging as well as emergency medicine. The close anatomical proximity of cervical organs, such as the thyroid gland, larynx, and carotid arteries, demands intimate knowledge to accurately interpret pathological findings and safely approach lesions. Anatomical anomalies or variations can be confused with each other, resulting in delayed diagnosis or inadvertent trauma during biopsy or airway management. In combination with vertebral anomalies, these also complicate procedures like tracheostomy or central line insertion, emphasizing the need for meticulous preoperative assessment. Overall, an understanding of the clinical significance of the structural and functional anatomy of the neck and cervical viscera is necessary to offer optimum patient care in a wide range of medical specialties.

Test Your Knowledge

1. What are the three parts of the pharynx based on anatomical location?
2. Why is the pharynx clinically significant in airway and infection management?

14.7. The Larynx

Learning Outcome

1. Describe the Structure of the Larynx
2. Know Functions of the Larynx
3. Focus on Disorders of the Larynx

Situated in the anterior neck, the larynx is a critical structure of the cervical viscera, fulfilling supreme functions of respiration, phonation, and airway protection. It is positioned anatomically above the trachea and is composed of cartilages, muscles, and ligaments that function in synergy to impart its dynamic functions. Its largest component, the thyroid cartilage, imparts structural strength to it and is easily palpable under the skin. Internally, it houses the vocal folds, whose vibration enables sound production. Its complex anatomy also allows this organ to act as a valve through occlusion of the airway to inhibit aspiration during swallowing.

Its relation to the surrounding cervical viscera is relevant in understanding pathologies relating to voice loss and respiratory difficulty, referring to its significance beyond mechanical function in the neck (Clark et al., 1906). The larynx's functional ability relies greatly on its complex MSK framework, which entails intrinsic and extrinsic muscles. The muscular attachments control tension and position of the vocal cords and have a direct influence on phonation and the control of breathing. Importantly, intrinsic muscles like the cricothyroid and thyroarytenoid have central roles in the modulation of pitch and voice intensity. The coordinated action of these muscles demonstrates the larynx's versatility to neuromuscular input, with precise calibration during speech. Furthermore, its innervation and blood supply, predominantly from the superior and recurrent laryngeal nerves' branches, demonstrates its susceptibility to neurological injury.

The cervical visceras continuity is observed here, with impairment of laryngeal nerve function leading to vocal cord paralysis and impacting respiratory and swallowing function (Clark et al., 1906). Comparative anatomically, laryngeal study across species gives insight into its adaptation for communication and airway protection in mammalian evolution. Mammalian research, such as that on rabbits, has established major structural components and physiological events of the larynx, guiding a general understanding of its function in vertebrate neck anatomy. These investigations enable medical students and researchers to put human laryngeal anatomy into functional perspective, with ease of understanding its complex relationships to the other cervical viscera. These teaching approaches, blending precise dissection and illustration methods, fill gaps in anatomical knowledge and serve clinical use relevant to laryngeal disorders (Figure 14.13).

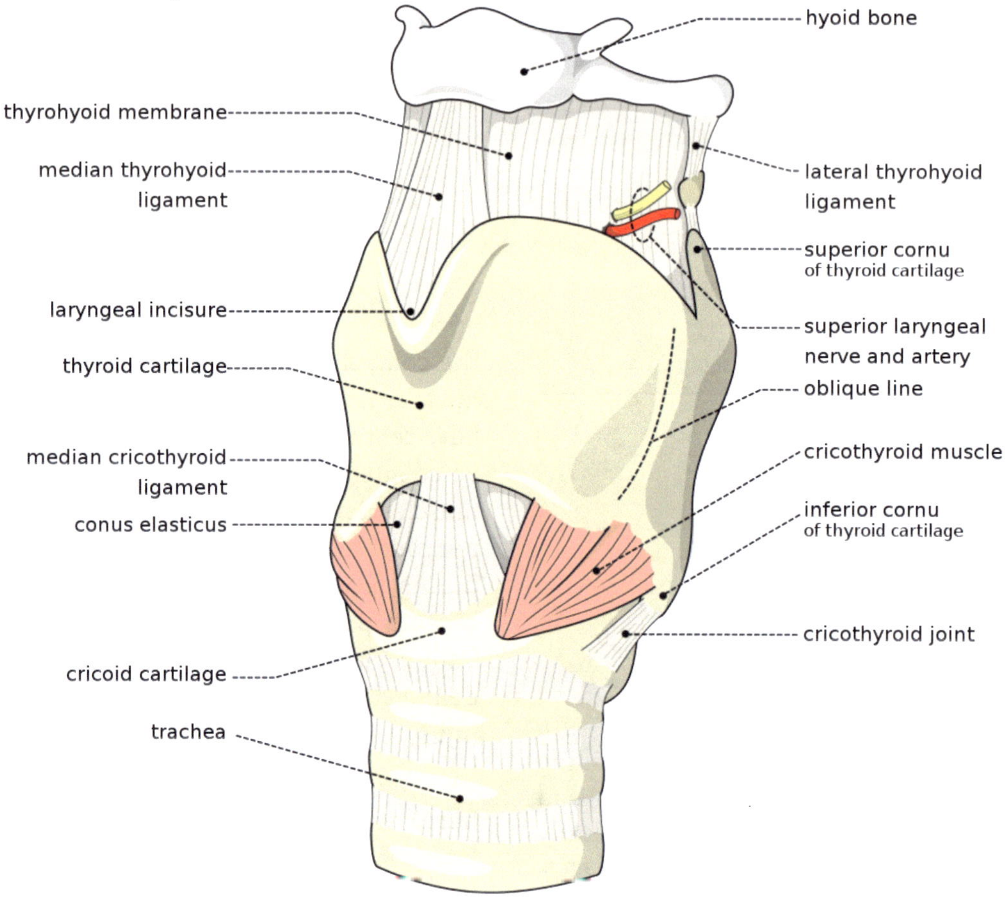

Figure 14.13. The larynx.

Source: By Olek Remesz (wiki-pl: Orem, commons: Orem) - Own work based on: Gray951.png, CC BY-SA 2.5, https://commons.wikimedia.org/w/index.php?curid=3492701

14.7.1. Structure of the Larynx

The fine anatomy of the neck holds numerous vital structures tastefully arranged with each other to enable vital functions such as breathing, swallowing, and making speech possible. Such a structure is the larynx, which is of highly significant importance, located anteriorly in the cervical area, suspended between the hyoid bone and the trachea. This cartilaginous framework is comprised of an array of individual cartilages, including the thyroid, cricoid, arytenoid, and epiglottic cartilages, each contributing in its own way to the larynx's structural strength and functional physiology. The thyroid cartilage forms the prominent anterior shield called the "Adam's apple," while the cricoid cartilage provides a complete ring that supports the airway from the underside. All these components combined create a channel that not only protects the lower respiratory system but also contributes to phonation and airway patency. Knowledge of layered arrangement and interrelationship of the neck is highly important, especially in the event of complications arising as a result of surgeries in this region (Palumbo et al., 2012). A further dive into anatomy reveals the larynx as an advanced organ made up of firm and elastic components with which it can carry out its dynamic functions. Two pyramid-shaped arytenoid cartilages are responsible for the function of the vocal folds and the glottis opening and closing during breathing and speaking. Supported by ligaments and muscles, the vocal cords are positioned within the laryngeal cavity and project across the external framework to facilitate voice production by vibration. The epiglottis is another critical protective mechanism that folds downward to cover the airway when swallowing and thus prevents aspiration.

This complex interaction of cartilage, muscle, and mucosa emphasizes the dual function of the larynx in respiration and voice adjustment, its position in the anterior neck requiring careful attention in both anatomical research and clinical practice (Clark et al., 1906). Clinical implications relative to the structure of the larynx emphasize the necessity of thorough anatomical knowledge, especially in surgical procedures relative to cervical viscera. Former techniques of cervical spine surgery, for instance, carry the risk of postoperative complications such as hematoma of the wound, which would press on the larynx and adjacent airway structures and consequently cause potentially fatal obstruction. This emphasizes the clinical significance of the positioning of the larynx within relatively limited anatomical spaces and vulnerability to postoperative trauma or edema. Prompt recognition and management of such complications depend heavily on understanding laryngeal anatomy and the three-dimensional spatial relationships of the larynx in the neck. Designing treatment strategies and preventive interventions is thus integrally linked to a thorough knowledge of laryngeal form and function, emphasizing the central position of the larynx within the neck and cervical viscera (Palumbo et al., 2012).

14.7.2. Functions of the Larynx

Neck structure coordination is an integral part of critical physiological functions such as respiration, phonation, and lower airway protection. Among these structures, the most critical is the larynx, which not only plays a central role in voice generation but also protects the respiratory tract during the act of swallowing. The larynx is an active valve, which closes to protect against aspiration of food and liquid into the trachea, a process whose maintenance is critical to ensuring pulmonary health. Neural control through cranial nerves and the cervical plexus helps to ensure the precise timing of such protective closure in synchrony with the act of swallowing controlled by sophisticated neurophysiological mechanisms. This defensive function highlights the larynx's intimate position in the neck and cervical viscera, extending its role beyond speech generation to airway protection and respiratory regulation (Melc, 2018). Speech generation is a basic and solitary laryngeal function that relies on the complex cooperation of its anatomical structures, such as the vocal folds and intrinsic muscles. The laryngeal muscles modify tension and length of the vocal folds, altering the pitch and volume of phonation. This subtle motor control is facilitated by the recurrent laryngeal nerve, a branch of the vagus nerve, which innervates most of the intrinsic laryngeal muscles. The superior laryngeal nerve also provides sensory input and motor innervation to the cricothyroid muscle, further refining vocal modulation. Degeneration of these neural tracts, which is a characteristic element in lower cranial nerve lesions, can cripple phonation, highlighting the larynx's dependence on intact neural integrity to produce an effective voice (Loidl et al., 2015). The adaptability of the larynx to function involves these neural and muscular components, positioning it as an essential organ of the cervical viscera. Besides the defense of the airway and phonation, the larynx is also responsible for regulating intrathoracic and intra-abdominal pressure through the Valsalva maneuver. Through glottic occlusion, the larynx enables pressure buildup required during defecation, parturition, and heavy lifting. This valvular function helps in the stabilization of the thoracic cavity and diaphragm, which facilitates effective muscular contractions. The role of the larynx in such pressure regulation thus demonstrates its involvement in more universal physiological processes based on coordinated motion in neck viscera. Its neural inputs, as being of a complex nature and originating from diverse cranial nerves and cervical spinal nerves, equip the larynx with precision and sensitivity in performing such functions (Loidl et al., 2015; Melc, 2018). Thus, the larynx is not only essential to facilitate communication but also to support the vital body functions dependent on controlled airway closure.

14.7.3. Disorders of the Larynx

The complex anatomy and physiology of the larynx are vital to phonation, protection of the airway, and respiration and, therefore, are prone to a variety of structural and functional disorders. These are often a consequence of trauma, infection, inflammation, or neoplastic change affecting the friable cartilaginous framework, intrinsic musculature, and mucous cover of the larynx. Dysfunctional abnormalities of laryngeal function not only alter voice quality but can compromise airway patency and threaten respiratory dysfunction. Working knowledge of the etiology of such alterations must include a complete understanding of cervical viscera and anatomical relations of the neck. Structural lesions causing laryngeal architectural distortion can therefore trigger a chain of impairments of function. This postulate accommodates the concept that structural changes are accountable for derangements of function, a theory highlighted in osteopathic literature that is focused on the importance of anatomical and physiological correlations in disease causation (Clark et al., 1906). Therefore, judicious assessment of laryngeal anatomy determines diagnosis and therapeutic management. Neoplasms, of which squamous cell carcinomas are the most disabling, are also the most common malignant lesions involving the neck and cervical viscera. These cancers occur following chronic exposure to irritants such as alcohol and tobacco, leading to mucosal dysplasia and malignant transformation. Laryngeal tumors can cause orofacial pain, dysphonia, and airway obstruction and have an important negative effect on patient QoL. In oncology, multidisciplinary therapy comprising surgical, medical, and dental teams is central to ensuring optimal patient outcomes. Dental specialists' involvement is particularly important when managing orofacial pain associated with head and neck cancer (HNC) treatment, demonstrating the complex interrelationship of laryngeal pathology and adjacent structures (Arantes et al., 2018).

Successful rehabilitation and pain control are crucial to the restoration of communication and airway function, emphasizing the role of multidisciplinary treatment strategies in laryngeal diseases. Infectious and inflammatory laryngitis and vocal cord nodules also have a marked impact on laryngeal function, usually manifesting as chronic cough, airway obstruction, or hoarseness. Environmental irritants, viral or bacterial infection, or mechanical trauma following misuse of laryngeal tissues are the etiologic factors for these conditions. The laryngeal tissues may undergo fibrosis and scarring due to chronic inflammation and develop permanent dysphonia or airway stenosis. The small anatomical compartments of the neck and cervical viscera mean that minor pathological changes in the larynx can have severe functional consequences. A profound understanding of the pathophysiological processes behind these conditions is thus essential to develop productive interventions. The osteopathic perspective favors the notion that anatomical dysfunction is a manifestation of deranged function and thus requires therapeutic intervention to restore structural integrity so that physiological homeostasis may be re-instituted (Clark et al., 1906). Disorder of the larynx, therefore, requires anatomical precision and functional awareness.

Test Your Knowledge

1. Which structure within the larynx is responsible for sound production?
2. What are two common disorders of the larynx and their symptoms?

14.8. The Esophagus

Learning Outcome

1. Discuss the Anatomy of the Esophagus
2. Focus on Functions of the Esophagus
3. Know Common Esophageal Disorders

Strategically positioned as a crucial passageway from stomach to pharynx, the esophagus is a muscular tube that facilitates controlled passage of ingested material. Its body running through the cervical area places it among the complex visceral structures of the neck, being situated behind the trachea and in front of the vertebral column. This location exposes the esophagus to contact with vital neurovascular structures, like recurrent laryngeal nerves of the vagus nerve. Esophageal wall is made up of distinct layers—mucosa, submucosa, muscularis externa, and adventitia—that allow smooth peristaltic movement to facilitate effective transit of bolus. Interestingly, the innervation of the esophagus bears witness to a complicated interaction of autonomic inputs necessary to both motor and secretory functions, emphasizing its integration into the broader cervical and thoracic nervous complex. Such neuroanatomical associations bear witness to the esophagus's significance beyond conduit functions, highlighting its contribution to autonomic control of the neck's visceral compartment (Ahmed et al., 2022). The musculature of the esophagus holds a zone of transition with unequivocal transition from cervical striated to thoracic smooth muscle, allowing for differential control needs of voluntary and involuntary phases of swallowing. This anatomical feature is an indicator of the flexibility of the esophagus to allow food to travel through the neck to the mediastinum. In addition, the cervical esophagus is most sensitive to neural regulation via the vagus nerve which has motor and sensory fibers important for peristaltic coordination. Recent developments in the comprehension of vagal nerve stimulation reveal potential therapeutic applications in disorders of esophageal motility, underlining the significance of precise neuromodulation in the visceral framework of the neck. Selective vagal fiber stimulation or inhibition may potentially increase esophageal function with fewer off-target effects, which is important in the context of the vagus nerve's generalized effect on cervical and thoracic viscera (Ahmed et al., 2022). The esophagus is exposed to pathophysiological influences due to its proximity to the respiratory apparatus and systemic inflammatory disease. For instance, vagus nerve stimulation has been emerging as a way to minimize inflammatory responses in disease states such as acute respiratory distress syndrome (ARDS), which compromises pulmonary and upper gastrointestinal functions. While non-selective VNS can produce side effects, such as augmented mucus secretion or altered airway muscle tone, the more selective means of stimulation of single fascicles of nerve does promise to modulate inflammatory processes with minimal interference with esophageal motility. This new knowledge is used to highlight the interplay between esophageal function and activity of the autonomic nervous system in the neck viscera and to suggest new directions for modulating esophageal and respiratory complications simultaneously using targeted neuromodulation strategies (Figure 14.14).

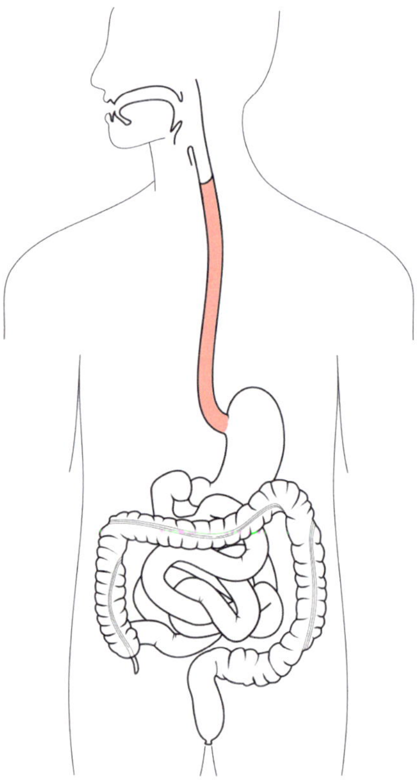

Figure 14.14. The esophagus.

Source: By Olek Remesz (wiki-pl: Orem, commons: Orem) - Own work, CC BY-SA 2.5, https://commons.wikimedia.org/w/index.php?curid=2599304

14.8.1. Anatomy of the Esophagus

Placed as a most important passageway between stomach and pharynx, the esophagus runs through this area of the neck and cervix and serves as a key component of the viscera in the cervical and neck areas. Its general topology is derived from the cricoid cartilage, which is positioned at the level of the sixth cervical vertebra, when the esophagus is let out from the pharyngeal constrictor muscles. The cervical part moves downward, posterior to the trachea and anterior to the vertebral column, before becoming the thoracic esophagus. This part measures approximately 4 to 6 centimeters and is characterized by the muscular composition, with the upper esophageal sphincter comprised largely of striated muscle fibers. Fascial planes covering it, such as the pretracheal fascia, provide essential structural support and both permit mobility and protection from mechanical trauma. Acknowledging this spatial arrangement in the neck highlights functional interaction among the esophagus and the adjacent cervical structures during swallowing processes. The histologic organization of the esophagus also assists its anatomical position among cervical viscera. The wall of the esophagus consists of four distinct layers: mucosa, submucosa, muscularis externa, and adventitia. The mucosa is lined with non-keratinized stratified squamous epithelium, which protects from mechanical abrasion of consumed food. Beneath this, the submucosa has important esophageal glands producing mucus for smooth bolus transit. Of notable interest, in the cervical region, the muscularis externa consists predominantly of striated muscle, transitioning to smooth muscle within the thoracic esophagus. This arrangement facilitates voluntary initiation of swallowing together with involuntary peristalsis more distally. The esophagus lacks a serosal coating in the neck but is enveloped by adventitia, which adheres it tightly to cervical connective tissue surrounding it, reflecting its unique adaptation to the cervical dynamic environment. Such morphological details reflect the esophagus's capacity to fulfill its dual role of propulsion and protection. Functional implications of anatomy of the esophagus in the cervical region are of major importance in physiological and pathological contexts. The upper esophageal sphincter also acts as a critical barrier against retrograde flow, keeping air out of the digestive tract during respiration. Furthermore, nociceptive receptors within the esophageal wall, regulated by transient receptor potential cation channel vanilloid subfamily member 1 (TRPV1), underscore its role in visceral pain detection and regulation of inflammatory processes, as evidenced by experimental use of capsaicin for modeling esophageal inflammation (Frias et al., 2016). Additionally, the intimate association of the cervical esophagus with lymphoid tissues suggests potential pathways for metastatic spread or involvement in lymphedema, a condition managed by surgical intervention with the use of lymph node transfer between cervical lymph basins (Mark et al., 2018). These functional considerations underscore the clinical significance of cervical esophageal anatomy, particularly surgical approach and pain relief strategies among neck and cervical viscera.

14.8.2. Functions of the Esophagus

Swallowing is a complex motor activity utilizing multiple neural pathways and muscle activity closely coordinated in the cervical region and neck. Central to the function is the esophagus, which forms the conduit for bolus transit from the pharynx to the stomach. The esophagus not only serves as a passive tube but rather an active one through coordinated muscular contractions. These peristalsis-coordinated contractions facilitate bolus propulsion despite gravity. The wall of the esophagus has a longitudinal and circular muscle layer whose coordination is critical for normal transit. Specifically, the longitudinal muscle coat in long-pitch spirals facilitates esophageal widening to reduce resistance on bolus passage, whereas short-pitch spiraled circular fibers generate propulsive force that moves contents distally. This anatomical and physiological coordination allows the esophagus to be part of smooth swallowing within the complex cervical viscera network (Melc, 2018). Besides bolus advancement, the esophagus plays a critical role in airway protection and reduction of reflux. The lower esophageal sphincter at the gastroesophageal junction maintains a constant tonic contraction that prevents gastric contents from moving back towards the esophagus and ultimately the respiratory system. In the cervical region, the upper esophageal sphincter, composed primarily of striated muscle, is tightly regulated to open for a moment during swallowing and remain closed at other times to prevent the airway from being aspirated into the esophagus. Such sphincters are an excellent example of the esophagus's function as a dynamic gatekeeper, ensuring unidirectional flow and preserving the distinct environments of the digestive and respiratory systems. These activities highlight the esophagus's crucial association with the neck's complex neural and muscular tissue, highlighting its key contributions to human survival and wellness (Melc, 2018). Besides its primary swallowing and guard roles, the esophagus also participates in more widespread physiological interactions with the cervical lymphatic system and contiguous viscera. While the esophagus itself is devoid of lymph nodes, its spatial location in relation to the cervical lymph node basins places it within an immunosurveillance and lymphatic drainage "hot spot." This association is especially significant in clinical situations of reconstructive surgery or disease management of the neck, where the cervical lymphatic topography, marked by developments like vascularized lymph node transfer (VATS), can impact esophageal recovery and function. The complex coordination among these structures shows the complex function of the esophagus in the viscera of the neck that brings together digestive function with immunologic and vascular mechanisms necessary to maintain homeostasis.

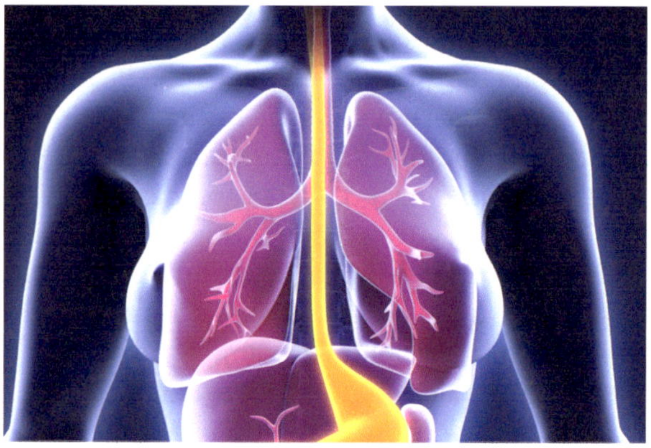

Source: Alina, A. (2016). Esophagus: Facts, functions and diseases. *Anatomy*. Live Science.

14.8.3. Common Esophageal Disorders

The intricacy of the cervical structures' relationship with visceral function emphasizes the importance of viewing esophageal disorders as part of the neck and cervical viscera. Very often, patients presenting with dysphagia, odynophagia, or pain in the cervical region may have underlying esophageal pathology with symptoms manifesting outside the thoracic cavity. Common esophageal conditions such as gastroesophageal reflux disease (GERD), esophageal motility disorders, and anatomical abnormalities may affect nearby cervical tissues through shared neural pathways and mechanical effects. Clinicians should know about these interactions because, on the odd occasion, esophageal dysfunction may be mistaken for MSK neck pain, complicating diagnosis and treatment. Thus, complete assessment of neck pain should consider these visceral causes to avoid diagnostic error and optimize patient outcomes (Oliva-Pascual-Vaca et al., 2019). This integrative approach acknowledges the multifactorial etiologies of cervical symptoms and validates multimodal intervention strategies. Chronic esophageal conditions may lead to significant morbidity via their indirect influence on nearby cervical structures. Inflammatory conditions like GERD will also regularly irritate the proximal esophagus and the adjacent pharyngeal structures, causing symptoms of chronic cough, throat clearing, and cervical pain. Additionally, esophageal motility disorders like achalasia or diffuse esophageal spasm can cause referred pain perceived in the cervical area, mimicking other visceral or somatic illness. This intricacy demands advanced diagnostic imaging and a high level of clinical suspicion for visceral etiologies in the evaluation of complaints of neck pain. Therapeutic interventions directed at visceral function—that is, visceral manipulation—have also demonstrated a potential benefit for symptom reduction by enhancing organ mobility and reducing periesophageal adhesions, with consequent symptom reduction and functional capacity improvement (Andoniki et al., 2020). These findings underscore the need for continued exploration of esophageal disease in the context of cervical and neck visceral health. The diagnostic challenge posed by the overlap of symptoms of both esophageal disease and cervical MSK disease is compounded by a general under-appreciation of visceral causes of neck pain. The literature indicates that clinical guidelines often do not mention visceral etiologies, although the literature proposes a high frequency of esophageal involvement in cervical pain (Oliva-Pascual-Vaca et al., 2019). Not doing this can lead to incomplete evaluation and inferior response to treatment. The inclusion of visceral evaluation in clinical practice enhances diagnostic accuracy and enables targeted intervention that addresses the symptom cause. Furthermore, manual therapies that target the cervical viscera have emerged as adjunct therapies that can optimize esophageal motility and reduce soft tissue constraints through the application of gentle mobilization techniques (Andoniki et al., 2020). Overall, a broadening of the diagnostic focus to include common esophageal disorders is necessary for the development of patient care in neck and cervical viscera disorders.

Test Your Knowledge

1. What are the three physiological constrictions of the esophagus?
2. What are two common esophageal disorders and their key symptoms?

14.9. The Thyroid Gland

Learning Outcome

1. Evaluate Anatomy of the Thyroid Gland
2. Know Hormonal Functions
3. Understand Thyroid Disorders

The complex neck anatomy of the front contains several important endocrine organs, with the thyroid gland being paramount in systemic metabolic regulation. Lying anterior to the trachea and inferior to the larynx is the thyroid gland, which consists of two lobes connected by an isthmus, often exhibiting morphological variations making surgical techniques more difficult. They highlight the importance of thorough anatomical familiarity in procedures like thyroidectomy, wherein the intraoperative injury to adjacent structures such as the recurrent laryngeal nerve or the parathyroid glands can lead to resultant morbidity. Clinicians need to be aware of these potential variations to prevent intraoperative issues and optimize the outcome for the patient. The clinical significance of anatomical variations to surgery practice has been established, with their influence on surgical strategy and complication rates, particularly in delicate regions like the neck and cervical viscera (Katarzyna et al., 2021). Besides its anatomical complexity, the thyroid gland is also an important endocrine gland that is responsible for the synthesis and secretion of thyroid hormones in the thyroxine (T4) and triiodothyronine (T3) forms. These hormones exert a very important effect on basal metabolic rate, thermoregulation, and development. Vascular supply of the gland by the superior and inferior thyroid arteries, and occasionally by a thyroid ima artery, highlights the significance of meticulous dissection in neck surgery to prevent hemorrhagic complications. Besides, the gland's relation with other surrounding cervical tissues, e.g., strap muscles, carotid sheath, and laryngeal nerves—demands a comprehensive understanding within the scope of accepted anatomical curricula to teach trainees the acquisition of operative competence. Educational models like the Anatomical Society's core syllabus ensure that clinical professionals possess rudimentary knowledge regarding the anatomy of the thyroid gland in the broad context of neck and cervical viscera (Smith et al., 2015). Surgery of the thyroid gland is not only concerned with the anatomical aspects of the organ but also its endocrine pathologic significance. Conditions such as goiter, thyroid nodule, and cancer require precise diagnostic and treatment planning that blends anatomical understanding with clinical acumen. The proximity of the gland to significant neurovascular bundles requires the surgeon to foresee and recognize variations to avoid postoperative complications such as paralysis of the vocal cords or hypoparathyroidism. The evolving appreciation of anatomical nuances in the thyroid region highlights the necessity of ongoing anatomical research and collaboration between surgical oncologists and anatomists. The dynamic interplay of anatomy and clinical practice in this way is a quintessential manifestation of the far-reaching relationship between accurate anatomical information and the safe control of neck and cervical viscera diseases (Katarzyna et al., 2021) (Figure 14.15).

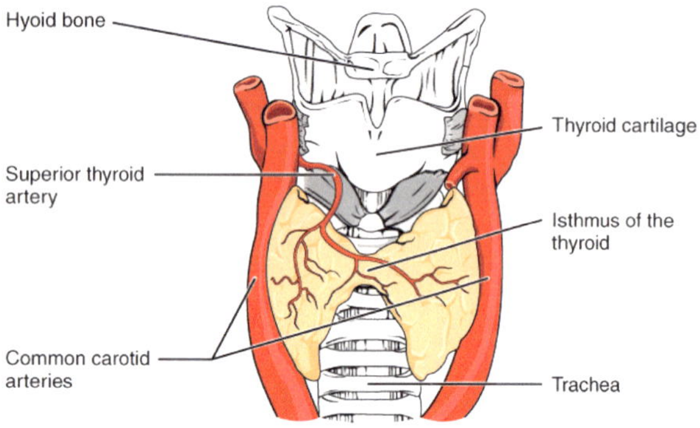

Figure 14.15. The thyroid gland.

Source: By CFCF - Own work, CC BY-SA 3.0, https://commons.wikimedia.org/w/index.php?curid=33190618

14.9.1. Anatomy of the Thyroid Gland

The anatomical structures of the neck are so complex that accurate modeling is required for both clinical and educational purposes, especially in the case of the thyroid gland. Advances in 3D printing and medical imaging have transformed the capability to reproduce these complex details, thus providing high-fidelity simulation for training and research. Using CT scans, individualized molds can be created to accurately represent the position of the thyroid with respect to the surrounding tissues, such as the trachea, carotid arteries, and jugular veins. The models not only visualize normal anatomic variation but also are beneficial in the development and testing of ultrasound-guided procedures. The echogenicity of these phantoms resembles that of real human tissue to ensure that the ultrasound practice is as realistic as possible. This is a breakthrough in the pursuit of improving the understanding of thyroid gland anatomy in general neck viscera (Aida et al., 2024). Historical and recent anatomical research offers vital information on the normal morphological characteristics of the thyroid gland necessary for surgical operations. Long-standing studies on both living subjects and cadaveric specimens have revealed significant variations in gland size, shape, and position relation. It is documented that morphological characteristics such as the presence or absence of the pyramidal lobe, retrothyroid processes, and Zuckerkandls tubercle exhibit high variability, which influences clinical procedures. Furthermore, the bilaterally symmetrical or asymmetrical character of the gland determines surgical strategy and underscores the requirement for meticulous dissection techniques to avoid neurovascular damage. These anatomical nuances refer to the necessity of a comprehensive, evidence-driven framework for endocrine surgeons to optimize patient outcomes and reduce intraoperative risk (Romashchenko et al., 2022). The complex vascular supply and neural relations of the thyroid gland create further difficulty within the confined space of the neck, pointing to the gland's clinical significance in the cervical viscera. The superior and inferior thyroid arteries and their variations must be clearly defined to prevent hemorrhagic complications during surgery. The close relationship of the recurrent laryngeal nerve with the posterior surface of the thyroid gland also requires careful preoperative mapping to preserve vocal cord function. Detailed anatomical knowledge allows the determination of risk areas in the operating field, enabling targeted visualization of the parathyroid glands and minimizing incidental injury. Incorporation of this kind of anatomical knowledge into surgical practice and master classes enhances the proficiency of endocrine surgeons, one such instance of translation of anatomical science into life-saving clinical practice (Romashchenko et al., 2022).

14.9.2. Hormonal Functions

The complex interaction of the endocrine organs within the cervical region underscores the critical hormonal functions regulated by the neck and cervical viscera. Among them, the thyroid gland is the most critical, which controls regulation of metabolism through its secretion of thyroxine (T4) and triiodothyronine (T3). These contribute to systemic metabolic rates, influencing virtually every tissue by controlling oxygen use and heat production. The parathyroid glands, located behind the thyroid, release PTH, which is essential in maintaining calcium homeostasis. It increases the serum calcium by activating osteoclastic activity, enhancing renal calcium reabsorption, and activating the intestinal absorption of calcium through vitamin D activation. This fine tuning of calcium concentration is essential to neuromuscular function and bone health. Moreover, the endocrine functions of the cervical viscera extend beyond individual glands because systemic effects illustrate integrating endocrine control with respiratory and cardiovascular controls. Such controls reflect the functional complexity embodied in the anatomy of the neck. The hormonal influence of the cervical area extends beyond developmental or metabolic activities but assumes a prominence in response to disease states. For instance, thyroid hormone secretion disturbances lead to overt clinical syndromes such as hypothyroidism or hyperthyroidism, with the wide range of systemic manifestations ranging from cardiovascular disorders to neuropsychiatric manifestations. Further, failure of the parathyroid glands to secrete parathyroid hormone results in hypocalcemia or hypercalcemia, which subsequently manifests as neuromuscular excitability or depression. Recent research shows that genetic and developmental defects in the endocrine elements of the cervical viscera also predispose to congenital conditions such as congenital diaphragmatic hernia, connecting defective diaphragmatic and endocrine development in complex etiologies (Cannata et al., 2021). These observations further elucidate hormonal functions by demonstrating their intrinsic association with anatomical development and potential multisystemic effects, further highlighting the homeostatic role of cervical viscera. Current advancements further demonstrate cervical viscera hormonal influence extends into neuroimmune and autonomic regulatory domains, particularly in aging and susceptibility to systemic disease. The vagus nerve, which runs through the neck, is a demonstration of this integration through its control of inflammation and cardiovascular function through the cholinergic anti-inflammatory pathway. This neural-hormonal interaction is essential in diseases like Alzheimer's and COVID-19, where autonomic dysfunction hastens mortality risk (Rangon et al., 2020). Brainstem autonomic nuclei, in turn modulated by cervical sensory input, regulate life-supporting rhythms and systemic inflammation levels, linking cervical visceral functions with larger neuroendocrine networks. Therapies targeting such pathways, like VNS, underscore the increasing recognition of cervical hormonal functions beyond conventional endocrine territories, putting the neck and cervical viscera in the spotlight for integrated system control and new medical approaches.

14.9.3. Thyroid Disorders

The complex anatomical position of the thyroid gland in the neck is a testament to its varied role in endocrine function and its vulnerability to a wide range of disorders. Lying anterior to the trachea and inferior to the larynx, the two lobes of the thyroid are connected by an isthmus, making it a prominent cervical viscus susceptible to structural and functional abnormalities. These disorders range from autoimmune-mediated hypothyroidism and hyperthyroidism to nodular goiter and cancer. With the gland's rich vascular supply and the proximity of vital structures like the recurrent laryngeal nerve, pathological process tends to present with symptoms beyond endocrine imbalance, such as dysphonia or airway compromise. Anatomical relationships of the neck necessitate a combined understanding of thyroid morphology and physiology that is essential for accurate diagnosis and effective management in clinical practice, as evident from anatomical curricula guiding medical education (Tiffany et al., 2019). A nuanced communication of thyroid disease must also consider the gland's physiological function in regulating systemic metabolic processes via thyroid hormones. Hyperthyroidism, such as in Graves' disease, leads to a hypermetabolic condition, whereas hypothyroidism, usually due to Hashimoto's thyroiditis, leads to slowing of systemic metabolism. These are accompanied by distinctive clinical presentations of tachycardia, loss or gain in weight, and temperature sensitivity, all mirroring the endocrine function derangement of the gland. Importantly, structural lesions like multinodular goiters or cancers of the thyroid can complicate these clinical presentations by calling forth local compressive symptoms through their expansion in the confined cervical space. Diagnostic imaging and function tests thus play a central part in assessing these variations, new neurophysiological investigations showing the interplay between systemic disease and neural change, the clinician being reminded of the complex, bidirectional nature of neck and cervical viscera relationships (Tiffany et al., 2019). Therapeutic strategies to thyroid disease must thus be intimately combined with an advanced knowledge of the anatomy and pathophysiology of the gland to prevent iatrogenic complications. Surgical interventions, such as thyroidectomy, require surgical precision in the preservation of adjacent neurovascular structures, namely the recurrent laryngeal nerve and parathyroid glands, whose injury may result in severe morbidity. In addition, pharmacological treatment directed at hormone synthesis or replacement therapy necessitates lifelong therapy with continual monitoring on a regular basis to titrate doses and prevent side effects. The multidisciplinary management of thyroid disease, combining endocrinology, surgery, and radiology, highlights the importance of good anatomical knowledge and clinical judgment. The incorporation of consensus-based anatomical syllabi into medical education ensures adequate preparation of practitioners for these challenges in neck and cervical viscus pathology (Smith et al., 2015).

Test Your Knowledge

1. What are two common functional disorders of the thyroid gland?
2. What are the symptoms of hyperthyroidism?

14.10. The Parathyroid Glands

Learning Outcome

1. Discuss the Anatomy of the Parathyroid Glands
2. Explain the Role in Calcium Regulation
3. Focus on Parathyroid Disorders

Within the complex neck anatomy, the parathyroid glands are diminutive but important endocrine glands, typically four in number, found on the posterior sides of the thyroid gland. Small but important, their diminutiveness belies their role in calcium homeostasis as they secrete PTH which regulates serum calcium and phosphate levels. The location of the glands presents a surgical challenge, most notably in thyroidectomies or neck dissections, in which accidental damage can lead to profound metabolic derangements. Anatomical variations most frequently encountered, e.g., ectopic site or variable numbers of glands—demand thoughtful operative planning and consideration. Surgeons must be well aware of these variations to avoid accidental damage, leading to hypocalcemia or needing autotransplantation. These differences serve to point to the bigger picture of anatomical variability in the neck and cervical viscera that will affect clinical presentations and surgical planning (Katarzyna et al., 2021). The blood supply to the parathyroid glands is provided by the branches of the inferior thyroid artery that stem from the thyrocervical trunk, emphasizing the importance of vascular anatomy in neck surgery. This vascular link not only supports gland functionality but also presents dangers in surgical procedures when jeopardized by the vessels. Endovascular therapies on the thyrocervical trunk highlight the critical need for proper comprehension of this vascular system because it is linked with cervical and upper limb circulations. Understanding potential anastomoses, especially with the anterior spinal artery, is essential to avoid ischemic complications during manipulation of nearby arteries in head and neck surgery. These vascular complications apply directly to parathyroid adenomas or hyperplasia excision procedures, where precision in arterial preservation and gland excision is paramount (Carlos et al., 2018). Other than anatomical and vascular complications, the physiological activity of the parathyroid glands integrates them closely with the rest of the endocrine and cervical system. Abnormal regulation of the glands causes illnesses such as hyperparathyroidism, which is caused by hypersecretion of PTH and consequent hypercalcemia, having a potential impact on bone mineral density and renal function. Conversely, hypoparathyroidism, typically iatrogenic secondary to surgical damage, necessitates lifelong control of calcium status. These clinical factors emphasize the need for careful preoperative imaging and intraoperative localization techniques to preserve gland function in treating pathological status. The parathyroids' involvement with adjacent cervical viscera, like the recurrent laryngeal nerve and thyroid gland, necessitates extreme care and anatomical consideration in operative intervention, once more depicting the interrelationship between structure and function within the cervical compartment (Carlos et al., 2018; Katarzyna et al., 2021) (Figure 14.16).

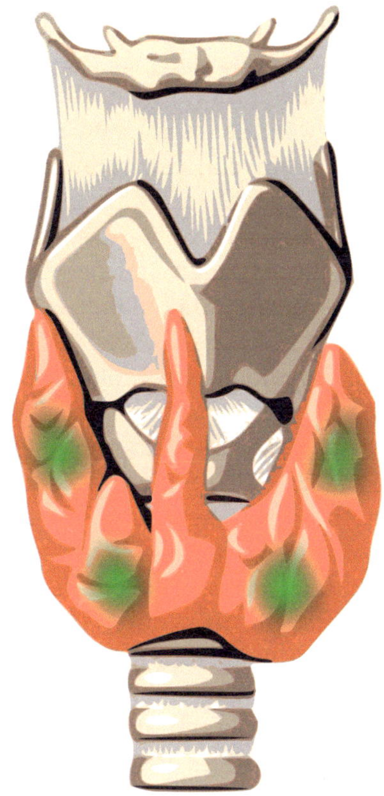

Figure 14.16. The parathyroid glands.

Source: By Busca tu equilibrio... (Namaste) 20:53, 18 December 2011 (UTC) - Own work, CC BY-SA 3.0, https://commons.wikimedia.org/w/index.php?curid=17720447

14.10.1. Anatomy of the Parathyroid Glands

The complex anatomical arrangement of the neck includes several vital structures, of which the parathyroid glands have a critical endocrine function. They are small, typically four in number, and are found on the posterior surface of the thyroid gland, either embedded in the connective tissue capsule or near it. The diameter of each gland measures approximately 3 to 5 millimeters. They occupy different locations that tend to be close to the inferior and superior poles of the thyroid lobes, hence calling for special care in operations such as thyroidectomy to avoid unintentional damage. This delicate balance stresses the importance of extensive understanding of the anatomy of the neck because parathyroid gland disruptions can profoundly influence calcium homeostasis, underlining their clinical relevance in the setting of neck and cervical viscus anatomy (Su et al., 2023). Apart from the area where they are located, the vascular and neural plexuses that provide parathyroid glands are integral to their functioning and upkeep. The superior and inferior thyroid arteries supply the arterial component in the majority of instances, with venous drainage in the same manner. A dual perfusion pattern is provided, which is critical for the synthesis and secretion of PTH, a vital regulator of systemic calcium homeostasis. The parathyroid innervation is mediated primarily through cervical ganglia sympathetic fibers with autonomic nervous system regulation involved in providing endocrine homeostasis. This neural incorporation is a testament to the complexity of the interrelationships of the cervical viscera and the importance of coordinated function in homeostatic control (Su et al., 2023). The structural composition of the parathyroid glands is reflective of their dedicated function in the endocrine system. Microscopically, they contain primarily chief cells that produce PTH and oxyphil cells, whose role is less definable. Located in connective tissue, these glands are still closely associated with the thyroid but are autonomously involved in regulating the metabolism of calcium. Familiarity with the anatomical and histological particularity of parathyroid glands is critical to clinicians who operate on pathology of the neck, most critically in the surgical context where a careless excision or damage leads to hypoparathyroidism and consequent hypocalcemia. Thus, parathyroid anatomy information not only helps in anatomical and physiological training but also enhances the success of neck surgery (Su et al., 2023).

14.10.2. Role in Calcium Regulation

The complex interaction between cervical and neck viscera is responsible for calcium homeostasis regulation, in significant part by way of the parathyroid glands that are positioned immediately adjacent to the thyroid gland. The small endocrine organs secrete PTH, which is a key controller of serum calcium through its effect on bone resorption, renal reabsorption of calcium, and intestinal absorption of calcium. The proximity of the parathyroid glands to the cervical region offers a rapid and efficient response to fluctuations in extracellular calcium concentration, which is essential for various physiological functions such as muscle contraction, neurotransmission, and blood coagulation. Neural circuits innervating these glands that may involve vagal inputs, may also regulate PTH secretion and hence be part of the overall autonomic regulation of calcium homeostasis in the body (Herrity et al., 2014). This complex interaction supports the importance of cervical viscera not only in local anatomical settings but also in systemic metabolic regulation. Calcium homeostasis within the body is interlocked with neural inputs which have their origin in the cervical area and extend through autonomic routes. The vagus nerve, which innervates many of the visceral organs, may be implicated in the perception and transmission of biochemical information affecting calcium metabolism, particularly after injury or systemic derangement. Plasticity of vagal afferents after injury has been observed in experimental models where modifications of neuronal properties reflect an adaptation process in homeostasis maintenance under compromised conditions. These electrophysiological and neurochemical changes in vagal sensory neurons can therefore modulate parathyroid function indirectly by changing visceral sensory feedback and autonomic output and thereby affect calcium levels systemically (Kowalczyk & Majewski, 2021). This neuro-visceral integration is an exemplary illustration of the integrative regulation of calcium, where cervical neural circuits are involved in the preservation of systemic mineral equilibrium essential for health. Apart from the direct endocrine action of cervical viscera, modulation of nociceptive and autonomic messages on calcium homeostasis is a task of complex central mechanisms between peripheral sensory input and brain centers responsible for homeostatic regulation. The cervical region serves as a center for carrying information from senses, like painful stimuli that indirectly affect calcium control by modulating hormonal secretions and autonomic tone. The interaction between nociceptive pathways and homeostatic processes highlights how visceral afferent input combined across cervical and neck neural networks might impact calcium balance, especially under conditions of stress or injury. Understanding these complex interactions between pain processing and calcium regulatory systems is significant, as it might inform therapeutic approaches to conditions in which disrupted calcium homeostasis and pain perception are implicated. This complex neuroanatomical system discloses the advanced function cervical viscera have in ensuring mineral balance via dynamic endocrine and neural interactions.

14.10.3. Parathyroid Disorders

The complex anatomy of the neck and cervical spine is essential in the management and comprehension of parathyroid disease. Surgery in this region, especially that affecting the thyroid and parathyroid glands, requires accurate anatomical understanding to reduce complications. The parathyroid glands, although small, are important structures located in proximity to the thyroid gland and are responsible for the regulation of calcium homeostasis via the secretion of PTH. Hyperparathyroidism is a condition caused by abnormal parathyroid tissue that often needs to be removed surgically. Since the parathyroid glands are intimately related to vital cervical structures, i.e., the recurrent laryngeal nerve and vascular structures, surgery needs to be performed with meticulous dissection. Avoiding injury to the nerves and surrounding structures is essential to prevent complications like hypoparathyroidism and nerve paresis, which are of serious concern in neck surgery on these glands (Pino, 2021). Thus, intimate knowledge of cervical anatomy assures safer manipulation and improved results in parathyroid diseases. Apart from the operative technique, the vascular anatomy of the neck significantly directs the course of management of parathyroid diseases, especially in preoperative embolization or in emergency situations. The thyrocervical trunk, which is a significant arterial branch of the subclavian artery, gives rise to vascular territories relevant to the parathyroid region. Its variable and complex pattern of branching is a major determinant in interventional procedures for hemorrhage control or tumor devascularization. Precision in operating in this "border land" between neuroradiology and vascular radiology is obligatory to avoid unintentional injury to neck structures and preserve blood supply essential for gland viability. This vascular data allows endovascular procedures to be safely performed, like preoperative embolizations of paragangliomas or atypical tumors near the parathyroid glands, to aid in global care of parathyroid pathology (Kowalczyk & Majewski, 2021). Parathyroid disease is a spectrum of clinical challenges that link with the overall anatomy of the neck viscera. Hyperparathyroidism, whether primary due to adenomas or secondary to systemic disease, manifests as hypercalcemia with its metabolic derangements, emphasizing the gland's systemic significance. Challenge in localizing ectopic or supernumerary parathyroid glands within the cervical region or mediastinum also complicates surgical procedures. Inadvertent excision or devascularization of normal parathyroid tissue during thyroid surgery is also a notable risk, often leading to postoperative hypocalcemia. These complexities underscore the necessity for surgeons to exercise caution during cervical lymphadenectomy or thyroidectomies to preserve parathyroid function, a delicate balance between endocrine preservation and oncologic adequacy (Pino, 2021). Through the melding of anatomic precision and clinical judgment, the surgery of parathyroid disease demonstrates the refined interaction of neck and cervical viscera in the operating field.

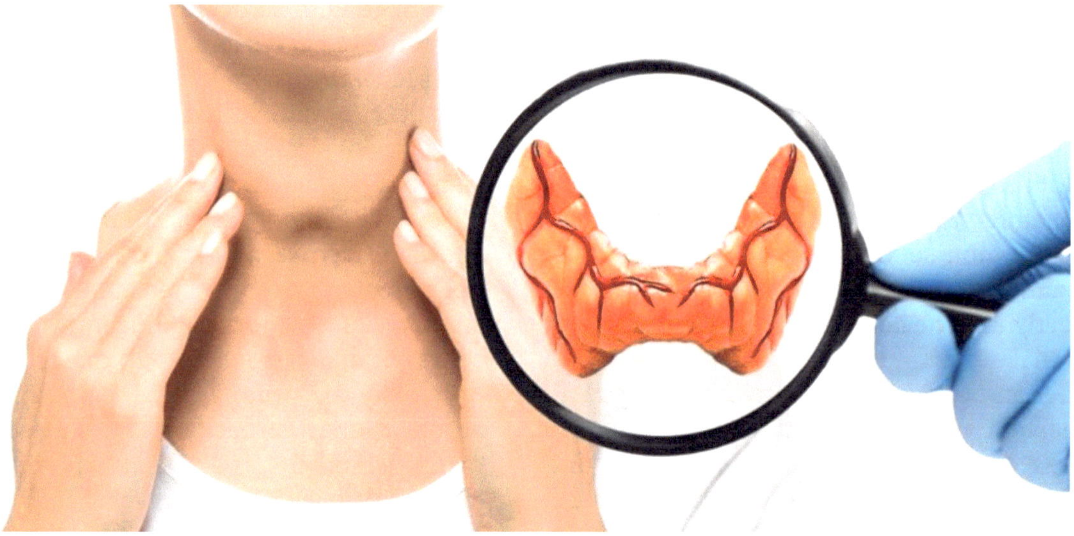

Source: Coastal Ear, Nose and Throat. (2021). *Parathyroid Gland Visualization*.

Test Your Knowledge

1. What hormone is secreted by the parathyroid glands to regulate calcium levels?
2. What is the effect of hyperparathyroidism on blood calcium levels?

SUMMARY

The complex neck and cervical viscera architecture demonstrates the delicate compromise among the structural complexity and functional unity required in human physiology. The understanding of these correlations makes clinical practice easier in the treatment of trauma, disease, and surgery in the region. The cervical viscera, which encompass significant structures such as the thyroid gland, pharynx, larynx, and the closely ramified vascular and nervous plexuses , play critical roles in respiration, endocrine regulation, and neurological transmission. Recent advancements in the use of therapeutic modalities, like VNS, have shown outstanding promise in inflammation modulation and treatment of cervical nervous system-associated disorders (Kowalczyk & Majewski, 2021). This growing body of research reiterates the paramount necessity of an in-depth knowledge of cervical anatomy to realize the highest degree of patient optimization and incorporation of how anatomical awareness must be followed by innovative management strategies to promote cervical health care. Furthermore, the neck lymphatic system along with cervical viscera has been known to be involved in immune regulation as well as pathological conditions such as lymphedema. The development of surgical techniques like VATS is a progressive step towards restoring lymphatic function and the prevention of chronic complications arising due to disruptions in the lymphatic network (Mark et al., 2018). This points to the importance of the cervical area not just as a conduit for nerve and vascular structures but as an active participant in systemic immune responses. The potential to utilize these anatomical and physiological observations for targeted surgical intervention underscores the coming together of accurate anatomy and innovative clinical practice, revealing new paths to the management of complex diseases including those of the neck and cervical viscera. Against this background, it becomes evident that sustained cross-disciplinary research is needed to fully untangle the complex nuances of the neck and cervical viscera. Advances in neurostimulation and microsurgical lymphatic reconstruction bear testimony to the translational potential of anatomy research linking basic science to therapeutic applications (Kowalczyk & Majewski, 2021). Such progress also highlights the dynamic nature of this field, where evolving technologies are to be integrated with fundamental anatomical knowledge. From the clinical viewpoint, the consequences are extensive, with possible growth in diagnostic precision, site-specific treatment possibilities, and improved QoL for sufferers of neck and cervical visceral disorders. It is this comprehensive knowledge on which future research and advances will be founded, opening the way for the next generation of cervical management.

The complex neck and cervical viscera anatomy is comprised of a number of organ systems and neurovascular structures whose integrative function is paramount to such fundamental physiological functions as respiration, swallowing, and circulation. In this complex region, the esophagus, trachea, thyroid gland, and concomitant lymphatic and vascular pathways intimately interact to provide homeostasis and accommodation to systemic needs. Advances in the knowledge of the neuronal components innervating these viscera have revealed the fine functions of single nerve fibers, particularly sensory afferent fibers that are involved in modulation of visceropain and reflex conduct. Current findings highlight that certain ion channels involved in the excitability of neurons, including voltage-gated sodium channel NaV 1.7, display differential functions within somatic versus visceral pathways of pain, validating the modality-specific nature of nociceptive transmission in cervical viscera (Baeyens et al., 2017). It is this variation that is critical to therapeutic treatment with directed therapies and adds to our knowledge of cervical viscera neurophysiology. The PNS is a critical intermediary that modulates motor and sensory transmission among the CNS and cervical viscera. Comparative detailed analysis of the brachial plexus and related neural structures presents significant variability not only among species but also in primates, suggesting evolutionary changes for different locomotor and functional demands (Kowalczyk & Majewski, 2021). Such morphologic heterogeneity of nerve networks is paralleled by the specialized viscera patterns of cervical innervation necessary for the delivery of fine motor control and autonomic control. An understanding of this plasticity offers greater insight into evolutionary pressures shaping cervical nervous architecture and into clinical approaches to the treatment of nerve injury and dysfunction in the cervical spine. The neural anatomy of the neck is therefore an integrative complex in which functional anatomy and evolutionary biology meet to explain the mechanism of critical cervical viscera functions. In general, the neck and cervical viscera are a complicated anatomical and physiological system governed by complex neurovascular dynamics. The specificity of sodium channel subtyping in pain response regulation points to a key aspect of visceral sensory processing not replicated in somatic design, informing pain treatment protocols (Bonaz et al., 2017). Concurrently, evolutionary studies of PNS anatomy, that is, the brachial plexus, suggest that structural variation is paired with functional adaptation essential to primate and human upper limb and cervical zone function (Kowalczyk & Majewski, 2021). Together, these arguments emphasize the importance of a multidisciplinary investigative methodology of cervical viscera which integrates neurophysiology, evolutionary biology, and clinical anatomy to promote more specific and effective treatments of cervical pathologies and better knowledge of upper body visceral integration.

KEY TERMS FROM THIS CHAPTER

- Tumor necrosis factor alpha (TNFα)
- Vascular disease
- Visceromotor interactions
- Osteochondromas
- Peripheral nervous system (PNS)
- Vagus nerve stimulation (VNS)
- Vascularized lymph node transfer (VLNT)
- Musculoskeletal (MSK) framework
- Parathyroid glands

CRITICAL THINKING QUESTIONS

1. **Which of the following structures is enclosed within the carotid sheath?**
   a. Subclavian vein
   b. Internal jugular vein
   c. External jugular vein
   d. Phrenic nerve
2. **The thyroid gland is located at which cervical vertebral level?**
   a. C1–C2
   b. C3–C5
   c. C5–T1
   d. T2–T4
3. **Which nerve runs within the carotid sheath along with the common carotid artery and internal jugular vein?**
   a. Phrenic nerve
   b. Hypoglossal nerve
   c. Vagus nerve
   d. Accessory nerve
4. **The infrahyoid muscles are primarily responsible for:**
   a. Elevating the hyoid bone
   b. Depressing the hyoid bone
   c. Flexing the neck laterally
   d. Rotating the head
5. **Which structure lies posterior to the trachea in the neck?**
   a. Thyroid gland
   b. Larynx
   c. Esophagus
   d. Internal jugular vein

Short Answer Questions

1. What are the major components of the cervical viscera?
2. Describe the anatomical position and function of the thyroid gland.
3. What is the role of the carotid sheath, and which structures does it enclose?
4. Differentiate between the infrahyoid and suprahyoid muscles in terms of function.
5. Explain the pathway and function of the vagus nerve in the cervical region.
6. Describe the location and clinical relevance of the cervical lymph nodes.
7. What is the anatomical relationship between the trachea and esophagus in the neck?
8. Briefly explain the blood supply to the thyroid gland.

Answers to Critical Thinking Questions

1. (b) 2. (c) 3. (c) 4. (b) 5. (c)

REFERENCES

1. Ahmed, U., Chang, Y. C., Zafeiropoulos, S., Nassrallah, Z., Miller, L. S., & Zanos, S. (2022). Strategies for precision vagus neuromodulation. *Bioelectronic Medicine, 8.* https://doi.org/10.1186/s42234-022-00091-1 (accessed on 8th May 2025).
2. Palumbo, M. A., Aidlen, J. P., Daniels, A. H., Thakur, N. A., & Caiati, J. (2012). Airway compromise due to wound hematoma following anterior cervical spine surgery. *The open orthopaedics journal*, *6*, 108–113. https://doi.org/10.2174/1874325001206010108 (accessed on 8th May 2025).
3. Andoniki, G. (2020). *The Role of Visceral Manipulation in Rehabilitation.* https://core.ac.uk/download/553380934.pdf (accessed on 8th May 2025).
4. Arantes, D., Costa, N., Resende, T., Mikulas, K., da Silva Júnior, P., Brito, R., Noronha, V., Pedras, R., & Corrêa, L. (2018). Dental approach of orofacial pain in head and neck cancer patients. *Journal of clinical and experimental dentistry*, *10*(11), e1082–e1090. https://doi.org/10.4317/jced.55311 (accessed on 8th May 2025).
5. Smith, C. F., Finn, G. M., Stewart, J., Atkinson, M. A., Davies, D. C., Dyball, R., Morris, J., Ockleford, C., Parkin, I., Standring, S., Whiten, S., Wilton, J., & McHanwell, S. (2016). The Anatomical Society core regional anatomy syllabus for undergraduate medicine. *Journal of anatomy*, *228*(1), 15–23. https://doi.org/10.1111/joa.12405on 8th May 2025).
6. Baker, S. J., & Porterfield, J. R. Jr. (2019). *The Endocrine System: Thyroid and Parathyroid.* DeckerMed Surgery. https://www.semanticscholar.org/paper/4583954d74215cd5974e28c919e8c50ca19c4583 (accessed on 8th May 2025).
7. Sienkiewicz-Zawilińska, J., Zawiliński, J., Kaythampilla, L. N., Jankiel, M., Urbaniak, J., Bereza, T., Kowalski, W., Loukas, M., & Walocha, J. (2018). Autonomic nervous system of the pelvis - general overview. *Folia medica Cracoviensia*, *58*(2), 21–44. https://doi.org/10.24425/fmc.2018.124656 (accessed on 8th May 2025).
8. Bonaz, B., Sinniger, V., & Pellissier, S. (2017). The vagus nerve in the neuro-immune axis: Implications in the pathology of the gastrointestinal tract. *Frontiers in Immunology, 8.* https://doi.org/10.3389/fimmu.2017.01452 (accessed on 8th May 2025).
9. Bordoni, B., & Zanier, E. (2013). Anatomic connections of the diaphragm: Influence of respiration on the body system. *Journal of Multidisciplinary Healthcare.* https://doi.org/10.2147/jmdh.s45443 (accessed on 8th May 2025).
10. Bordoni, B., & Zanier, E. (2013). Skin, fascias, and scars: Symptoms and systemic connections. *Journal of Multidisciplinary Healthcare.* https://doi.org/10.2147/jmdh.s52870 (accessed on 8th May 2025).
11. Chirica, M., Kelly, M. D., Siboni, S., Aiolfi, A., Riva, C. G., Asti, E., Ferrari, D., et al. (2019). Esophageal emergencies: WSES guidelines. *World Journal of Emergency Surgery, 14.* https://doi.org/10.1186/s13017-019-0245-2 (accessed on 8th May 2025).
12. Damineni, V. (2022). *Potential Differences in Male Versus Female Lymph Nodes.* https://core.ac.uk/download/539277148.pdf (accessed on 8th May 2025).
13. Falk, S. (1998). Thyroid disease: Endocrinology, surgery, nuclear medicine, and radiotherapy. *Endocrinologist, 8*, 105, 106. https://www.semanticscholar.org/paper/b9e449a8481ee49555f9add85fdccddd127a3195 (accessed on 8th May 2025).

14. Feigl, G., Hammer, G., Litz, R. J., & Kachlík, D. (2020). The intercarotid or alar fascia, other cervical fascias, and their adjacent spaces – A plea for clarification of cervical fascia and spaces terminology. *Journal of Anatomy, 237*, 197–207. https://doi.org/10.1111/joa.13175 (accessed on 8th May 2025).

15. Oliva-Pascual-Vaca, Á., González-González, C., Oliva-Pascual-Vaca, J., Piña-Pozo, F., Ferragut-Garcías, A., Fernández-Domínguez, J. C., & Heredia-Rizo, A. M. (2019). Visceral Origin: An Underestimated Source of Neck Pain. A Systematic Scoping Review. *Diagnostics (Basel, Switzerland), 9*(4), 186. https://doi.org/10.3390/diagnostics9040186 (accessed on 8th May 2025).

16. Frias, A. M. (2016). Capsaicin, nociception and pain. *Molecules, 21*, 797–797. https://doi.org/10.3390/molecules21060797 (accessed on 8th May 2025).

17. Gerritsen, R. J. S., & Band, G. P. H. (2018). Breath of life: The respiratory vagal stimulation model of contemplative activity. *Frontiers in Human Neuroscience, 12*. https://doi.org/10.3389/fnhum.2018.00397 (accessed on 8th May 2025).

18. Ochieng J, Ibingira CBR. Sternal Anomalies with Supernumerary and Subnumerary Vertebrae and Ribs – Case Reports. *East Cent Afr J Surg*. 2007;12(1):99-104. (accessed on 8th May 2025).

19. Kaniušas, E., Kampusch, S., Tittgemeyer, M., Panetsos, F., Fernandez, G. R., Papa, M., Kiss, A., et al. (2019). Current directions in the auricular vagus nerve stimulation I – A physiological perspective. *Frontiers in Neuroscience, 13*. https://doi.org/10.3389/fnins.2019.00854 (accessed on 8th May 2025).

20. Koeller, K. K., & Shih, R. (2019). Intradural extramedullary spinal neoplasms: Radiologic-pathologic correlation. *Radiographics, 39*, 468–490. https://doi.org/10.1148/rg.2019180200 (accessed on 8th May 2025).

21. Kowalczyk, K. A., & Majewski, A. (2021). Analysis of surgical errors associated with anatomical variations clinically relevant in general surgery: Review of the literature. *Translational Research in Anatomy, 23*, 100107. https://doi.org/10.1016/j.tria.2020.100107 (accessed on 8th May 2025).

22. Mastitskaya, S., Thompson, N., & Holder, D. (2021). Selective vagus nerve stimulation as a therapeutic approach for the treatment of ARDS: A rationale for neuro-immunomodulation in COVID-19 disease. *Frontiers in Neuroscience, 15*. https://doi.org/10.3389/fnins.2021.667036 (accessed on 8th May 2025).

23. Meyers, C. A., Lisiecki, J., Miller, S., Levin, A. S., Fayad, L. M., Ding, C., Sono, T., et al. (2019). Heterotopic ossification: A comprehensive review. *JBMR Plus, 3*. https://doi.org/10.1002/jbm4.10172 (accessed on 8th May 2025).

24. Pino, A. (2021). Lymph node dissection morbidity in thyroid cancer: An integrative review. *Şişli Etfal Hastanesi Tıp Bülteni / The Medical Bulletin of Sisli Hospital*. https://doi.org/10.14744/semb.2021.33401 (accessed on 8th May 2025).

25. Qi, F., Wang, Z., Cai, P., Zhao, L., Gao, J., Kokudo, N., Li, A., et al. (2013). Traditional Chinese medicine and related active compounds: A review of their role on hepatitis B virus infection. *Drug Discoveries & Therapeutics, 7*. https://doi.org/10.5582/ddt.2013.v7.6.212 (accessed on 8th May 2025).

26. Rangon, C. M., Krantic, S., Moyse, E., & Fougère, B. (2020). The vagal autonomic pathway of COVID-19 at the crossroad of Alzheimer's disease and aging: A review of knowledge. *Journal of Alzheimer's Disease Reports, 4*, 537–551. https://doi.org/10.3233/adr-200273 (accessed on 8th May 2025).
27. Rueda-Lopes, F. (2021). The cranial nerves: Extensions of the central nervous system or components of the peripheral nervous system – How should we evaluate them? *Radiologia Brasileira, 54*, V–VI. https://www.semanticscholar.org/paper/726a87af3ac8ed81ea18fed949aed98b0545d9f6 (accessed on 8th May 2025).
28. Salvador, J. C., Coutinho, M. P., Venâncio, J. M., & Viamonte, B. (2019). Dynamic magnetic resonance imaging of the female pelvic floor—A pictorial review. *Insights into Imaging, 10*. https://doi.org/10.1186/s13244-019-0687-9 (accessed on 8th May 2025).
29. Schaverien, M. V., Badash, I., Selber, J. C., Cheng, M. H., & Patel, K. M. (2018). Vascularized lymph node transfer for lymphedema. *Seminars in Plastic Surgery, 32*, 028–035. https://doi.org/10.1055/s-0038-1632401 (accessed on 8th May 2025).
30. Smith, C. F., Finn, G. M., Stewart, J. A., Atkinson, M., Davies, D. C., Dyball, R. E. J., Morris, J. F., et al. (2015). The anatomical society core regional anatomy syllabus for undergraduate medicine. *Journal of Anatomy, 228*, 15–23. https://doi.org/10.1111/joa.12405 (accessed on 8th May 2025).
31. Su, D., Zhang, Z., Xia, F., & Li, X. (2023). The safety, benefits and future development of overnight and outpatient thyroidectomy. *Frontiers in Endocrinology, 14*. https://doi.org/10.3389/fendo.2023.1110038 (accessed on 8th May 2025).
32. Vermeiren, S., Bellefroid, E., & Desiderio, S. (2020). Vertebrate sensory ganglia: Common and divergent features of the transcriptional programs generating their functional specialization. *Frontiers in Cell and Developmental Biology, 8*. https://doi.org/10.3389/fcell.2020.587699 (accessed on 8th May 2025).

BACK AND SPINE REGION

15

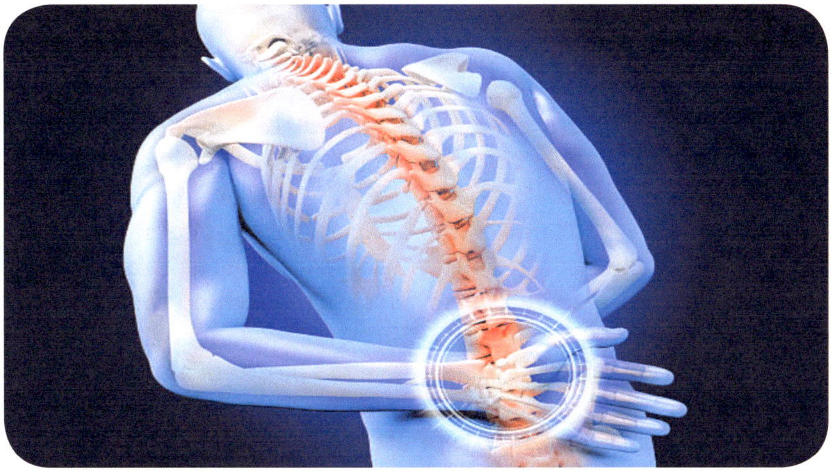

LEARNING OBJECTIVES

After studying this chapter, you will be able to:

1. Discuss the Anatomy of the Spine
2. Explain the Common Back and Spine Disorders
3. Focus on Diagnostic Techniques
4. Understand Treatment and Management

Introduction

The human body's complex structure is beautifully designed to enable motion, protect inner organs, and provide overall well-being. Among its many components, the back and spine region plays a very crucial role, as it serves as the pillar of physical mobility and strength. The region not only enables humans to walk on two legs but also provides flexibility and support during the course of various activities, from mere walking to competitive sports. It is important to know the spine's anatomy and physiology to realize its significance in daily life. The backbone, which consists of vertebrae, intervertebral discs (IVDs), and surrounding muscles, performs many functions, such as protecting the spinal cord while permitting a range of motion. Through studying the spine and back area, one can reap good information on how it aids human activity, assists in overall health, and highlights how it is essential to ensure a healthy spinal posture for efficient functioning.

Definition of the Back and Spine Region

The back and spine is a complex anatomical structure essential to many body functions, including mobility, support, and integrity of the central nervous system (CNS) protection. The vertebral column, formed by a series of bones named vertebrae, with interspersed discs allowing cushioning and flexibility, constitutes it. This region is also separated anatomically into definite regions: the cervical, thoracic, lumbar, sacral, and coccygeal segments, each with its own special function. The significance of the back is not just in the structural support; it also plays a very significant role in the overall body biomechanics, influencing posture and mobility. As medical imaging and analysis have progressed, as indicated in current research, a comprehension of the intricacies of the spine can enable improved diagnostics and therapies for spinal injury disorders and back pain (Liu & Sabatini, 2020). Anatomical knowledge of this area is critical, especially with the increasing prevalence of spine issues in modern society (Liu & Sabatini, 2020) (Figure 15.1).

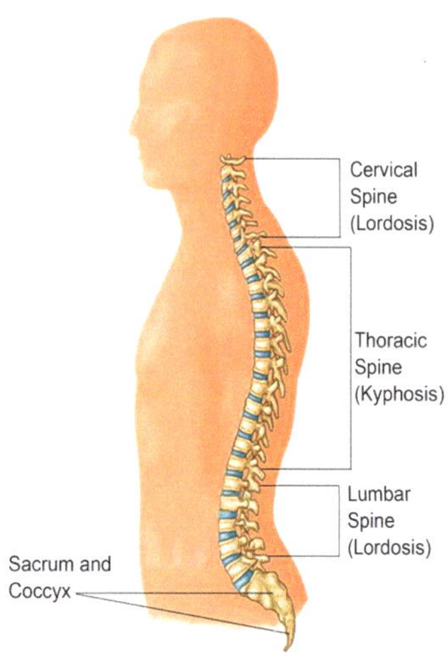

Figure 15.1. Regions of the spine.

Source: American Academy of Orthopedic Surgeons. (n.d.). *Spinal Curvature Anatomy*.

Importance of the Back and Spine in Human Anatomy

Outside of their role as stabilizing structures, back and spine also perform a secondary role in the overall functioning and mobility of the body. Possessing 33 vertebrae in a stable yet flexible structure, the spinal column has to accommodate the spinal cord, which is responsible for transmitting the nerve impulses throughout the body. This multi-dimensional process aims at the potential of good spinal health to prevent a cascade of musculoskeletal (MSK) ailments, including back pain, which is becoming more prevalent across people of all ages (Yao et al., 2011; Rajan and Koti, 2013). Additionally, education regarding back and spine health is essential, especially in the school setting. To pay attention to posture and ergonomics in children not only prevents future back problems but also allows for success in learning through the assurance of improved physical health, echoing the significance the back's health holds in leading a healthy and productive life (Liu & Sabatini, 2020). In attending to the spine, we set the stage for healthier generations to come.

Overview of the Structure of the Spine

The spinal column, or backbone, is a complex structure that is both required for support and movement. Composed of 33 individual vertebrae, the backbone contains five distinct regions: cervical, thoracic, lumbar, sacral, and coccygeal. Each region possesses its own specific functions, with the cervical vertebrae providing movement for the head, and the lumbar region supporting the upper weight of the body and helping to provide bending and twisting. The vertebrae are separated by intervertebral discs (IVDs), which act as shock absorbers and permit flexibility. This complex structure not only provides a stable framework to enclose the spinal cord but also allows a range of movement necessary for daily function. Disorder may arise from dysfunction within this structure, and it is therefore crucial to maintain optimum spine health by ensuring proper alignment and mobility exercises. Overall, the spinal anatomy is a very significant aspect of human function and anatomy, and it illustrates the need for adequate care and understanding.

Common Issues Related to the Back and Spine

Bad posture and too much sedentary life are common reasons for recurrent back and spine issues, leading to a range of MSK conditions.

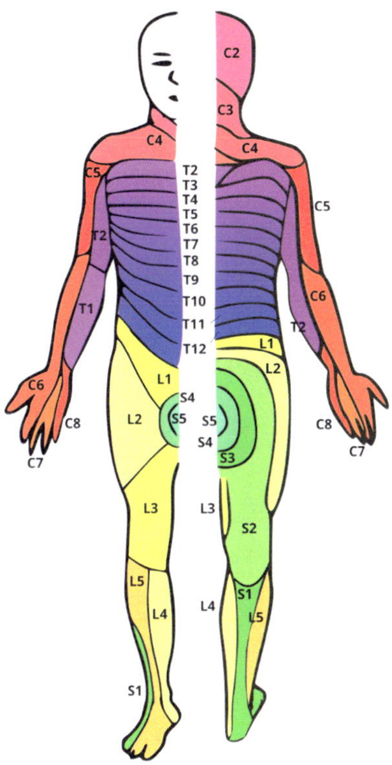

Source: By Ralf Stephan (mailto:ralf@ark.in-berlin.de) - altered from File:Dermatoms.svg. Colors changed, a couple corrections. original source: http://www.ark.in-berlin.de/senszonen.svgz(https://web.archive.org/web/20080525104214/www.ark.in-berlin.de/neuropics.html), Public Domain, https://commons.wikimedia.org/w/index.php?curid=46154280

For instance, the majority of individuals do not keep good ergonomics when working at desks or on computing devices, resulting in perpetual pain, particularly in the lower back and neck regions. Studies show that these MSK conditions are prevalent not only among the general population but also among some groups of workers, including dental workers who tend to experience discomfort due to the nature of their working environment (Liu & Sabatini, 2020). Additionally, other factors like heavy lifting, repetitive motions, and poor body mechanics add to existing problems with the back, leading to conditions like herniated discs and sciatica. At a larger level, prevention of such issues through improved ergonomic standards and education can help a great deal in enhancing spinal health and reducing the incidence of related disorders, towards a healthier workforce.

Brief Outline of the Topics to be Covered

The structure of the back and spinal region is complex, including anatomy, overall disease, and treatment. As a precursor, an extensive study of the anatomical structure will give the foundation, separating the region into vertebral column, surface muscle tissue, and spinal cord, all necessary to understanding the structure of how these parts are outlined and function. Second, the focus will shift to those disorders that are prevalent in this region, i.e., herniated discs and scoliosis, and how and in what way they pose a threat to mobility and overall quality of life (QoL). Finally, treatments may be discussed, alternatively ranging from physical therapy to surgery and cutting-edge medical technology, to illustrate the range of options patients can pursue to bring about an end to the agony and recovery. By presenting a step-by-step account of the same, the essay will be able to offer an informed opinion regarding the extent to which well-being is guaranteed through the preservation of back and spine health, along with the prevention and intervention elements as well.

Relevance of Back and Spine Health

The importance of back and spine health cannot be emphasized enough because these areas are central to general well-being and function in day-to-day life. Low back pain (LBP) has been established as the most prevalent global cause of disability, affecting millions and taxing health care systems globally. Interestingly enough, in 2015, LBP contributed to 60.1 million disability-adjusted life-years, a considerable 54% increase from 1990, and these levels were especially high in low-income and middle-income countries (Malfliet et al., 2019). This increase in the incidence of back pain highlights not just the subsequent burden of back pain but also the subsequent economic impact, with health expenditures skyrocketing; in the United States alone, low back and neck pain expenditures totaled a staggering $134.5 billion in 2016 (Liu & Sabatini, 2020). Spine health is thus an important concern, as mobility, QoL, and socioeconomic stability in general significantly hinge on it. Successful prevention and management would reduce individual suffering and healthcare expenditure, also underlining the importance of emergent public consciousness and intervention concerning spinal health.

Historical Perspective on Back and Spine Studies

Spinal and back research through the ages demonstrates the richness of scientific curiosity and treatment innovation across centuries. The genesis of spinal anatomy and relevance was traced to ancient times, when primitive observations formed the foundation for modern understanding. As the science developed, attention shifted from exterior level anatomical description to inquiries concerning spinal health and contribution toward improved human well-being in general. For example, developments in nanotechnology recently uncovered promising prospects for therapeutic uses, demonstrating how research pushes our practice of medical interventions beyond diagnostic functions to new drug delivery pathways (Liu & Sabatini, 2020). Further, previous successes with neuromodulation, such as vagus nerve stimulation (VNS), unveil the intricacy of spinal and nerve dynamics, demonstrating the far-reaching implications for spinal health-related disorders (Liu & Sabatini, 2020). Together, these innovations constitute a dialogue between the past record and current advances in the practice of medicine that continue to influence our understanding of the back and spine (Figure 15.2).

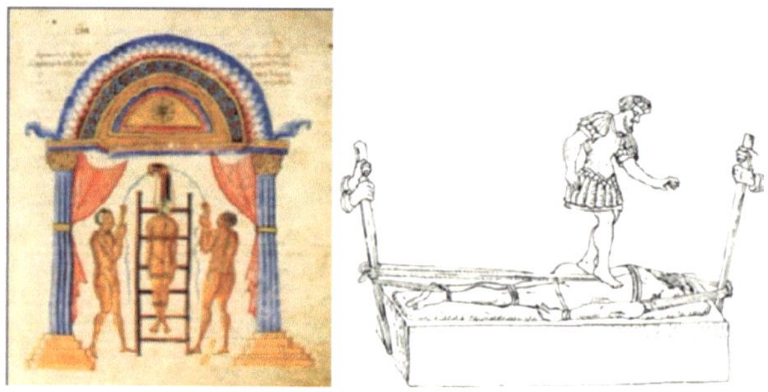

Figure 15.2. Historical perspective on back and spine studies.

Source: Bettany-Saltikov, J., Villagrasa, M., Ferrer, M., Negrini, S., Rigo, M., & Wood, G. (2017). Management of spinal deformities and evidence of treatment effectiveness. *The Open Orthopedics Journal, 11*, 1521–1547.

15.1. Anatomy of the Spine

Learning Outcome

1. Describe the Structure of Vertebrae
2. Explain the Types of Vertebrae: Cervical, Thoracic, Lumbar, Sacrum and coccyx
3. Focus on Intervertebral Discs and their Function
2. Understand Spinal Cord and Protective Role of Vertebrae
3. Focus on Spinal Nerves and their Significance
4. Know Curvatures of the Spine: Lordosis, Kyphosis, Scoliosis
5. Understand Ligaments and Muscles Supporting the Spine
6. Explain the Role of the Pelvis in Spinal Alignment
7. Explain the Blood Supply and Innervation of the Spine

The spine is a complex structure comprised of vertebrae, intervertebral discs (IVDs), ligaments, and nerves that all function together to protect the spinal cord and ensure the body's posture. Composed of 33 individual vertebrae segmented into five regions—cervical, thoracic, lumbar, sacral, and coccygeal—the spine offers a degree of motion and pliability required to perform day-to-day tasks. There are some parts of the spine which are susceptible to various disorders; e.g., low back pain (LBP) is a prevalent disorder with significant public health consequences, leading to gigantic economic cost and disability (Laxmaiah et al., 2015).

Anatomy also reveals varied risk factors for pain, including mechanical stress and psychosocial stressors, that are causative of chronic conditions like myelomeningocele when the neural anatomy is interfered with during development (Liu & Sabatini, 2020). The spine's complex structure is important to learn about the proper assessment, prevention and management of spinal pathology.

15.1.1. Structure of Vertebrae

The vertebrae comprise a compound structure with both protective and functional functions in the human body. The vertebral body, the arch, and the processes are some of the many critical parts that constitute all vertebrae and provide points of attachment for muscles and ligaments. Of particular interest, the IVDs between the vertebrae provide flexibility and shock absorption, which plays a crucial part in guaranteeing mobility and lessening impact, particularly during activities. There have also been advances in imaging technologies such as digital video fluoroscopy (DVF) that have increased understanding of spine mechanics so that clinicians can visualize motion and diagnose issues more effectively (Liu & Sabatini, 2020). Such insights are particularly valuable in both diagnostic and therapeutic applications. Additionally, understanding the vertebrae biomechanics can be utilized to engineer interventions and supports required to protect against the long-term effects of vibration and impacts, particularly in hostile environments, and improve the efficacy of spinal health screening (Malfliet et al., 2019) (Figure 15.3).

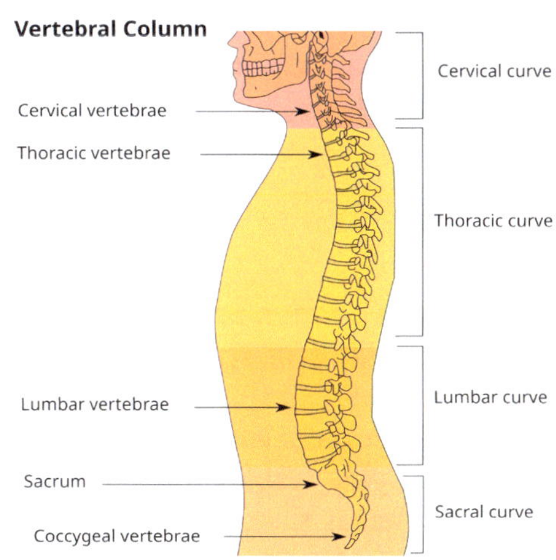

Figure 15.3. Vertebral column.

Source: Wikimedia Commons. (n.d.). *Vertebral Column Illustration*.

15.1.2. Types of Vertebrae: Cervical, Thoracic, Lumbar, Sacrum and coccyx

The human spine is made up of vertebrae that each have unique functions: cervical, thoracic, and lumbar, sacral and coccyx. Cervical vertebrae, located at the upper part of the spine, contain seven bones that support the weight of the head and allow for great mobility, including rotating and tilting. Such a degree of flexibility is needed for daily movement and neck function. Below the cervical spine, the 12 thoracic vertebrae fuse with the ribs to form a cage for the thoracic organs and stabilization of the upper body. The five lumbar vertebrae, the largest and strongest of the spine, which bear a considerable amount of weight and enable extension and flexion. The triangular bone at the base of the spine ,the sacrum, formed by fusion of five sacral vertebrae and connects the spine with the pelvis. The coccyx also known as the tail bone, made of fused vertebrae (4-5) located at the very end of the spine. These regions of the spine communicate with one another to have balance, offer posture support, and facilitate movement, making it crucial to comprehend them in diagnosing spinal conditions and creating efficient treatment methods, as researched in vertebral segmentation and identification processes (Clark, 1906).

15.1.3. Intervertebral Discs and their Function

The complex organization and function of IVDs are a major regulator of spinal flexibility and well-being. Between the vertebrae, the discs serve as shock absorbers with cushioning during movement and spine stabilization. Their tough outer layer known as the annulus fibrosus and gelatinous center known as the nucleus pulposus enable them to absorb and distribute loads effectively. Yet as implied in recent research, disc-vertebra interface injury is generally linked with disc herniation and chronic back pain. Such vulnerability arises as a result of cartilage endplate and vertebra structural breakdown, rendering them fragile and susceptible to breaking (Malfliet et al., 2019). Moreover, age degeneration in these discs can be a significant cause of pain, and this emphasizes their crucial role in spinal function as a whole and the need for their integrity to be preserved (Malfliet et al., 2019). Finally, IVDs are crucial to spinal function and thus worthy of consideration for discussion on back health.

15.1.4. Spinal Cord and Protective Role of Vertebrae

The spinal cord is a vital link between the brain and the rest of the body. Enclosed within the vertebral column, it is supported and protected by an elaborate system of the spinal meninges, CSF, and the vertebrae themselves. All these elements combined absorb impact force, which significantly diminishes the risk of injury from everyday activities and accidents (Liu & Sabatini, 2020).

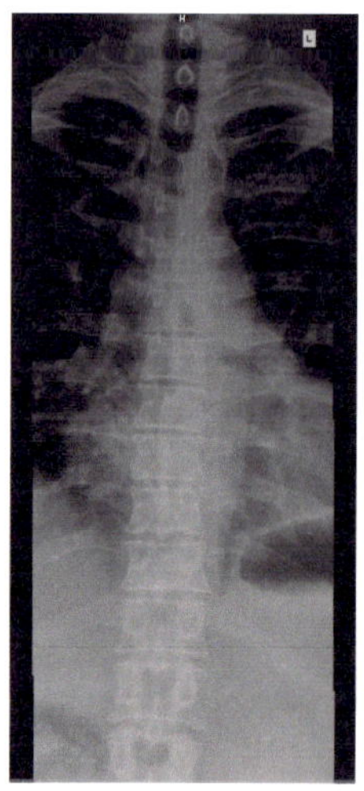

Figure 15.4. Spinal cord.

Source: By Whoisjohngalt - Taken with a Optima XR646Previously published: Never Before Published, CC BY-SA 4.0, https://commons.wikimedia.org/w/index.php?curid=64398006

Such a robust protective mechanism despite, the spinal cord is prone to severe injury, which is far-reaching with consequences involving paralysis (Malfliet et al., 2019). It is thus crucial in clinics and everyday life to be aware of the fine relationship between external forces and spinal integrity. By maintaining the spinal column and coverings in good health, people may be preventing the onset of serious spinal disease, reaffirming the importance of spine health for overall well-being (Figure 15.4).

15.1.5. Spinal Nerves and their Significance

The spinal nerves play a very vital role in the nervous system of the body as they serve as major pathways for the transmission of information between the brain and various parts of the body. A pair of spinal nerves emanates from the spinal cord, for every particular region of the body, and is responsible for transmitting sensory and motor impulses. This complex network of nerves makes possible such important functions as voluntary muscle movement and the senses of touch, temperature, and pain. Spinal nerves have significant medical uses, with damage potentially leading to life-altering consequences like paralysis or loss of sensation. For instance, in the assessment of spinal cord injury, proper documentation is critical to determine the severity of impairments and design rehabilitation interventions, as indicated by enhanced assessment tools like the American Spinal Injury Association (ASIA) Impairment Scale (Rüdiger et al., 2021). Such emphasis on spinal nerve integrity indicates their significance not only in mobility but also in quality of life (QoL).

15.1.6. Curvatures of the Spine: Lordosis, Kyphosis, Scoliosis

It is necessary to comprehend the curvatures of the spine so that one can diagnose and treat many disorders of the spine. Lordosis, or concavity of the lumbar spine, and kyphosis, or convexity of the thoracic spine, are both required to allow for the normal posture and equilibrium of the human body. Scoliosis, as a lateral spinal curvature, is a more complex deformity that has the potential to interfere with these natural alignments and lead to pain and dysfunction in the body. Studies have demonstrated that individuals with scoliosis exhibit decreased lumbar lordosis compared to individuals with typical spinal alignments, which suggests the connection between such curvatures and general spine health (Grzanka et al., 2018). Moreover, new non-invasive measuring techniques, i.e., the tangential calculation method, have been introduced to measure these deformities in a more reliable way without the hazard of radiation exposure using X-rays (Jáger et al., 2018). This is essential for long-term follow-up and effective treatment planning (Figure 15.5).

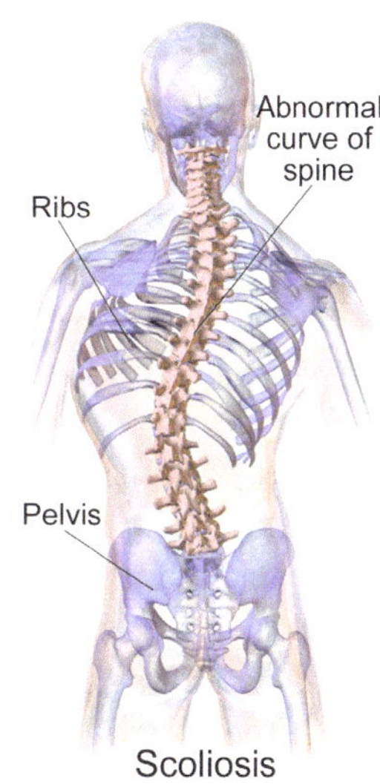

Figure 15.5. Normal and abnormal spinal curvature.

Source: By BruceBlaus. When using this image in external sources it can be cited as:Blausen.com staff (2014). "Medical gallery of Blausen Medical 2014". WikiJournal of Medicine 1 (2). DOI:10.15347/wjm/2014.010. ISSN 2002-4436. - Own work, CC BY 3.0, https://commons.wikimedia.org/w/index.php?curid=27796966

15.1.7. Ligaments and Muscles Supporting the Spine

The structural integrity and functionality of the spine are largely maintained by a sophisticated network of muscles and ligaments. Ligaments, such as the anterior and posterior longitudinal ligaments, provide crucial stability by connecting vertebrae and inhibiting inappropriate movement that could lead to damage. On the other hand, the paraspinal muscles are in charge of spinal motion and posture, stabilizing the spine during various motions, including bending and twisting. Research highlights the significance of such muscle contributions; the flexion-relaxation phenomenon (FRP), for instance, illustrates how the force of gravity and muscle fatigue can affect lumbar stability (Clark, 1906). It is significant to know individual muscle forces as well, since increased loading may cause tissue overload and pain, but this justifies the need for an integrated approach to spinal health (Clark, 1906). Hence, a balanced assessment of the ligaments and muscles provides insights essential to appreciating the mechanisms of the spine and preventing injury.

15.1.8. Role of the Pelvis in Spinal Alignment

The pelvis also serves as a significant foundation for the proper positioning of the spine, dictating how forces travel through the torso and lower body. An out-of-position pelvis can potentially create compensatory alterations in the lumbar spine, often resulting in pain or discomfort. For instance, chronic tightening of the adjacent muscles, such as the tensor fascia Lata (TFL), can result in an anterior pelvic tilt, thus negatively affecting the lumbar posture and vertebral alignment, exacerbating conditions such as LBP (Clark, 1906). Furthermore, the literature indicates that some chair designs, i.e., pelvic-support chairs, have the potential to enhance lumbar lordosis and sacral alignment, and through this, promote a healthier sitting posture and potentially decrease pain in those suffering from non-specific LBP (Kyue-Nam et al., 2022). Thus, optimal alignment of the pelvis is not only paramount to overall spine health but also to effective management and prevention of LBP.

15.1.9. Blood Supply and Innervation of the Spine

There is a complex system of innervation and blood supply that must be maintained to maintain the spine's integrity and function. The lumbar spine, for example, is innervated and supplied with vascular support by the lumbar arteries and their branches, which supply the vertebral bodies and related structures.

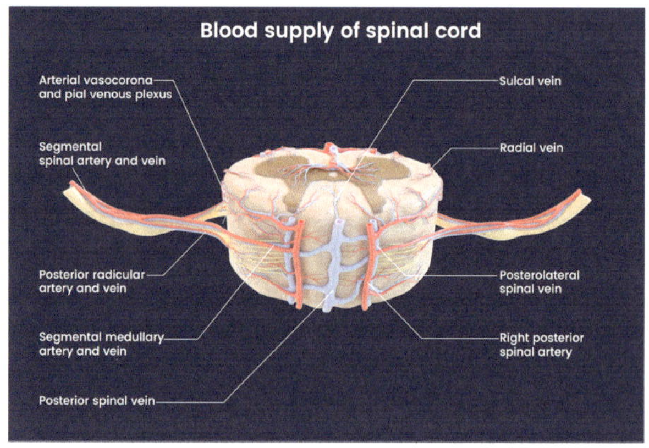

Figure 15.6. Blood supply and innervation of the spine.

Source: Anatomy.app. (n.d.). *Blood Supply of Spinal Cord.*

Further, the spinal nerves exiting the vertebral column at every segment play a crucial role in the maintenance of proprioception and in facilitating transmission between the spinal cord and the peripheral structures. According to the patterns of innervation, there are two different types of nerve supplies: segmental innervation by spinal nerves and non-segmental contributions from the sympathetic trunk, with a revealed complex interaction that can influence spinal well-being in general and perception of pain (Higuchi et al., 2002). Lastly, an integrated understanding of this spinal neural and vascular architecture underlies the significant correlation between structural integrity and functional performance of the spine (Clark, 1906) (Figure 15.6).

Test Your Knowledge

1. Discuss the Role of the Pelvis in Spinal Alignment
2. Focus on Blood Supply and Innervation of the Spine

15.2. Common Back and Spine Disorders

Learning Outcome

1. Describe the Herniated Discs and their Impact
2. Explain the Sciatica: Causes and Symptoms
3. Know Osteoarthritis and Spinal Degeneration
4. Understand Scoliosis: Types and Treatment Options
5. Evaluate Spinal Stenosis and Its Effects
6. Define the Muscle Strains and Sprains in the Back
7. Know Osteoporosis and its Relation to Spine Health
8. Describe the Chronic Back Pain: Causes and Management
9. Discuss the Impact of Lifestyle on Back Disorders

There are many disorders that are accountable for the high prevalence of spine and back disorders, significantly impacting individuals' QoL. Among those disorders is lumbar disc herniation (LDH), which is frequently presented as LBP radiating down the legs, sensory impairment, and even urinary dysfunction in critical cases. Surgery is contemplated if conservative treatment fails, yet open surgery may cause appreciable trauma to the surrounding ligaments and muscles, with loss of spinal stability (Clark, 1906). Such physical ailments are often accompanied by psychological comorbidities like depression and anxiety, as in the case of young patients with osteochondrosis of the lumbar spine, which can exacerbate pain perception and distort the outcomes of treatment (Krychun et al., 2021). It is important to know the interplay of physical and psychological factors to create effective treatment strategies for patients with these widespread disorders of the back and spine region.

15.2.1. Herniated Discs and their Impact

The impact of herniated discs is far more than mere body pain; it can severely disturb day-to-day life, work efficiency, and general health. A herniated disc refers to the situation where the soft material within the disc bulges out, putting pressure on the adjacent nerves and causing pain, numbness, or weakness along the nerve paths of the offending nerves. It is a major cause of LBP, a condition that is increasingly prevalent in today's world. Of special note, recent studies emphasize that surgical interventions, such as spinal fusion, can result in significant relief for patients suffering from chronic back pain caused by disc degeneration (Binch et al., 2015). Further, advances in medical research introduce new treatments into the limelight, for example, stem cell therapies aimed at recovering from defective disc tissue and minimizing pain, which highlights the relevance of the examination of the cellular process of disc degeneration (Haq et al., 2015). Last but not least, the management of the consequences of herniated discs is necessary to optimize patient QoL and design effective treatments (Figure 15.7).

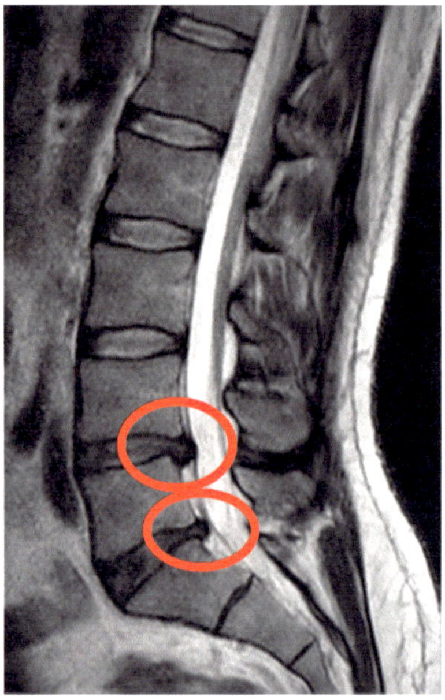

Figure 15.7. Herniated disk.

Source: By Miguel Tremblay - Own work, CC0, https://commons.wikimedia.org/w/index.php?curId=137827133

15.2.2. Sciatica: Causes and Symptoms

Characterized by severe, stabbing pain that radiates along the path of the sciatic nerve, sciatica can significantly interfere with normal functioning. Its primary cause is a herniated disc, where the soft tissue of the disc bulges out and compresses adjacent spinal nerves, which in turn results in numbness and muscle weakness in the affected limb (Venes, 2011). The other causes are stenosis of the spine, in which the canal of the spine narrows, and degenerative disc disease, as the hydration and elasticity of discs diminish over time increasing friction and inflammation. The presentation of sciatica will be highly variable, but apart from pain in the back of the leg, it will be tingling or burning (Venes, 2011). Understanding the complex relationship between these causes and their individual symptoms is important in developing successful treatment plans, which may involve physical therapy, medication, or in the case of severe injuries, surgery (Figure 15.8).

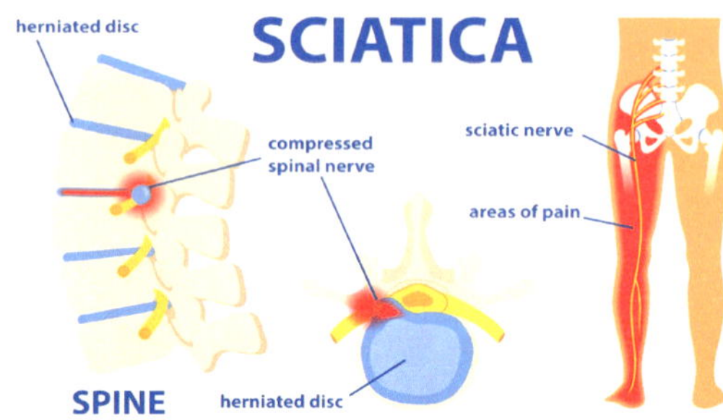

Figure 15.8. Sciatica.

Source: St.Louis Brain & Spine. (2021). *Sciatica: Herniated Disc Compressing Spinal Nerve and Pain Distribution.*

15.2.3. Osteoarthritis and Spinal Degeneration

Spinal decay, more so due to osteoarthritis, contributes significantly to an individual's QoL. The degenerative condition is mainly responsible for chronic pain, reduced mobility, and other neurological features, which might originate from structural changes in the spinal column. Surgical interventions, such as spinal decompression, may address some of these issues by improving function and decreasing the levels of pain, as evidenced in studies where better results were found for lower limb function following the procedures (Liu & Sabatini, 2020). But also, the transition to non-surgical approaches to treatment, such as intramuscular and intraosseous lidocaine trigger point injections, has also been given attention. Such interventions have been shown to have differential success in alleviating post-surgical residual pain, with intraosseous injection being much more potent as an analgesic than intramuscular injections

(Al-Zamil et al., 2024). Treating osteoarthritis and spinal degeneration overall is a treatment strategy that is multidimensional and tailored to the individual's unique condition.

15.2.4. Scoliosis: Types and Treatment Options

A common spinal disease, scoliosis is very difficult and unique in individuals. There are different types of scoliosis, of which adolescent idiopathic scoliosis, occurring primarily at growth spurts, affects a large proportion of children, particularly adolescent girls. Degenerative scoliosis, on the contrary, typically occurs later in life due to degeneration of spinal discs, more commonly among those over the age of 65, as highlighted by the prevalence of chronic pain for this type of scoliosis (Husejko et al., 2019). Treatment depends on severity and type of curvature; for instance, curvatures less than 30° can be managed without treatment, while bracing may be applied for some adolescents with minimal curves to prevent progression (Janse et al., 2008). For severe curvature, surgery may be required, especially for those with curves greater than 50°. In most cases, early detection and timely treatment can enhance QoL for the affected to a great extent.

15.2.5. Spinal Stenosis and Its Effects

A readily overlooked condition, spinal stenosis can significantly impair QoL by its effects on mobility and activities of daily living. Characterized as the narrowing of the spinal canal, the condition can lead to incapacitating symptoms such as lower back pain, which has been shown to be responsive to interventions like vitamin D supplementation, especially in patients with documented deficiency (Liu & Sabatini, 2020).

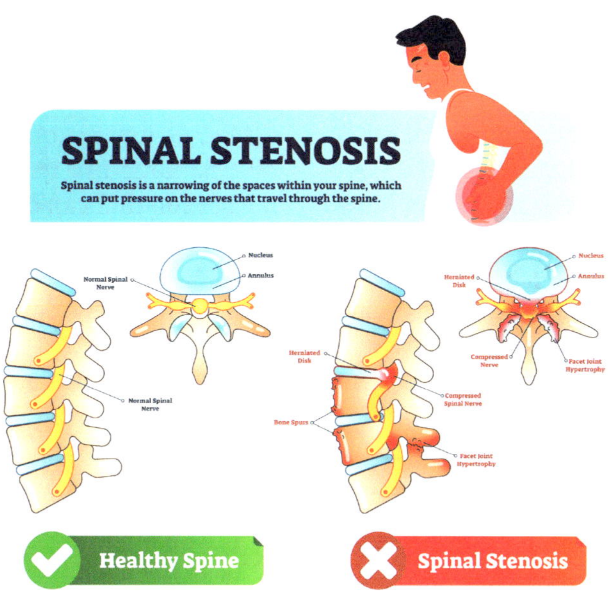

Figure 15.9. Spinal stenosis.

Source: Premia Spine. (2024). Grades and treatment options for spinal stenosis severity. *Spinal Stenosis*.

In addition, outcomes following surgical interventions, such as posterior decompression, indicate that individuals with spinal stenosis may experience varied results based on their preoperative sagittal alignment. The literature reveals that patients with malalignment experience worse health-related quality of life (HRQOL) scores post-surgery than those without malalignment, demonstrating the importance of meticulous assessment and personalized management approaches (Momotaro et al., 2023). Thus, familiarity with the multifaceted effects of spinal stenosis is essential for effective treatment and rehabilitation (Figure 15.9).

15.2.6. Muscle Strains and Sprains in the Back

Back injuries, such as muscle strain and sprain, are prevalent conditions that may severely impact an individual's mobility and QoL. They typically develop due to acute and forced motion or repetitive stress, resulting in the overstretching or tearing of muscle fibers and ligaments. The lumbosacral region is more vulnerable, as it carries most of the body's weight and provides protection against the shock of everyday activity and sports. According to several reports, the primary symptom is LBP and spasms of the muscles, which, unless effectively managed, run the risk of becoming chronic complications that can impede active life participation (Dalen et al., 2007). For example, in sporting activities such as surfing, muscle trauma is frequent secondary to violent contractions in dynamic maneuvers (Climstein et al., 2020). An understanding of the mechanism of these sprains and strains is critical to the design of effective prevention and rehabilitation strategies, ultimately decreasing their occurrence in both sporting and daily contexts.

15.2.7. Osteoporosis and its Relation to Spine Health

The correlation of osteoporosis with spinal health has extreme implications for the elderly. As bone density worsens, one is increasingly at risk of spine fracture that can significantly impair mobility and QoL. For instance, a new Swedish pilot study highlights the fact that fractures of the spine may have higher costs and a worse Quality of Life (QoL) than earlier understood, the clear need for comprehensive health economic evaluations in this area (Borgström et al., 2002). Furthermore, exercise programs to enhance bone density have been shown to have a profound positive effect on the health of the spine. It was found in a research that compliance with a multi-component exercise program led to an increase in bone mineral density at the femoral neck, which highlights the importance of exercise in preventing osteosporosis damaging effects (Shiva Prasad et al., 2023). These findings cumulatively highlight the importance of early prevention of osteoporosis in ensuring spinal health and general well-being in the elderly.

15.2.8. Chronic Back Pain: Causes and Management

Chronic low back pain is a frequent complaint of ill health and often the consequence of a variety of causative factors such as muscular strain, degeneration of the intervertebral discs, or traumatic injury. One such condition is disc herniation that can cause pain and disability and hence must be understood in their pathogenesis and treatments. Management of chronic low back pain must be a comprehensive process that may involve physical therapy, medical management, and lifestyle modifications. For instance, Pilates training has proved to enhance pain sensitivity and stabilometric indices in patients with nonspecific LBP, emphasizing the importance of individually tailored physical activity during rehabilitation (Jinks et al., 2014). Furthermore, careful examination of disc disease, including internal disc disruption and annular tears, is critical in developing tailored treatment protocols (Jinks et al., 2014). Lastly, an understanding of the multifaceted nature of chronic back pain allows clinicians to employ more effective, individualized treatment, which can result in improved patient outcomes.

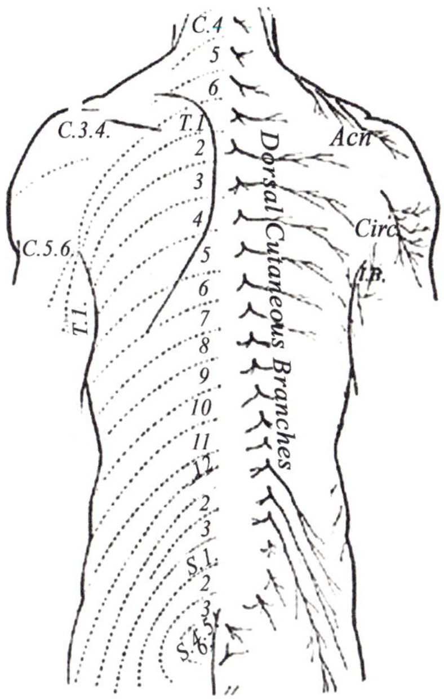

Source: By Henry Gray (1827–1861) - Cropped and trimmed version of File:Gray798.png, from Henry Gray (1918) Anatomy of the Human Body., Public Domain, https://commons.wikimedia.org/w/index.php?curid=77508331

15.2.9. Impact of Lifestyle on Back Disorders

Lifestyle contributes significantly to the prevalence and severity of back disorders, and hence, there is a call for comprehensive health interventions. Sedentary way of life, poor posture, and lack of exercise on a regular basis result in musculoskeletal (MSK) conditions like chronic pain and discomfort. Evidence indicates that exercising through non-impact activities contributes to a decrease in the symptoms of conditions like ankylosing spondylitis (AS), and this again points towards the necessity of proactive lifestyle modifications (Owen et al., 2017). Also, emotional status is involved; individuals with distress associated with their neck pain have more disability. For patients with neck pain, in one study, those with emotional problems, such as sleeping difficulties or chronic tearfulness, were found to have high levels of disability compared to their healthier counterparts (Frank et al., 2004). Therefore, adopting a life of physical well-being and mental well-being can significantly minimize the likelihood of back disorders with overall improved well-being.

Test Your Knowledge

1. What is the difference between a muscle strain and a ligament sprain in the back?
2. How can poor posture contribute to back disorders?

15.3. Diagnostic Techniques

Learning Outcome

1. Discuss the Physical Examination Methods
2. Explain the Imaging Techniques: X-Rays, MRIs, CT Scans
3. Focus on Electromyography (EMG) and Nerve Conduction Studies
4. Discuss the Role of Ultrasound in Spine Assessment
5. Explain the Diagnostic Injections for Pain Relief
6. How to Importance of Patient History in Diagnosis
7. Differential Diagnosis of Back Pain
8. Understand Emerging Technologies in Spinal Diagnostics
9. How to Limitations of Current Diagnostic Methods

Effective diagnostic procedures are essential to properly identify disorders involving the back and spine. The traditional methods are prone to beginning with a thorough clinical assessment, whereby practitioners conduct patient histories and physical examinations to highlight symptoms. Imaging procedures, such as X-rays and MRIs, are valuable sources of information regarding structural issues, especially documenting details of disc conditions, including herniations or degenerative changes, which may manifest as long-term pain (Walker et al., 1993). In addition, emerging technologies, including state-of-the-art MRI techniques that assess inflammatory processes, enhance detection capability for diagnoses like AS, which involve complex autoimmune interactions in the spine (Owen et al., 2017). These diagnostic tools not only provide accurate diagnosis but also feed into successful treatment strategies, which enable practitioners to tailor interventions to individual patient profiles. Hence, a multidisciplinary diagnostic strategy ensures improved outcomes in the management of back and spine conditions.

15.3.1. Physical Examination Methods

In the assessment of patients presenting with back and spine issues, physical examination methods are crucial in determining the etiology of pain and dysfunction. Physical examination begins with a thorough patient history, then the physical evaluation of individual areas such as the lumbar, thoracic, and cervical spines. Techniques such as palpation, observation of posture, and functional movement analysis demonstrate the areas of tenderness and mechanical dysfunction. Notably, research showed that clinicians place greater emphasis on other screening processes when they are considering the application of thrust joint manipulation (TJM) in the cervical spine, a reflection of concern about safety and effectiveness in contrast to the thoracic and lumbar regions (Reilly et al., 2016). Moreover, consideration of subjective symptoms like pain or tenderness over the buttock area of the sciatic notch is valuable because such aspects can play a determining role in the diagnosis and management of conditions like piriformis syndrome (Chantraine et al., 2010). Overall, formal approach-based physical examination enhances diagnostic accuracy and informs effective treatment planning.

15.3.2. Imaging Techniques: X-Rays, MRIs, CT Scans

In evaluation of the back and spine region, imaging procedures such as X-rays, MRIs, and CT scans play a crucial role in diagnosis and treatment of conditions. X-rays provide a quick outline of bones, easily identifying fractures or improper alignment, but have limitations in identifying soft tissues and inflammatory processes. On the other hand, MRIs are optimum in giving clear pictures of the soft tissues, disc herniations, and nerve root compressions, making them a goldmine in assessing conditions such as AS that can lead to incapacitating pain and stiffness (Venes, 2011). Apart from that, CT scans are utilized to provide a better overview, particularly in complex cases that have a history of previous spinal surgery or trauma. Above all else, integration of advanced imaging techniques like SPECT/CT has been shown to enhance diagnostic specificity, revealing pain-generating structures that would otherwise be undetected by traditional imaging modalities (Kelechi et al., 2024). United, they are instrumental in evidence-based clinical decision-making in spinal conditions (Figure 15.10).

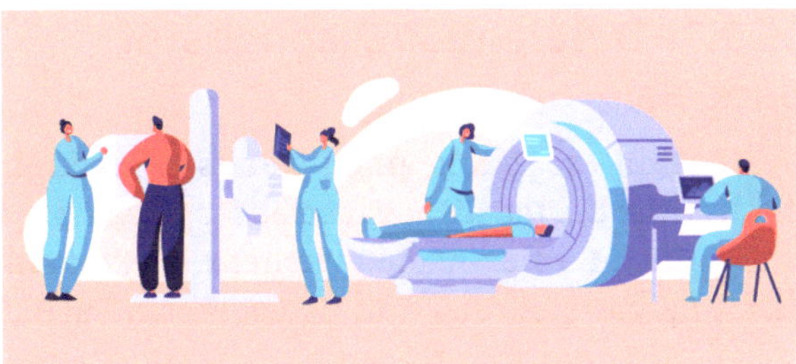

Figure 15.10. Imaging techniques: X-rays, MRIs, CT scans.

Source: Juhi, M. (2022). *X-Ray vs. CT Scan vs. MRI: Understanding the Differences in Imaging.*

15.3.3. Electromyography (EMG) and Nerve Conduction Studies

Understanding EMG and nerve conduction studies' uses and meanings is crucial in the diagnosis of back and spine neuromuscular disorders. In addition to the diagnostic tests measuring electrical muscle activity as well as nerve signal speed, they also provide a good approximation of muscle function and any disease within it. For instance, in back pain, EMG can detect underlying issues of neuropathic pain and muscle dysfunction so that individualized treatment can be directed. Moreover, while pain has been noted as a symptom of these tests, several interventions such as vapocoolant sprays and ibuprofen are available to minimize pain during the test (London et al., 2016). This is crucial for patient compliance and accurate outcomes. In this way, the effective use of EMG and nerve conduction studies is at the core of advancements in treatment techniques for spinal and back disorders (Liu & Sabatini, 2020).

15.3.4. Role of Ultrasound in Spine Assessment

In the past ten years, ultrasound has proven to be a promising modality in spinal condition evaluation, with clinicians acquiring a non-invasive, real-time imaging tool. The technique, specifically ultrasound elastography, gives the possibility of examining the characteristics of soft tissues, including IVDs' mechanical behavior. For example, research has shown that shear wave speed measurements obtained using elastography have been beneficial in the understanding of the mechanical properties of IVDs and hence in their diagnosis and follow-up of degenerative diseases (Bonneau et al., 2014). Moreover, ultrasounds' capability to image cervical IVDs has proven to be valuable in the assessment of macroscopic degeneration, therefore its use in detecting structural imperfections that are not apparent on standard imaging modalities like MRI (Back et al., 2019). With continued research, the use of ultrasound in routine spinal exams can prove to enhance diagnostic performance and improve patient outcomes.

15.3.5. Diagnostic Injections for Pain Relief

Pain relief diagnostic injections are a valuable resource in the treatment of spine and back disease, particularly when all other treatments have been exhausted. These injections, such as epidural steroid injections or facet joint blocks, serve both therapeutic and diagnostic purposes by treating a specific pain generator in the lumbar spine. By locating the origin of distress, they can distinguish between various types of LBP, such as nociceptive or neuropathic, and hence make more personalized treatment plans. Because of the complexity of the conditions manifest in the back, as outlined in the biopsychosocial model, the employment of diagnostic injections allows clinicians to create an interdisciplinary treatment plan that addresses the biological, psychological, and social factors that contribute to pain (Nebojša et al., 2021). Such overall approaches are necessary, as undiagnosed pain in the back can cause permanent disability as well as increasing healthcare costs (Liu & Sabatini, 2020). Therefore, modern pain treatment must involve such injections to achieve maximum outcomes.

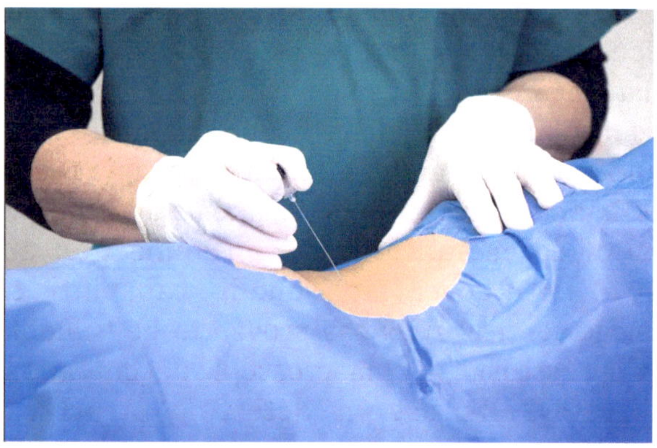

Source: Spine & Orthopedic Center. (2022). *Spine Injection Procedure.*

15.3.6. Importance of Patient History in Diagnosis

A good patient history is one of the pillars of sound diagnosis, particularly in complex areas like the back and spine region. Obtaining detailed information about the patient's previous injuries, patterns of pain, and lifestyle allows clinicians to identify underlying issues that are not readily apparent with diagnostic imaging alone. For instance, because pelvic osteoporosis can lead to vertebral fractures, information on a patient's risk factors—i.e., age, history, and occurrence of previous fractures—is vital in preventing future complications because unmanaged osteoporosis puts one at risk of further fracture, thereby escalating the possibility of disability and healthcare costs (Liu & Sabatini, 2020). Further, information on a patient's emotional and psychological state can give insight into perpetuating factors to his/her pain experience. Clinicians who have a full history are better able to individualize interventions, with final results being enhanced patient outcomes and solidarity during patient-provider communication, an essential ingredient in developing trust and adherence to treatment regimens.

15.3.7. Differential Diagnosis of Back Pain

Evaluation of back pain needs thorough differential diagnosis because etiology can play a significant role in management. Herniated discs, spinal stenosis, and osteoarthritis are a few of the conditions that need to be considered when assessing lumbar pain, but other less common conditions should not be forgotten. For instance, spontaneous spinal epidural hematoma (SSEH) is characterized by acute severe pain and neurologic impairment and highlights the need for early diagnostic imaging, particularly for unexplained weakness or pain, such as in case series where accurate identification led to early treatment (Venes, 2011). Other rare etiologies, such as tumor-induced osteomalacia in association with phosphaturic mesenchymal tumors, illustrate diagnostic complexity. These tumors are capable of causing systemic symptoms and may require surgical intervention, making an interdisciplinary approach a key for effective management (Shuzhong et al., 2020). A comprehensive diagnostic evaluation is therefore central to appropriate treatment outcomes in patients with back pain.

15.3.8. Emerging Technologies in Spinal Diagnostics

Spinal diagnostics have been evolving and revolutionizing how doctors diagnose and treat scoliosis, among other spinal deformities. Some emerging technologies, like the MAGEC system, are at the forefront with magnetically distractible rods that provide for incremental lengthening of the spine without exposing the patient to further surgeries, thus rendering the patient more comfortable and reducing recovery times (Andrew et al., 2014). Additionally, new products in the market, such as the Vertebral Metrics technology, are further expanding the promise of spinal assessment by accurately measuring the spatial coordinates of individual vertebrae. The technology finds application not just in scoliosis assessment, but also in other wellness and healthcare applications, a sign of its versatility and promise for widespread adoption (Venes, 2011). Integrating these technologies can lead to more precise diagnosis, individualized treatment planning, and improved long-term outcomes for patients with spinal disorders. As these technologies continue to evolve, they represent a new era in spine treatment.

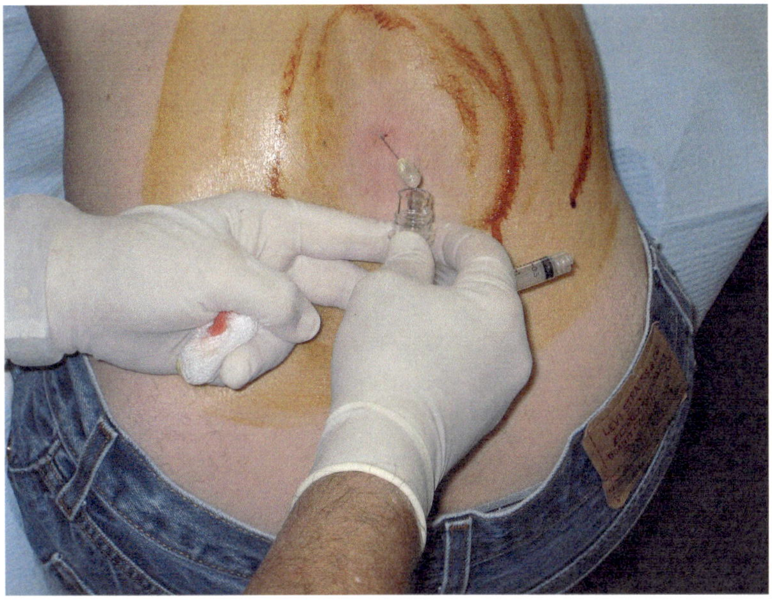

Source: By Brainhell - English Wikipedia, CC BY-SA 3.0, https://commons.wikimedia.org/w/index.php?curid=865889

15.3.9. Limitations of Current Diagnostic Methods

The present diagnosis of back and spine disorders often fails to provide complete evaluations. The traditional imaging techniques, such as X-rays and MRIs, while useful, have significant limitations in recognizing subtle changes in the spine and soft tissues surrounding the spine. These tests can miss early signs of conditions like osteoporosis that are crucial in preventing future fractures and problems (Venes, 2011). Furthermore, reliance on these imaging results can lead to delayed therapy or incorrect diagnosis because they primarily deal with structural lesions rather than functional deficits or pain mechanisms. The complexity of spine disease also impedes the interpretation of findings because the symptoms can vary significantly in various patients, and it is challenging to establish a clear correlation between imaging findings and clinical presentations. Developing increasingly complex diagnostic tools that integrate imaging and functional assessments has the potential to improve patient outcomes and lead to timely and effective interventions (Venes, 2011).

Test Your Knowledge

1. What is one emerging technology improving spinal diagnostics?
2. What is a major limitation of traditional X-rays in spinal diagnosis?

15.4. Treatment and Management

Learning Outcome

1. Focus on Physical Therapy and Rehabilitation
2. Explain the Medications for Pain Relief
3. Discuss the Surgical Options for Severe Conditions
4. Understand Alternative Therapies: Acupuncture, Chiropractic Care
5. Know Lifestyle Modifications for Prevention
6. Explain the Role of Exercise in Back Health
7. Give details Ergonomics and Workplace Adjustments
8. Focus on Importance of Maintaining a Healthy Weight
9. Explain the Psychological Aspects of Chronic Back Pain Management

Effective treatment and management of back and spine disorders depend on a multi-modal strategy to suit specific needs. These typically begin with conservative management, such as physical therapy and medication, to reduce pain and improve mobility. In cases where these prove to be inadequate, more invasive options like steroid injections or surgery can be utilized. For instance, thermal radiofrequency ablation has proven to be an effective option for chronic thoracic back pain due to costotransverse joint arthropathy, underscoring the significance of accurate diagnosis of pain generators (Venes, 2011). Furthermore, novel evidence suggests the potential involvement of dietary factors in response to treatment of inflammatory spine diseases, and higher fiber intake and lower intake of red meat could improve the response to biologic therapy in rheumatoid arthritis patients (Overgaard et al., 2022). Personalized treatment regimens including both medical and lifestyle therapies are then required to optimize patient outcomes (Figure 15.11).

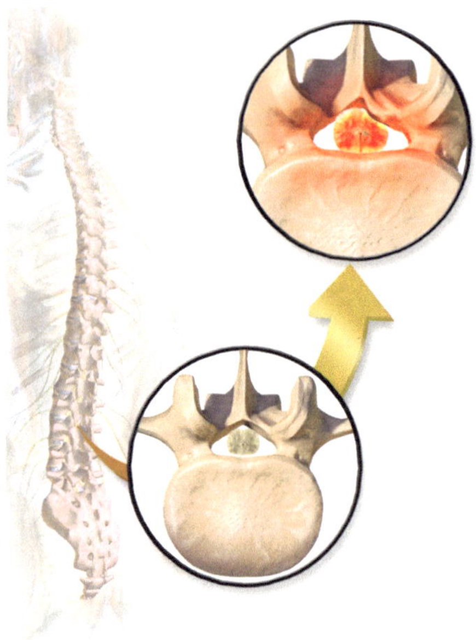

Figure 15.11. Effective treatment and management of back and spine conditions require a multifaceted approach tailored to individual needs.

Source: By BruceBlaus. When using this image in external sources it can be cited as:Blausen.com staff (2014). "Medical gallery of Blausen Medical 2014". WikiJournal of Medicine 1 (2). DOI:10.15347/wjm/2014.010. ISSN 2002-4436. - Own work, CC BY 3.0, https://commons.wikimedia.org/w/index.php?curid=27796936

15.4.1. Physical Therapy and Rehabilitation

Treatment of back and spine disorders today relies more on physical therapy and rehabilitation, which are an integral component of the healing process and also in complication prevention. Rehabilitation techniques, as suitable for the individual case, help restore function and also help to alleviate pain, with the use of devices like biofeedback machines. One such innovation is Lumbatex, a composite system that employs inertial sensors to monitor lumbar curvature with the potential to provide real-time feedback to both patients and clinicians (Juan et al., 2019).

As LBP is a leading cause of disability globally, its multifactorial etiology—ranging from occupational hazards to socioeconomic determinants—becomes important to decipher (Jan et al., 2018). Through personalized exercise programs and education in body mechanics, physical therapy not only eliminates existing pain but also creates resistance to future incidents. Last but not least, a comprehensive approach to rehabilitation enhances QoL, giving individuals the power to play an active role in keeping their spine healthy.

15.4.2. Medications for Pain Relief

Pain relief is a critical component of treatment of back- and spine-related conditions, given the high prevalence of pain-related disorders such as LBP and sciatica. Medications are a central aspect of pain relief and improvement in QoL among those affected by the condition. Non-steroidal anti-inflammatory drugs (NSAIDs) are the most frequent form of treatment since they can potentially inhibit inflammation as well as provide pain relief. But in chronic diseases, for example, those affecting sciatica, other types of treatment become necessary. For example, treatments such as Ayurvedic therapies Erand-Mooladi Basti proved to be effective in Gridharsi, a condition similar to sciatic pain, resulting in spectacular relief from symptoms (Venes, 2011). Moreover, medical shared decision-making promotes the importance of patient autonomy to select the appropriate pain treatment methods and foster an interdisciplinary approach that enhances treatment efficacy (Venes, 2011). Lastly, integration of varied medicinal approaches forms the basis for effective pain management for back and spinal disorders.

15.4.3. Surgical Options for Severe Conditions

Whenever the patients suffer from severe conditions in the spine and back, surgery is unavoidable in providing pain relief and restoring function. Surgical consideration tends to be based on severity of symptoms, the presence of structural abnormality, and the overall health of patients. Proper understanding of various existing surgical operations is essential for optimizing outcomes.

For instance, spinal canals can be decompressed microsurgically, as seen in the case of lumbar ganglion cysts wherein gross cystectomy has been demonstrated to lead to significant symptomatic improvement regardless of initial necessity for stabilization (London, 2017). Likewise, elective surgical indications vary according to region, where there is a need for shared decision-making to tailor treatment alternatives to patients' conditions to allow for informed decisions (Venes, 2011). Thus, selectively chosen surgical procedures not only cure the direct pathological problems but also empower the patients by engaging them in treatment planning.

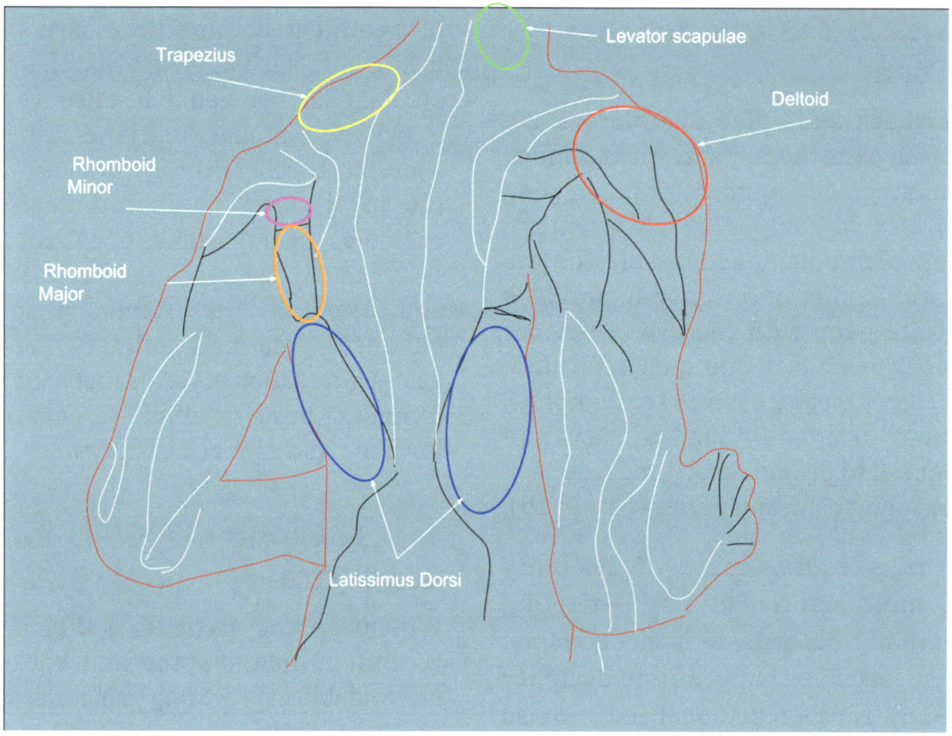

Source: By Angel.Nolasc - Own work, CC BY-SA 4.0, https://commons.wikimedia.org/w/index.php?curid=132052328

15.4.4. Alternative Therapies: Acupuncture, Chiropractic Care

In the past several years, more and more individuals have turned to alternative therapies such as chiropractic and acupuncture for back and spine conditions. These treatments offer a different philosophy from conventional medical practices. Acupuncture, based on traditional Chinese medicine, is reported to ease pain by stimulating body points, and has been found to reduce pain intensity. Similarly, chiropractic care focuses on spinal manipulation to improve alignment, often providing relief for LBP. Patients also reported a perceived need for these interventions, particularly chiropractic care, as they appreciated the one-on-one attention and hands-on approach. There is, however, a need to acknowledge the need for further research to determine long-term effectiveness and safety completely. By assessing patient experiences along with clinical outcomes, healthcare providers are better able to integrate these alternative therapies into the management of back and spine disorders.

15.4.5. Lifestyle Modifications for Prevention

Mindful lifestyle modification plays a crucial role in averting back and spine issues, particularly as one ages or has pre-existing medical issues. Exercise on a regular basis not only strengthens the muscles that support the spine but also improves flexibility and balance, thereby reducing the risk of falls and attendant injuries. Structured exercise programs, such as progressive resistance training and balance exercises, have been found to be particularly useful for older adults or those at risk of osteoporosis as they can successfully build up strength with less room for side effects (Skelton & Mavroeidi, 2018). Additionally, rehabilitation interventions aimed at addressing lifestyle risk factors can lead to considerable improvement in both general well-being and particular orthopedic conditions, making them invaluable to overall health management (Shiva Prasad et al., 2023).). By prioritizing these lifestyle changes, an individual can have a healthy spine and back, ultimately leading to improved QoL.

15.4.6. Role of Exercise in Back Health

Engagement in exercise regularly helps maintain and improve the health of the back as it significantly enhances strength, flexibility, and stability of the spinal region. Exercise specifically targeting the core muscles is capable of easing the strain on the spine and reducing the risk of injury.

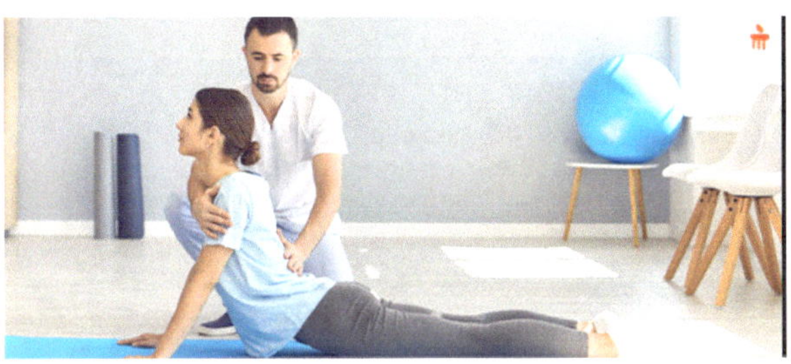

Source: Ishwar, K. (2025). *Exercises to Strengthen Your Back and Spine.*

As indicated by Edries (2009), many dancers get back injuries due to the lack of prevention education for injuries, highlighting the necessity of available resources advocating for healthy movement practices. In addition, a study of workplace wellness programs confirms that behavioral modification, including exercise, is an important factor in improving HRQOL, particularly in risk groups for back problems (Edries, 2009). Through developing individualized exercise routines with strengthening and flexibility exercises, individuals can be proactive in back health, thereby producing reduced pain and improved general QoL.

15.4.7. Ergonomics and Workplace Adjustments

Effective workplace adjustments play a critical role in ensuring employee well-being, particularly in the prevention of back and spine issues. The beginning of remote work due to the COVID-19 pandemic exposed the majority of employees to bad ergonomics at home offices, and they reported back pain, neck tension, and eye strain (Furness et al., 2016). Addressing these requirements necessitates conscious modifications, such as preparing the working environment, acquiring ergonomic tools, and employing appropriate technology. Furthermore, information regarding the body's requirement for lifting activity is essential, since research involving the correlation of lifting energy consumption (LEC) with lifting index (LI) and forces at the L5-S1 joint validates (Ranavolo et al., 2017). Incorporating ergonomics not only aids physical wellbeing but can increase productivity and mental wellbeing by creating a supportive working environment. As such, an organization has a responsibility to give prominence to ergonomic checks and periodic modifications to maintain a long-term harmony between efficiency and workers' health, specifically for the back and spinal area.

15.4.8. Importance of Maintaining a Healthy Weight

Proper weight management is key to overall health and has a significant impact on the health of the spine and back. Being overweight can lead to additional stress on the MSK system, and in particular the spine, potentially exacerbating or causing conditions such as osteoporosis and chronic back pain. It has been understood by studies that patients with untreated osteoporosis can experience recurrent fractures, which progress towards a cycle of disability along with poor QoL (Furness et al., 2016). Moreover, eating a healthy diet along with regular exercise is essential in maintaining weight management and bone health. The mTOR pathway that regulates cell growth and metabolism is also controlled by nutritional status, which shows the importance of good lifestyle and dietary habits in maintaining not just weight but also the health of bone density (Haq, 2015). Ultimately, maintaining a healthy weight is an active process that can prevent excessive health issues and provide a robust spine.

15.4.9. Psychological Aspects of Chronic Back Pain Management

Apart from physical therapy, chronic back pain management also requires knowledge of psychological issues that may affect patient outcomes. Patients with chronic pain are likely to be assailed by anxiety and depression, which exacerbate the condition and make the recovery process even harder. Such psychological issues may arise from a simple fear of re-injury or from a belief in loss of physical ability, which subconsciously reinforces the cycle of pain and psychological distress that obstructs the treatment. Also, as noted by research, psychosocial factors can be pivotal in the success of interventions for chronic LBP, and, therefore, physical therapy alone is not sufficient (Frank et al., 2005). Evidence also discovers that chronic back pain can result in structural brain changes, thereby suggesting that a neurological rationale could exist for the psychological distress experienced by patients (Venes, 2011). Therefore, the incorporation of psychological assessment and intervention into treatment routines could be crucial to facilitate effective control and improve overall QoL in affected individuals (Rensburg, 2008).

Test Your Knowledge

1. How can ergonomic workplace adjustments help prevent back pain?
2. What are common ergonomic tools used to support spinal health at work?

SUMMARY

We can simply note that syndromes such as lumbosacral radiculopathy are extremely harmful to one's health, particularly to specific groups of people. According to research, it is shown that nearly one in six people with LBP may also have radiculopathy, and has a high incidence in females and people between the ages of 40-50-years (Furness et al., 2016). It is evident from risk group statistics here that the need exists for prevention and intervention measures against prevention measures that are risk group-specific. The intricacy of treatment protocols, such as manual therapy, further emphasizes the need to come up with high-quality evidence supporting clinical practice. Although much research has been done, just one study of high quality was reviewed, which highlights the need for large studies in this field (Malfliet et al., 2019). These findings validate ongoing research into back and spinal disorders, justifying the necessity for further research and the development of treatment to further improve patient outcomes.

A conclusion regarding the interactive dynamics of the back and spinal region yields several key conclusions about function as well as health. First, the high incidence of lumbo pelvic pain (LPP) in postpartum participants emphasizes the need for adequate intervention procedures, as highlighted in recent systematic reviews (Furness et al., 2016). Physical training is one of the most important interventions, but no solid evidence exists for optimal exercise protocols to prevent LPP. Furthermore, understanding charged particle mechanics as an analog to magnetic reconnection is a captivating example, of demarcating boundaries of energy redistribution in restructuring a broad variety of circumstances (Haq, 2015). Lastly, the advanced interaction between physical treatment methods and physiological forces at play is essential to informed strategies for spine and back wellness, deserving of additional examination to identify the most efficacious interventions across diverse populations.

KEY TERMS FROM THIS CHAPTER

- American Spinal Injury Association (ASIA)
- Ankylosing spondylitis (AS)
- Back pain
- Bad posture
- Diagnostic Techniques
- Digital video fluoroscopy (DVF)
- Flexion-relaxation phenomenon (FRP)
- Health-related quality of life (HRQOL)
- Lordosis
- Lumbar disc herniation (LDH)

CRITICAL THINKING QUESTIONS

1. **Which of the following is the normal curvature of the cervical spine?**
   a. Kyphosis
   b. Lordosis
   c. Scoliosis
   d. Straight
2. **The vertebral foramen is formed by which structures?**
   a. Body and spinous process
   b. Pedicles and laminae
   c. Transverse and spinous processes
   d. Articular processes
3. **Which of the following vertebrae has a bifid spinous process?**
   a. T1
   b. L1
   c. C3
   d. S1
4. **The intervertebral disc is composed of:**
   a. Bone and cartilage
   b. Nucleus pulposus and annulus fibrosus
   c. Synovial fluid and capsule
   d. Ligaments and tendons
5. **Which ligament prevents hyperextension of the vertebral column?**
   a. Posterior longitudinal ligament
   b. Ligamentum flavum
   c. Anterior longitudinal ligament
   d. Interspinous ligament

Short Answer Questions

1. Describe the normal curvatures of the vertebral column and their functional significance.
2. What are the main components of a typical vertebra?
3. What is the function of the intervertebral discs?
4. Describe the structure and function of the spinal cord.
5. What is the clinical significance of the cauda equina?
6. Explain what scoliosis is and how it affects the spine.

Answers to Critical Thinking Questions

1. (b) 2. (b) 3. (c) 4. (b) 5. (c)

REFERENCES

1. Aljanakh, M., Shaikh, S., Siddiqui, A. A., Al-Mansour, M., & Hassan, S. S. (2015). Prevalence of musculoskeletal disorders among dentists in the Ha'il Region *of Saudi Arabia. Saudi Medical Journal, 35, 456–461. https://doi.org/10.5144/0256-4947.2015.456 (accessed on 8th May* 2025).
2. Allen, R., Nixon, M. S., & Zheng, Y. (2001). Automatic Lumbar Vertebrae Segmentation in Fluoroscopic Images via Optimized Concurrent Hough transform. https://core.ac.uk/download/pdf/7097926.pdf (accessed on 8th May 2025).
3. Alqahtani, T., & Konbaz, *F. (2021). Scoliosis Sec*ondary to Lumbar Spine Herniated Nucleus Pulposus in Adolescents: A Case Report. https://www.semanticscholar.org/paper/a463d4686*c839548d512d9b500568125000fa348 (accessed on 8th May 2025).*
4. *Back, W., Bergmann, W., Nielen, M., van de*n Belt, A. J. M., Veraa, S., Vernooij, H., & Wijnberg, I. D. (2019). Equine Cervical Intervertebral Disc Degen*eration is Associated with Location and MRI Malfliet, A., Ickmans, K., Huysmans, E., Coppie*ters, I., Willaert, W., Bogaert, W. V., Rheel, E., Bilterys, T., Wilgen, P. V., & Nijs, J. (2019). Best Evidence Rehabilitation for Chronic Pain Part 3: Low Back Pain. Journal of clinical medicine, 8(7), 1063. https://do*i.org/10.3390/jcm8071063 (accessed on 8th May 2025).*
5. *Borgström, F., Zethraeus, N., Jo*hnell, O., Lidgren, L., Ponzer, S., Svensson, O., Abdon, P., Ornstein, E., Lunsjö, K., Thorngren, K. G., Sernbo, I., Rehnberg, C., & Jönsson, B. (2006). Costs and quality of life associated with osteoporosis-related *fractures in Sweden. Osteopo*rosis international : a journal established as result of cooperation between the European Foundation for Osteoporosis and the National Osteoporosis Foundation of the USA, 17(5), 637–650. https://doi.org/10.1007/s00198-005-0015-8(accessed on 8th May 2025).
6. Broshek, D. K., Pardini, J., & Herring, S. A. (2022). Persisting symptoms after concussion*: Time for a paradigm shift. PM&R, 14, 1509–1513. https://doi.org/10.1002/pmrj.12884 (accessed on 8th May 2025).*
7. *Böttcher, E., Grote, V., Puff, H., & Unger, A. (2019). What to* Expect: Medical Quality Outcomes and Achievements of a Multidisciplinary Inpatient Musculoskeletal System Rehabilitation. IntechOpen. https:/*/core.ac.uk/download/322444944.pdf (accessed on 8th May 2025).*
8. *Callejón, F. Á. J., Gómez, G. M., López, A. L., & López, L. R. (20*17). Applications of the Standardized Nordic Questionnaire: A Review. MDPI AG. https://core.ac.uk/download/286590648.pdf (accessed on 8th May 2025).
9. Caplan, N., Debuse, D., & Gibbon, K. (2013). Low Impac*t Weight-*Bearing Exercise in an Upright Posture Achieves Greater Lumbopelvic Stability than Overground Walking. Elsevier BV. https://core.ac.uk/download/*9990838.pdf (accessed on 8th May 2025).*
10. *Clark, M. E. (1906). Appl*ied Anatomy: Designed for the Use of Osteopathic Students and Practitioners as an Aid in the Anatomical Exploration of Disease *from an Osteopathic Viewpoint. The Journal Printing Company. https://core.ac.uk/download/234130026.pdf (accessed on 8*th May 2025).
11. Climstein, M., Furness, J., Jorgensen, D., & McArthur, K. (2020). Epidemiology of Acute Inj*uries in Surfing: Type, Location, Mechanism, Severity, and Incidence: A Systematic Review. MDPI AG. https://core.ac.uk/download/322824648.pdf (accessed on 8th* May 2025).

12. Coe, T., Shenoi, R. A., & Xing, J. T. (2006). A human Body Model for Dynamic Response Analysis of an Integrated Human-Seat-Controller-High Speed Marine Craft *Interaction System. Institute of Sound and Vibration Research. https://core.ac.uk/download/234130026.pdf (accessed* on 8th May 2025).

13. Cook, W. H., & Baker, J. (2022). Incidental finding of arachnoiditis ossificans in the lumbar spine. Spine, *92, 3063, 3064. https://www.semanticscholar.org/paper/3252a0cf29ad3a1d57 0139e2512f62e30ba59a5c (accessed on 8th May 2025).*

14. *Copp, A.* J., Adzick, N. S., Chitty, L. S., Fletcher, J. M., Holmbeck, G. N., & Shaw, G. M. (2015). Spina bifida. Nature Reviews Disease Primers, 1. https://doi.org/10.1038/nrdp.2015.7 (accessed on 8th May 2025).

15. Coppack, R. J., Karageorghis, C. I., & Kristensen, J. (2012). Use of a Goal Setting Intervention to Increase Adherence to Low Back Pai*n Rehabilitation:* A *R*andomized Controlled Trial. SAGE Publications. https://core.ac.uk/download/29410054.pdf (accessed on 8th May 2025).

16. Cortell-Tormo, J. M., García-Jaén, M., Ruíz, F. D., & Fuster-Lloret, V. *(2019).* Lumbatex: A wearable monitoring system based on inertial sensors to measure and control the lumbar spine motion. IEEE Transactions on Neural Systems and Rehabilitation Engineering, 27, 1644–1653. https://doi.org/10.1109/tnsre.2019.292*7083 (accessed on 8th May 2025).*

17. Delfini, R., Domenicucci, M., Marruzzo, D., Miscusi, M., Missori, P., Ramieri, A., & Tarantino, R. (2017). Lumbar Ganglion Cyst: *Nosology, Surgical Management and Proposal of a New Classification Based on 34 Personal Cases and Literature Review. B*aishideng Publishing Group Inc. https://core.ac.uk/download/153367188.pdf (accessed on 8th May 2025).

18. De Souza, L. H., & Frank, A. O. (2001). Conservative Management of Low Back Pain. Blackwell Publishing Ltd. https://core.ac.uk/download/333411.pdf (accessed on 8th May 2025).

19. Edries*, N. (2009). Employee wellness programme in clothing/textile manufactu*ring companies: what are the effects?. Unpublished Dissertation for Master of Science in Physiotherapy. Cape Town: The Univer*sity of Cape Town.(accessed on 8th May* 2025).

20. Fiani, B., Jarr*ah, R*., Fiani, N. J., & Runnels, J. (2021). Spontaneous cervical epidural hematoma: Insight into this occurrence with case examples. Surgical Neurology International, 12, 79–79. https://doi.org/10.25259/sni_15_2021 (accessed on 8th May 2025).

21. FM dos Santos Venes (2011). *A Go-to-Market Strategy for Vertebral Metri*cs. FCT-UNL. Dissertação para obtenção do Grau de Mestre em Engenharia Biomédica. https://core.ac.uk/download/157623817.pdf (accessed on 8th May 2025).

22. Frank, A. O., De Souza, L. H., & Frank, C. A. (2*005). Neck pain and disability: a cross-sectional survey of the demographic and clinical characteristics of neck pain seen in a rheumatol*ogy clinic. International journal of clinical practice, 59(2), 173–182. https://doi.org/10.1111/j.1742-1241.2004.00237.x (accessed on 8th May 2025).

23. Furness, J., Climstein, M., Sheppard, J. M., Abbott, A., & Hing, W. (2016). Clinical methods to quantify trunk mobility in an elite male surfing population. Physical therapy in sport : official journal of the Association of Chartered Physiotherapists in Sports Medicine, 19, 28–35. https://doi.org/10.1016/j.ptsp.2015.09.003 (accessed on 8th May 2025).

24. *Grilli, S. L. (1997). Spinal Model*ling to Investigate Postural Loading and Stability. https://core.ac.uk/download/288390817.pdf (a*ccessed on 8th May 2025).*

25. Haq, Rabia. "Multi-Surface Simplex Spine Segmentation for Spine Surgery Simulation and Planning" (2015). Doctor of Philosophy (PhD), Dissertation, Computational Modeling & Simulation Engineering, Old Dominion University, DOI: 10.25777/93jp-zw72 https://digitalcommons.odu.edu/msve_etds/23(accessed on 8th May 2025).

26. Heng, W., Solomon, S. A., & Gao, W. (2021). Flexible electronics and devices as human–machine interfaces for medical robotics. Advanced Materials, 34. https://doi.org/10.1002/adma.202107902 (accessed on 8th May 2025).

27. Higuchi, K., & Sato, T. (2002). Anatomical Study of Lumbar Spine Innervation. Salvia Medical Sciences Ltd. https://core.ac.uk/download/268450791.pdf (accessed on 8th May 2025).

28. Janse van Rensburg, A. H. (2008). A study to determine the incidence of scoliosis in school children within the metropolis of Johannesburg, South Africa [University of Johannesburg]. https://ujcontent.uj.ac.za/esploro/outputs/doctoral/A-study-to-determine-the-incidence/9912301607691#file-0(accessed on 8th May 2025).

29. Jenks, M., Craig, J., Higgins, J., Willits, I., Barata, T., Wood, H., Kimpton, C., & Sims, A. (2014). The MAGEC system for spinal lengthening in children with scoliosis: A NICE Medical Technology Guidance. Applied health economics and health policy, 12(6), 587–599. https://doi.org/10.1007/s40258-014-0127-4(accessed on 8th May 2025).

30. Knežević, N. N., Candido, K. D., Vlaeyen, J. W. S., Van Zundert, J., & Cohen, S. P. (2021). Low back pain. The Lancet, 398, 78–92. https://doi.org/10.1016/s0140-6736(21)00733-9 (accessed on 8th May 2025).

31. Ko, S., Kim, H. C., & Kwon, J. (2023). The effectiveness of vitamin D3 supplementation in improving functional outcome of non-surgically treated symptomatic lumbar spinal stenosis: Randomized controlled clinical trial - Pilot study. Medicine, 102(40), e32672. https://doi.org/10.1097/MD.0000000000032672 (accessed on 8th May 2025).

32. Kokkula Shiva Prasad, et al. (2023). An Overview of Inflammatory Spondylitis for Biomedical Imaging Using Deep Neural Networks. International Journal on Recent and Innovation Trends in Computing and Communication, 11(9), 4506–4515. https://doi.org/10.17762/ijritcc.v11i9.9957(accessed on 8th May 2025).

33. Litjens, G., Kooi, T., Ehteshami, B. B., et al. (2017). A survey on deep learning in medical image analysis. Medical Image Analysis, 42, 60–88. https://doi.org/10.1016/j.media.2017.07.005 (accessed on 8th May 2025).

34. Liu, G. Y., & Sabatini, D. M. (2020). mTOR at the nexus of nutrition, growth, ageing and disease. Nature Reviews Molecular Cell Biology, 21, 183–203. https://doi.org/10.1038/s41580-019-0199-y (accessed on 8th May 2025).

35. London Z. N. (2017). Safety and pain in electrodiagnostic studies. Muscle & nerve, 55(2), 149–159. https://doi.org/10.1002/mus.25421llowed=y (accessed on 8th May 2025).

36. Ranavolo, A., Varrecchia, T., Rinaldi, M., Silvetti, A., Serrao, M., Conforto, S., & Draicchio, F. (2017). Mechanical lifting energy consumption in work activities designed by means of the "revised NIOSH lifting equation". Industrial health, 55(5), 444–454. https://doi.org/10.2486/indhealth.2017-0075 (accessed on 8th May 2025).

37. Skelton, D. A., & Mavroeidi, A. (2018). Which strength and balance activities are safe and efficacious for individuals with specific challenges (osteoporosis, vertebral fractures, frailty,

dementia)?: A Narrative review. Journal of frailty, sarcopenia and falls, 3(2), 85–104. https://doi.org/10.22540/JFSF-03-085(accessed on 8th May 2025).

38. Thompson, S., O'Leary, G. H., Austelle, C. *W., Gruber, E., Kahn, A. T.,* Manett, A. J., Short, B., & Badran, B. W. (2021). A review of parameter settings for invasive and n*on-invasive vagus nerve stimulation (VNS) ap*plied in neurological and psychiatric disorders. Frontiers in Neuroscience, 15. https://doi.org/10.3389/fnins.2021.709436 (accessed on 8th May 2025).

INDEX

C

D

K

L

M

U

V

X